Gastrointestinal Disease (Fifth Series) Test and Syllabus

Dennis M. Balfe, M.D.
Section Chairman

Judith L. Chezmar, M.D.
R. Brooke Jeffrey, M.D.
Robert E. Koehler, M.D.
Marc S. Levine, M.D.
David H. Stephens, M.D.

 American College of Radiology
Reston, Virginia 1995

Sets Published
Chest Disease
Bone Disease
Genitourinary Tract Disease
Gastrointestinal Disease
Head and Neck Disorders
Pediatric Disease
Nuclear Radiology
Radiation Pathology and
    Radiation Biology
Chest Disease II
Bone Disease II
Genitourinary Tract Disease II
Gastrointestinal Disease II
Head and Neck Disorders II
Nuclear Radiology II
Cardiovascular Disease
Emergency Radiology
Bone Disease III
Gastrointestinal Disease III
Chest Disease III
Pediatric Disease II
Nuclear Radiology III
Head and Neck Disorders III
Genitourinary Tract Disease III
Diagnostic Ultrasound

Breast Disease
Bone Disease IV
Pediatric Disease III
Chest Disease IV
Neuroradiology
Gastrointestinal Disease IV
Nuclear Radiology IV
Magnetic Resonance
Radiation Bioeffects and
    Management
Genitourinary Tract Disease IV
Head and Neck Disorders IV
Pediatric Disease IV
Breast Disease II
Musculoskeletal Disease
Diagnostic Ultrasonography II
Gastrointestinal Disease V

Sets in Preparation
Chest Disease V
Neuroradiology II
Emergency Radiology II
Genitourinary Tract Disease V
Nuclear Radiology V
Body MRI
Head and Neck Disorders V

Note: While the American College of Radiology and the editors of this publication have attempted to include the most current and accurate information possible, errors may inadvertently appear. Diagnostic and interventional decisions should be based on the individual circumstances of each case.

SET 39:
Gastrointestinal Disease (Fifth Series) Test and Syllabus

Editor in Chief
BARRY A. SIEGEL, M.D., Professor of Radiology and Medicine and Director, Division of Nuclear Medicine, Mallinckrodt Institute of Radiology, Washington University School of Medicine, St. Louis, Missouri

Associate Editor
DAVID H. STEPHENS, M.D., Professor of Radiology, Mayo Medical School; Department of Diagnostic Radiology, Mayo Clinic, Rochester, Minnesota

Section Chairman
DENNIS M. BALFE, M.D., Professor of Radiology and Director, Diagnostic Radiology Residency Program, Mallinckrodt Institute of Radiology, Washington University School of Medicine, St. Louis, Missouri

Co-Authors
JUDITH L. CHEZMAR, M.D., Associate Professor of Radiology and Director, Division of Abdominal Imaging, Emory University School of Medicine, Atlanta, Georgia

R. BROOKE JEFFREY, M.D., Professor of Radiology and Chief of Abdominal Imaging, Stanford University School of Medicine, Stanford, California

ROBERT E. KOEHLER, M.D., Professor and Vice Chairman of Radiology, University of Alabama Hospital, Birmingham, Alabama

MARC S. LEVINE, M.D., Professor of Radiology, University of Pennsylvania School of Medicine; Gastrointestinal Radiology Section, Hospital of the University of Pennsylvania, Philadelphia, Pennsylvania

DAVID H. STEPHENS, M.D., Professor of Radiology, Mayo Medical School; Department of Diagnostic Radiology, Mayo Clinic, Rochester, Minnesota

AMERICAN COLLEGE OF RADIOLOGY
PROFESSIONAL SELF-EVALUATION PROGRAM

Publishing Coordinators:	*G. Rebecca Haines and Thomas M. Rogers*
Administrative Assistant:	*Beth Meehan*
Production Editor:	*Sean M. McKenna*
Copy Editors:	*Yvonne Strong and John N. Bell*
Index:	*EEI, Inc., Alexandria, Va.*
Image Scanning:	*Cadmus Color Center, Richmond, Va*
Typesetting:	*Pubication Technology Corp., Fairfax, Va..*
Printing:	*John D. Lucas Printing, Baltimore, Md.*

Library of Congress Cataloging-in-Publication Data

Gastrointestinal disease (fifth series) test and syllabus / Dennis M. Balfe, section chairman ; [coauthors] Judith L. Chezmar ... [et al.].
    p. cm. — (Professional self-evaluation program; set 39)
    "Committee on Professional Self-Evaluation, Commission on Education, American College of Radiology"—Cover.
    Includes bibliographical references and index.
    ISBN 1-55903-039-9 : $200.00. — ISBN 1-55903-000-3 (series)
    1. Gastrointestinal system—Radiography—Examinations, questions, etc. 2. Gastrointestinal system—Diseases—Diagnosis. I. Balfe, Dennis M. II. Chezmar, Judith L. III. American College of Radiology. Commission on Education. Committee on Professional Self-Evaluation. IV. Series.
    [DNLM: 1. Gastrointestinal diseases—radiography—examination questions. W1 PR606 set 39 1995 / WI 18.2 G257 1995]
    RC804.R6G358   1995
    616.3'307572'076—dc20
    DNLM/DLC   95-20536
    for Library of Congress   CIP

Additional Contributors

KAY M. HAMRICK, M.D., Assistant Professor of Radiology, University of Alabama Hospital, Birmingham, Alabama

DAVID S. MEMEL, M.D., Assistant Professor of Radiology, University of Alabama Hospital, Birmingham, Alabama

DESIREE E. MORGAN, M.D., Assistant Professor of Radiology, University of Alabama Hospital, Birmingham, Alabama

SHAWN P. QUILLIN, M.D., Instructor in Radiology, Mallinckrodt Institute of Radiology, Washington University School of Medicine, St. Louis, Missouri

ELLEN M. WARD, M.D., Assistant Professor of Radiology, Mayo Medical School; Department of Radiology, Mayo Cinic, Rochester, Minnesota

Section Chairman's Preface

During the past 20 years, the practice of gastrointestinal radiology has undergone remarkable changes. New technologies, such as computed tomography and magnetic resonance imaging, have emerged; older ones, such as sonography, have evolved to become nearly unrecognizable to radiologic practitioners of two decades ago. This surge of technical wizardry has engendered an enormous amount of literature that today's radiologist must understand and master. A single disease now has many faces, one for each imaging method, and the expert consultant must recognize them all. Moreover, he or she must also try to assess which of the powerful (and expensive) array of tools is the most appropriate place to start in evaluating a given medical problem.

At the same time, there have been sweeping changes in both clinical gastroenterology and gastrointestinal surgery. Radiologists are now presented with new problems related to interventional endoscopic techniques, liver transplantation, or laparoscopic cholecystectomy. In addition, immune suppression, either iatrogenic or acquired, is now associated with an ever-broadening spectrum of unusual diseases, or of strange manifestations of common diseases.

It is the aim of this, the fifth Self-Evaluation Test and Syllabus in Gastrointestinal Radiology, to reflect the recent growth of scientific information by presenting new concepts in the diagnosis and treatment of gastrointestinal diseases, by outlining sensible approaches for effective utilization of imaging methods, and by reviewing the current state of scientific opinion with regard to specific disease entities. I had the good fortune to be associated with a talented and hard-working committee: Drs. Judith Chezmar, Marc Levine, Brooke Jeffrey, Robert Koehler, and David Stephens were tireless in researching and preparing the manuscripts that comprise this volume. In some cases, committee members turned to their colleagues for assistance in the preparation of manuscripts, and we are consequently very grateful to Drs. Ellen Ward, David Memel, Shawn Quillin, Kay Hamrick, and Desiree Morgan for their quality efforts. One member of the committee, Dr. David Stephens, who was the Section Editor for the fourth *Gastrointestinal Disease Test and Syllabus*, has now taken on the duties of Associate Editor. Despite these added responsibilities, David read every word of this syllabus and repeatedly came to our aid with insightful comments and crucial references. In addition to being highly talented, productive people, this team was a joy to work with. The friendly give-and-take of our group meetings was, for me, a highlight of this project and serves to remind me to thank the many family members and friends who were deprived of their company during the book's preparation.

Each institution represented by our team has contributed not only a committee member, but also a good part of its resources in secretarial staff, photography, and communication equipment. These largely uncredited individuals are hereby gratefully acknowledged. For my own part, Ms. Lynn Losse has served as Unofficial Deputy Editor, all the while trying to carry out her paid duties as Abdominal Section Secretary; she has been a mainstay in completing this project.

The publication staff of the American College of Radiology—specifically, Ms. G. Rebecca Haines and Mr. Thomas Rogers—have endured our chronic tardiness from the inception of this syllabus. They have been responsible for planning our group meetings, organizing the flow of manuscripts, and copy-editing every word of the text you now hold in your hands.

We were also fortunate to have had the direction of the Editor in Chief of the Self-Evaluation Syllabus series, Dr. Barry Siegel. Barry was the "reader's advocate" for this project. No unsupported statement and no unreferenced opinion escaped his notice; no imprecise word and no ill-conceived question was allowed to long abide within the manuscript pages.

It would, of course, be a mistake to consider the discussions accompanying our case material, however thoughtful and well-researched, to be the "final word." They are intended to reflect the authors' views on a particular topic that he or she considers important. Such topics tend to be related to areas in which there is the most rapid growth in scientific information. If the discussions in *Gastrointestinal Disease (Fifth Series) Test and Syllabus* are truly successful, they will cause our readers to think critically and creatively about the pathophysiology underlying the various radiologic images presented here. It is through these readers that the specialty of gastrointestinal radiology will continue to expand.

Dennis M. Balfe, M.D.
Section Chairman

Editor's Preface

On behalf of the editors of the American College of Radiology Professional Self-Evaluation (PSE) Program, I am pleased to introduce the *Gastrointestinal Disease (Fifth Series) Test and Syllabus* to program participants. This volume represents the 39th in the College's series of diagnostic radiology exercises, as the PSE Program continues into its 24th year. Like its predecessors, this book addresses key recent advances in gastrointestinal radiology, with particular emphasis on the roles of ultrasonography, computed tomography, and interventional techniques. As is pointed out by Dr. Dennis M. Balfe in his Section Chairman's Preface, this test and syllabus deals with important clinical issues that most diagnostic radiologists are likely to face in their daily practices.

Despite many years of evolution, the educational goals and basic structure of a PSE package remain unchanged. The self-evaluation test consists of a series of cases. Each of these cases generally begins with a diagnostic exercise that requires program participants to analyze one or more images and relevant clinical data from an individual patient and then to select the most likely diagnosis from a carefully chosen list of alternatives. These primary questions are artfully crafted by the authors to test the observational and analytical skills used by diagnostic radiologists in their own reading rooms. Accompanying the primary question in each case, there typically are several satellite questions, which are designed to probe a participant's fund of knowledge relevant to the issues addressed by the case, and particularly in relation to the disorders that comprise its differential diagnosis. The syllabus discloses the answers to the test questions, but far more importantly, it attempts to capture and explain to readers the thought process used by the experts in assessing the evidence and reaching a diagnosis. The syllabus discussions of satellite questions are intended to represent short topical reviews that will help participants keep abreast of the rapidly expanding body of radiologic information. Because the audience for each PSE package consists of both practicing radiologists and radiologists in training, an effort is made to include some questions that will be challenging even to subspecialists, while ensuring that the syllabus discussions are sufficiently thorough to be of instructional value even to neophytes.

The development and production of a self-evaluation test and its companion syllabus is an arduous process. It begins with a series of intensive but intellectually stimulating meetings of the authors at which the package's educational goals are established, the cases are selected, and the questions are scrutinized and edited to ensure that they reflect the consensus of the experts. The syllabus discussions represent the individual efforts of one or two principal authors, but the entire volume is subjected to rigorous editorial review by the Section Chairman and by the series editors. Most manuscripts experience at least one revision cycle before finalization. The goal of this process is to ensure that the information in each syllabus is current and clearly presented so that participants will derive maximal educational benefit.

As our readers work through this volume, they will surely recognize the tremendous effort expended on their behalf by Dr. Dennis Balfe, who served as Section Chairman for this self-evaluation package. The College was extremely fortunate to have garnered the services of such an expert clinician, teacher, editor, and leader for this project. Our gratitude is also due to Dennis' principal co-authors for this volume—Drs. Judith L. Chezmar, R. Brooke Jeffrey, Robert E. Koehler, Marc S. Levine, and David H. Stephens—who, along with several additional contributors, devoted long hours of voluntary service to this project and to the PSE Program. Special thanks are due to David Stephens, who also served as the Associate Editor for this book. Working with these talented and devoted radiologists was a great personal pleasure for me.

Thanks are also due to the many other individuals who contributed directly or indirectly to the successful fruition of this project. As chairman of the College's Committee on Professional Self-Evaluation, Dr. Anthony V. Proto guides the development of each package and helps to maintain the momentum of the entire program. The continuing support and encouragement of Dr. Robert Hattery and of the Commission on Education, as well as that of the entire ACR Board of Chancellors, are gratefully acknowledged. The highly professional and efficient staff of the ACR Publications Department, under the able direction of G. Rebecca Haines, make the whole process possible. As always, my special thanks go to Becky and to her colleague, Thomas M. Rogers, who has principal responsibility for the production of the PSE volumes. Their consummate attention to detail and continuing innovation to improve the efficiency of syllabus production are critical to the high quality of each volume.

The editors hope that this self-evaluation package will prove as palatable and as popular as the volumes that preceded it. The enthusiastic endorsement of the PSE Program for nearly a quarter century by radiologists is the sole reason the program continues and thrives. Since the inception of this program, the total number of recorded subscriptions is nearly 198,000. As series editors, we hope that we can continue to contribute beneficially to the overall education of radiologists.

Finally, we would like to recognize the enormous contributions made to the PSE program by its founder, Dr. Elias P. G. Theros, whose death in November 1994 saddened all whose lives had ever been touched by this legendary radiologist. The College's program arose out of teaching concepts first developed by Lee during his tenure as Chairman of the Department of Radiologic Pathology at the Armed Forces Institute of Pathology and first presented as scientific exhibits at the meetings of the Radiological Society of North America and the American Roentgen Ray Society in 1969 and 1970. The success of these exhibits led to the preparation of the first *Chest Disease Syllabus*, published in 1972 under his direction and editorial guidance. Lee served as Chairman of the Committee on Professional Self-Evaluation and Continuing Education until 1985, as Editor in Chief until 1988, and as Editor Emeritus until his death. The current editors of the PSE program learned the art of self-evaluation "at his feet." Lee was widely acknowledged as an exceptional teacher of radiology. This program was a special labor of love for him and is one small part of the giant legacy he leaves to all radiologists and to our specialty.

Barry A. Siegel, M.D.
Editor in Chief

Gastrointestinal Disease (Fifth Series)

Program Objective

After completing this program, the diagnostic radiologist should be able to successfully answer the questions that comprise the program's evaluation component. The intent of the course is to provide the reader with recent scientific information relating to the radiologic diagnosis and treatment of gastrointestinal disease, including the presentation of issues relating to the effective use of various imaging methods. This course should also provide the reader with a review of the current state of scientific opinion relating to specific disease entities.

CME Credit Award: 20 Credit Hours

The American College of Radiology (ACR) is accredited by the Accreditation Council for Continuing Medical Education to sponsor continuing medical education for physicians.

The ACR designates the following continuing medical education activity as meeting the criteria for up to 20 credit hours in Category 1 of the Physician's Recognition Award of the American Medical Association.

The *Gastrointestinal Disease (Fifth Series)* program has been approved for ACR and AMA/PRA Category 1 CME credit for the period from October 1995 through October 1998.

CME Credit Award Process

To receive the Category 1 credit, participants must complete the accompanying *answer sheet* and return it to the ACR.

Within 40 days of receipt of the answer sheet, the ACR will provide you with a credit award letter. The letter will indicate your score, the date it was recorded, and a credit award statement. You may also request a report which provides you with a ranking of all the test scores from all the tests completed within the first 6 months of the course. This will allow you to compare your score with those of your peers. To place yourself on the mailing list to receive the report, contact the ACR's Educational Services Division at 1-800-227-5463, ext. 4986.

This CME activity was planned and produced in accordance with the ACCME Essentials. Category 1 CME for this program is not transferable. Only the purchaser may apply for and receive Category 1 credit.

Gastrointestinal Disease (Fifth Series) Test

For you to derive the maximum benefit from this program, you should complete the following test, and send your answer sheet to the ACR for scoring, before you proceed to the syllabus.

If for any reason you refer to the syllabus material, or any other references, in answering the questions, please be sure to so indicate when answering Question 97, the first demographic question. Your score will then not be used in developing the norm tables.

CASE 1: Questions 1 through 3

This 50-year-old woman has dysphagia. You are shown an esophagram (Figure 1-1).

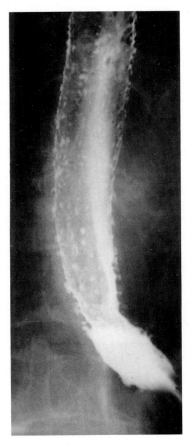

Figure 1-1

1. Which *one* of the following is the MOST likely diagnosis?

   (A) Herpes esophagitis
   (B) Radiation esophagitis
   (C) Crohn's disease
   (D) Barrett's esophagus
   (E) Intramural pseudodiverticulosis

QUESTIONS 2 AND 3: MARK YOUR ANSWER SHEET TRUE (T) OR FALSE (F) FOR EACH OF THE RESPONSE CHOICES.

2. Concerning Barrett's esophagus,

    (A) it occurs in about 10% of patients with endoscopically proven reflux esophagitis
    (B) it is associated with an increased risk of squamous cell carcinoma
    (C) it is characterized by a continuous area of columnar metaplasia in the lower esophagus
    (D) patients with scleroderma are at increased risk of developing this condition
    (E) it is a common cause of midesophageal strictures

3. Concerning esophageal intramural pseudodiverticula,

    (A) they are dilated excretory ducts of deep mucous glands in the esophagus
    (B) patients are usually immunocompromised
    (C) they usually cause odynophagia
    (D) they often occur in the region of a peptic stricture
    (E) when viewed in profile, they cannot be differentiated radiographically from esophageal ulcers

CASE 2: Questions 4 through 6

You are shown esophagrams of three patients. For each numbered image listed below (Questions 4 through 6), select the *one* lettered diagnosis (A, B, C, D, or E) that is MOST closely associated with it. Each lettered diagnosis may be used once, more than once, or not at all.

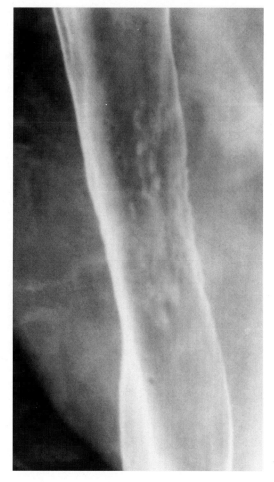

Figure 2-1

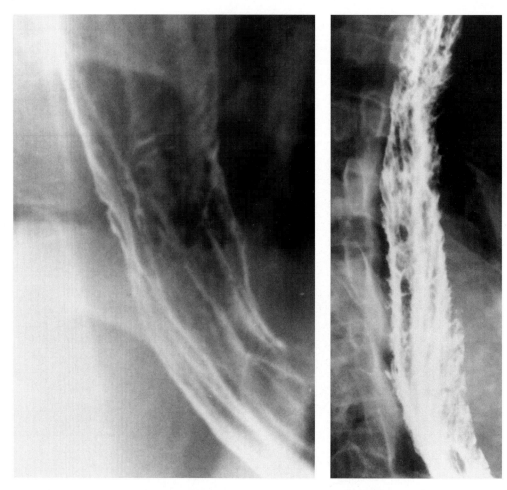

Figure 2-2   Figure 2-3

4. Figure 2-1
5. Figure 2-2
6. Figure 2-3

    (A) Reflux esophagitis
    (B) *Candida* esophagitis
    (C) Drug-induced esophagitis
    (D) Glycogenic acanthosis
    (E) Superficial spreading carcinoma

CASE 3: Questions 7 through 9

This 42-year-old woman has nausea and vomiting of recent onset. You are shown two radiographs from an upper gastrointestinal examination (Figure 3-1). Both were obtained 10 minutes after ingestion of barium.

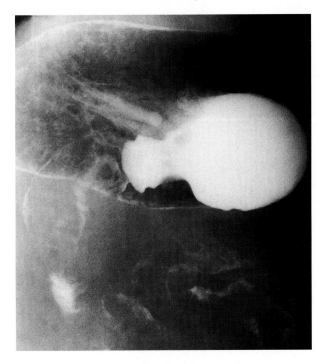

Figure 3-1

7. Which *one* of the following is the MOST likely diagnosis?

   (A) Pancreatic inflammatory mass
   (B) Adenocarcinoma of the duodenum
   (C) Leiomyosarcoma (stromal cell tumor)
   (D) Duodenal hematoma
   (E) Amyloidosis

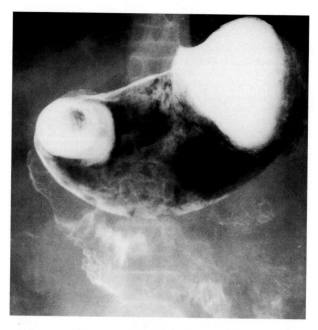

Figure 3-1 *(Continued)*

QUESTIONS 8 AND 9: MARK YOUR ANSWER SHEET TRUE (T) OR FALSE (F) FOR EACH OF THE RESPONSE CHOICES.

8. Concerning tumors of the duodenum,

   (A) most in the duodenal bulb are benign
   (B) gastrinomas rarely cause Zollinger-Ellison syndrome in the absence of hepatic metastases
   (C) the duodenum is the most common site of involvement by lymphoma in the gastrointestinal tract
   (D) most carcinomas are located at or distal to the papilla of Vater
   (E) villous tumors have a much lower rate of malignant transformation than do those in the colon
   (F) leiomyosarcoma typically presents as an annular stricture

CASE 3 (Cont'd)

9. Concerning amyloidosis,

   (A) the gastrointestinal tract is a common site of involvement
   (B) esophageal involvement causes both dilatation and loss of peristalsis
   (C) it causes impaired gastric emptying
   (D) the finding of duodenal amyloidosis should trigger the search for underlying carcinoma
   (E) small bowel involvement causes diffuse fold thickening

CASE 4: Questions 10 through 13

This 70-year-old man presented with metabolic alkalosis and abdominal pain and distension. You are shown three images from a CT study of the abdomen and pelvis (Figure 4-1).

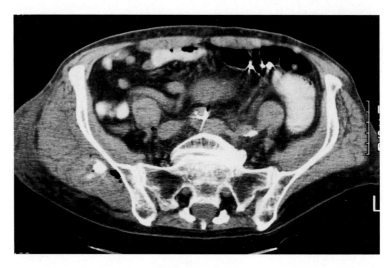

Figure 4-1

10. Which *one* of the following is the MOST likely diagnosis?

   (A) Diverticulitis
   (B) Metastatic tumor
   (C) Small bowel obstruction by adhesion
   (D) Crohn's disease
   (E) Strangulated hernia

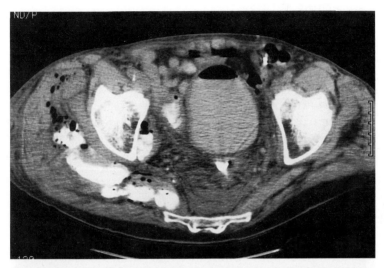

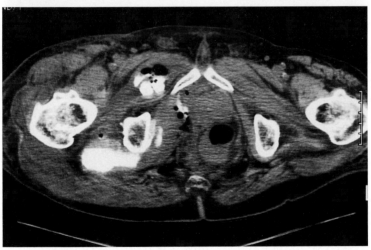

CASE 4 (Cont'd)

QUESTIONS 11 THROUGH 13: MARK YOUR ANSWER SHEET TRUE (T) OR FALSE (F) FOR EACH OF THE RESPONSE CHOICES.

11.   Concerning hernias,

    (A)   spigelian hernias always occur just lateral to the margin of the rectus abdominis muscle

    (B)   obturator hernias typically occur in elderly women

    (C)   sciatic hernias are rarely associated with bowel obstruction

    (D)   incarcerated Richter hernias are nearly always associated with bowel obstruction

    (E)   direct inguinal hernias are less likely to strangulate than are indirect inguinal hernias

12.   Concerning CT of small bowel obstruction,

    (A)   ileal dilatation (exceeding 2.5 cm) is a specific sign

    (B)   if it shows no apparent cause, adhesions are usually responsible for the obstruction

    (C)   air-fluid levels in the small intestine strongly suggest mechanical obstruction

    (D)   it is both more sensitive and more specific than abdominal radiography

    (E)   in patients with a history of cancer, it is likely to identify the specific cause of the obstruction

13.   Concerning CT findings in closed-loop obstruction,

    (A)   if strangulation occurs, the wall of the affected bowel loop is stretched thin as it worsens

    (B)   the presence of edema and hemorrhage within the affected mesentery suggests strangulation

    (C)   a U-shaped loop of bowel is characteristic

    (D)   the diagnosis of strangulation is based on the detection of intramural or portal venous gas

    (E)   the finding of two collapsed loops adjacent to the site of obstruction suggests the diagnosis

CASE 5: Questions 14 through 17

This 39-year-old woman has abdominal pain. You are shown pre-contrast (A) and postcontrast (B) CT scans of the abdomen (Figure 5-1).

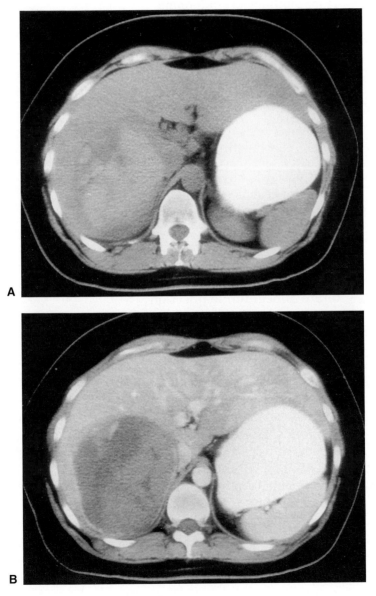

Figure 5-1

CASE 5 (Cont'd)

14. Which *one* of the following is the MOST likely diagnosis?

   (A) Focal nodular hyperplasia
   (B) Cavernous hemangioma
   (C) Hepatocellular adenoma
   (D) Hepatobiliary cystadenoma
   (E) Mesenchymal hamartoma

QUESTIONS 15 THROUGH 17: MARK YOUR ANSWER SHEET TRUE (T) OR FALSE (F) FOR EACH OF THE RESPONSE CHOICES.

15. Concerning focal nodular hyperplasia,

   (A) most patients have a solitary lesion
   (B) a central scar is specific for this lesion
   (C) a stellate central scar is consistently identified on dynamic contrast-enhanced CT scans
   (D) on T2-weighted MR images, the lesion is typically hypointense relative to normal liver
   (E) on MRI, the lesion does not enhance following gadopentetate dimeglumine injection

16. Concerning cavernous hemangiomas of the liver,

   (A) they are encapsulated
   (B) small lesions are typically both hyperechoic and homogeneous sonographically
   (C) nodular peripheral enhancement on contrast-enhanced dynamic CT is a characteristic feature
   (D) on delayed postcontrast CT images, complete fill-in is essential for establishing the diagnosis
   (E) the specificity of SPECT with Tc-99m erythrocytes is less than 50%
   (F) the specificity of MRI for diagnosing lesions is about 90%

17. Concerning hepatocellular adenoma,

 (A) use of anabolic steroids is a risk factor
 (B) cirrhosis is a risk factor
 (C) it does not demonstrate uptake of Tc-99m sulfur colloid
 (D) sonographically, the lesion often appears identical to focal nodular hyperplasia
 (E) pathologically, it has no distinct surrounding capsule

This 62-year-old man on chronic hemodialysis has vague abdominal pain. You are shown a spot radiograph of the duodenum from an upper gastrointestinal examination (Figure 6-1).

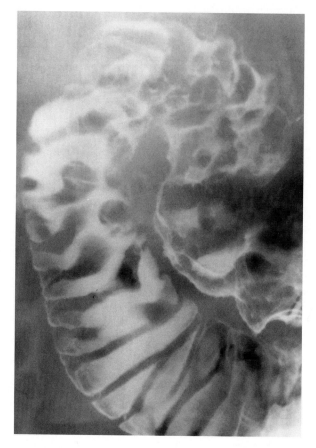

Figure 6-1

18. Which *one* of the following is the MOST likely cause of the findings?

(A) Renal failure
(B) Pancreatitis
(C) Ischemia
(D) Lymphoma
(E) Crohn's disease

This 53-year-old man has epigastric discomfort. You are shown a spot radiograph from an upper gastrointestinal examination (Figure 7-1).

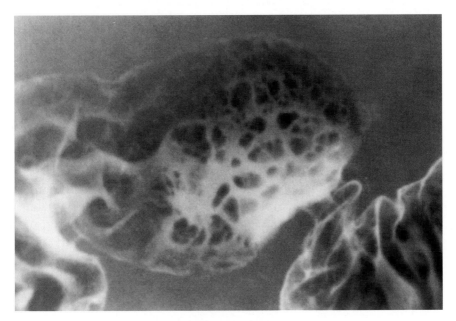

Figure 7-1

19. Which *one* of the following is the MOST likely diagnosis?

(A) Duodenitis
(B) Lymphoid hyperplasia
(C) Brunner's gland hyperplasia
(D) Heterotopic gastric mucosa
(E) Crohn's disease

CASE 7 (Cont'd)

QUESTIONS 20 AND 21: MARK YOUR ANSWER SHEET TRUE
(T) OR FALSE (F) FOR EACH OF THE RESPONSE CHOICES.

20. Concerning Brunner's gland hyperplasia,

   (A) it occurs in response to increased gastric acid secretion
   (B) it is often associated with duodenitis
   (C) it is confined to the duodenal bulb
   (D) it is a premalignant condition
   (E) lymphoid hyperplasia produces similar radiographic findings

21. Concerning heterotopic gastric mucosa in the duodenum,

   (A) it is a premalignant condition
   (B) it commonly causes epigastric pain
   (C) endoscopic biopsies should be performed to confirm the diagnosis when barium studies suggest this condition
   (D) it tends to be located near the base of the duodenal bulb
   (E) prolapsed gastric mucosa produces similar radiographic findings

This 60-year-old man with chronic active hepatitis is being evaluated for possible liver transplantation. You are shown T1-weighted (A) and T2-weighted (B) MR images (Figure 8-1).

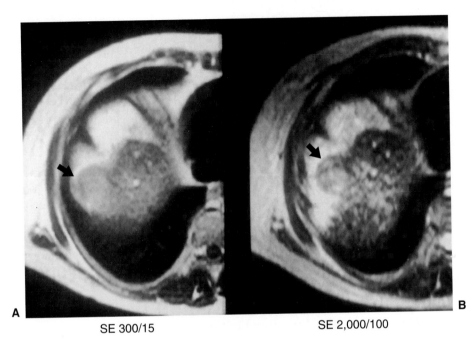

SE 300/15   SE 2,000/100

Figure 8-1

22. The hepatic lesion (arrow) in the test images MOST probably represents:

    (A) regenerative nodule
    (B) adenomatous hyperplasia (macroregenerative nodule)
    (C) nodular regenerative hyperplasia
    (D) hepatocellular carcinoma
    (E) fibrolamellar hepatocellular carcinoma

QUESTIONS 23 THROUGH 25: MARK YOUR ANSWER SHEET TRUE (T) OR FALSE (F) FOR EACH OF THE RESPONSE CHOICES.

23.   Concerning regenerative nodules,

(A) they are invariably present in the cirrhotic liver
(B) they are composed of hepatocytes surrounded by fibrosis
(C) they are easily identified on contrast-enhanced CT scans
(D) their low signal intensity on T2-weighted MR images is due to iron deposition

24.   Imaging features suggestive of hepatocellular carcinoma include:

(A) venous invasion
(B) encapsulation
(C) intratumoral septation
(D) intratumoral arterial flow
(E) arterioportal shunting

25.   Concerning fibrolamellar hepatocellular carcinoma,

(A) it occurs most commonly in elderly patients
(B) it is associated with cirrhosis
(C) it is usually multifocal
(D) central calcification is a characteristic feature
(E) the prognosis is favorable compared with that for typical hepatocellular carcinoma

CASE 9: Question 26

This 47-year-old woman has epigastric discomfort and heme-positive stool samples. You are shown a radiograph from an upper gastrointestinal examination (Figure 9-1).

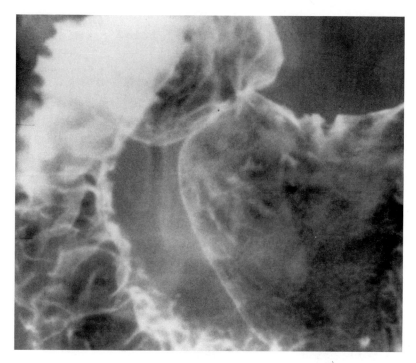

Figure 9-1

26. Which *one* of the following is the MOST likely cause of the findings?

(A) *Helicobacter pylori*
(B) Cytomegalovirus
(C) Nonsteroidal anti-inflammatory drugs
(D) Crohn's disease
(E) Zollinger-Ellison syndrome

This 35-year-old HIV-positive man presented with odynophagia. You are shown double-contrast (A) and single-contrast (B) radiographs from an esophagram (Figure 10-1).

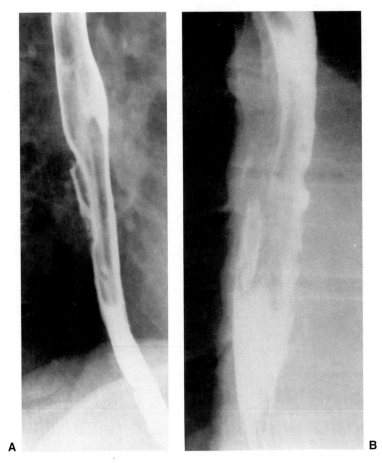

Figure 10-1

27. Which *one* of the following is the MOST likely diagnosis?

(A) *Candida* esophagitis
(B) Herpes esophagitis
(C) HIV esophagitis
(D) Lymphoma
(E) Kaposi's sarcoma

CASE 10 (Cont'd)

QUESTIONS 28 THROUGH 30: MARK YOUR ANSWER SHEET TRUE (T) OR FALSE (F) FOR EACH OF THE RESPONSE CHOICES.

28. Concerning *Candida* esophagitis,

   (A) it is the most common type of opportunistic esophagitis
   (B) about 90% of patients have associated oropharyngeal candidiasis
   (C) plaques are seen on double-contrast esophagrams in about 90% of endoscopically proven cases
   (D) a shaggy esophageal contour is characteristic of early candidiasis
   (E) an infiltrating esophageal carcinoma produces similar radiographic findings

29. Concerning herpes esophagitis,

   (A) it is characterized by discrete, superficial ulcers
   (B) it occasionally occurs as an acute, self-limited syndrome in otherwise healthy patients
   (C) eosinophilic intranuclear inclusions are characteristic
   (D) it often leads to the formation of esophageal strictures
   (E) drug-induced esophagitis produces similar radiographic findings

30. Concerning HIV esophagitis,

   (A) not all affected individuals have AIDS at the time of presentation
   (B) it can be associated with a maculopapular rash on the upper half of the body
   (C) cytomegalovirus esophagitis produces similar radiographic findings
   (D) treatment with oral steroids is recommended

CASE 11: Questions 31 through 33

This 22-year-old man with AIDS has fever, leukocytosis, right lower quadrant pain, and bloody diarrhea. You are shown two images from an abdominal CT scan (Figure 11-1).

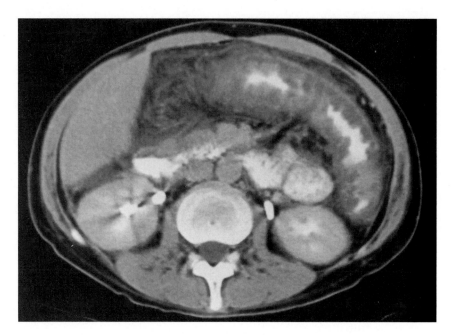

Figure 11-1

31. Which *one* of the following is the MOST likely diagnosis?

   (A) Lymphoma
   (B) Cytomegalovirus colitis
   (C) Herpes simplex colitis
   (D) Pseudomembranous colitis
   (E) Gonococcal colitis

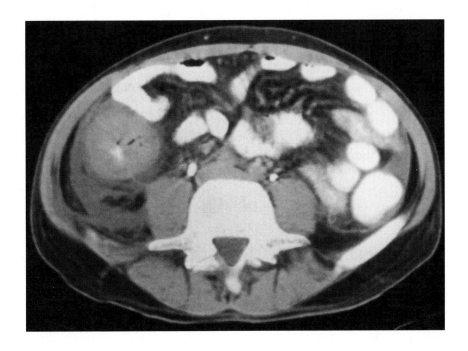

QUESTIONS 32 AND 33: MARK YOUR ANSWER SHEET TRUE (T) OR FALSE (F) FOR EACH OF THE RESPONSE CHOICES.

32. Concerning gastrointestinal infections in patients with AIDS,

   (A) symptomatic infection occurs in most patients with AIDS

   (B) a specific pathogen is identified in fewer than 50% of patients with diarrhea

   (C) there is little geographic variation in causative pathogens

   (D) mucosal biopsy is usually necessary to establish a diagnosis of viral infection

   (E) infections of the small bowel usually have nonspecific radiologic findings

33. Concerning gastrointestinal tumors in patients with AIDS,

   (A) lymphoma arises more commonly in the stomach than in the duodenum
   (B) bowel involvement with lymphoma is infrequent in the absence of nodal disease
   (C) most patients with Kaposi's sarcoma involving the bowel have skin lesions
   (D) submucosal nodules are the characteristic radiologic finding in patients with gastrointestinal Kaposi's sarcoma
   (E) there is a high incidence of anal cancer

CASE 12: Questions 34 through 36

This 47-year-old man has fever and right lower quadrant pain. You are shown a postcontrast CT scan of the lower abdomen (Figure 12-1).

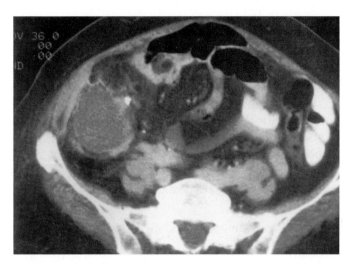

Figure 12-1

34. Which *one* of the following is the MOST likely diagnosis?

   (A) Ruptured cecal carcinoma
   (B) Ruptured cecal diverticulum
   (C) Periappendiceal phlegmon
   (D) Periappendiceal abscess
   (E) Mucocele of the appendix

CASE 12 (Cont'd)

QUESTIONS 35 AND 36: MARK YOUR ANSWER SHEET TRUE (T) OR FALSE (F) FOR EACH OF THE RESPONSE CHOICES.

35. Concerning periappendiceal inflammatory masses,

    (A) percutaneous drainage of periappendiceal phlegmons is contraindicated
    (B) small (1- to 2-cm) periappendiceal abscesses can be treated successfully with broad-spectrum intravenous antibiotics
    (C) percutaneous drainage of periappendiceal abscesses has a complication rate of less than 10%
    (D) fistulas to the cecum or base of the appendix are commonly demonstrated on immediate post-drainage abscess sinograms
    (E) fistulas to the cecum or base of the appendix rarely close without operative intervention

36. Concerning mucoceles of the appendix,

    (A) they are found in approximately 5% of all appendectomy specimens
    (B) the most common CT appearance is a tubular low-density mass
    (C) they are a cause of enteroenteric intussusception
    (D) they are associated with pseudomyxoma peritonei

This 64-year-old alcoholic man has abnormal liver function tests. You are shown an oblique color Doppler sonogram of the porta hepatis (Figure 13-1).

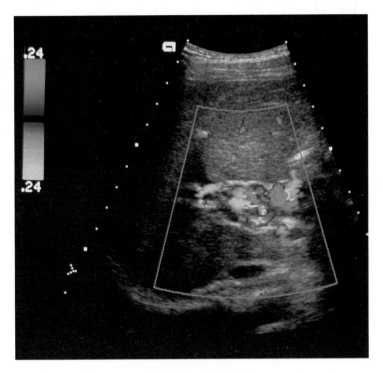

Figure 13-1

37. Which *one* of the following is the MOST likely diagnosis?

   (A) Cavernous transformation of the portal vein
   (B) Acute portal vein thrombosis
   (C) Hepatic artery aneurysm
   (D) Pylephlebitis
   (E) Periportal adenopathy

CASE 13 (Cont'd)

QUESTION 38: MARK YOUR ANSWER SHEET TRUE (T) OR
FALSE (F) FOR EACH OF THE RESPONSE CHOICES.

38.   Concerning portal vein thrombosis,

    (A) septic thrombosis is associated with *Bacteroides fragilis* septicemia

    (B) signal within the portal vein on spin-echo MR images is diagnostic for thrombosis

    (C) duplex sonography demonstrating arterial flow within a portal vein thrombus suggests tumor thrombosis

    (D) its high intensity on T2-weighted spin-echo MR images is due to extracellular methemoglobin

    (E) on noncontrast CT, acute thrombus in the portal vein has an attenuation lower than flowing blood

CASE 14: Questions 39 through 41

This 27-year-old man sustained blunt abdominal trauma in a motor vehicle accident. You are shown a CT scan obtained after both oral and intravenous administration of contrast medium (Figure 14-1).

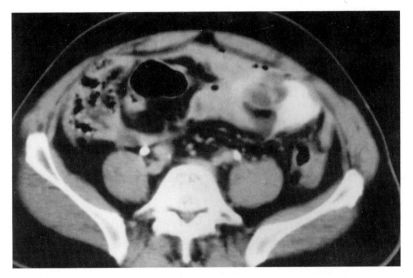

Figure 14-1

39. Which *one* of the following is the MOST likely diagnosis?

    (A) Intraperitoneal hemorrhage
    (B) Mesenteric hematoma
    (C) Small bowel obstruction
    (D) Colonic hematoma
    (E) Jejunal perforation

CASE 14 (Cont'd)

QUESTIONS 40 AND 41: MARK YOUR ANSWER SHEET TRUE (T) OR FALSE (F) FOR EACH OF THE RESPONSE CHOICES.

40. Concerning CT of blunt abdominal trauma,

   (A) the most common site of gastrointestinal injury is the jejunum
   (B) free air is nearly always noted if the jejunum is perforated
   (C) interloop blood is a common finding in patients with splenic lacerations
   (D) focal bowel wall thickening is a sign of intramural hematoma
   (E) water-density interloop fluid is a sign of small bowel perforation

41. Concerning intra-abdominal hemorrhage on CT scans of blunt abdominal trauma,

   (A) the fluid attenuation value with acute hemoperitoneum is typically greater than 30 HU
   (B) the fluid attenuation value with acute hemoperitoneum is lower in patients with severe anemia than in patients who are not anemic
   (C) clotted blood has a higher attenuation value than free lysed blood does
   (D) the "sentinel clot" sign refers to the observation that blood has higher attenuation values closer to the site of injury
   (E) on precontrast studies, areas of active arterial extravasation are often isodense with adjacent major arterial structures

Four patients referred for evaluation of obstructive jaundice underwent cholangiography and CT studies (Figures 15-1 through 15-4). For each numbered set of images listed below (Questions 42 through 45), select the *one* lettered diagnosis (A, B, C, D, or E) that is MOST closely associated with it. Each lettered diagnosis may be used once, more than once, or not at all.

42. Figure 15-1
43. Figure 15-2
44. Figure 15-3
45. Figure 15-4

(A) Carcinoma of the bile duct
(B) AIDS cholangiopathy
(C) Nodal metastases to the porta hepatis
(D) Carcinoma of the gallbladder
(E) Mirizzi's syndrome

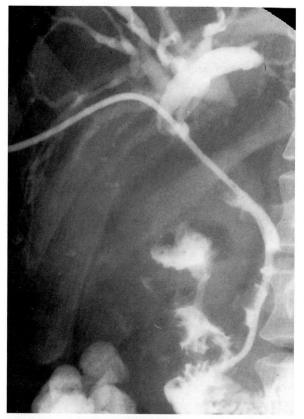

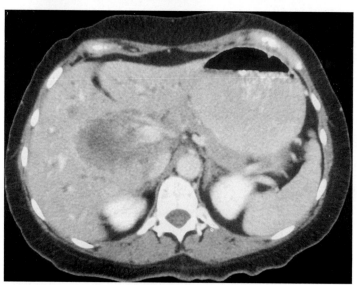

Figure 15-1

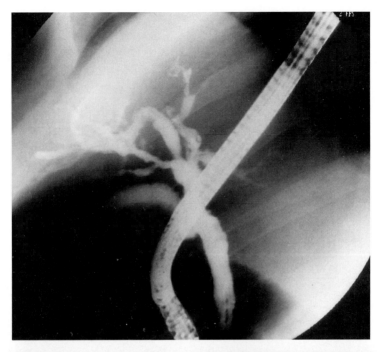

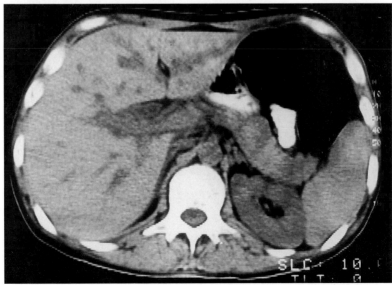

Figure 15-2

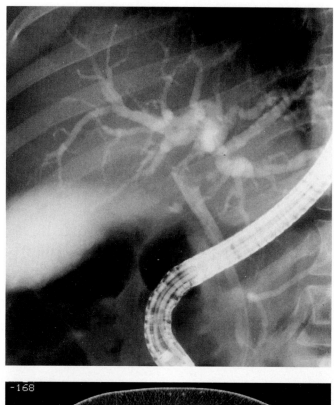

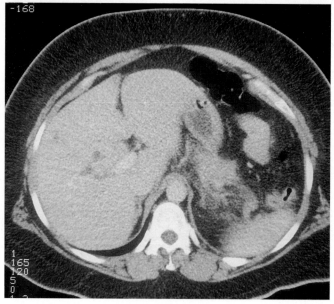

Figure 15-3

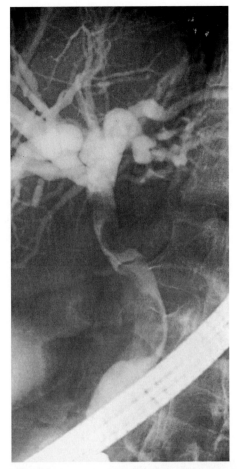

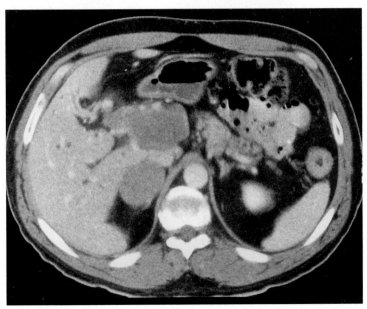

Figure 15-4

CASE 15 (Cont'd)

QUESTION 46: MARK YOUR ANSWER SHEET TRUE (T) OR
FALSE (F) FOR EACH OF THE RESPONSE CHOICES.

46. Concerning percutaneous biliary drainage,

   (A) direct drainage of the left hepatic duct is contraindicated

   (B) it is important to attempt placement of an internal (duodenal) drainage catheter during the initial procedure

   (C) in patients with multiple obstructed segments, all hepatic segments should be drained

   (D) in patients with distal obstruction, endoscopic drainage is preferable

   (E) in patients undergoing catheter drainage who develop hemobilia, a cholangiogram is the first radiologic examination that should be performed

This 50-year-old woman has fever, right upper quadrant abdominal pain, and pleuritic left chest pain. You are shown two images from an abdominal CT scan (Figure 16-1).

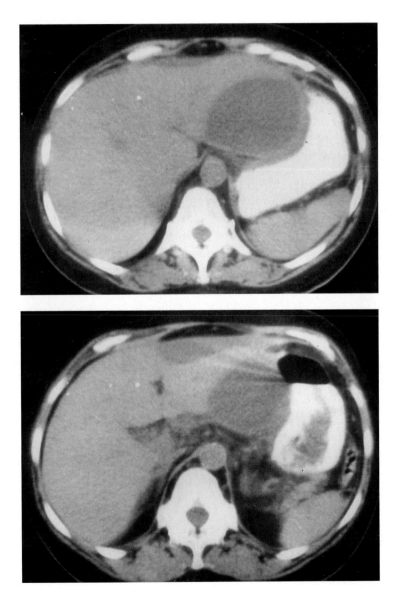

Figure 16-1

47. Which *one* of the following is the MOST likely diagnosis?

   (A) Pyogenic liver abscess
   (B) Amebic liver abscess
   (C) Echinococcosis
   (D) Abscess in the greater peritoneal sac
   (E) Abscess in the lesser peritoneal sac

QUESTIONS 48 THROUGH 52: MARK YOUR ANSWER SHEET TRUE (T) OR FALSE (F) FOR EACH OF THE RESPONSE CHOICES.

48. Concerning the lesser peritoneal sac,

   (A) a needle can be placed into a collection in the inferior recess without traversing any structure except properitoneal fat
   (B) collections in the inferior recess occasionally extend into the greater omentum
   (C) in draining collections in the superior recess, a catheter traversing the left lobe of the liver is acceptable
   (D) part of the anterior border of the inferior recess is formed by the lesser omentum
   (E) abscesses within the superior recess usually extend into the hepatorenal recess (Morison's pouch)

49. Concerning intrahepatic infectious lesions,

   (A) pyogenic abscesses are solitary in over 95% of patients
   (B) in immunocompetent patients, most abscesses result from seeding of the portal vein from appendicitis
   (C) in immunocompromised patients, multiple small (<2-cm) collections are most likely to be caused by *Candida albicans*
   (D) hydatid cysts can be successfully treated by percutaneous aspiration
   (E) peripheral calcification is a characteristic of hydatid cysts

50. Contraindications to percutaneous abscess drainage include:

   (A) multiple loculations
   (B) ascites
   (C) lack of a safe access route
   (D) bleeding diathesis
   (E) infected pseudoaneurysms

51. Concerning percutaneous abscess drainage,

   (A) successful drainage of a pleural space collection requires a larger-diameter catheter than does drainage of an abdominal abscess
   (B) routine irrigation of the abscess cavity with an antibiotic solution is beneficial
   (C) an enteric fistula is a cause of therapeutic failure
   (D) complete distension of the abscess cavity is potentially hazardous

52. Concerning injection of contrast agent into an abscess cavity (abscess sinography),

   (A) it is indicated when CT, ultrasonography, or clinical evaluation suggests the presence of a residual cavity
   (B) it is essential before removal of the drainage catheter
   (C) it is helpful in evaluating patients with persistent or increasing drainage
   (D) in conjunction with CT, it is useful in detecting residual pockets not drained by the abscess catheter

This 32-year-old HIV-positive man has vague right upper quadrant pain. You are shown transverse sonograms of the liver (Figure 17-1).

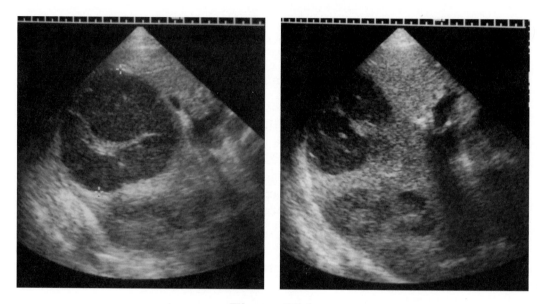

Figure 17-1

53. Which *one* of the following is the MOST likely diagnosis?

    (A) Pyogenic abscess
    (B) Lymphoma
    (C) Kaposi's sarcoma
    (D) Mycobacterial infection
    (E) *Pneumocystis carinii* infection

CASE 17 (Cont'd)

QUESTIONS 54 THROUGH 56: MARK YOUR ANSWER SHEET TRUE (T) OR FALSE (F) FOR EACH OF THE RESPONSE CHOICES.

54. Concerning lymphadenopathy in patients with HIV infection,

    (A) mild enlargement of retroperitoneal lymph nodes (less than 1.5 cm) is often due to reactive hyperplasia
    (B) Kaposi's sarcoma is a cause of bulky retroperitoneal lymphadenopathy
    (C) on postcontrast CT, low-attenuation areas within the lymph nodes are typically due to Kaposi's sarcoma
    (D) percutaneous fine-needle aspiration biopsy of enlarged lymph nodes often yields a specific diagnosis

55. Concerning AIDS-related lymphomas,

    (A) they are aggressive histologic subtypes of non-Hodgkin's lymphoma
    (B) most patients present with advanced disease
    (C) there is a predilection for extranodal sites of involvement
    (D) the liver is a commonly involved extranodal site

56. Features of extrapulmonary *Pneumocystis carinii* infection in patients with AIDS include:

    (A) punctate calcifications in the liver and spleen
    (B) generalized renal hypoechogenicity
    (C) splenic abscesses
    (D) biliary obstruction
    (E) association with prophylactic pentamidine inhalation therapy

This 52-year-old man has vague abdominal discomfort 6 months after an episode of pancreatitis. You are shown a transverse sonogram of the upper abdomen (A), a corresponding color Doppler sonogram (B), and a spectral Doppler waveform tracing at the same level (C) (Figure 18-1).

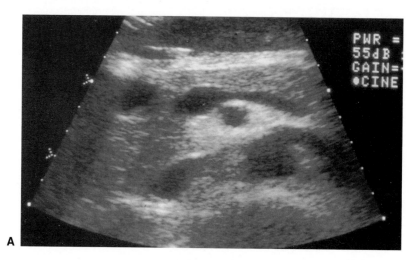

Figure 18-1

57. Which *one* of the following is the MOST likely diagnosis?

    (A) Arteriovenous malformation
    (B) Pseudocyst
    (C) Neuroendocrine tumor
    (D) Pseudoaneurysm
    (E) Varix

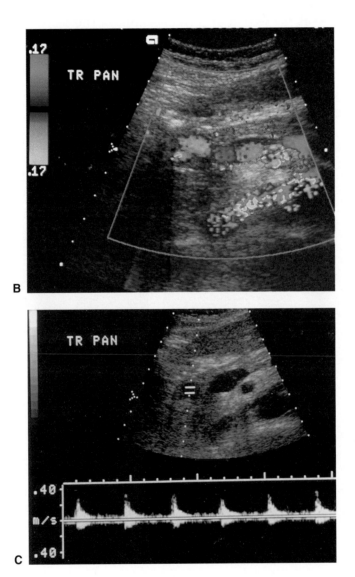

This 64-year-old man underwent total laryngectomy 13 months ago for a large epiglottic carcinoma. He now complains of slowly progressive dysphagia for solid food. You are shown solid-column (A) and air-contrast (B) lateral radiographs of the pharynx (Figure 19-1).

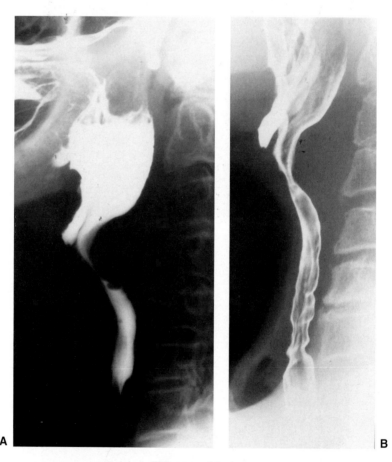

A   B

Figure 19-1

58. Which *one* of the following is the MOST likely diagnosis?

    (A) Ulceration of the neopharynx
    (B) Recurrent carcinoma of the posterior pharyngeal mucosa
    (C) Expected postoperative appearance of the pharynx after total laryngectomy
    (D) Benign stricture of the neopharynx
    (E) Abscess within the soft tissues at the base of the neck

QUESTION 59: MARK YOUR ANSWER SHEET TRUE (T) OR FALSE (F) FOR EACH OF THE RESPONSE CHOICES.

59. Concerning the complications of total laryngectomy,

    (A) pharyngeal ulceration is a common early postoperative complication
    (B) fistulas and sinus tracts originate most often from the lower margin of the surgical suture line
    (C) preoperative radiation therapy increases the frequency of fistulas and sinus tracts
    (D) recurrent carcinoma occurs more commonly in the soft tissues of the neck than in the remaining pharyngeal mucosa
    (E) about 15% of patients will develop dysphagia

This 50-year-old man has vague upper abdominal discomfort. You are shown pre- and postcontrast CT images (Figure 20-1) and T1- and T2-weighted MR images (Figure 20-2).

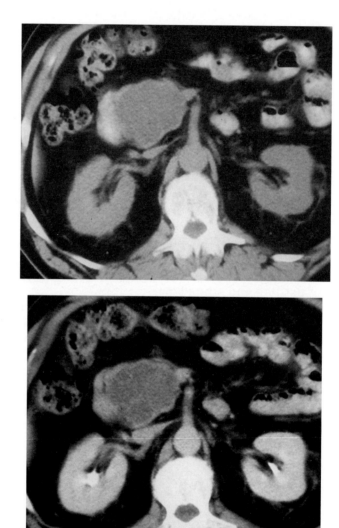

Figure 20-1

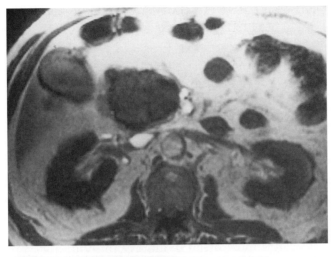

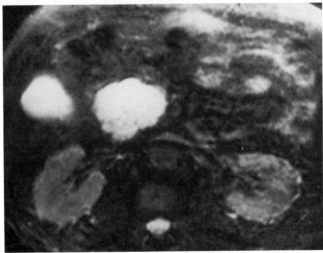

Figure 20-2

60. Which *one* of the following is the MOST likely diagnosis?

   (A) Mucinous cystic neoplasm
   (B) Adenocarcinoma
   (C) Serous cystadenoma
   (D) Solid and papillary epithelial neoplasm
   (E) Mucin-hypersecreting tumor of the pancreatic duct

QUESTIONS 61 THROUGH 63: MARK YOUR ANSWER SHEET TRUE (T) OR FALSE (F) FOR EACH OF THE RESPONSE CHOICES.

61. Concerning serous cystadenoma,

    (A) it usually arises in the pancreatic tail
    (B) calcification is typically central
    (C) its epithelium is rich in glycogen
    (D) the septa are well vascularized
    (E) its malignant potential is high

62. Concerning solid and papillary epithelial neoplasm,

    (A) it occurs most often in elderly individuals
    (B) it is associated with von Hippel-Lindau disease
    (C) cystic degeneration is common
    (D) calcification is typically central
    (E) metastasis is usual at the time of discovery

63. Concerning mucin-hypersecreting tumors of the pancreatic duct,

    (A) they rarely involve ductal side branches
    (B) histologically, they resemble mucinous cystic neo-plasms
    (C) most are surgically resectable when discovered
    (D) pancreatitis is a common clinical presentation
    (E) intraductal filling defects are a characteristic finding on endoscopic retrograde pancreatography

This 60-year-old man has dysphagia and heme-positive stools. You are shown a radiograph from an upper gastrointestinal examination (Figure 21-1).

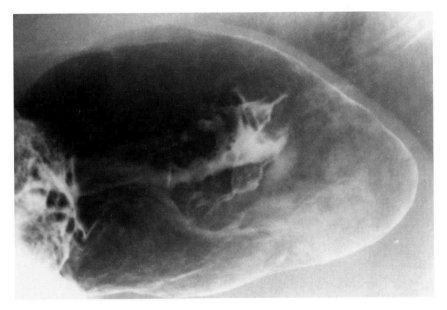

Figure 21-1

64. Which *one* of the following is the MOST likely diagnosis?

   (A) Lymphoma
   (B) Varices
   (C) Carcinoma of the cardia
   (D) Metastatic squamous cell carcinoma
   (E) Benign gastric ulcer

CASE 21 (Cont'd)

QUESTIONS 65 AND 66: MARK YOUR ANSWER SHEET TRUE
(T) OR FALSE (F) FOR EACH OF THE RESPONSE CHOICES.

65. Concerning carcinoma arising at the cardia,

    (A) it makes up less than 10% of all gastric cancers

    (B) it is more common in men than in women

    (C) at surgery, the esophagus is involved by tumor in less than 10% of patients

    (D) referred dysphagia to the upper esophagus or pharynx is a symptom

    (E) affected individuals have a better prognosis than patients with carcinoma arising in a Barrett's esophagus that invades the gastroesophageal junction

66. Concerning gastric metastases from squamous cell carcinoma of the esophagus,

    (A) they are found at autopsy in about 50% of patients who die of esophageal carcinoma

    (B) they are caused by tumor emboli that seed the gastric fundus via submucosal esophageal lymphatics

    (C) they rarely occur in patients with carcinoma of the upper esophagus or midesophagus

    (D) barium studies usually demonstrate multiple lesions

    (E) they are often indistinguishable from gastric leiomyomas

This 48-year-old man with idiopathic cirrhosis underwent a trans-jugular intrahepatic portosystemic shunt (TIPS) procedure for intractable variceal bleeding 6 months ago. You are shown a color Doppler sonogram (Figure 22-1) performed as a routine follow-up study to evaluate the shunt.

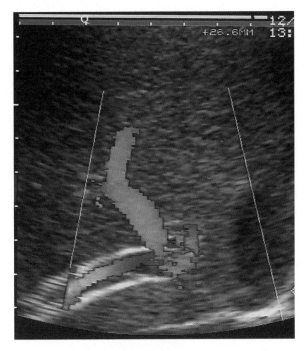

Figure 22-1

QUESTIONS 67 AND 68: MARK YOUR ANSWER SHEET TRUE (T) OR FALSE (F) FOR EACH OF THE RESPONSE CHOICES.

67. Concerning this patient,

    (A) flow within the shunt is in the normal direction

    (B) the direction of flow in the portal vein branches suggests shunt malfunction

    (C) there is evidence of pseudointimal hyperplasia within the shunt

    (D) the patient is at risk for recurrent variceal bleeding

68. Concerning Doppler sonography of the portal vein,

   (A) the normal waveform is triphasic in nature
   (B) flow reversal is an early sign of portal hypertension
   (C) a hepatic mass is a cause of focal flow reversal
   (D) flow within intrahepatic branches adjacent to the shunt is reversed (hepatofugal) after TIPS placement
   (E) flow velocity in the main portal vein is expected to increase after a successful TIPS procedure

You are shown a CT scan (Figure 23-1) of a 50-year-old man with abdominal pain and distension 1 week after laparoscopic cholecystectomy.

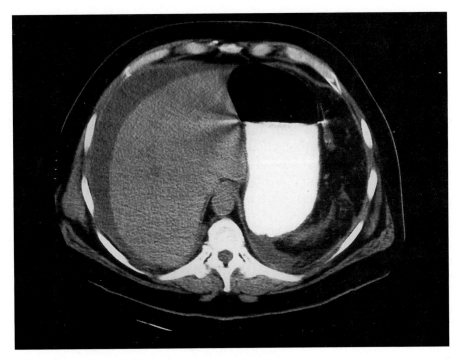

Figure 23-1

69. Which *one* of the following complications is the MOST likely cause of the CT findings in the test patient?

   (A) Duodenal perforation
   (B) Intraperitoneal hematoma
   (C) Intraperitoneal abscess
   (D) Bile leakage from the cystic duct remnant
   (E) Ligation of the common hepatic bile duct

CASE 23 (Cont'd)

QUESTION 70: MARK YOUR ANSWER SHEET TRUE (T) OR FALSE (F) FOR EACH OF THE RESPONSE CHOICES.

70. Concerning laparoscopic cholecystectomy and its complications,

    (A) the site of a bile duct injury can usually be determined by CT

    (B) most bile duct injuries involve the proximal extrahepatic bile ducts (within 2 cm of the confluence of the right and left hepatic ducts)

    (C) most bile duct injuries occur in patients with anomalous bile duct anatomy

    (D) intraoperative cholangiography is technically possible in less than 50% of laparoscopic cholecystectomies

    (E) hepatobiliary scintigraphy is useful to distinguish cystic duct remnant leak from common hepatic duct injury

    (F) leaks from the cystic duct remnant usually require surgical repair

    (G) ligation of the hepatic artery rarely leads to hepatic infarction

This 70-year-old man has a chronically sore throat. He received full-course radiation therapy for an epidermoid cancer of the right true vocal cord 7 years ago and continued to smoke and drink alcohol after therapy. You are shown a lateral radiograph (Figure 24-1) from an air-contrast barium pharyngogram.

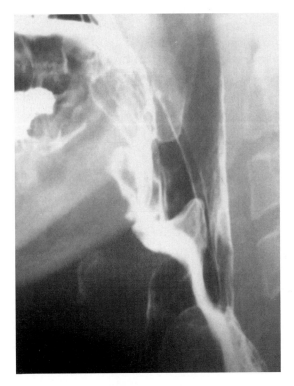

Figure 24-1

71. Which *one* of the following is the MOST likely diagnosis?

(A) Expected appearance of the pharynx after irradiation
(B) Recurrent carcinoma
(C) New primary epidermoid carcinoma
(D) Radiation-induced ulceration
(E) Pharyngeal diverticulum

CASE 24 (Cont'd)

QUESTION 72: MARK YOUR ANSWER SHEET TRUE (T) OR
FALSE (F) FOR EACH OF THE RESPONSE CHOICES.

72.   Concerning the pharynx after radiation therapy,

    (A) chondronecrosis is a frequent complication of full-
course therapy

    (B) asymmetry of the mucosa overlying the arytenoid carti-
lage is a sign of recurrent carcinoma

    (C) aspiration often occurs without associated coughing

    (D) the epiglottis often exhibits reduced motility

    (E) mucosal biopsy is not completely reliable in diagnosing
recurrent cancer within an irradiated field

CASE 25: Questions 73 through 76

This 42-year-old woman received an orthotopic liver transplant 3 months ago. She now has abnormal liver function tests. You are shown a longitudinal oblique abdominal sonogram through the porta hepatis (Figure 25-1) and a T-tube cholangiogram (Figure 25-2).

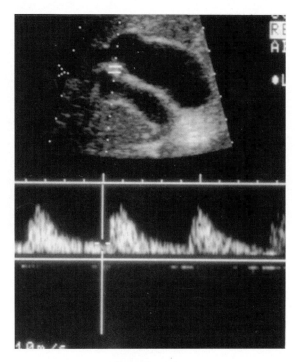

Figure 25-1

73. Which *one* of the following is the MOST likely cause of the finding?

(A) Hepatic artery stenosis
(B) Chronic rejection
(C) Cytomegalovirus infection
(D) Postsurgical fibrosis
(E) Sclerosing cholangitis

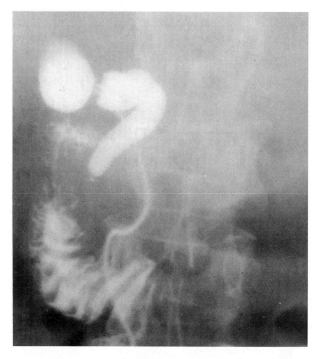

Figure 25-2

QUESTIONS 74 THROUGH 76: MARK YOUR ANSWER SHEET TRUE (T) OR FALSE (F) FOR EACH OF THE RESPONSE CHOICES.

74. Concerning the portal vein in liver transplant recipients,

(A) a normal Doppler sonographic examination demonstrates continuous flow with variation due to respiration

(B) thrombosis of this vessel is the most common vascular complication after transplantation

(C) the site of anastomosis cannot be visualized by ultrasonography

(D) stenosis at the anastomosis is characterized on Doppler sonography by low-velocity blood flow in the main portal vein distal to the anastomosis

CASE 25 (Cont'd)

75. Concerning hepatic artery thrombosis in liver transplant re-
    cipients,

    (A) it is more common in adults than in children
    (B) massive hepatic necrosis is the most common initial
        clinical presentation
    (C) retransplantation is often necessary
    (D) it occasionally presents clinically with bile leakage

76. Concerning post-transplantation lymphoproliferative disor-
    der,

    (A) it is related to Epstein-Barr virus infection
    (B) it affects less than 1% of transplant recipients
    (C) it is more likely to occur following liver transplantation
        than following heart-lung transplantation
    (D) the mean interval between transplantation and devel-
        opment of the disease is 5 years
    (E) treatment is the same as that for classic non-Hodgkin's
        lymphoma

Four patients underwent postcontrast CT for evaluation of abnormal liver function tests. For each numbered image listed below (Figures 26-1 through 26-4), select the *one* lettered explanation for the CT appearance (A, B, C, D, or E) that is MOST likely. Each lettered explanation may be used once, more than once, or not at all.

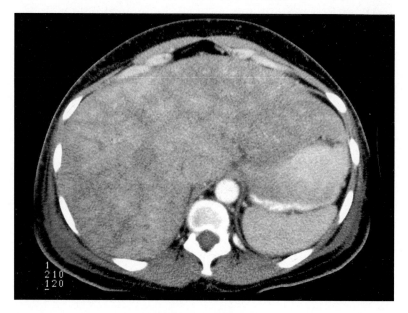

Figure 26-1

77. Figure 26-1
78. Figure 26-2 (Note: this patient has a known metastasis [M])
79. Figure 26-3
80. Figure 26-4

    (A)   Preferential segmental arterial flow
    (B)   Thrombosis of the main portal vein
    (C)   Hepatic venous outflow impairment
    (D)   Superior vena cava obstruction
    (E)   Focal fatty infiltration

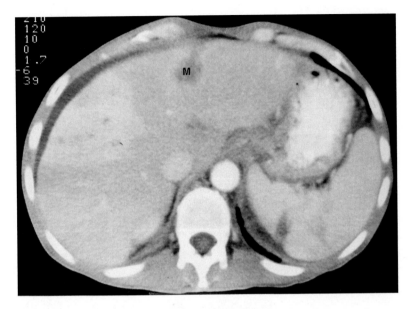

Figure 26-2

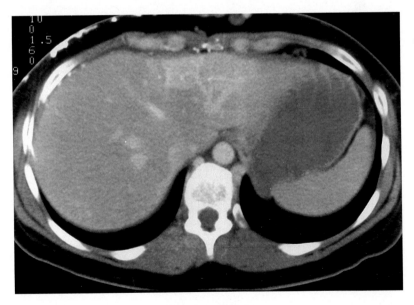

Figure 26-3

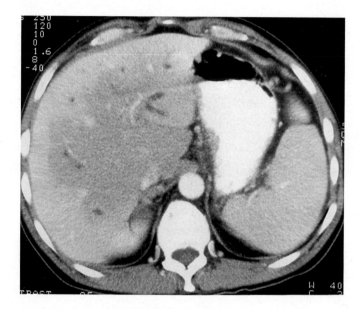

Figure 26-4

This 65-year-old man has recent onset of dysphagia and weight loss. You are shown a radiograph from an esophagram (Figure 27-1). There was no esophageal peristalsis at fluoroscopy.

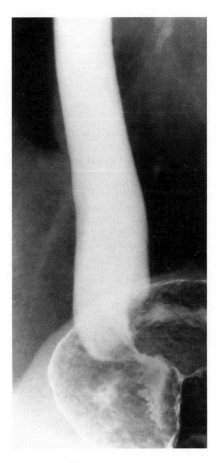

Figure 27-1

81. Which *one* of the following is the MOST likely diagnosis?

(A) Primary achalasia
(B) Secondary achalasia (pseudoachalasia)
(C) Peptic stricture
(D) Esophageal carcinoma
(E) Scleroderma

This 48-year-old woman with adenocarcinoma of the colon is being evaluated for possible resection of hepatic metastatic disease. You are shown one image from a CT arterial portogram (Figure 28-1).

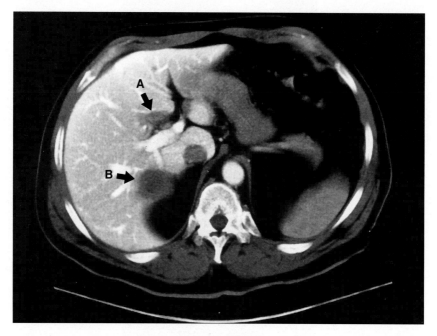

Figure 28-1

82. Which *one* of the following is the MOST likely explanation for the finding indicated by the arrow labeled A?

(A) Metastasis
(B) Hemangioma
(C) Benign perfusion defect
(D) Hepatic cyst
(E) Portal vein occlusion

CASE 28 (Cont'd)

QUESTIONS 83 AND 84: MARK YOUR ANSWER SHEET TRUE
(T) OR FALSE (F) FOR EACH OF THE RESPONSE CHOICES.

83. Concerning the lesion marked with the arrow labeled B on
     the test image,

     (A) it is located in the anterior segment of the right hepatic
          lobe
     (B) it is located in Couinaud's segment VIII
     (C) it involves the inferior vena cava
     (D) its appearance excludes cavernous hemangioma

84. Concerning surgical resection of hepatic metastases from a
     primary colorectal carcinoma,

     (A) approximately 30% of patients with newly diagnosed
          colorectal cancer meet the criteria for hepatic resection
     (B) only patients with solitary metastatic lesions are con-
          sidered candidates
     (C) lymph node metastases are a contraindication to he-
          patic resection
     (D) the post-resection liver volume must be at least 50% of
          the preoperative volume
     (E) the 5-year survival rate is about 60%

This 44-year-old woman has recurrent gastrointestinal hemor-rhage. You are shown three radiographs from a superior mesen-teric arteriogram (Figure 29-1).

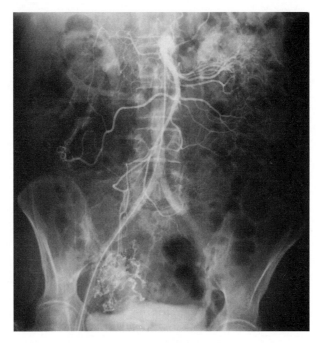

Figure 29-1

85. Which *one* of the following is the MOST likely diagnosis?

(A) Angiodysplasia
(B) Adenocarcinoma
(C) Leiomyosarcoma
(D) Small bowel diverticulum
(E) Carcinoid tumor

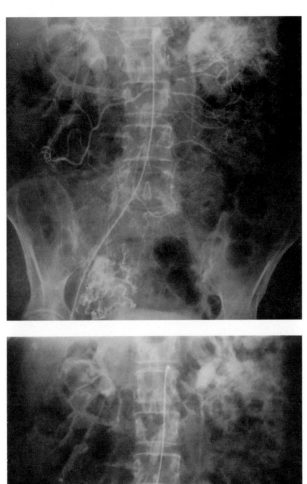

Figure 29-1 *(Continued)*

QUESTIONS 86 AND 87: MARK YOUR ANSWER SHEET TRUE (T) OR FALSE (F) FOR EACH OF THE RESPONSE CHOICES.

86. Concerning gastrointestinal angiodysplasia,

    (A) most occur in the descending colon

    (B) arteriography shows late opacification of the ileocolic vein

    (C) venous varices often lie adjacent to the lesion

    (D) it is a common cause of gastrointestinal bleeding in young adults

    (E) in individuals with Rendu-Osler-Weber syndrome, telangiectasias occur most often in the stomach and colon

87. Concerning patients with recurrent episodes of acute gastrointestinal bleeding with no etiology found by endoscopy or conventional barium studies,

    (A) arteriography is diagnostic only during periods of active bleeding

    (B) the small bowel is the most common location for an identifiable bleeding site

    (C) if the patient is actively bleeding, scintigraphy with Tc-99m erythrocytes is sensitive in localizing the site of bleeding

    (D) enteroclysis will identify the responsible lesion in about 20% of patients

88. Which *one* of the following is LEAST appropriate in a patient with acute hematochezia?

    (A) Placement of a nasogastric tube

    (B) Barium studies

    (C) Colonoscopy

    (D) Arteriography

    (E) Tc-99m erythrocyte scintigraphy

QUESTION 89: MARK YOUR ANSWER SHEET TRUE (T) OR FALSE (F) FOR EACH OF THE RESPONSE CHOICES.

89. Concerning transcatheter treatment of gastrointestinal hemorrhage,

   (A) the treatment of choice in patients with acute colonic bleeding is usually pharmacologic therapy
   (B) embolization is indicated for the treatment of hemorrhage due to duodenal ulcer
   (C) metallic coils are not indicated for embolization of the upper gastrointestinal tract
   (D) the standard intra-arterial dose of vasopressin is 20 to 40 U/minute
   (E) unstable angina is a contraindication to vasopressin infusion

This 72-year-old man underwent a Billroth II procedure 31 years ago for peptic ulcer disease. He now has nausea and vomiting. You are shown two radiographs from an upper gastrointestinal study (Figure 30-1).

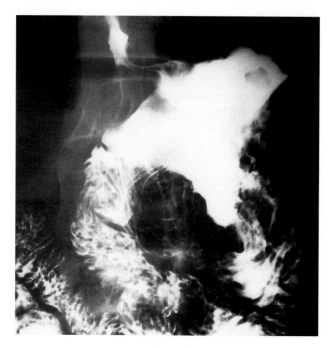

Figure 30-1

90. Which *one* of the following is the MOST likely diagnosis?

   (A) Lymphoma
   (B) Carcinoma
   (C) Bile reflux gastritis
   (D) Bezoar
   (E) Jejunogastric intussusception

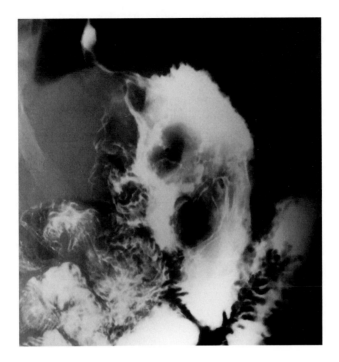

QUESTIONS 91 AND 92: MARK YOUR ANSWER SHEET TRUE (T) OR FALSE (F) FOR EACH OF THE RESPONSE CHOICES.

91. Concerning combined vagotomy and antrectomy,

(A) over 90% of the acid-producing (parietal) cells of the stomach are typically removed

(B) the gastrin level in serum rises markedly in the postoperative period

(C) frequent vomiting in the first 10 days after operation usually indicates the presence of alkaline gastritis

(D) it virtually eliminates reflux esophagitis in patients prone to gastroesophageal reflux

CASE 30 (Cont'd)

92. Concerning postoperative complications of vagotomy and antrectomy,

    (A) dumping syndrome can be diagnosed by radiographic evaluation of gastric emptying
    (B) barium evaluation can distinguish alkaline gastritis from recurrent acid-peptic inflammation
    (C) afferent loop syndrome can be caused by narrowing of either the afferent or efferent jejunal loop
    (D) the most likely site of marginal ulcer after a Billroth II procedure is on the jejunal side of the anastomosis
    (E) the retained antrum syndrome is due to hyperplasia of gastrin-producing cells (G-cells) in the gastric remnant

CASE 31: Questions 93 through 96

For each of the numbered barium enema radiographs from four different patients (Figures 31-1 through 31-4), select the *one* lettered diagnosis (A, B, C, D, or E) that is MOST closely associated with it. Each lettered diagnosis may be used once, more than once, or not at all.

93. Figure 31-1
94. Figure 31-2
95. Figure 31-3
96. Figure 31-4

    (A) Ischemic colitis
    (B) Radiation colitis
    (C) Ulcerative colitis
    (D) Granulomatous colitis
    (E) Pseudomembranous colitis

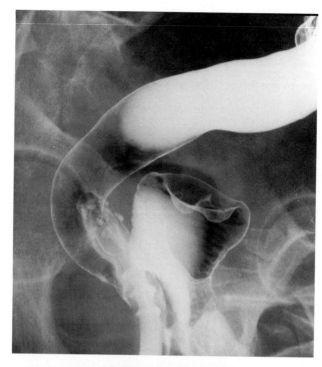

Figure 31-1

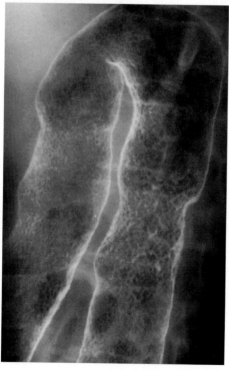

Figure 31-2

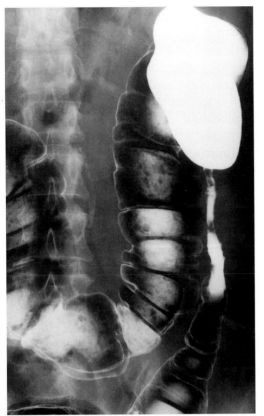

Figure 31-3

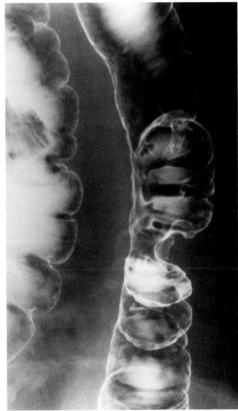

Figure 31-4

DEMOGRAPHIC DATA QUESTIONS

Please answer all of the questions below. The data you provide will be used to supply information that will allow you to compare your performance on the examination with that of others at similar levels of training and with similar backgrounds, and for purposes of planning continuing education projects. Please answer each question as accurately and as objectively as possible. Please mark the *one* BEST response for each question. Recall, of course, that we do *not* want individual names. Our analyses will reflect only categories and groups; everything will remain completely anonymous, and no attempt will be made to identify any specific individual.

97. The ACR will be evaluating the questions in this examination to determine their degree of difficulty and to determine the success of the examination as an instrument of self-evaluation and continuing education. To assist the ACR, please indicate in which of the following ways you took this examination.

    (A) Used reference materials or read the syllabus portion of this book to assist in answering some portion of the examination
    (B) Did not use reference materials and did not read the syllabus portion of this book while taking the examination

98. How much residency and fellowship training in Diagnostic Radiology have you completed?

    (A) None
    (B) Less than 1 year
    (C) 1 year
    (D) 2 years
    (E) 3 years
    (F) 4 or more years

DEMOGRAPHIC DATA QUESTIONS (Cont'd)

99. When did you finish your residency training in Radiology?

   (A) More than 10 years ago
   (B) 5 to 10 years ago
   (C) 1 to 5 years ago
   (D) Less than 1 year ago
   (E) Not yet completed
   (F) Radiology is not my specialty

100. Have you been certified by the American Board of Radiology in Diagnostic Radiology?

   (A) Yes
   (B) No

101. Have you completed fellowship training in Abdominal Imaging?

   (A) Yes
   (B) No

102. Which one of the categories listed below BEST describes the setting of your practice in the immediate past 3 years? (For residents and fellows, in which one did you or will you spend the major portion of your residency or fellowship?)

   (A) Community or general hospital—less than 200 beds
   (B) Community or general hospital—200 to 499 beds
   (C) Community or general hospital—500 or more beds
   (D) University-affiliated hospital
   (E) Office practice

DEMOGRAPHIC DATA QUESTIONS (Cont'd)

103. In which *one* of the following general areas of Radiology do you consider yourself MOST expert?

   (A) Breast imaging
   (B) Cardiovascular radiology
   (C) Chest radiology
   (D) Gastrointestinal radiology
   (E) Genitourinary radiology
   (F) Head and neck radiology
   (G) Musculoskeletal radiology
   (H) Neuroradiology
   (I)   Pediatric radiology
   (J) Other

104. In which *one* of the following radiologic modalities do you consider yourself MOST expert?

   (A) Computed tomography
   (B) General angiography
   (C) Interventional radiology
   (D) Magnetic resonance imaging
   (E) Nuclear radiology
   (F) Ultrasonography
   (G) Radiation oncology
   (H) Other

Gastrointestinal Disease
(Fifth Series)

Table of Contents

The Table of Contents is placed in this unusual location so that the reader will not be distracted by the answers before completing the test. A detailed index of the areas considered in this syllabus is provided (beginning on p. 587) for further reference.

Case 1   **Esophageal Intramural Pseudodiverticulosis**. 2
Marc S. Levine, M.D.

Case 2   **Esophagitis** 18
Marc S. Levine, M.D.

Case 3   **Duodenal Hematoma**. 28
Robert E. Koehler, M.D.

Case 4   **Strangulated Hernia**. 54
D. S. Memel, M.D., and Robert E. Koehler, M.D.

Case 5   **Hepatocellular Adenoma** 86
Judith L. Chezmar, M.D.

Case 6   **Duodenitis Secondary to Renal Failure**. 108
Marc S. Levine, M.D.

Case 7   **Heterotopic Gastric Mucosa** 114
Marc S. Levine, M.D.

Case 8   **Hepatocellular Carcinoma** 124
Judith L. Chezmar, M.D.

Case 9   **Erosive Gastritis Caused by Nonsteroidal Anti-Inflammatory Drugs** 142
Marc S. Levine, M.D.

Case 10   **HIV Esophagitis** 152
Marc S. Levine, M.D.

Case 11   **Cytomegalovirus Colitis**. 166
Judith L. Chezmar, M.D.

Case 12   **Periappendiceal Abscess**. 182
R. Brooke Jeffrey, M.D.

Case 13   **Cavernous Transformation of the Portal Vein**. 198
R. Brooke Jeffrey, M.D.

Case 14   **Traumatic Small Bowel Perforation** 212
R. Brooke Jeffrey, M.D.

Case 15   **Suprapancreatic Biliary Obstruction** 224
Dennis M. Balfe, M.D.

Case 16   **Abscess in the Greater Peritoneal Cavity** 252
Dennis M. Balfe, M.D.

Case 17   **AIDS-Related Lymphoma** 280
R. Brooke Jeffrey, M.D.

Case 18   **Pseudoaneurysm of the Gastroduodenal Artery** 298
R. Brooke Jeffrey, M.D.

Case 19   **Benign Stricture after Total Laryngectomy** 314
Dennis M. Balfe, M.D.

Case 20   **Serous Cystadenoma** 332
David H. Stephens, M.D.

Case 21   **Carcinoma of the Cardia** 364
Marc S. Levine, M.D.

Case 22   **Transjugular Intrahepatic Portosystemic Shunt** 376
Shawn P. Quillin, M.D., and Dennis M. Balfe, M.D.

Case 23   **Laparoscopic Cholecystectomy** 390
Ellen M. Ward, M.D.

Case 24   **Pharynx after Radiation** 410
Dennis M. Balfe, M.D., and Shawn P. Quillin, M.D.

Case 25   **Anastomotic Biliary Stricture** .426
Judith L. Chezmar, M.D.

Case 26   **Time-Related Contrast Enhancement Effects
on Liver CT** 442
Dennis M. Balfe, M.D.

Case 27   **Secondary Achalasia** 478
Marc S. Levine, M.D.

Case 28   **Nontumorous Perfusion Defect** 486
Judith L. Chezmar, M.D.

Case 29   **Bleeding Small Intestinal Leiomyosarcoma** 500
Kay M. Hamrick, M.D., and Robert E. Koehler, M.D.

Case 30   **Gastric Remnant Carcinoma** .530
Robert E. Koehler, M.D.

Case 31   **Colitis** 550
Desiree E. Morgan, M.D., and Robert E. Koehler, M.D.

Index 587

Gastrointestinal Disease (Fifth Series) Syllabus

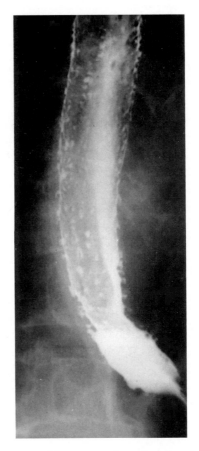

Figure 1-1. This 50-year-old woman has dysphagia. You are shown an esophagram.

Case 1: Esophageal Intramural Pseudodiverticulosis

Question 1

Which *one* of the following is the MOST likely diagnosis?

(A) Herpes esophagitis
(B) Radiation esophagitis
(C) Crohn's disease
(D) Barrett's esophagus
(E) Intramural pseudodiverticulosis

The test patient's esophagram (Figure 1-1) shows multiple tiny outpouchings in longitudinal rows parallel to the long axis of the esophagus. Note that many of the outpouchings are wider at the base than at the neck. These outpouchings could be mistaken *en face* for ulcers; however, their appearance in profile is characteristic of esophageal intramural pseudodiverticulosis **(Option (E) is correct).** Most reported cases of diffuse esophageal intramural diverticulosis have been associated with strictures, usually in the upper one-third of the esophagus (Figure 1-2). Patients can present with dysphagia because of the underlying stricture. Despite their dramatic appearance, pseudodiverticula have no significance, so dilation of the stricture usually alleviates the patient's symptoms. When pseudodiverticula are seen in patients with high esophageal strictures, they often extend above and below the level of the stricture (Figure 1-2).

Herpes esophagitis (Option (A)) is often manifested by multiple shallow ulcers in the middle or, less commonly, distal one-third of the esophagus (see Case 10, Figure 10-5). When viewed in profile, however, the ulcers would not have the appearance of the outpouchings seen in the test image.

Radiation esophagitis (Option (B)) is sometimes manifested radiographically by superficial ulceration of the mucosa within 1 to 4 weeks of radiotherapy. These ulcers can be recognized as small, shallow collec-

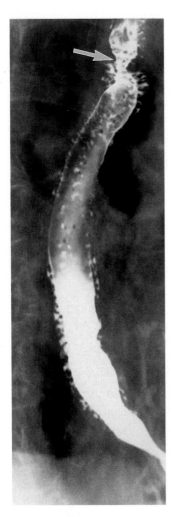

Figure 1-2. Esophageal intramural pseudodiverticulosis. An esophagram shows diffuse pseudodiverticulosis with an associated stricture (arrow) in the upper thoracic esophagus. This patient presented with dysphagia because of the underlying stricture. (Reprinted with permission from Levine [7].)

tions of barium on the esophageal mucosa within a preexisting radiation portal. In other patients, acute radiation esophagitis can produce a granular appearance of the mucosa associated with decreased distensibility of the irradiated segment (Figure 1-3A). In patients with more-severe disease, the esophagus can have a grossly irregular contour as a result of larger areas of ulceration and mucosal sloughing. Not infrequently, radiation esophagitis leads to the development of radiation strictures 4 to 8 months after completion of radiotherapy (Figure 1-3B). The strictures typically appear as relatively smooth, tapered areas of narrowing in the upper esophagus or midesophagus.

As in the small bowel or colon, aphthous ulcers are the earliest morphologic lesions of esophageal Crohn's disease (Option (C)). Esophageal

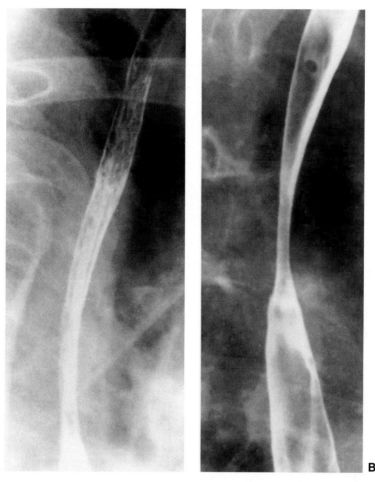

A   B

Figure 1-3. Acute radiation esophagitis with the development of a radiation stricture. (A) An esophagram obtained 3 weeks after radiotherapy
for bronchogenic carcinoma shows mucosal granularity and decreased
distensibility of the upper thoracic esophagus. (B) A repeat esophagram
obtained 6 months later shows a smooth, tapered stricture within the
radiation portal. (Reprinted with permission from Gore RM, Levine MS,
Laufer I, eds. Textbook of gastrointestinal radiology. Philadelphia: WB
Saunders; 1994.)

aphthous ulcers are seen on double-contrast esophagrams in about 3% of
patients with granulomatous ileocolitis. Aphthous ulcers typically
appear as punctate or slit-like collections of barium surrounded by radiolucent mounds of edema (Figure 1-4). More-advanced esophageal Crohn's
disease can be manifested by a localized or diffuse esophagitis with ulceration, thickened folds, pseudomembranes, and, rarely, a cobblestone
appearance. Other patients can develop transverse or longitudinal intra-

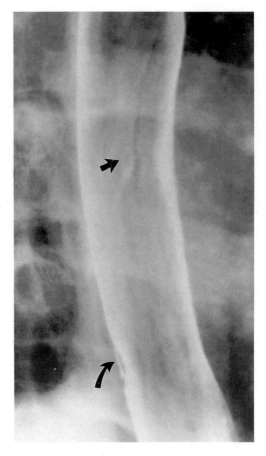

Figure 1-4. Esophageal Crohn's disease with aphthous ulcers. Several widely separated aphthous ulcers are seen *en face* (straight arrow) and in profile (curved arrow) due to early esophageal involvement by Crohn's disease. (Reprinted with permission from Gohel et al. [22].)

mural tracks similar to those found in the colon in patients with granulomatous colitis. Subsequent scarring can lead to the development of strictures, most commonly in the distal esophagus. However, esophageal intramural pseudodiverticula are rarely seen in patients with Crohn's disease.

Barrett's esophagus (Option (D)) is often associated with high esophageal strictures or ulcers, but no such lesions are visible in the test image. Furthermore, most cases of Barrett's esophagus are not associated with extensive intramural pseudodiverticulosis in the thoracic esophagus.

Question 2

Concerning Barrett's esophagus,

- (A) it occurs in about 10% of patients with endoscopically proven reflux esophagitis
- (B) it is associated with an increased risk of squamous cell carcinoma
- (C) it is characterized by a continuous area of columnar metaplasia in the lower esophagus
- (D) patients with scleroderma are at increased risk of developing this condition
- (E) it is a common cause of midesophageal strictures

Barrett's esophagus is an acquired condition in which there is progressive columnar metaplasia of the distal esophagus as a result of long-standing gastroesophageal reflux and reflux esophagitis. Many investigators now believe that Barrett's esophagus is much more common than was previously recognized. In various studies, the prevalence of Barrett's esophagus is about 10% in patients with endoscopically proven reflux esophagitis **(Option (A) is true).** Despite its frequency, Barrett's esophagus would not be important if it were a benign entity. However, there is considerable evidence that it is a premalignant condition associated with a significantly increased risk of esophageal adenocarcinoma. The risk of squamous cell carcinoma is not increased, however **(Option (B) is false).** It is widely believed that adenocarcinoma evolves through a sequence of progressively more severe epithelial dysplasia, eventually leading to the development of invasive adenocarcinoma. In various studies, the overall prevalence of adenocarcinoma in patients with Barrett's esophagus is about 15%. Prevalence data can exaggerate the risk of cancer; however, prospective studies have found that the annual incidence of malignant transformation in patients with Barrett's esophagus is 1 to 2%. Many investigators therefore advocate periodic endoscopic surveillance at 6-month or 1-year intervals to detect dysplastic or carcinomatous changes at the earliest possible stage in patients with Barrett's esophagus.

Barrett's esophagus can be recognized at endoscopy by velvety, pinkish islands or tongues of columnar epithelium extending more than 2 cm above the gastroesophageal junction. Endoscopy has a sensitivity of greater than 90% in diagnosing Barrett's esophagus simply on the basis of the endoscopic appearance. However, a definitive diagnosis can be made only on the basis of histologic criteria. The columnar epithelium in patients with Barrett's esophagus is not simply gastric mucosa but a mosaic of intimately admixed cell types from the stomach and small bowel, including a gastric-fundic-type epithelium with parietal and chief cells, a junctional-type epithelium with cardiac mucous glands, and a specialized columnar-type epithelium with a villiform surface, mucous glands, and intestinal-like goblet cells (i.e., intestinal metaplasia). These areas of metaplasia often occur as islands or tongues of columnar mucosa, so they can be separated by residual areas of squamous epithelium in the esophagus. Thus, Barrett's esophagus is not generally characterized by a continuous area of columnar metaplasia in the lower esophagus **(Option (C) is false).**

Scleroderma, a connective tissue disease characterized by smooth muscle atrophy and fibrosis, affects the esophagus in about 75% of patients. Esophageal involvement is manifested by a patulous, incompetent lower esophageal sphincter and absent esophageal peristalsis with poor clearance of refluxed peptic acid from the esophagus once reflux has occurred. As a result, patients often develop severe reflux esophagitis and have an even higher risk of developing Barrett's esophagus than do other patients with reflux disease **(Option (D) is true).** In one study, 37% of patients with scleroderma who underwent endoscopy for reflux symptoms were found to have Barrett's mucosa in the esophagus. Scleroderma should be considered an indirect premalignant condition in the esophagus, because Barrett's esophagus predisposes to esophageal adenocarcinoma.

The classic radiologic findings of Barrett's esophagus are a midesophageal stricture or ulcer, usually associated with a sliding hiatal hernia or gastroesophageal reflux. The strictures can appear as smooth, tapered areas of narrowing or, more commonly, as ringlike constrictions in the midesophagus (Figure 1-5). Other causes of midesophageal strictures include mediastinal irradiation, caustic ingestion, primary or metastatic tumors, and, rarely, esophageal involvement by dermatologic disorders such as epidermolysis bullosa dystrophica and benign mucous membrane pemphigoid. However, these conditions can usually be differentiated from Barrett's esophagus by the clinical history and presentation. Since Barrett's esophagus is a comparatively common condition and since midesophageal strictures are frequently observed in these patients, Barrett's esophagus is a common cause of midesophageal strictures **(Option (E) is true).**

Barrett's ulcers typically appear as relatively deep ulcer craters within the columnar mucosa at a discrete distance from the gastroesophageal junction (Figure 1-6). These findings are unusual in patients with uncomplicated reflux esophagitis; therefore, the presence of a midesophageal stricture or ulcer, particularly if associated with a hiatal hernia or gastroesophageal reflux, should be strongly suggestive of Barrett's esophagus. However, strictures are actually more common in the distal esophagus in patients with Barrett's esophagus, so most cases do not fit the classic description of a midesophageal stricture or ulcer.

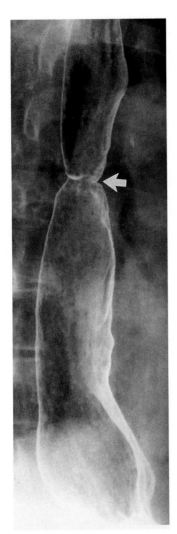

Figure 1-5. Barrett's esophagus with a midesophageal stricture. A focal ringlike constriction (arrow) is present in the midesophagus near the level of the left main bronchus. In the presence of a hiatal hernia and gastroesophageal reflux, a midesophageal stricture is virtually pathognomonic of Barrett's esophagus. (Reprinted with permission from Levine [7].)

A reticular mucosal pattern has also been described as a relatively specific sign of Barrett's esophagus, particularly if located adjacent to the distal aspect of a midesophageal stricture. This reticular pattern is characterized radiographically by innumerable barium-filled grooves or crevices on the esophageal mucosa, often extending distally a variable distance from the stricture (Figure 1-7). This distinctive reticular pattern is highly suggestive of Barrett's esophagus, but it has been observed in only 5 to 30% of patients with this condition. Thus, most cases of Barrett's esophagus will be missed on double-contrast esophagography if the diagnosis is made only in patients who have classic radiologic findings such

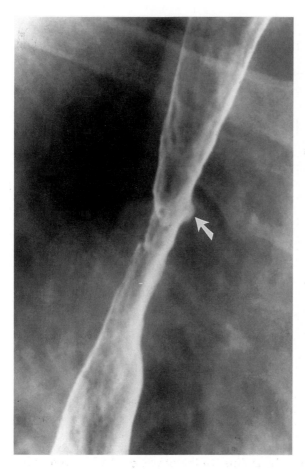

Figure 1-6. Barrett's esophagus with a mid-esophageal stricture and ulcer. A segmental stricture is present in the midesophagus, with a discrete ulcer (arrow) in the region of the stricture. (Reprinted with permission from Gore RM, Levine MS, Laufer I, eds. Textbook of gastrointestinal radiology. Philadelphia: WB Saunders; 1994:379.)

as a midesophageal stricture or ulcer or a reticular pattern of the mucosa.

Barrett's esophagus develops as the sequela of chronic reflux esophagitis; therefore, affected patients often have radiographic evidence of hiatal hernias, gastroesophageal reflux, reflux esophagitis, and peptic strictures. However, such findings can also occur in patients with uncomplicated reflux disease. Thus, radiographic findings that are relatively specific for Barrett's esophagus are not sensitive, and findings that are sensitive are not specific. Many investigators therefore believe that esophagography has limited value as a screening examination for Barrett's esophagus and that endoscopy and biopsy are required to diagnose this condition.

Gilchrist et al. have suggested an alternative approach to radiologic screening for Barrett's esophagus in which patients are classified into

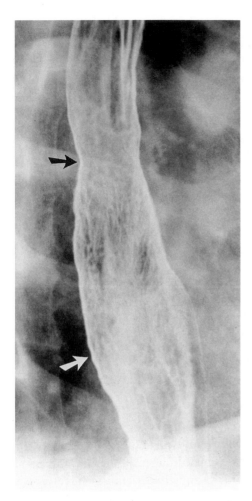

Figure 1-7. Barrett's esophagus with a reticular mucosal pattern. A mild stricture (black arrow) is present in the midesophagus, with a reticular pattern extending distally a considerable distance from the stricture (approximately to the level of the white arrow). This reticular pattern is highly suggestive of Barrett's esophagus, particularly if it is adjacent to the distal aspect of a midesophageal stricture. (Reprinted with permission from Levine et al. [33].)

groups at high, moderate, and low risk for Barrett's esophagus on the basis of the findings at double-contrast esophagography. Patients are classified as being at high risk if the radiographs reveal the classic findings of a high stricture or ulcer or a reticular mucosal pattern, at moderate risk if the radiographs reveal a distal peptic stricture or reflux esophagitis, and at low risk if there is no evidence of esophagitis or stricture formation. In the study by Gilchrist et al., Barrett's esophagus was present in 90% of patients at high risk for Barrett's esophagus, 16% of those at moderate risk, and less than 1% of those at low risk. On the basis of these findings, it seems reasonable to conclude that patients who are at high risk for Barrett's esophagus because of a high stricture or ulcer or a reticular mucosal pattern should undergo early endoscopy and biopsy for a definitive diagnosis. A larger group of patients are at moderate risk for Barrett's esophagus because of reflux esophagitis or peptic strictures, so clinical judgment should be used regarding the decision for endoscopy in these patients. However, most patients with reflux symptoms have no radiologic evidence of esophagitis or strictures, and their risk for Barrett's esophagus is so low that endoscopy does not appear to be warranted. Thus, the major value of double-contrast esophagography is its ability to separate patients into high-, moderate-, and low-risk groups for Barrett's esophagus to determine the relative need for endoscopy and biopsy.

Question 3

Concerning esophageal intramural pseudodiverticula,

    (A) they are dilated excretory ducts of deep mucous glands in the esophagus
    (B) patients are usually immunocompromised
    (C) they usually cause odynophagia
    (D) they often occur in the region of a peptic stricture
    (E) when viewed in profile, they cannot be differentiated radiographically from esophageal ulcers

Esophageal intramural pseudodiverticula are believed to represent dilated excretory ducts of deep mucous glands in the esophagus **(Option (A) is true).** The explanation for this ductal dilatation is unclear. Some patients with esophageal intramural pseudodiverticulosis have associated *Candida* esophagitis, but most investigators believe that the fungal organism is probably a secondary esophageal invader and not an important etiologic factor in the development of this condition. It has also been postulated that ductal dilatation results from plugging and obstruction of the ducts by inspissated mucus and inflammatory material. Alternatively, the ducts may be extrinsically compressed by periductal inflammation and fibrosis associated with chronic esophagitis. In various studies, as many as 90% of patients with esophageal intramural pseudodiverticulosis have had endoscopic or histologic evidence of esophagitis.

Most patients with esophageal intramural pseudodiverticulosis are not immunocompromised **(Option (B) is false).** However, between 15 and 20% of patients with esophageal intramural pseudodiverticulosis are diabetic or alcoholic. Affected individuals often present with dysphagia as a result of the high prevalence of associated strictures. Treatment in such cases is usually directed toward the stricture because the pseudodiverticula themselves rarely cause symptoms **(Option (C) is false).**

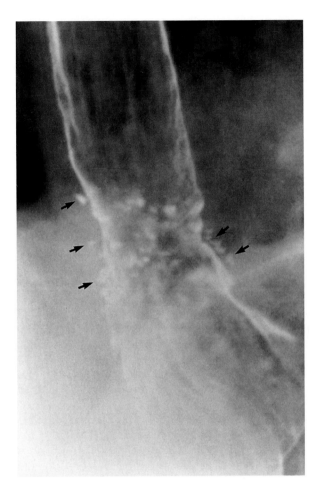

Figure 1-8. Localized esophageal intramural pseudodiverticulosis in the region of a peptic stricture. Note that many of the pseudodiverticula seen in profile (arrows) do not appear to communicate with the lumen. This is a characteristic feature of pseudodiverticula. (Reprinted with permission from Levine [7].)

Mechanical dilatation of the strictures produces a satisfactory clinical response in almost all symptomatic patients.

There are many anecdotal reports of diffuse pseudodiverticulosis involving the entire thoracic esophagus with associated strictures, usually in the upper one-third of the esophagus (Figure 1-2). However, one study found that most patients with esophageal intramural pseudodiverticulosis had isolated involvement of the distal esophagus, with a focal cluster of pseudodiverticula in the region of a peptic stricture (Figure 1-8) **(Option (D) is true).** It should therefore be recognized that esophageal intramural pseudodiverticulosis often occurs in the distal esophagus as a localized phenomenon associated with scarring from reflux esophagitis.

When viewed *en face*, intramural pseudodiverticula can be mistaken for multiple discrete ulcers associated with various types of esophagitis.

When viewed in profile, however, intramural pseudodiverticula often seem to be floating outside the esophageal wall without any apparent communication with the lumen (Figure 1-8), whereas true ulcers almost always communicate directly with the lumen. The characteristic appearance of the pseudodiverticula in profile should therefore differentiate these structures from true ulcers **(Option (E) is false)**.

Marc S. Levine, M.D.

SUGGESTED READINGS

ESOPHAGEAL INTRAMURAL PSEUDODIVERTICULOSIS

1. Beauchamp JM, Nice CM, Belanger MA, Neitzschman HR. Esophageal intramural pseudodiverticulosis. Radiology 1974; 113:273–276
2. Boyd RM, Bogoch A, Greig JH, Trites AE. Esophageal intramural pseudodiverticulosis. Radiology 1974; 113:267–270
3. Bruhlmann WF, Zollikofer CL, Maranta E, et al. Intramural esophageal pseudodiverticulosis of the esophagus: report of seven cases and literature review. Gastrointest Radiol 1981; 6:199–208
4. Castillo S, Aburashed A, Kimmelman J, Alexander LC. Diffuse intramural esophageal pseudodiverticulosis. New cases and review. Gastroenterology 1977; 72:541–545
5. Cho SR, Sanders MM, Turner MA, Liu CI, Kipreos BE. Esophageal intramural pseudodiverticulosis. Gastrointest Radiol 1981; 6:9–16
6. Culver GJ, Chaudhari KR. Intramural esophageal diverticulosis. AJR 1967; 99:210–211
7. Levine MS. Radiology of the esophagus. Philadelphia: WB Saunders; 1989:106–110
8. Levine MS, Moolten DN, Herlinger H, Laufer I. Esophageal intramural pseudodiverticulosis: a reevaluation. AJR 1986; 147:1165–1170
9. Sabanathan S, Salama FD, Morgan WE. Oesophageal intramural pseudodiverticulosis. Thorax 1985; 40:849–857
10. Troupin RH. Intramural esophageal diverticulosis and moniliasis. A possible association. AJR 1968; 104:613–616
11. Umlas J, Sakhuja R. The pathology of esophageal intramural pseudodiverticulosis. Am J Clin Pathol 1976; 65:314–320

HERPES ESOPHAGITIS

12. Levine MS, Laufer I, Kressel HY, Friedman HM. Herpes esophagitis. AJR 1981; 136:863–866
13. Levine MS, Loevner LA, Saul SH, Rubesin SE, Herlinger H, Laufer I. Herpes esophagitis: sensitivity of double-contrast esophagography. AJR 1988; 151:57–62
14. Shortsleeve MJ, Gauvin GP, Gardner RC, Greenberg MS. Herpetic esophagitis. Radiology 1981; 141:611–617

RADIATION ESOPHAGITIS

15. Goldstein HM, Rogers LF, Fletcher GH, Dodd GD. Radiological manifestations of radiation-induced injury to the normal upper gastrointestinal tract. Radiology 1975; 117:135–140
16. Lepke RA, Libshitz HI. Radiation-induced injury of the esophagus. Radiology 1983; 148:375–378
17. Northway MG, Libshitz HI, West JJ, et al. The opossum as an animal model for studying radiation esophagitis. Radiology 1979; 131:731–735

ESOPHAGEAL CROHN'S DISEASE

18. Cynn WS, Chon H, Gureghian PA, Levin BL. Crohn's disease of the esophagus. AJR 1975; 125:359–364
19. Degryse HR, De Schepper AM. Aphthoid esophageal ulcers in Crohn's disease of ileum and colon. Gastrointest Radiol 1984; 9:197–201
20. Dyer NH, Cook PL, Kemp Harper RA. Oesophageal stricture associated with Crohn's disease. Gut 1969; 10:549–554
21. Ghahremani GG, Gore RM, Breuer RI, Larson RH. Esophageal manifestations of Crohn's disease. Gastrointest Radiol 1982; 7:199–203
22. Gohel V, Long BW, Richter G. Aphthous ulcers in the esophagus with Crohn colitis. AJR 1981; 137:872–873
23. Tishler JM, Helman CA. Crohn's disease of the esophagus. J Can Assoc Radiol 1984; 35:28–30

BARRETT'S ESOPHAGUS

24. Agha FP. Radiologic diagnosis of Barrett's esophagus: critical analysis of 65 cases. Gastrointest Radiol 1986; 11:123–130
25. Chen YM, Gelfand DW, Ott DJ, Wu WC. Barrett esophagus as an extension of severe esophagitis: analysis of radiologic signs in 29 cases. AJR 1985; 145:275–281
26. Chernin MM, Amberg JR, Kogan FJ, Morgan TR, Sampliner RE. Efficacy of radiologic studies in the detection of Barrett's esophagus. AJR 1986; 147:257–260
27. Gilchrist AM, Levine MS, Carr RF, et al. Barrett's esophagus: diagnosis by double-contrast esophagography. AJR 1988; 150:97–102
28. Glick SN, Teplick SK, Amenta PS. The radiologic diagnosis of Barrett esophagus: importance of mucosal surface abnormalities on air-contrast barium studies. AJR 1991; 157:951–954
29. Haggitt RC, Tryzelaar J, Ellis FH, Colcher H. Adenocarcinoma complicating columnar epithelium-lined (Barrett's) esophagus. Am J Clin Pathol 1978; 70:1–5
30. Hameeteman W, Tytgat GN, Houthoff HJ, van den Tweel JG. Barrett's esophagus: development of dysplasia and adenocarcinoma. Gastroenterology 1989; 96:1249–1256
31. Harle IA, Finley RJ, Belsheim M, et al. Management of adenocarcinoma in a columnar-lined esophagus. Ann Thorac Surg 1985; 40:330–336
32. Levine MS, Caroline D, Thompson JJ, Kressel HY, Laufer I, Herlinger H. Adenocarcinoma of the esophagus: relationship to Barrett mucosa. Radiology 1984; 150:305–309

33. Levine MS, Kressel HY, Caroline DF, Laufer I, Herlinger H, Thompson JJ. Barrett esophagus: reticular pattern of the mucosa. Radiology 1983; 147:663–667

34. Paull A, Trier JS, Dalton D, Camp RC, Loeb P, Goyal RK. The histologic spectrum of Barrett's esophagus. N Engl J Med 1976; 295:476–480

35. Robbins AH, Hermos JA, Schimmel EM, Friedlander DM, Messian RA. The columnar-lined esophagus—analysis of 26 cases. Radiology 1977; 123:1–7

36. Robbins AH, Vincent ME, Saini M, Schimmel EM. Revised radiologic concepts of the Barrett esophagus. Gastrointest Radiol 1978; 3:377–381

37. Robertson CS, Mayberry JF, Nicholson DA, James PD, Atkinson M. Value of endoscopic surveillance in the detection of neoplastic change in Barrett's oesophagus. Br J Surg 1988; 75:760–763

38. Sanfey H, Hamilton SR, Smith RR, Cameron JL. Carcinoma arising in Barrett's esophagus. Surg Gynecol Obstet 1985; 161:570–574

39. Sarr MG, Hamilton SR, Marrone GC, Cameron JL. Barrett's esophagus: its prevalence and association with adenocarcinoma in patients with symptoms of gastroesophageal reflux. Am J Surg 1985; 149:187–193

40. Shapir J, DuBrow R, Frank P. Barrett oesophagus: analysis of 19 cases. Br J Radiol 1985; 58:491–493

41. Sjogren RW Jr, Johnson LF. Barrett's esophagus: a review. Am J Med 1983; 74:313–321

42. Spechler SJ, Goyal RK. Barrett's esophagus. N Engl J Med 1986; 315:362–371

43. Thompson JJ, Zinsser KR, Enterline HT. Barrett's metaplasia and adenocarcinoma of the esophagus and gastroesophageal junction. Hum Pathol 1983; 14:42–61

Notes

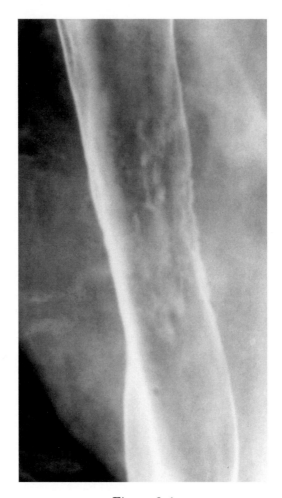

Figure 2-1

Case 2: Esophagitis

Questions 4 through 6

4. Figure 2-1
5. Figure 2-2
6. Figure 2-3

    (A) Reflux esophagitis
    (B) *Candida* esophagitis
    (C) Drug-induced esophagitis
    (D) Glycogenic acanthosis
    (E) Superficial spreading carcinoma

Figure 2-1, a double-contrast esophagram, shows multiple punctate and linear areas of superficial ulceration clustered in the midesophagus below the level of the left main bronchus. Note that the more distal esophageal mucosa appears normal (Figure 2-4). Reflux esophagitis (Option (A)) is the most common cause of ulceration in the esophagus, but it almost always involves the distal esophagus; it would be extremely unusual to have an isolated area of ulceration in the midesophagus with sparing of the mucosa below in patients with reflux disease. The most common causes of superficial ulceration in the upper esophagus or midesophagus are herpes esophagitis and drug-induced esophagitis. Herpes esophagitis typically occurs in immunocompromised patients with odynophagia, but it occasionally develops in otherwise healthy patients who have no underlying immunologic problems. Some patients have several discrete ulcers in the esophagus, whereas others have multiple areas of ulceration. Herpes esophagitis tends to occur as a more diffuse process than that illustrated in Figure 2-1, but localized herpes esophagitis is sometimes encountered. However, herpes esophagitis is not listed as an option. Thus, drug-induced esophagitis is the most likely diagnosis **(Option (C) is the correct answer to Question 4)**. Ulceration can occur in *Candida* esophagitis (Option (B)), but the ulcers are almost always superimposed on a background of diffuse plaque formation. Finally, glycogenic acanthosis (Oprion (D)) and superficial spread-

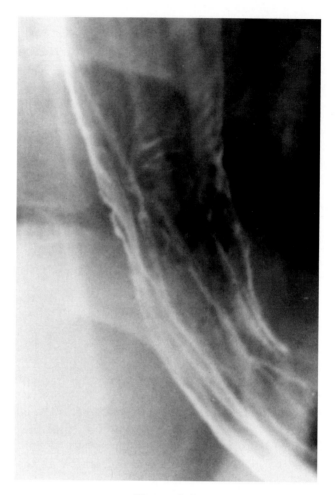

Figure 2-2

ing carcinoma (Option (E)) can be associated with mucosal nodules or plaques, but these conditions rarely cause ulceration (see below).

The findings on barium studies in patients with drug-induced esophagitis depend on the nature of the offending medication. Doxycycline and tetracycline usually cause superficial ulceration in the esophagus without permanent sequelae. The patient whose esophagram is illustrated in Figure 2-1 was taking doxycycline. Affected individuals can have a solitary ulcer, several discrete ulcers, or a localized cluster of tiny ulcers distributed circumferentially on a normal background mucosa (Figure 2-4). The ulcers are usually located in the midesophagus, near the level of the aortic arch or left main bronchus. When esophageal ulcers are drug induced, a repeat esophagram 7 to 10 days after withdrawal of the offending agent often shows dramatic healing of the ulcers.

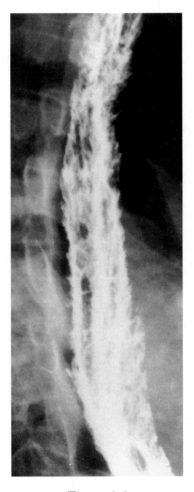

Figure 2-3

Other drugs such as potassium chloride and quinidine tend to be associated with areas of deeper ulceration; therefore, they can lead to the development of esophageal strictures. The strictures often appear as areas of segmental narrowing above the level of an enlarged left atrium. Occasionally, these large ulcers or strictures are mistaken radiographically for esophageal carcinoma. However, the possibility of drug-induced esophagitis or stricture formation should be suspected in patients with cardiomegaly who have a history of taking potassium chloride or quinidine.

Other, less common causes of ulceration in the midesophagus include caustic ingestion, mediastinal irradiation, Crohn's disease, Behçet's disease, epidermolysis bullosa dystrophica, and benign mucous membrane

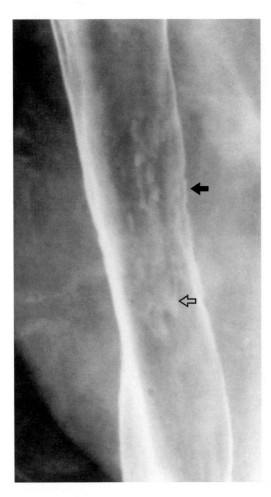

Figure 2-4 (Same as Figure 2-1). Drug-induced esophagitis. Multiple punctate and linear ulcers are seen *en face* (open arrow) and in profile (solid arrow) in the midesophagus below the level of the left main bronchus. Herpes esophagitis can produce similar findings; however, this patient was taking doxycycline. The correct diagnosis can therefore be suggested on the basis of the clinical and radiographic findings.

pemphigoid. The correct diagnosis of these diseases can be suspected on the basis of the clinical history and presentation.

Reflux esophagitis is by far the most common cause of ulceration in the distal esophagus, so it is the most likely diagnosis for the patient whose esophagram is illustrated in Figure 2-2 **(Option (A) is the correct answer to Question 5).** In contrast, drug-induced and *Candida* esophagitis tend to involve the upper esophagus and midesophagus. Glycogenic acanthosis and superficial spreading carcinoma can involve the distal esophagus, but they are usually manifested by nodules or plaques rather than by ulcers. Some patients with reflux esophagitis can have a solitary ulcer in the distal esophagus at or near the gastroesophageal junction. More commonly, however, reflux esophagitis is manifested radiographically by multiple shallow ulcers and erosions in the distal

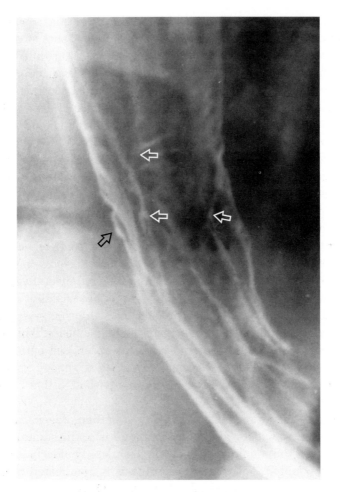

Figure 2-5 (Same as Figure 2-2).   Reflux esophagitis. Small, shallow ulcers are seen both *en face* (white arrows) and in profile (black arrow) in the distal esophagus near the gastroesophageal junction. Also note the radiating folds and deformity of the adjacent esophageal wall. These findings are characteristic of reflux esophagitis.

esophagus (Figure 2-5). Some ulcers have an irregular appearance, but others have a linear configuration with their long axis oriented perpendicular to the gastroesophageal junction. As in the patient whose esophagram is illustrated in Figure 2-2, the ulcers are often associated with radiating folds and puckering or deformity of the adjacent esophageal wall. Occasionally, longitudinally oriented ulcers have a serpentine appearance with multiple transverse folds straddling the ulcers.

When superficial ulceration is detected in patients with reflux esophagitis, the correct diagnosis is usually suggested by the distal location of the ulcers, the presence of an associated hiatal hernia or gastroesophageal reflux, and the clinical presentation. Some patients have relatively diffuse ulceration involving the distal one-third or one-half of the thoracic esophagus, but ulceration in patients with reflux esophagitis generally occurs as a continuous area of disease extending proximally from the gastroesophageal junction. Therefore, the presence of superficial ulcers in the midesophagus with distal esophageal sparing should suggest another diagnosis.

The esophagram in Figure 2-3 shows the classic "shaggy" esophagus of advanced *Candida* esophagitis in a patient with AIDS **(Option (B) is the correct answer to Question 6).** This appearance results from extensive plaque and pseudomembrane formation, with barium trapped between these lesions. This fulminant form of candidiasis is found predominantly in patients with AIDS. Superimposed areas of ulceration can also be seen in these patients as a result of mucosal sloughing. Advanced herpes esophagitis may occasionally be manifested by a shaggy esophagus. However, other types of esophagitis rarely produce this appearance. Occasionally, patients with AIDS present with the shaggy esophagus of candidiasis as the initial manifestation of their disease. This degree of esophagitis rarely occurs in other immunocompromised patients, so the possibility of AIDS should be suspected when a shaggy esophagus is detected on barium studies, particularly in a patient with a high risk for HIV infection.

Glycogenic acanthosis (Option (D)) is a benign, degenerative condition in which cytoplasmic glycogen accumulates in the squamous epithelial cells lining the esophagus. Patients are usually elderly and have no esophageal symptoms. Glycogenic acanthosis is manifested radiographically by nodules or plaques similar to those of *Candida* esophagitis (Figure 2-6). However, it would not produce the grossly irregular or shaggy esophageal contour associated with severe candidiasis. A superficial spreading carcinoma (Option (E)) can produce diffuse mucosal nodularity in the esophagus, but such tumors also would not produce the grossly irregular esophageal contour seen in Figure 2-3.

Marc S. Levine, M.D.

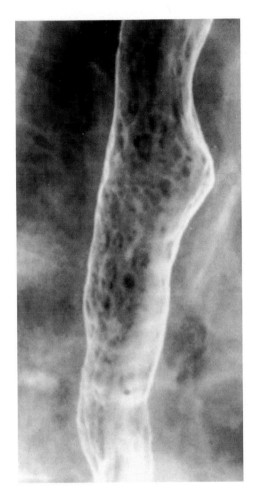

Figure 2-6. Glycogenic acanthosis. Multiple discrete nodules and plaques are present in the midesophagus. *Candida* esophagitis could produce identical findings; however, this patient was elderly and had no esophageal symptoms. (Reprinted with permission from Levine MS. Radiology of the esophagus. Philadelphia: WB Saunders; 1989.)

SUGGESTED READINGS

REFLUX ESOPHAGITIS

1. Creteur V, Thoeni RF, Federle MP, et al. The role of single and double-contrast radiography in the diagnosis of reflux esophagitis. Radiology 1983; 147:71–75

2. Graziani L, Bearzi I, Romagnoli A, Pesaresi A, Montesi A. Significance of diffuse granularity and nodularity of the esophageal mucosa at double-contrast radiography. Gastrointest Radiol 1985; 10:1–6

3. Graziani L, De Nigris E, Pesaresi A, Baldelli S, Dini L, Montesi A. Reflux esophagitis: radiologic-endoscopic correlation in 39 symptomatic cases. Gastrointest Radiol 1983; 8:1–6

4. Kressel HY, Glick SN, Laufer I, Banner M. Radiologic features of esophagitis. Gastrointest Radiol 1981; 6:103–108
5. Laufer I. Radiology of esophagitis. Radiol Clin North Am 1982; 20:687–699
6. Levine MS, Goldstein HM. Fixed transverse folds in the esophagus: a sign of reflux esophagitis. AJR 1984; 143:275–278
7. McDermott P, Wallers KJ, Holden R, James WB. Double-contrast examination of the oesophagus: the radiological changes of peptic oesophagitis. Clin Radiol 1982; 33:259–264
8. Ott DJ, Gelfand DW, Wu WC. Reflux esophagitis: radiographic and endoscopic correlation. Radiology 1979; 130:583–588
9. Wolf BS, Marshak RH, Som ML. Peptic esophagitis and peptic ulceration of the esophagus. AJR 1958; 79:741–759

CANDIDA ESOPHAGITIS

10. Levine MS, Macones AJ Jr, Laufer I. *Candida* esophagitis: accuracy of radiographic diagnosis. Radiology 1985; 154:581–587
11. Levine MS, Woldenberg R, Herlinger H, Laufer I. Opportunistic esophagitis in AIDS: radiographic diagnosis. Radiology 1987; 165:815–820

DRUG-INDUCED ESOPHAGITIS

12. Agha FP, Wilson JA, Nostrand TT. Medication-induced esophagitis. Gastrointest Radiol 1986; 11:7–11
13. Bova JG, Dutton NE, Goldstein HM, Hoberman LJ. Medication-induced esophagitis: diagnosis by double-contrast esophagography. AJR 1987; 148:731–732
14. Creteur V, Laufer I, Kressel HY, et al. Drug-induced esophagitis detected by double-contrast radiography. Radiology 1983; 147:365–368
15. Kikendall JW, Friedman AC, Oyewole MA, Fleischer D, Johnson LF. Pill-induced esophageal injury. Case reports and review of the medical literature. Dig Dis Sci 1983; 28:174–182
16. Teplick JG, Teplick SK, Ominsky SH, Haskin ME. Esophagitis caused by oral medication. Radiology 1980; 134:23–25

GLYCOGENIC ACANTHOSIS

17. Bender MD, Allison J, Cuartas F, Montgomery C. Glycogenic acanthosis of the esophagus: a form of benign epithelial hyperplasia. Gastroenterology 1973; 65:373–380
18. Berliner L, Redmond P, Horowitz L, Ruoff M. Glycogen plaques (glycogenic acanthosis) of the esophagus. Radiology 1981; 141:607–610
19. Ghahremani GG, Rushovich AM. Glycogenic acanthosis of the esophagus: radiographic and pathologic features. Gastrointest Radiol 1984; 9:93–98
20. Glick SN, Teplick SK, Goldstein J, Stead JA, Zitomer N. Glycogenic acanthosis of the esophagus. AJR 1982; 139:683–688
21. Rywlin AM, Ortega R. Glycogenic acanthosis of the esophagus. Arch Pathol 1970; 90:439–443

22. Itai Y, Kogure T, Okuyama Y, Akiyama H. Diffuse finely nodular lesions of the esophagus. AJR 1977; 128:563–566
23. Itai Y, Kogure T, Okuyama Y, Akiyama H. Superficial esophageal carcinoma. Radiological findings in double-contrast studies. Radiology 1978; 126:597–601
24. Levine MS, Dillon EC, Saul SH, Laufer I. Early esophageal cancer. AJR 1986; 146:507–512
25. Sato T, Sakai Y, Kajita A, et al. Radiographic microstructures of early esophageal carcinoma: correlation of specimen radiography with pathologic findings and clinical radiography. Gastrointest Radiol 1986; 11:12–19

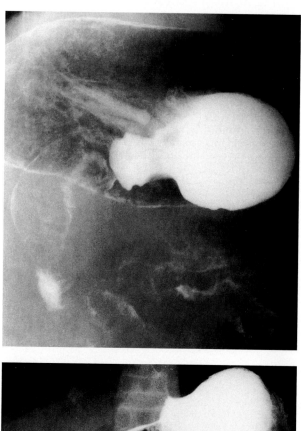

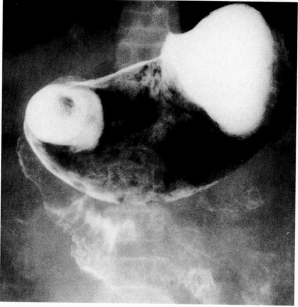

Figure 3-1. This 42-year-old woman has nausea and vomiting of recent onset. You are shown two radiographs from an upper gastrointestinal examination. Both were obtained 10 minutes after ingestion of barium.

Case 3:   Duodenal Hematoma

Question 7

Which *one* of the following is the MOST likely diagnosis?

(A) Pancreatic inflammatory mass
(B) Adenocarcinoma of the duodenum
(C) Leiomyosarcoma (stromal cell tumor)
(D) Duodenal hematoma
(E) Amyloidosis

The two radiographs from an upper gastrointestinal examination (Figure 3-1) show nearly complete obstruction of the duodenum by a mass that extends from the pyloric channel to the mid-descending portion and virtually fills the lumen (Figure 3-2A). The smooth, ovoid, well-demarcated appearance of the mass is typical of an intramural process that bulges into the lumen. The valvulae conniventes in the portion of the duodenum just distal to the filling defect are thickened and straightened (Figure 3-2B). These folds have the stacked-coin appearance characteristic of intramural bowel hemorrhage. The radiographic findings, taken together with the history of vomiting of recent onset, are typical of a duodenal hematoma **(Option (D) is correct).**

Intramural hematomas of the duodenum also have a characteristic CT appearance. Even when they are large, they typically remain within the confines of the serosa (Figure 3-3A). This gives them a smooth, sharp outline. There is usually an element of bowel obstruction, but some oral contrast material typically gets through the affected area (Figure 3-3B). Hematomas between a few hours and several days old contain areas of clotted blood that are identifiable by their characteristically high attenuation on CT. This is most evident on CT scans obtained without intravenously administered contrast material. As the weeks pass, the clot is lysed and the hematoma becomes a seroma with fluid density contents.

A pancreatic inflammatory mass (Option (A)) can have a profound effect on the duodenum. Most often such a mass is due to enlargement of

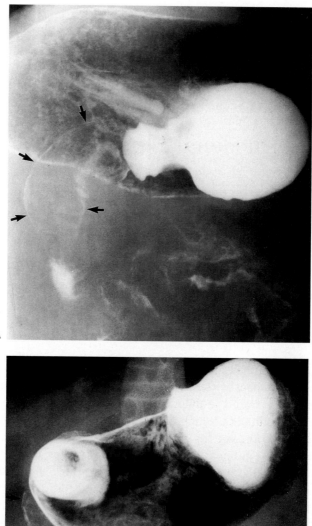

A

B

Figure 3-2 (Same as Figure 3-1).   Duodenal obstruction by intramural hematoma. The intramural hemorrhage was due to thrombocytopenia related to systemic lupus erythematosus. (A) The hematoma (arrows) extends from the duodenal bulb to the mid-descending portion of the duodenum. It is sharply outlined and smooth in contour. (B) Note the "stacked coin" appearance of the thickened valvulae conniventes (arrow-heads) in the segment of duodenum just distal to the intramural mass (arrows).

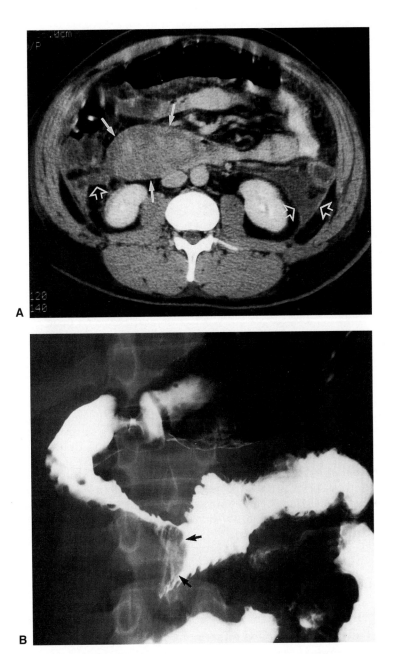

Figure 3-3. Traumatic hematoma of the second and third portions of the duodenum in a 33-year-old man involved in a motor vehicle accident. (A) A CT scan on the day of the injury shows a large intramural mass (solid arrows) confined by the duodenal serosa. The ill-defined areas of higher CT attenuation within the hematoma represent recently formed clot. Fluid in the anterior pararenal spaces (open arrows) is related to associated traumatic pancreatitis. (B) A radiograph from an upper gastrointestinal series performed 8 days later reveals narrowing of the duodenal lumen and a sharply demarcated margin (arrows) at the distal end of the hematoma.

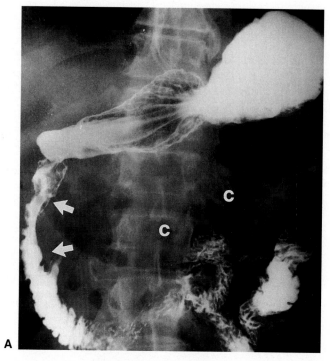

Figure 3-4. Duodenal effacement by pancreatic inflammatory mass in a patient with acute pancreatitis. (A) A radiograph from an upper gastrointestinal series demonstrates an extrinsic mass impression, or pad sign (arrows), on the medial aspect of the descending duodenum. Note also the wide separation of the greater curvature of the gastric antrum from the gas-filled transverse colon (c) as a result of thickening of the transverse mesocolon. (B) A CT scan shows an inflammatory pancreatic and peripancreatic mass (m) composed of fluid and necrotic tissue. Note that the descending duodenum (arrows) lies in contact with the mass and is displaced laterally.

the pancreatic head by a pseudocyst (Figure 3-4). Unlike the smooth, well-demarcated intramural mass seen in the test patient, there tends to be asymmetric flattening and effacement of the mucosal folds on the side of the duodenum in contact with the pseudocyst, contrasted with the unaffected folds on the opposite duodenal wall. When the inflammatory mass involves the pancreatic tail, similar abnormalities affect the fourth (ascending) portion of the duodenum, which shows effacement on its superior aspect and is displaced anteriorly and inferiorly. The enlarged pancreatic head often widens the duodenal C-loop, but this finding is not diagnostic, since the size of the duodenal loop varies so much from person to person. Findings on upper gastrointestinal series suggesting a

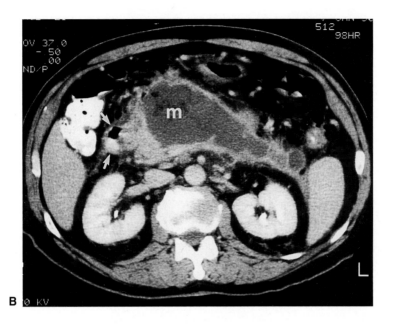

pancreatic inflammatory mass are invariably clarified on CT, which provides a direct view of the mass itself.

Adenocarcinoma of the duodenum (Option (B)) almost always occurs at or distal to the papilla of Vater, unlike the lesion in the test patient, which involves the duodenal bulb. Like primary carcinomas elsewhere in the gastrointestinal tract, adenocarcinoma of the duodenum is an annular or polypoid mass. When in the form of a polypoid mass, duodenal carcinoma is lobulated and has an irregular surface. Ulceration is a prominent feature (Figure 3-5). When present, mucosal fold thickening adjacent to the tumor mass is nodular and irregular, not of the straight, stacked-coin variety typical of intramural hematoma.

Duodenal leiomyosarcoma (Option (C)) presents as a well-circumscribed mass that is spherical or ovoid (Figure 3-6). It can grow into or out of the lumen. Intraluminal leiomyosarcoma appears on barium studies or CT as a filling defect with more lobulation than is seen in the test images. It tends not to cause obstruction despite its sometimes large size. Macroscopic infiltration of the adjacent bowel wall is not typical, and so mucosal fold thickening is not likely to be seen radiographically. CT may show extension into the pancreas and other periduodenal tissues.

Amyloidosis (Option (E)) can affect the duodenum in a variety of patterns. In one form, amyloid protein accumulates focally as a polypoid mass that mimics the appearance of primary carcinoma and can cause duodenal obstruction (Figure 3-7). This form of gastrointestinal amyloid

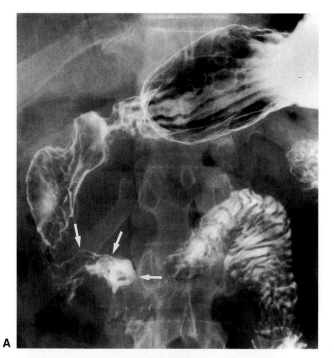

A

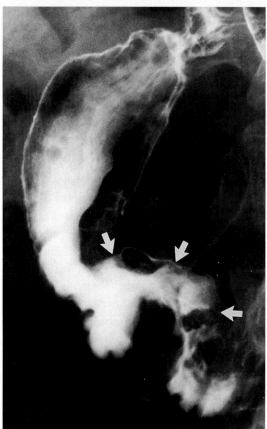

B

Figure 3-5. Adenocarci-
noma of the duodenum.
The tumor extends from
about the level of the papilla of Vater to the third
portion. In addition to
narrowing and irregular-
ity of the lumen, there is
a large ulcer (arrows) in
the tumor.

34

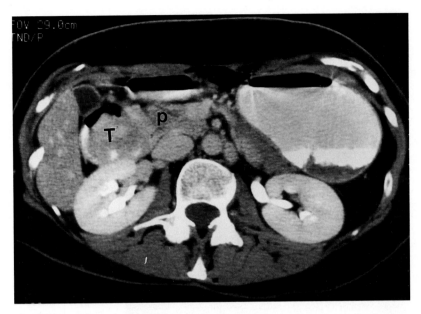

Figure 3-6. Leiomyosarcoma of the descending duodenum in a 58-year-old woman with nausea, vomiting, and occult gastrointestinal bleeding. The tumor (T) arises from the medial duodenal wall and bulges into the lumen. It has a lobulated contour and extends into the adjacent pancreatic head (p).

deposition has a predilection for the gastric antrum and proximal duodenum. The amyloidoma is usually lobulated and can cause obstruction. It does not typically present with the smooth, ovoid appearance shown in the test images.

Hematomas of the duodenum and small intestine typically occur in three clinical settings: hypocoagulable states, blunt abdominal trauma, and mesenteric veno-occlusive disease. The test patient had systemic lupus erythematosus for many years, and hematologic evaluation during her present illness revealed pancytopenia with thrombocytopenia. Other hypocoagulable states include anticoagulant overdose and congenital clotting-factor deficiencies, such as hemophilia.

Traumatic duodenal hematomas are almost always located in the second or third portion, or in both portions, of the duodenum (Figure 3-3). This segment of the bowel is particularly susceptible to injury because it is retroperitoneal and therefore fixed in position. Rapid deceleration in a motor vehicle accident can cause impact with the steering wheel. Alternatively, the patient can injure the upper abdomen by falling over a hard object. The same mechanisms put the pancreas at risk of injury, and traumatic pancreatitis can accompany a duodenal hema-

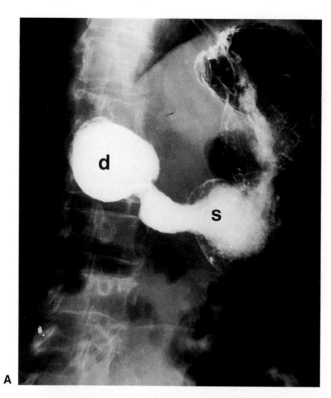

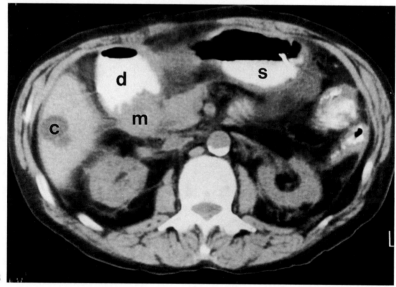

Figure 3-7. Type AL (primary) amyloidosis presenting as an obstructing mass (amyloidoma) of the postbulbar portion of the duodenum. (A) A radiograph from an upper gastrointestinal series taken 15 minutes after the ingestion of barium shows duodenal obstruction. No barium passed beyond the postbulbar region. (B) A CT scan shows an irregular duodenal mass (m). d = duodenum; s = stomach; c = incidental hepatic cyst.

toma. The CT scan in Figure 3-3A shows that the right and left anterior pararenal spaces and mesenteric root contain fluid related to an associated traumatic pancreatitis. Transection of the pancreas can also occur.

Characteristically this appears as a midline discontinuity in the gland, with marked inflammation of the surrounding tissues.

Occlusion of the superior mesenteric vein or one of its major branches can cause ischemia of the affected segments of the bowel. The local elevation of venous pressure causes intramural hemorrhage and edema, which can be so severe that they occlude the lumen. The venous thrombus is often demonstrated on CT or ultrasonography. The condition often responds to conservative treatment with anticoagulants, hydration, and bowel rest.

In approaching a patient suspected of having obstruction of the proximal gastrointestinal tract, one should first look closely at abdominal radiographs taken in the supine and upright (or left lateral decubitus) positions. In patients with high-grade obstruction, there is dilatation of gas- and fluid-filled stomach and duodenum with a paucity or even absence of gas in the bowel distal to the point of obstruction.

If no free intraperitoneal gas is seen, a contrast-enhanced examination of the upper gastrointestinal tract can be done safely with barium administration via a nasogastric tube after the gastric fluid has been aspirated through the tube. The barium study will confirm or exclude the presence of obstruction and can suggest a specific etiology. Further characterization of most obstructing lesions proximal to the junction of the second and third portions of the duodenum is best provided by endoscopy and biopsy. CT is most useful for (1) characterizing lesions distal to this point, (2) assessing the spread of neoplasms confirmed endoscopically, and (3) imaging patients in whom the clinical and radiographic findings suggest duodenal involvement by an extrinsic mass, such as one of pancreatic origin.

Question 8

Concerning tumors of the duodenum,

    (A) most in the duodenal bulb are benign
    (B) gastrinomas rarely cause Zollinger-Ellison syndrome in the absence of hepatic metastases
    (C) the duodenum is the most common site of involvement by lymphoma in the gastrointestinal tract
    (D) most carcinomas are located at or distal to the papilla of Vater
    (E) villous tumors have a much lower rate of malignant transformation than do those in the colon
    (F) leiomyosarcoma typically presents as an annular stricture

Tumors of the duodenum vary widely in histologic type and clinical significance. This is in sharp contrast to tumors of adjacent anatomic structures, which are more common, are almost always adenocarcinoma, and have a very poor prognosis. In the Michelassi et al. study of 647 primary tumors of the duodenum, pancreas, ampulla, and distal common bile duct, 98% of all tumors were adenocarcinoma and patients with these tumors had a 5-year survival rate of only 2%. Considering only the 29 duodenal tumors in the series, 16 (55%) were adenocarcinomas, 7 (24%) were sarcomas, and 6 (21%) were carcinoid tumors. Two-thirds of patients with duodenal carcinoid tumor and one-half of those with duodenal sarcoma lived 5 years or longer.

The great majority of duodenal tumors proximal to the papilla of Vater are benign **(Option (A) is true).** Tumors of the duodenal bulb tend to be asymptomatic and are usually discovered incidentally. They typically appear as solitary, polypoid, spherical, intraluminal filling defects on barium studies or CT. They can be sessile or pedunculated. Some are lobulated in contour. The differential diagnosis includes adenomas, Brunner's gland hamartomas, neuroendocrine tumors, and a variety of mesenchymal neoplasms. With the exception of lipomas, their radiographic features do not indicate their specific histologic type. Lipomas are often confidently identified by CT because they contain fatty tissue of uniformly low attenuation.

When multiple polypoid tumors of the duodenum are found, the possibility of a familial condition should be considered. The polyps of the familial adenomatous polyposis syndromes, juvenile polyposis, and Peutz-Jeghers syndrome can all occur in this area. Duodenal adenomas are particularly common in patients with the familial adenomatous polyposis sydromes, which include familial polyposis coli and Gardner syndrome, two conditions that may be part of a single disease spectrum. In an endoscopic surveillance program, Church et al. found duodenal adenomas in 66 to 88% of patients with familial polyposis coli studied. They

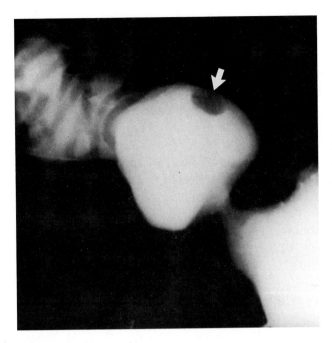

Figure 3-8. Nonfunctional carcinoid tumor (arrow) in the duodenal bulb, discovered incidentally on an upper gastrointestinal series in an 84-year-old woman. The smooth, rounded, sessile appearance and small size are typical.

performed biopsies of normal-appearing papillae of Vater and showed that 50% of specimens contained adenomatous tissue. They encountered no carcinomas in this series. Harned et al. reviewed the cases of familial polyposis coli and Gardner syndrome from the Armed Forces Institute of Pathology and reported that 60 to 100% had adenomatous polyps of the duodenum. These premalignant lesions tend to be small and multiple and are hard to detect radiographically.

Neuroendocrine tumors of the duodenum are submucosal and occur most often in the duodenal bulb and postbulbar region. They appear as smooth, rounded, sessile, polypoid lesions (Figure 3-8) and can have an irregular central depressed area. They vary in size from 1 mm to 2 cm at the time of discovery. These tumors are usually of the carcinoid type. They vary considerably in histologic pattern, and 85% exhibit argyrophilic staining properties. Burke et al. found that 56% of argyrophilic neuroendocrine tumors of the duodenum produce gastrin. These are commonly referred to as gastrinomas. Other hormones elaborated by these tumors include serotonin (47%), calcitonin (19%), and insulin (5%). Many tumors produce multiple hormones. Patients with multiple endocrine neoplasia type 1 commonly develop gastrin-producing tumors of this type.

The 15% of duodenal carcinoid tumors that are nonargyrophilic tend to occur in the periampullary region and usually produce somatostatin.

They have a glandular histologic appearance, often contain psammoma bodies, and can be difficult to distinguish histologically from adenocarcinoma. These nonargyrophilic carcinoid tumors of the duodenum are linked to neurofibromatosis type 1 (von Recklinghausen's disease).

Gastrinomas of the duodenum and pancreas frequently lead to the clinical manifestations of hypergastrinemia known as the Zollinger-Ellison (ZE) syndrome. The search for a gastrinoma should begin in the pancreas, but if that search proves negative, the duodenum should be examined. Duodenal gastrinomas accounted for 38% of the cases of ZE syndrome reported by Kaplan et al. and for 37% of the cases reported by Thom et al. in 1991. At least 90% are located in the first and second portions of the duodenum. Most are single, but cases of multiple duodenal carcinoid tumors are common enough to warrant a careful search for a second lesion. About 50% of symptomatic duodenal gastrinomas exhibit malignant behavior, usually in the form of spread to regional lymph nodes. Metastasis to the liver is not a necessary condition for symptomatic hypergastrinemia (unlike the carcinoid syndrome) and is seen in fewer than 10% of patients with ZE syndrome **(Option (B) is false)**.

Detection of duodenal gastrinomas presents a significant challenge. Clinically significant hypergastrinemia is common with tumors as small as 2 mm, sometimes called microgastrinomas. The average tumor size in the 1991 series of Thom et al. was only 6 mm. Duodenal microgastrinomas probably account for most cases of failed operations for ZE syndrome. Some duodenal gastrinomas can be detected endoscopically. CT is advocated by some, but it is likely to detect only larger duodenal lesions and nodal metastasis. In 1992, Thom et al. reported a sensitivity of 78% in the detection of duodenal gastrinoma by using selective intra-arterial injection of secretin with simultaneous venous sampling for gastrin. Ko et al. used selective injection of methylene blue into the gastroduodenal artery in a patient whose 2-mm gastrinoma had eluded detection by other means. Thompson et al. reported detecting gastrinomas in 45 of 46 patients by using a combination of percutaneous transhepatic venous sampling of gastrin and aggressive surgical exploration including duodenotomy and inspection of the everted duodenal mucosa.

Recently, endoscopic ultrasonography has proven to be a useful technique for preoperative localization of small gastrinomas in the duodenum and pancreas. In their extensive experience with examination of the upper gastrointestinal tract with this technique, Lightdale et al. report finding endocrine tumors of the pancreas in nine patients and two small endocrine tumors in the duodenal wall in another patient. The duodenal tumors were submucosal and were 6 and 10 mm in size.

Radionuclide imaging with ^{111}In-pentetreotide, a radiolabeled form of the somatostatin analog octreotide, has recently proven useful in detecting a variety of neuroendocrine tumors. Krenning et al. detected 15 of 18 islet cell tumors in this way, while none of the 18 pancreatic carcinomas in their patients showed positive uptake. Interestingly, all 19 of the carcinoid tumors they studied with ^{111}In-pentetreotide were also visualized. In another study of somatostatin receptor scintigraphy, Kerviler et al. found abnormal tracer uptake in 39 (81%) of 48 patients with ZE syndrome and correctly localized 50 of 60 gastrinomas. Scintigraphy was significantly more sensitive than endoscopic ultrasonography in their study.

Although the gastrointestinal tract is a common extranodal site of involvement by non-Hodgkin's lymphoma, the duodenum *per se* is rarely involved **(Option (C) is false)**. In a series of 58 patients with primary non-Hodgkin's lymphoma of the gastrointestinal tract, Cirillo et al. reported involvement of the stomach in 47 (81%), the ileum in 7 (15%), the colon in 3 (6%), and the duodenum in only 1 (2%). Radiographic features include duodenal wall thickening, which can be concentric or asymmetric. Such tumors often contain a large area of ulceration (Figure 3-9). Enlargement of regional lymph nodes is common. Differentiation from adenocarcinoma or metastatic disease is not possible on the basis of radiographic findings.

Adenomas of the duodenum are uncommon in patients without familial polyposis coli. Duodenal villous adenomas occur most often in the second and third portions, often near the papilla. Most have villous histologic features. They have a propensity to bleed, and occult gastrointestinal blood loss is a common presenting feature. Obstruction is rare. Their irregular surface gives rise to a characteristic radiologic appearance on barium studies described as a "frondlike" or "soap bubble" appearance. Most are sessile and broad based, but occasionally a pedunculated villous adenoma is attached by a long stalk that allows it to move with peristalsis from the second to the fourth portion of the duodenum (Figure 3-10).

As with villous adenomas of the colon, duodenal villous adenomas have a high frequency of malignant change **(Option (E) is false)**. Infiltrating carcinoma or carcinoma *in situ* is variably reported as being found at operation in 30 to 78% of cases. The fact that foci of carcinoma are typically intermixed with benign adenomatous tissue leads to unreliable findings on endoscopic biopsy and frozen section. For this reason, many authors recommend pancreaticoduodenectomy as the treatment of choice even when preoperative biopsies show only benign tissue.

Adenocarcinoma of the small intestine usually originates in the portion of the bowel between the mid-duodenum and mid-jejunum **(Option (D) is true)**. Local extension is usually present at the time of diagnosis and involves mainly spread to regional lymph nodes, pancreas, and the

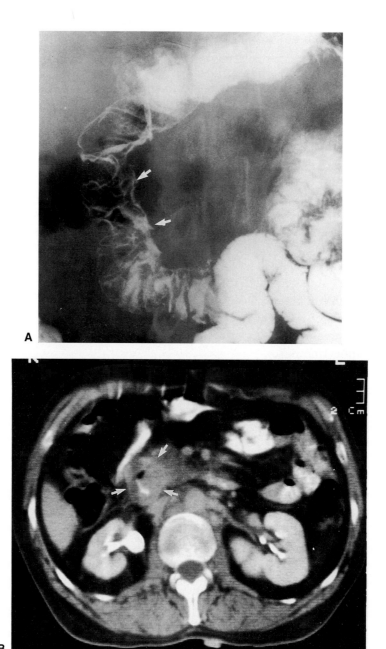

Figure 3-9. Non-Hodgkin's lymphoma of the duodenum. (A) A barium study shows a polypoid mass encasing and narrowing the descending duodenum. There is a large ulcer (arrows) within the mass. (B) A CT scan demonstrates concentric thickening of the duodenal wall (arrows). The duodenal lumen is opacified with oral contrast medium and is narrowed to a slit.

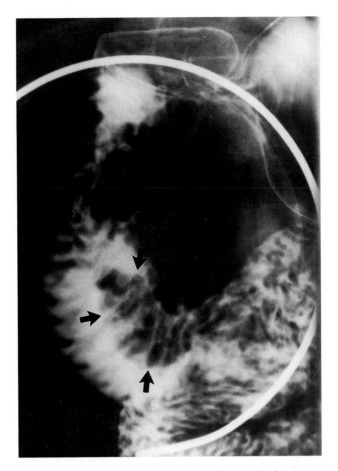

Figure 3-10. Benign villous adenoma. A radiograph from an upper gastrointestinal series in an asymptomatic 30-year-old woman with occult gastrointestinal blood loss and anemia shows a polypoid intraluminal filling defect (arrows) in the distal descending duodenum. The adenoma was pedunculated and was observed fluoroscopically to move back and forth from this position to the duodenojejunal junction. Its finely irregular surface texture is barely visible.

mesenchymal tissues of the anterior pararenal space. The prognosis is poor but not as bad as that of pancreatic adenocarcinoma. Kim et al. reported a 50% resectability rate for duodenal carcinoma and only a 21% resectability rate for pancreatic cancer. Of that select group of patients found to be resectable, the 5-year survival rate was 21% for duodenal cancer and 11% for pancreatic cancer. Overall 5-year survival rates for both types of tumor were much lower. On barium studies, duodenal carcinoma is polypoid or annular. Ulceration and obstruction are common. CT shows thickening of the duodenal wall, an irregularly narrowed lumen, and extramural spread.

Leiomyomas and leiomyosarcomas represent rare but interesting tumors of the duodenum, where they occur with one-tenth the frequency that they do in the stomach. By light microscopy they show epithelioid and spindle cell elements, and they were thought to be of smooth muscle origin. Lately, ultrastructural and immunohistochemical analyses have revealed features more consistent with neural or Schwann cell origin. For this reason the more generic terms "stromal cell tumor" and "stromal cell sarcoma" are now used by some authors when referring to these tumors. Paraganglionoma is another rare duodenal tumor that may fit under the same heading. It is difficult to characterize stromal cell tumors of the upper gastrointestinal tract as malignant or benign. Both tumor size and the number of mitotic figures have some prognostic value, but the only reliable indicators of malignancy are the presence of metastatic spread and aggressive local recurrence after surgical resection. Even patients with large, invasive, duodenal stromal cell sarcomas, however, have a better prognosis than do patients with duodenal adenocarcinoma.

Duodenal leiomyomas and leiomyosarcomas often involve the descending portion and are more or less spherical in most patients (Figure 3-11). They appear radiographically as intraluminal masses. They vary from 1 to 10 cm in diameter at the time of discovery (Figure 3-6). Barium or orally administered CT contrast material tends to flow freely around them even when they appear to fill the bowel lumen. They do not grow in annular fashion **(Option (F) is false).** Their tendency to develop surface ulceration is responsible for the high rate at which they present clinically with occult gastrointestinal blood loss.

Finally, metastatic tumors should also be considered when dealing with mass lesions in the duodenum. Malignant melanoma and bronchogenic carcinoma head the list of tumors that spread to the duodenum, but any number of primary malignant tumors can involve this portion of the gastrointestinal tract. Metastatic lesions can be single or multiple. They typically involve the bowel wall asymmetrically, and ulceration is common. As with most other malignant duodenal tumors, occult gastrointestinal blood loss is the usual presenting sign.

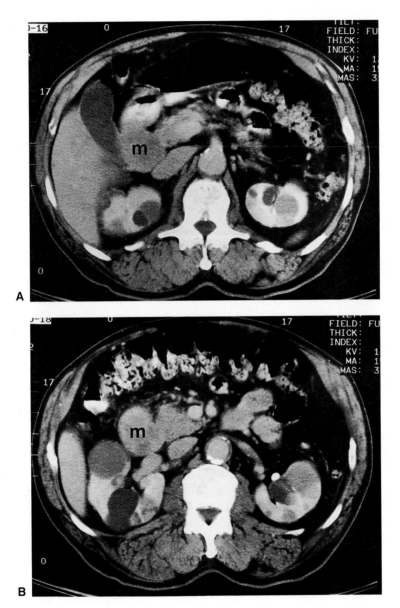

Figure 3-11. Well-circumscribed stromal cell sarcoma (m) in the descending duodenum in an elderly man with weight loss and gastrointestinal bleeding. Multiple renal masses are incidental cysts of different CT attenuation.

Question 9

Concerning amyloidosis,

    (A) the gastrointestinal tract is a common site of involvement
    (B) esophageal involvement causes both dilatation and loss of peristalsis
    (C) it causes impaired gastric emptying
    (D) the finding of duodenal amyloidosis should trigger the search for underlying carcinoma
    (E) small bowel involvement causes diffuse fold thickening

The term amyloidosis refers to a set of conditions, all characterized by extracellular deposition of proteinaceous material. The various types of amyloidosis have different underlying causes and are associated with tissue deposition of amyloid protein of several biochemical types. All amyloid proteins share a similar fibrillar structure and histopathologic appearance. Amyloid deposits can be strictly localized or systemic and diffuse. They can develop in areas where they have little clinical consequence or in tissues where the resultant organ dysfunction causes overt signs and symptoms. The clinical course can vary from a benign (or even asymptomatic) one to a rapidly progressive and fatal illness. Conceptually, Buxbaum has likened amyloidosis to a symptom rather than a disease. Like anemia, it is an ultimate manifestation of a variety of underlying conditions. In histologic sections, Congo red stain causes tissue deposits of amyloid to show a characteristic green birefringence when viewed with a polarizing microscope.

Amyloidosis commonly affects the gastrointestinal tract **(Option (A) is true).** The kidneys and the gastrointestinal tract are the most common sites of clinically significant involvement. The types of amyloidosis that most often show gastrointestinal tract involvement are primary or multiple myeloma-associated amyloidosis (type AL) and secondary or reactive amyloidosis (type AA) (Table 3-1). Amyloidosis associated with chronic hemodialysis (type AH) also affects the gastrointestinal tract in some patients. Direct involvement of the gastrointestinal tract by various forms of familial amyloidosis (type AF) is rare. Localized amyloidosis (type AE) affects endocrine organs and spares the gastrointestinal tract.

Type AL amyloidosis (L stands for light chain) is the form most often reported with clinically evident gastrointestinal involvement. It is a disease of older adults, almost never occurring in persons under age 40. It is rapidly progressive; Gertz and Kyle reported a 5-year survival rate of 20%. Most deaths are due to renal and cardiovascular involvement. The amyloid protein in this condition is composed of immunoglobulin light-chain protein fragments. The light-chain fragments are produced by a monoclonal population of plasma cells that can originate from a malig-

Table 3-1: Biochemical and clinical features of amyloidosis types most likely to affect the gastrointestinal tract

Abbreviation	Type(s)	Amyloid fibril composition	Usual areas affected
AL	Primary and multiple myeloma associated	Immunoglobulin light-chain fragments	Heart, tongue, nodes, gastrointestinal tract, joints, ligaments
AA	Secondary	Amyloid A protein	Kidneys, gastrointestinal tract, liver, spleen
AH	Dialysis associated	β_2-Microglobulin	Joints, carpal tunnel, gastrointestinal tract
AF	Familial amyloid polyneuropathy	Transthyretin (prealbumin)	Peripheral nerves (neuropathy can cause gastrointestinal tract hypomotility)

nant clone (multiple myeloma) or from nonmalignant plasma cells (primary amyloidosis). This distinction is sometimes difficult to make and is usually based on the presence or absence of the clinical features of multiple myeloma: lytic skeletal lesions, anemia, hypercalcemia, and a monoclonal spike of serum immunoglobulin.

Type AA amyloidosis (A refers to amyloid A protein, the first amyloid protein to be characterized) is seen in patients with long-standing infectious or inflammatory conditions. It is also referred to as secondary or reactive amyloidosis. Unlike type AL amyloidosis, this condition usually follows a long, indolent course. In former years, the inciting inflammatory condition was typically tuberculosis, empyema, or osteomyelitis. Now that those diseases are better controlled by antibiotic therapy and are seldom active for long periods, type AA amyloidosis is much more likely to be seen in patients with chronic, noninfectious inflammatory conditions.

Rheumatoid arthritis is currently the most common underlying condition in patients with type AA amyloidosis. Buxbaum reported that amyloid deposits were found at autopsy in the tissues of up to 20% of patients with rheumatoid arthritis, although clinical signs of amyloidosis were seen in only 3 to 5%. Type AA amyloidosis also occurs in patients with ankylosing spondylitis or psoriatic arthritis and in bedridden patients with chronic decubitus ulcers. In their 1991 series of 64 patients with secondary amyloidosis, Gertz and Kyle found that inflammatory bowel disease was the underlying condition in 6 (9%). Crohn's disease was the predisposing inflammatory condition in 5 (15%) of the 34 patients with type AA amyloidosis in the 1994 series of Tada et al. There is no particular association between amyloidosis and underlying carcinoma **(Option (D) is false);** only a few case reports several years ago describe the coexistence of the two conditions.

An interesting feature of type AA amyloidosis is that disappearance of the underlying inflammatory condition sometimes leads to a reduction in the deposits of amyloid protein and reversal of signs and symptoms of amyloidosis. Donaldson described an improvement in amyloidosis after resection of bowel affected by Crohn's disease. A similar reversal has been documented in patients with chronic osteomyelitis whose infection was eliminated by antibiotics or resection of the infected part.

Type AH amyloidosis is due to the deposition of ß$_2$-microglobulin fibrils. It presents as arthropathy or carpal tunnel syndrome in most patients. Gastrointestinal tract involvement is less common but does occur, and the development of malabsorption or chronic diarrhea in a patient on chronic hemodialysis should suggest the possibility of type AH amyloidosis.

Type AF amyloidosis rarely involves the gastrointestinal tract directly, but it does affect peripheral nerves. Orthostatic hypotension and bowel hypomotility (with resulting malabsorption) are the two most common clinical manifestations. Autonomic nerve involvement can cause hypomotility of any level of the gastrointestinal tract. Affected nerves are characteristically extrinsic to the gastrointestinal tract, and there is sparing of intrinsic gastrointestinal tract nerves.

The first step in establishing the diagnosis of amyloidosis is to suspect the condition from the clinical clues so that an appropriate biopsy can be performed. Aspiration biopsy of subcutaneous abdominal wall fat and proctoscopic biopsy of a rectal valve yield high rates of positive results. Amyloidosis should come to mind as an explanation for diarrhea, malabsorption, or gastrointestinal tract bleeding in patients with multiple myeloma, rheumatoid arthritis, or renal failure on long-term hemodialysis. In patients with long-standing Crohn's disease, the development of proteinuria or hepatosplenomegaly should trigger the suspicion of amyloidosis.

Amyloidosis of the gastrointestinal tract can have a variety of clinical and radiographic manifestations. Hypomotility is often a dominant feature and can be due to direct infiltration of the smooth muscle of the gut wall or to amyloid involvement of autonomic nerves with resulting denervation. The hypomotility can be severe and can be accompanied by malabsorption. Abdominal distension, nausea, and vomiting occur, particularly in patients with type AL amyloidosis. Diarrhea and gastrointestinal blood loss are more common in patients with type AA amyloidosis.

In 1990 Tada et al. reported that 36 (80%) of 45 patients with amyloidosis of the gastrointestinal tract had type AA amyloidosis, but others have reported a preponderance of the AL type. Menke et al. reviewed the records of 769 patients with type AL amyloidosis and found that 8% had histologically documented gastrointestinal tract involvement. In the series of Tada et al., the small intestine was involved in 80% of patients, the duodenum in 61%, the stomach in 53%, the colon in 32%, and the esophagus in 14%. In other series the duodenum has been found to be the site of greatest accumulation of amyloid protein in the gastrointestinal tract.

In the esophagus, diminished peristalsis causes dilatation and impaired transit **(Option (B) is true).** Wald et al. reported failure of relaxation of the lower esophageal sphincter. Incompetence of the lower esophageal sphincter is also known to occur. Amyloid infiltration of the esophageal submucosa can thicken the esophageal folds (Figure 3-12) or narrow the lumen with masslike accumulation of amyloid protein (amyloidoma).

Gastric involvement can be associated with gastroparesis **(Option (C) is true).** The rugae are typically thickened, but, paradoxically, Legge et al. also reported loss of rugal folds. Large submucosal masses of amyloid-infiltrated tissue can occur, especially in the antrum, duodenal bulb, and descending duodenum (Figure 3-7), where they mimic the appearance of adenocarcinoma. Such masses can ulcerate and can block gastric emptying. Primary (type AL) amyloidosis is the type in which gastric and duodenal amyloidomas most often develop. Dastur and Ward described a patient with an ulcerated antral amyloidoma that resembled gastric carcinoma but was more pliable. Similar masslike deposits can occur in the colon and rectum as well.

The duodenum, jejunum, and ileum are the portions of the gastrointestinal tract most frequently affected by amyloidosis. Matsumoto found prolonged small intestinal transit time and bacterial overgrowth. Legge et al. reported intestinal pseudo-obstruction, sometimes severe, in 7% of patients with systemic amyloidosis. The valvulae conniventes can be diffusely thickened and nodular **(Option (E) is true).** Cozzi et al., Pandarinath et al., and others have reported multiple polypoid nodules, in the range of 0.5 to 1.5 cm in diameter, throughout the intestine. This pattern is seen most often in patients with type AL amyloidosis. The nodules can be widely scattered or so numerous as to be confluent. Erosion and ulceration can occur on their overlying mucosa and can bleed. In 1991, Tada et al. reported the frequent occurrence in patients with type

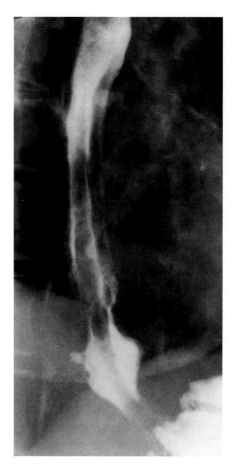

Figure 3-12. Amyloid deposition in the esophageal submucosa in a patient with type AL amyloidosis. The mucosal folds of the distal esophagus are strikingly thickened.

AA amyloidosis of a finely granular mucosal surface that is visible endoscopically and on high-quality, double-contrast barium studies.

In 1994, Tada et al. showed clear correlations between the chemical composition of the amyloid protein, the layer of the gut wall in which it is deposited, and the specific radiographic findings. Amyloid A protein was found principally in the lamina propria and appeared as a coarse gastrointestinal mucosal pattern characterized by innumerable tiny, granular, mucosal elevations. In patients with type AL amyloidosis, light-chain protein was found primarily in the muscularis mucosae and submucosa. This caused radiographically demonstrable thickening of mucosal folds and nodular or polypoid protrusions into the lumen. Deposition of ß_2-microglobulin in the muscularis propria produced intestinal dilatation and prolonged transit.

Choi et al. have emphasized that the tendency for amyloid protein to be deposited in and around blood vessels sometimes leads to intestinal ischemia and infarction. This is probably the basis for most cases of perforation and bleeding. However, although ulceration or ischemia is sometimes seen, bleeding and perforation can occur in areas in which bowel wall infiltration is the only pathologic finding.

Robert E. Koehler, M.D.

SUGGESTED READINGS

DUODENAL HEMATOMAS

1. Kunin JR, Korobkin M, Ellis JH, Francis IR, Kane NM, Siegel SE. Duodenal injuries caused by blunt abdominal trauma: value of CT in differentiating perforation from hematoma. AJR 1993; 160:1221–1223
2. Sadry F, Hauser H. Fatal pancreatitis secondary to iatrogenic intramural duodenal hematoma: a case report and review of the literature. Gastrointest Radiol 1990; 15:296–298

DUODENAL TUMORS

3. Attanoos R, Williams GT. Epithelial and neuroendocrine tumors of the duodenum. Semin Diagn Pathol 1991; 8:149–162
4. Beckwith PS, van Heerden JA, Dozois RR. Prognosis of symptomatic duodenal adenomas in familial adenomatous polyposis. Arch Surg 1991; 126:825–827
5. Burke AP, Federspiel BH, Sobin LH, Shekitka KM, Helwig EB. Carcinoids of the duodenum. A histologic and immunohistochemical study of 65 tumors. Am J Surg Pathol 1989; 13:828–837
6. Chappuis CW, Divicenti FC, Cohn I Jr. Villous tumors of the duodenum. Ann Surg 1989; 209:593–598
7. Church JM, McGannon E, Hull-Boiner S, et al. Gastroduodenal polyps in patients with familial adenomatous polyposis. Dis Colon Rectum 1992; 35:1170–1173
8. Cirillo M, Federico M, Curci G, Tamborrino E, Piccinini L, Silingardi V. Primary gastrointestinal lymphoma: a clinicopathological study of 58 cases. Haematologica 1992; 77:156–161
9. Cwikiel W, Andren-Sandberg A. Diagnostic difficulties with duodenal malignancies revisited: a new strategy. Gastrointest Radiol 1991; 16:301–304
10. Delcore R Jr, Cheung LY, Friesen SR. Characteristics of duodenal wall gastrinomas. Am J Surg 1990; 160:621–623
11. Eaton SB, Ferrucci JT Jr. Radiology of the pancreas and duodenum. Philadelphia: WB Saunders; 1973:289–303
12. Harned RK, Buck JL, Olmsted WW, Ros PR. Extracolonic manifestations of the familial adenomatous polyposis syndromes. AJR 1991; 156:481–485
13. Kaplan EL, Horvath K, Udekwu A, et al. Gastrinomas: a 42-year experience. World J Surg 1990; 14:365–375

14. Kerviler E, Cadiot G, Lebtahi R, Guludec DL, Mignon M. Somatostatin receptor scintigraphy in forty-eight patients with Zollinger-Ellison syndrome. Eur J Nucl Med 1994; 21:1191–1197

15. Kim SM, Kim SH, Choi SY, Kim YC. Surgical treatment of periampullary cancer—review of 766 surgical experiences of 8 hospitals. J Korean Med Sci 1992; 7:297–303

16. King CM, Reznek RH, Dacie JE, Wass JA. Imaging islet cell tumours. Clin Radiol 1994; 49:295–303

17. Ko TC, Flisak M, Prinz RA. Selective intra-arterial methylene blue injection: a novel method of localizing gastrinoma. Gastroenterology 1992; 102:1062–1064

18. Krenning EP, Kwekkeboom DJ, Reubi JC, et al. ^{111}In-octreotide scintigraphy in oncology. Metabolism 1992; 41(9 Suppl 2):83–86

19. Lightdale CJ, Botet JF, Woodruff JM, Brennan MF. Localization of endocrine tumors of the pancreas with endoscopic ultrasonography. Cancer 1991; 68:1815–1820

20. Michelassi F, Erroi F, Dawson PJ, et al. Experience with 647 consecutive tumors of the duodenum, ampulla, head of the pancreas, and distal common bile duct. Ann Surg 1989; 210:544–554

21. Pipeleers-Marichal M, Somers G, Willems G, et al. Gastrinomas in the duodenums of patients with multiple endocrine neoplasia type 1 and the Zollinger-Ellison syndrome. N Engl J Med 1990; 322:723–727

22. Thom AK, Norton JA, Axiotis CA, Jensen RT. Location, incidence, and malignant potential of duodenal gastrinomas. Surgery 1991; 110:1086–1091

23. Thom AK, Norton JA, Doppman JL, Miller DL, Chang R, Jensen RT. Prospective study of the use of intraarterial secretin injection and portal venous sampling to localize duodenal gastrinomas. Surgery 1992; 112:1002–1008

24. Thompson NW, Vinik AI, Eckhauser FE. Microgastrinomas of the duodenum. A cause of failed operations for the Zollinger-Ellison syndrome. Ann Surg 1989; 209:396–404

AMYLOIDOSIS

25. Buxbaum JN. The amyloid diseases. In: Wyngaarden JB, Smith LH Jr, Bennett JC (eds), Cecil textbook of medicine, 19th ed. Philadelphia: WB Saunders; 1992:1141–1145

26. Choi HS, Heller D, Picken MM, Sidhu GS, Kahn T. Infarction of intestine with massive amyloid deposition in two patients on long-term hemodialysis. Gastroenterology 1989; 96:230–234

27. Cozzi G, Ballardini G, Colombi R, Bellomi M, Frigerio LF, Severini A. Double contrast small bowel enema in a case of selective duodeno-jejunal amyloidosis. Acta Radiol 1990; 31:355–356

28. Dastur KJ, Ward JF. Amyloidoma of the stomach. Gastrointest Radiol 1980; 5:17–20

29. Donaldson RM Jr. Crohn's disease. In: Sleisinger MH, Fordtran JS (eds), Gastrointestinal disease. Pathophysiology, diagnosis, management, 4th ed. Philadelphia: WB Saunders; 1989:1327–1358

30. Gertz MA, Kyle RA. Primary systemic amyloidosis—a diagnostic primer. Mayo Clin Proc 1989; 64:1505–1519

31. Gertz MA, Kyle RA. Secondary systemic amyloidosis: response and survival in 64 patients. Medicine (Baltimore) 1991; 70:246–256

32. Legge DA, Carlson HC, Wollaeger EE. Roentgenologic appearance of systemic amyloidosis involving gastrointestinal tract. AJR 1970; 110:406–412

33. Menke DM, Kyle RA, Fleming CR, Wolfe JT III, Kurtin PJ, Oldenburg WA. Symptomatic gastric amyloidosis in patients with primary systemic amyloidosis. Mayo Clin Proc 1993; 68:673–677

34. Pandarinath GS, Levine SM, Sorokin JJ, Jacoby JH. Selective massive amyloidosis of the small intestine mimicking multiple tumors. Radiology 1978; 129:609–610

35. Seliger G, Krassner RL, Beranbaum ER, Miller F. The spectrum of roentgen appearance in amyloidosis of the small and large bowel: radiologic-pathologic correlation. Radiology 1971; 100:63–70

36. Shipps FC, Brennan DD. Roentgen findings in amyloidosis of the stomach—case report. AJR 1952; 68:204–208

37. Tada S. Diagnosis of gastrointestinal amyloidosis with special reference to the relationship with amyloid fibril protein. Fukuoka Igaku Zasshi 1991; 82:624–647

38. Tada S, Iida M, Iwashita A, et al. Endoscopic and biopsy findings of the upper digestive tract in patients with amyloidosis. Gastrointest Endosc 1990; 36:10–14

39. Tada S, Iida M, Matsui T, et al. Amyloidosis of the small intestine: findings on double-contrast radiographs. AJR 1991; 156:741–744

40. Tada S, Iida M, Yao T, et al. Gastrointestinal amyloidosis: radiologic features by chemical types. Radiology 1994; 190:37–42

41. Urban BA, Fishman EK, Goldman SM, et al. CT evaluation of amyloidosis: spectrum of disease. RadioGraphics 1993; 13:1295–1308

42. Wald A, Kichler J, Mendelow H. Amyloidosis and chronic intestinal pseudoobstruction. Dig Dis Sci 1981; 26:462–465

43. Yousuf M, Akamatsu T, Matsuzawa K, et al. AL-type generalized amyloidosis showing a solitary duodenal tumor. Hepatogastroenterology 1992; 39:267–269

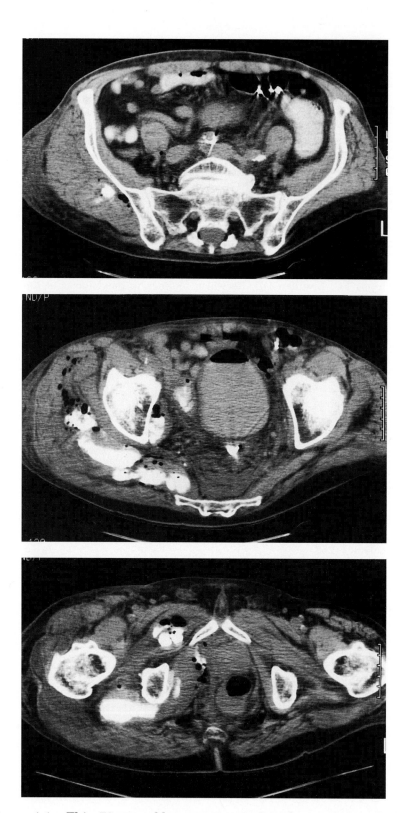

Figure 4-1. This 70-year-old man presented with metabolic alkalosis and abdominal pain and distension. You are shown three images from a CT study of the abdomen and pelvis.

Case 4:   Strangulated Hernia

Question 10

Which *one* of the following is the MOST likely diagnosis?

    (A) Diverticulitis
    (B) Metastatic tumor
    (C) Small bowel obstruction by adhesion
    (D) Crohn's disease
    (E) Strangulated hernia

    The three CT images through the lower abdomen and pelvis (Figure 4-1) show orally administered contrast material opacifying the lumen of the small intestine. A loop of gas-containing sigmoid colon of normal caliber lies in the left anterior abdomen (Figure 4-2A). A trace of residual dense barium in a few sigmoid colonic diverticula is the result of a barium enema done a few weeks earlier. Opacified distal ileal loops in the right lower abdomen are also of normal caliber; however, there is a mildly dilated loop of more-proximal ileum, with a caliber of 3 cm, lying in the left iliac fossa (Figure 4-2A). This discrepancy between the dilated mid-ileum and the nondilated distal ileum and colon indicates the presence of mechanical obstruction at the level of the mid-ileum. The presence of oral contrast material in the nondilated distal ileum indicates that the obstruction is partial rather than complete.
    Extraluminal gas and oral contrast material lie between the right gluteus minimus and medius muscles, adjacent to the right piriformis muscle, and in the periprostatic area (Figure 4-2). The bladder, prostate, and rectum are displaced to the left, and the right gluteus, piriformis, and obturator muscles and the tissues surrounding them are swollen. A loop of bowel is seen coursing through the right obturator canal, along the superior margin of the obturator internus muscle (Figure 4-2B). On the lowest of the three images (Figure 4-2C), a herniated loop of ileum lies just outside the right obturator foramen, between the superior and middle fasciculi of the obturator externus muscle, deep to the pectineus muscle. These findings are typical of an obturator hernia containing

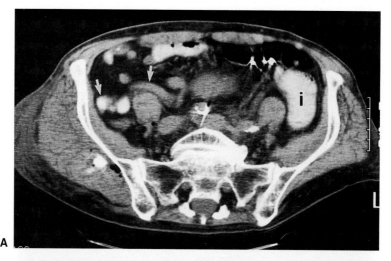

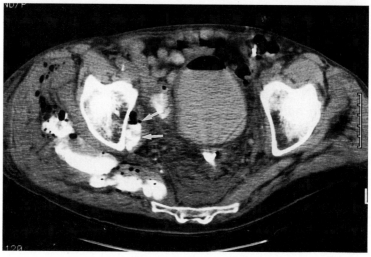

Figure 4-2 (Same as Figure 4-1). Strangulated obturator hernia. Three CT scans obtained after administration of an oral contrast agent. (A) A dilated segment of small intestine (i) containing orally administered contrast material lies in the left iliac fossa. Note the nondilated distal ileum (arrows), also opacified with contrast agent, in the right lower abdominal quadrant. This discrepancy in bowel caliber indicates mechanical small bowel obstruction. Also note the leaked oral contrast agent and gas bubbles between the gluteus muscles and right iliac bone. (B) In addition to the extensive extraluminal gas and bowel contrast agent between the layers of the right gluteus muscles, there is edema of these muscles and of the presacral-space soft tissues. Leaked contrast agent also lies in the right perivesical area. A loop of bowel (arrows) lies in the right obturator canal. (C) A loop of ileum (arrows) lies between the fascicles of the right obturator externus muscle, just outside the right obturator foramen. Extraluminal gas is also present in the right periprostatic area.

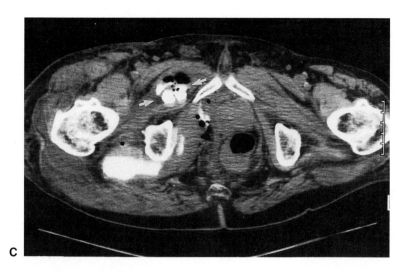

C

small intestine. As commonly occurs in patients with an obturator hernia, the blood supply to the involved segment of bowel has been compromised (strangulated) with resulting infarction and perforation **(Option
(E) is correct).** At operation, the segment of ileum within the hernia
was necrotic and perforated.

Diverticulitis (Option (A)) is characterized by inflammation associated with perforation of a diverticulum. The prevalence of diverticulosis
in western countries increases from 5% by 40 years of age to greater than
50% by 80 years of age. Diverticulitis occurs in 4 to 5% of all people who
have diverticulosis and in 10 to 20% of patients with a known diagnosis
of diverticulosis. Diverticulitis almost always occurs in the colon,
although diverticula of other parts of the bowel can be affected (Figure
4-3). Most cases of colonic diverticulitis involve the sigmoid portion of the
colon. The perforation or microperforation is usually walled off, and
symptoms are largely due to inflammation of the pericolic tissues. It is
unlikely that an abscess associated with diverticulitis would spread to
the obturator or gluteal regions, as in the test patient. Left lower quadrant abdominal pain and tenderness are the most common presenting
symptom and sign and are often constant in intensity. In addition to
localized left lower quadrant pain and tenderness, patients can present
with leukocytosis, fever, a palpable lower abdominal or pelvic mass, or
signs of diffuse peritoneal inflammation. Bowel obstruction (colon or
small bowel) occurs in approximately 10% of patients with diverticulitis.
Diverticulitis would not be expected to cause herniation of small intestine outside the normal confines of the abdominal and pelvic cavity, as
seen in the test patient. Until recently, barium enema was considered
the most reliable radiologic procedure for detecting the presence of

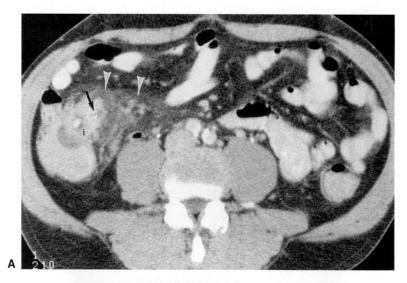

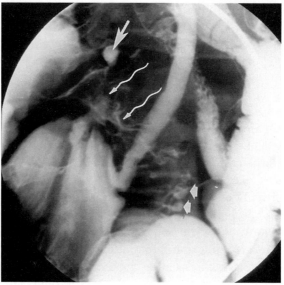

Figure 4-3. Ileal diverticulitis in a 60-year-old man presenting with right lower quadrant pain and fever. (A) A CT scan through the right lower quadrant shows infiltration of the ileal mesentery (arrowheads) and marked thickening of the ileal wall (i). At the periphery of the ileal wall is a small focus of fluid and barium (arrow). (B) A spot radiograph from a small bowel barium examination. Multiple diverticula (short arrows) are evident in the distal ileum. A persistent collection of barium (long arrow), corresponding to the intramural collection seen in panel A, is accompanied by inflammatory fold thickening in the terminal ileum (wavy arrows).

colonic diverticulitis. On barium enema examinations, the affected segment of the colon shows haustral fold thickening and narrowing as a result of edema and muscular spasm. These findings are not specific, however, and the diagnosis is more firmly established if extravasation of barium, impression by a paracolic inflammatory mass, or both are visible.

Recent studies have shown that CT is more sensitive than barium enema in the diagnosis of diverticulitis, and it is increasingly being used as the first or only radiologic examination. In addition to showing the abnormalities seen on barium enema, CT demonstrates even mild peridiverticular inflammation, which appears as a subtle, localized increase in the CT attenuation of the mesenteric or omental fat surrounding the perforated diverticulum (Figure 4-4A). Even tiny bubbles of extraluminal gas are clearly demonstrated by CT (Figure 4-4B). CT is also superior to barium enema for demonstrating the full extent of a peridiverticular abscess (Figure 4-5). CT can be used to guide percutaneous catheter drainage as an alternative to immediate surgical treatment of a peridiverticular abscess too large to treat by conservative measures alone. Catheter drainage of peridiverticular abscesses allows surgeons to perform a one-step resection and reanastomosis of the diseased segment of bowel after resolution of the abscess and initial inflammation, rather than performing an immediate operative abscess drainage, creating a temporary colostomy, and subsequently taking the colostomy down during a second operative procedure. Because perforated colon carcinoma can mimic diverticulitis with a peridiverticular abscess on CT, the possibility of missing an underlying neoplasm can be minimized by performing a barium enema or sigmoidoscopy after drainage of the abscess and resolution of the acute inflammation.

Metastatic tumor of various types can involve the small intestine. The most common primary tumors producing metastases involving the small bowel include melanoma and carcinomas of the lung, colon, stomach, pancreas, breast, and ovary. Metastatic melanoma and bronchogenic carcinoma typically disseminate to the small bowel hematogenously and present as one or more mural nodules or masses that protrude into the lumen. Bleeding or bowel obstruction is the usual presenting sign. The nodules can develop a central ulcer, giving them a "target" appearance on barium studies, and they can be a source of bleeding or the nidus of intussusception and subsequent small bowel obstruction. Strangulation and subsequent perforation secondary to infarction are uncommon in patients with obstruction due to small bowel metastases (Option (B)). Enteroclysis is more sensitive in detecting these nodules than is the conventional small-bowel follow-through examination. Even with enteroclysis, most of these metastases escape radiographic detection.

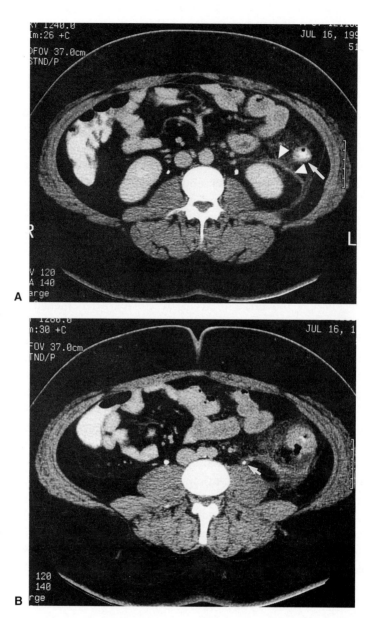

Figure 4-4. Diverticulitis of descending colon with localized perforation. (A) A CT scan shows that the wall of the descending colon (arrow) is slightly thickened. There is edema of the pericolonic tissues in this area and inflammatory thickening of the anterior leaf of the renal fascia (arrowheads). (B) A CT scan 4 cm inferiorly shows marked thickening of the descending colon wall and gas within the colonic wall and pericolonic tissues. Note the thickening of the wall of the left ureter (arrow).

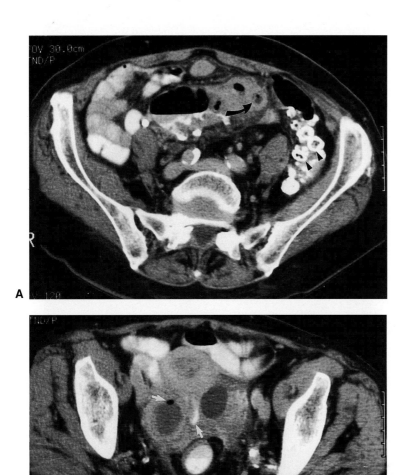

Figure 4-5. Diverticular abscess. CT scan of the abdomen and pelvis performed with oral, rectal, and intravenous contrast. (A) Scattered contrast-filled diverticula (arrowheads) are present along the proximal sigmoid colon. Note the eccentric wall thickening of the more distal sigmoid colon and the adjacent extraluminal fluid collection (curved arrow). (B) A CT image 2 cm inferiorly shows two larger extraluminal pericolonic fluid collections due to the perforated sigmoid diverticulum. One of the collections contains gas and rectal contrast material (arrows), suggesting communication with the bowel.

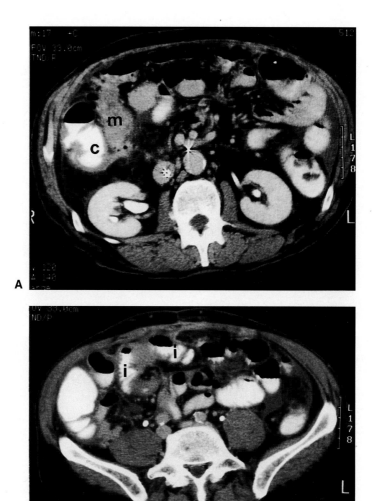

Figure 4-6. Partial small bowel obstruction due to peritoneal carcinomatosis in a patient with recurrent pancreatic carcinoma. (A) A CT scan shows an ill-defined mass (m) medial to the ascending colon (c). Note the hazy infiltration of the mesenteric fat surrounding the posterior portion of the mass. (B) Tumor encases distal ileum (i) in the right lower abdomen. The affected bowel is kinked and shows straightening and thickening of its valvulae in a pattern sometimes described as a "transverse stretch" appearance. Note the dilated small bowel segments in the left mid-abdomen.

Carcinomas of the pancreas, colon, stomach, ovary, and breast tend to seed the peritoneum and mesentery (Figures 4-6 and 4-7). They generally cause ascites and can encase the bowel, causing partial or complete

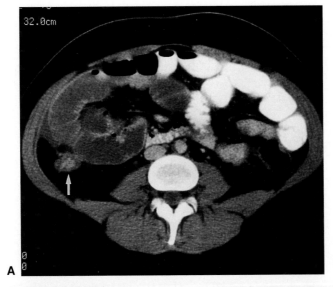

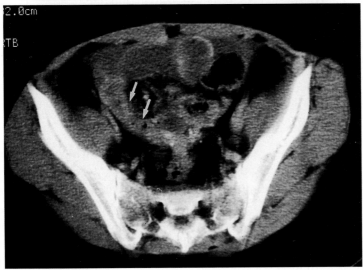

Figure 4-7. Small bowel obstruction due to intraperitoneal spread of ovarian carcinoma. (A) A CT scan shows mildly dilated small bowel segments filled with orally administered contrast medium in the left abdomen and unopacified intestinal fluid in the right mid-abdomen. The presence of the collapsed right colon (arrow) indicates that the small bowel dilatation is due to obstruction. (B) Lower in the pelvis, tumor encases a distal ileal segment (arrows), which is narrowed and has a thickened wall as a result of serosal implants.

obstruction. Associated fibrosis causes fixation, kinking, and angulation. The valvulae conniventes take on a transversely stretched appearance.

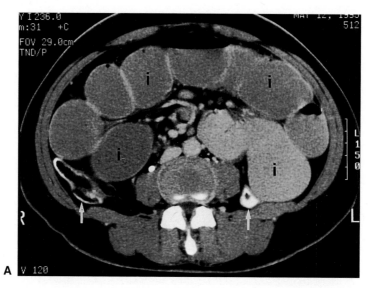

Figure 4-8. High-grade small bowel obstruction due to adhesions follow-ing hysterectomy in a 47-year-old woman. (A) A CT scan shows marked distension of multiple small bowel loops (i) and collapsed ascending and descending colon (arrows). This combination of findings is diagnostic of mechanical small bowel obstruction. (B) A CT scan through the mid-pel-vis shows narrowed, kinked ileum (curved arrow) at the site of adhesions in the bed of the uterus.

The same radiographic abnormalities can be seen with benign adhesions on barium studies, but patients with metastasis to the small intestine often show, in addition, the more characteristic finding of intestine stretched over round, serosal masses.

Adhesions (Option (C)) are strands of fibrous tissue that attach seg-ments of intestine to one another, adjacent structures, or both. Intraperi-toneal adhesions usually form in response to peritoneal inflammation in patients who have had laparotomy, peritoneal dialysis, peritonitis, or bowel perforation. Occasionally, fibrotic bands are congenital in origin. Adhesions are not directly seen on barium studies, but they are detected by virtue of their effects on the bowel. Bowel fixation and angulation, stretched folds, and partial mechanical obstruction form a readily recog-nizable pattern on CT or barium studies (Figure 4-8). Although adhe-sions are one of the most common causes of strangulating obstruction, they, as with diverticulitis, would not be expected to cause herniation of small intestine outside the normal confines of the abdominal and pelvic cavity. When adhesions are not widespread, radiographic studies may show only obstruction with no sign of the cause.

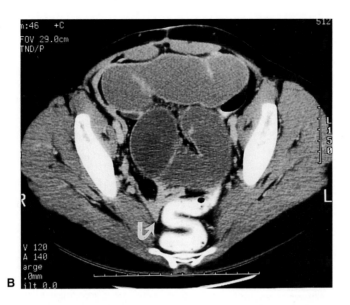

Crohn's disease (Option (D)) most often involves the small bowel. It involves the small bowel only in 29% of patients, the small bowel and colon in 50% of patients, the colon only in 19% of patients, and the anorectal area only in 2% of patients. Affected segments are thick walled, have narrow lumens, and lack the normal mucosal-fold pattern. The surrounding mesenteric fat can proliferate into a space-occupying mass that displaces adjacent bowel loops and can be quite striking (Figure 4-9). The fat surrounding an affected segment of bowel can have a normal CT attenuation value (−80 to −100 HU) or can exhibit hazy or streaky increased CT attenuation. There can also be enlarged lymph nodes in the region of fatty proliferation. CT can show bands of soft tissue density connecting affected loops to one another, to an abscess, or to the adjacent body wall. These bands can represent nonspecific inflammatory tissue, fistulas, or sinus tracts. Gas or oral contrast material within these soft tissue bands indicates that they are communicating with the bowel lumen. Although abscesses and diseased bowel can communicate with the body wall in patients with Crohn's disease, herniation of the bowel outside of the abdominal or pelvic cavity is not a common finding in these patients.

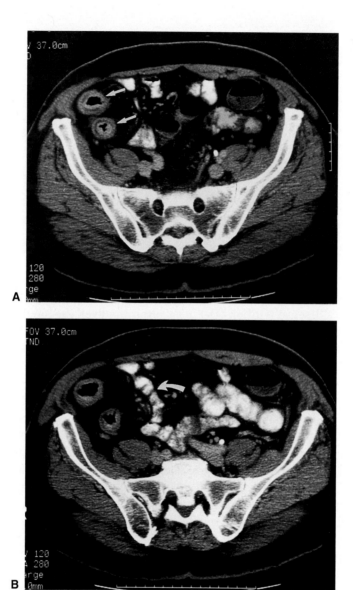

Figure 4-9. Crohn's disease of the distal ileum. (A) There is thickening of the ileum (arrows) in the right lower abdomen, with a "halo" appearance of the bowel wall. (B) In addition to the bowel wall thickening, note the proliferation of the mesenteric fat, which is displacing normal-appearing bowel loops (curved arrow) away from the affected loops.

Question 11

Concerning hernias,

    (A) spigelian hernias always occur just lateral to the margin of the rectus abdominis muscle

    (B) obturator hernias typically occur in elderly women

    (C) sciatic hernias are rarely associated with bowel obstruction

    (D) incarcerated Richter hernias are nearly always associated with bowel obstruction

    (E) direct inguinal hernias are less likely to strangulate than are indirect inguinal hernias

External hernias are abnormal protrusions of intra-abdominal structures through a normal opening or through a congenital or acquired defect in the fascia that normally confines the protruding structures to the abdominal cavity. The protruding structures of a hernia consist of a peritoneal sac with or without intra-abdominal fat, bowel, or solid viscera. In contrast to external hernias, internal hernias are confined to the abdominal or thoracic cavity. Internal hernias are protrusions of intra-abdominal structures (usually bowel) through a developmental or surgically created defect in the peritoneum or mesentery. These hernias usually occur in the region of the ligament of Treitz (paraduodenal), through the foramen of Winslow, or through postoperative or posttraumatic tears in the omentum, mesentery, or diaphragm.

Hernias can be reducible or irreducible. Reducible hernias are ones in which the contents of the hernia sac return to the abdomen spontaneously or with manual pressure. The contents of irreducible hernias (also called incarcerated hernias) cannot be returned to the abdomen, usually because of a narrow hernia opening at the site of protrusion of the peritoneal sac. Incarceration of a hernia can lead to obstruction or strangulation, or both, of the hernia sac and its contents. For strangulation to occur, the blood supply of the hernia contents must be compromised. Strangulation of the hernia results in ischemia and, if not recognized and treated early, infarction of the herniated peritoneal sac and its contents. Strangulation generally occurs only in incarcerated hernias associated with bowel obstruction. However, a Richter hernia, an uncommon type of external hernia that can occur in any location and in which only one wall of the bowel becomes incarcerated, often results in strangulation without obstruction **(Option (D) is false).** Furthermore, obstruction does not always lead to strangulation.

External hernias can occur in the groin (inguinal and femoral), pelvis (obturator, sciatic, perineal), abdominal wall (incisional, spigelian, umbilical, paraumbilical, epigastric), and lumbar regions. Approximately 75% of external hernias occur in the groin region, 10% are incisional her-

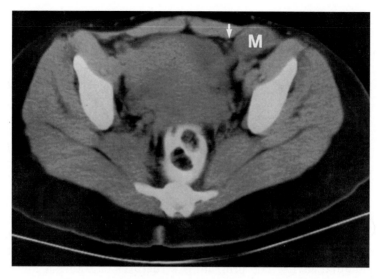

Figure 4-10. Desmoid tumor (M) lying in the inguinal canal and simulating a left inguinal hernia. Note the location of the inferior epigastric vessels (arrow); hernias lateral to the epigastric vessels are referred to as indirect inguinal hernias. (Case courtesy of Richard J. Wechsler, M.D., Thomas Jefferson University Hospital, Philadelphia, Penn.)

nias of the abdominal wall, and less than 3% occur in each of the other locations. The diagnosis of external hernia is usually made easily by obtaining a careful medical history and performing a physical examination. However, in obese patients, patients with thick scars, or patients with hernias that remain undetectable by dissecting between muscle or fascial layers, an accurate clinical diagnosis of hernia can be difficult. CT can be very helpful in the diagnosis in these patients. In addition, abdominal wall masses such as tumors, abscesses, seromas, or hematomas can mimic hernias (Figure 4-10).

The morbidity and mortality associated with external hernias are often related to delays in presentation and diagnosis. Up to 15% of cases of small bowel obstruction are reported to be caused by hernias (72% external, 28% internal). Of the cases of small bowel obstruction caused by hernia, approximately 28% progress to strangulation of the hernia. The occurrence of strangulation in small bowel obstruction as a result of hernia appears to be related to the delay between clinical presentation and operative intervention. Cross-sectional imaging, including CT and sonography, is useful in evaluating patients with abdominal pain or symptoms of small bowel obstruction who are suspected of having external hernias but have no mass apparent on physical examination or have a confusing clinical presentation.

Spigelian hernias are acquired hernias of the ventral abdominal wall; they represent less than 2% of all anterior abdominal wall hernias. The hernias occur at the lateral aspect of the rectus abdominis muscle **(Option (A) is true)** through the spigelian fascia, which is the portion of the transversus abdominis aponeurosis just lateral to the edge of the rectus sheath and medial to the linea semilunaris (also called the spigelian line). The linea semilunaris is the point of transition of the transversus abdominis muscle to its aponeurotic tendon and can be seen on the external abdominal wall as the groove that parallels the lateral margin of the rectus muscle. Spigelian hernias usually occur at the point where the arcuate line (also called the semicircular line or line of Douglas) crosses the spigelian line. The arcuate line is the level at which the aponeuroses of the internal oblique and transversus abdominis muscles no longer pass posterior to the rectus muscles. This line marks the lower border of the posterior layer of the rectus sheath and is usually located just below the level of the umbilicus. Below the level of the arcuate line, the peritoneum is separated from the anterior abdominal wall only by the extraperitoneal fat and the transversalis fascia (Figure 4-11). This anatomic arrangement creates a weak point in the anterior abdominal wall through which a hernia can occur. Spigelian hernias are associated with a high frequency of incarceration and strangulation as a result of the small size of the associated fascial defect.

The sac of a spigelian hernia usually dissects laterally and remains deep to the external oblique muscle, resulting in an interstitial type of hernia that can be difficult to feel on physical examination. A spigelian hernia can be identified on CT by the protrusion of a hernia sac at the lateral border of the rectus abdominis muscle (Figure 4-12). If the patient has had previous surgery in that area, it can be difficult to differentiate a true spigelian hernia from an incisional hernia (Figure 4-13). Sonography of a spigelian hernia shows a complex gas- or fluid-containing mass in the appropriate area of the abdominal wall.

Obturator hernias account for less than 1% of external hernias. These hernias occur through the obturator canal, which is bordered superiorly by the obturator groove of the superior pubic ramus and inferiorly by the superior margin of the obturator membrane and the obturator internus and externus muscles. The canal is approximately 2 to 3 cm long and 1 cm in diameter. The obturator artery, vein, and nerve pass through this canal, which runs obliquely anteriorly, medially, and inferiorly to end in the obturator region of the thigh. Obturator hernias occur six times more frequently in women than in men and are more common on the right side than the left. Most patients are between 70 and 90 years old **(Option (B) is true)**. Emaciation is thought to be the most important predisposing factor, although laxity of the pelvic soft tissues,

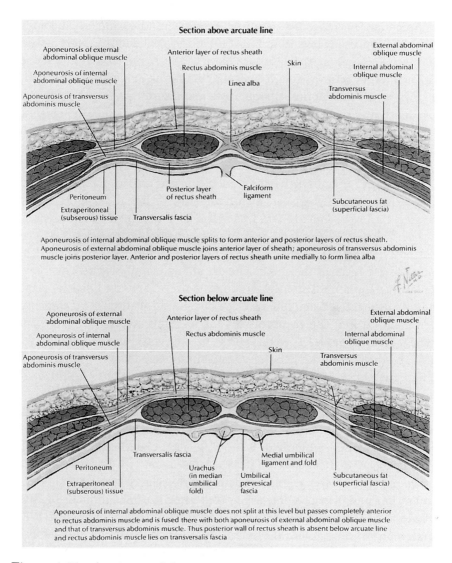

Section above arcuate line

Aponeurosis of external abdominal oblique muscle

Anterior layer of rectus sheath

Rectus abdominis muscle

Skin

External abdominal oblique muscle

Aponeurosis of internal abdominal oblique muscle

Linea alba

Internal abdominal oblique muscle

Aponeurosis of transversus abdominis muscle

Transversus abdominis muscle

Peritoneum

Posterior layer of rectus sheath

Falciform ligament

Subcutaneous fat (superficial fascia)

Extraperitoneal (subserous) tissue

Transversalis fascia

Aponeurosis of internal abdominal oblique muscle splits to form anterior and posterior layers of rectus sheath. Aponeurosis of external abdominal oblique muscle joins anterior layer of sheath; aponeurosis of transversus abdominis muscle joins posterior layer. Anterior and posterior layers of rectus sheath unite medially to form linea alba

Section below arcuate line

Aponeurosis of external abdominal oblique muscle

Anterior layer of rectus sheath

Rectus abdominis muscle

External abdominal oblique muscle

Aponeurosis of internal abdominal oblique muscle

Internal abdominal oblique muscle

Skin

Aponeurosis of transversus abdominis muscle

Transversus abdominis muscle

Transversalis fascia

Medial umbilical ligament and fold

Peritoneum

Urachus (in median umbilical fold)

Umbilical prevesical fascia

Subcutaneous fat (superficial fascia)

Extraperitoneal (subserous) tissue

Aponeurosis of internal abdominal oblique muscle does not split at this level but passes completely anterior to rectus abdominis muscle and is fused there with both aponeurosis of external abdominal oblique muscle and that of transversus abdominis muscle. Thus posterior wall of rectus sheath is absent below arcuate line and rectus abdominis muscle lies on transversalis fascia

Figure 4-11. Anatomy of the anterior abdominal wall above and below the level of the arcuate line. (Reprinted with permission from Netter FH. Rectus sheath: cross sections. In: Colacino S (ed), Atlas of human anatomy. Summit, NJ: CIBA-GEIGY Corp.; 1989:235.)

which develops after multiple pregnancies, is also thought to contribute to the development of these hernias. The sac in obturator hernias usually contains small bowel, especially ileum. There have also been reports of obturator hernias containing colon, appendix, Meckel's diverticulum, omentum, bladder, ovary, and uterus.

The peritoneal sac of obturator hernias can follow any of three potential pathways: (1) most commonly the sac emerges from the obturator

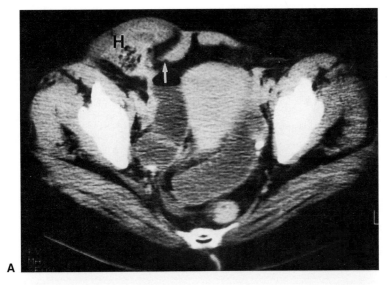

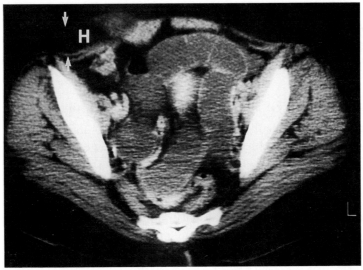

Figure 4-12. Spigelian hernia at the lateral border of the right rectus abdominis muscle about halfway between the inguinal canal and the arcuate line. (A) A CT scan shows that the bowel within the hernia (H) passes just lateral to the border of the rectus muscle (arrow) and is contained by the aponeurosis of the external oblique muscle. (B) A CT scan 2 cm superiorly shows the hernia (H) dissecting cephalad between the aponeuroses of the internal and external oblique muscles (arrows).

canal, follows the anterior division of the obturator nerve, and lies between the obturator externus muscle posteriorly and pectineus muscle anteriorly; (2) alternatively, the sac emerges from the canal, follows the

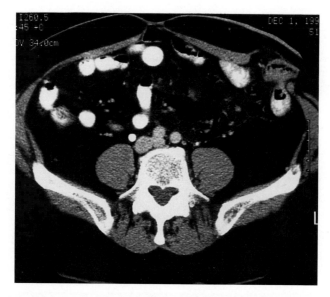

Figure 4-13. Incisional hernia of the left anterior abdominal wall. If it were not known that this was the site of a previous surgical incision, the appearance could be mistaken for that of a spigelian hernia.

posterior division of the obturator nerve, and extends between the superior and middle fasciculi of the obturator externus muscle; or (3) rarely, the sac emerges from the canal and dissects between the obturator internus and externus muscles.

Obturator hernias have a high frequency of incarceration, obstruction, and strangulation. It has been reported that 80 to 90% of patients with obturator hernias present with signs of small bowel obstruction. Obturator hernias account for approximately 0.4% of cases of mechanical small bowel obstruction. The clinical diagnosis of obturator hernia is often difficult because of the lack of specific signs and symptoms. The Howship-Romberg sign, which is said to be pathognomonic of incarcerated obturator hernia, occurs only in approximately one-third of patients with obturator hernias. This sign, which consists of pain that radiates down the medial aspect of the thigh and is relieved by flexion and increased by extension, abduction, or medial rotation, is due to compression of the obturator nerve in the canal by the hernia sac. The high frequency of serious complications from obturator hernias and the relatively low frequency of specific signs and symptoms mean that cross-sectional imaging plays an important role in the care of these patients. On CT these hernias are seen as masses, which may or may not contain loops of bowel, passing through the obturator canal (Figure 4-2).

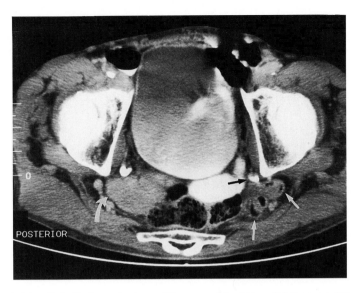

Figure 4-14. Sciatic hernia in a 65-year-old man with intermittent constipation. A CT scan of the pelvis at the level of the acetabular roof shows a portion of the sigmoid colon (straight white arrows) herniating through the left sciatic foramen. The left ureter (black arrow) is just medial to the bowel but not quite through the foramen. Also note the beginning of a right sciatic foramen hernia containing a loop of small bowel (curved white arrow).

Sciatic hernias are the rarest of all external hernias. These hernias exit from the pelvis through the greater or lesser sciatic foramen. They can contain bowel, ureter, bladder, or ovary. They have a high association with incarceration, obstruction, and strangulation **(Option (C) is false).** Cross-sectional imaging shows a sciatic hernia as a mass posterior to the posterior inferior iliac spine or the ischial spine (Figure 4-14).

Inguinal hernias are the most common of the external hernias. The hernia sac can contain intra-abdominal fat, bowel, or ascites. Depending on their relationship to the inferior epigastric vessels, inguinal hernias are classified as either indirect or direct.

Most inguinal hernias in infants, children, and young adults are indirect. Indirect inguinal hernias occur in the setting of failure of obliteration of the processus vaginalis. The hernia sac passes lateral to the inferior epigastric vessels through the deep inguinal ring into the inguinal canal. Depending on the degree of patency of the processus vaginalis, the hernia can exit the canal through the superficial inguinal ring and pass into the scrotum in men or follow the course of the round ligament of the uterus into the labium in women (Figure 4-15).

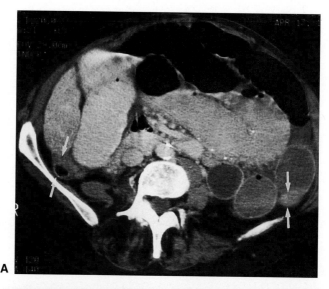

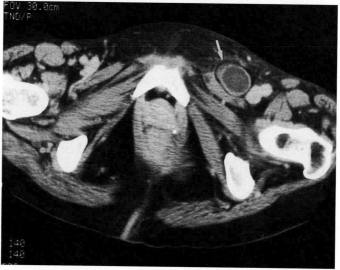

Figure 4-15. Small bowel obstruction due to left inguinal hernia in a 66-year-old woman. (A) A CT scan through the level of the mid-abdomen shows marked distension of numerous gas- and fluid-filled small intestinal loops. Note the collapsed ascending and descending colon (arrows). (B) Fluid-filled ileum (arrow) lies outside the abdomen in the left inguinal canal.

Direct inguinal hernias are acquired as a result of the development of a region of weakness in the transversalis fascia in Hesselbach's triangle, the region bounded inferiorly by the medial half of the inguinal ligament, laterally by the inferior epigastric vessels, and medially by the conjoined tendon, which runs along the inferolateral edge of the rectus abdominis muscle and attaches to the pubic tubercle. Direct inguinal hernias generally do not actually pass through any preformed inguinal ring or focal fascial defect. Instead, the direct inguinal hernia sac bulges anteriorly, pushing the transversalis fascia, which forms the floor of the inguinal canal, ahead of it. These hernias generally do not traverse the inguinal canal.

Most inguinal hernias do not produce symptoms until the patient notices a mass in the groin region. Occasionally these hernias cause a nagging pain, which can radiate into the scrotum in men. They are often detected incidentally during a routine physical examination. Direct inguinal hernias generally cause fewer symptoms and are less likely to incarcerate, obstruct, or strangulate than indirect inguinal hernias **(Option (E) is true).**

Question 12

Concerning CT of small bowel obstruction,

(A) ileal dilatation (exceeding 2.5 cm) is a specific sign
(B) if it shows no apparent cause, adhesions are usually responsible for the obstruction
(C) air-fluid levels in the small intestine strongly suggest mechanical obstruction
(D) it is both more sensitive and more specific than abdominal radiography
(E) in patients with a history of cancer, it is likely to identify the specific cause of the obstruction

The evaluation of patients suspected of having small bowel obstruction should be directed toward answering the following four key questions. (1) Is obstruction present? (2) If so, what is the level and cause of obstruction? (3) Is the obstructed bowel strangulated? (4) Is immediate surgical treatment needed, or is a trial of nonoperative management indicated?

Small bowel obstruction can be low-grade partial, high-grade partial, or complete. The obstruction can be acute, chronic, or intermittent. It can be caused by a variety of entities including adhesions, internal or external hernia, primary or metastatic tumor, abscess, and inflammatory bowel disease. A 3-year retrospective study of 289 patients with small bowel obstruction at the Mayo Clinic showed that 80% of all small bowel obstructions are caused by adhesions (50%), hernias (15%), and neoplasms (15%) (mainly metastatic disease from abdominal primary tumors). In that series, more than one-third of the patients had multiple causes of their obstruction.

The diagnosis of small bowel obstruction can usually be made on the basis of clinical history, physical examination, and abdominal radiography. Abdominal radiography in patients with small bowel obstruction demonstrates conclusive evidence of small bowel obstruction in 50 to 60% of cases, is equivocal in 20 to 30% of cases, and is normal in 10 to 20% of cases. Many patients with ischemic or metabolic disturbances have a plain film pattern resembling that of small bowel obstruction. Abdominal radiography has been reported to have a specificity of 58 to 80%. Until recently, if the diagnosis of small bowel obstruction was not confirmed on the basis of the history, physical examination, and radiographs of the abdomen, the next step in the radiologic examination was the performance of either small-bowel follow-through examination or enteroclysis. CT has now also become accepted as a useful radiologic modality in the evaluation of these patients.

CT has been shown to have a sensitivity of 90 to 94% and a specificity of 96% for diagnosing small bowel obstruction **(Option (D) is true).** Maglinte et al. showed this high sensitivity to be valid primarily in patients with long-standing or high-grade small bowel obstruction. In patients with early or low-grade partial small bowel obstruction, the bowel can be only minimally dilated or not dilated at all. This limits the utility of CT in making a diagnosis of small bowel obstruction, which is based on the demonstration of a transition zone in the bowel with dilated bowel proximal to the transition and collapsed bowel distal to it.

There are several advantages to using CT instead of small bowel contrast studies in the evaluation of patients with suspected small bowel obstruction. In addition to correctly identifying the presence of obstruction, the ability of CT to identify the cause of the obstruction (73% of cases in the series by Megibow et al.) exceeds that of either radiography or small bowel contrast studies. This is due to the ability of CT to directly demonstrate extraluminal and bowel wall abnormalities. CT is particularly useful in patients with a history of malignancy, due to its ability to detect tumor masses in the mesentery, omentum, or bowel serosa in the region of the transition zone **(Option (E) is true)** (Figure 4-16). When no mass, abscess, bowel wall abnormality, or other cause of obstruction is apparent in the transition zone, adhesions are the likely cause **(Option (B) is true)** (Figure 4-17). CT is also the most useful modality for identifying patients with strangulating small bowel obstruction.

Pitfalls in the use of CT for diagnosing small bowel obstruction include the false assumptions that bowel loops in the pelvis are necessarily more distal to bowel loops in the upper abdomen and that small bowel dilatation greater than 2.5 cm is a specific sign of obstruction **(Option (A) is false).** Fukuya et al. used receiver-operating-characteristic analysis to show that bowel with a diameter greater than 2.5 cm should be

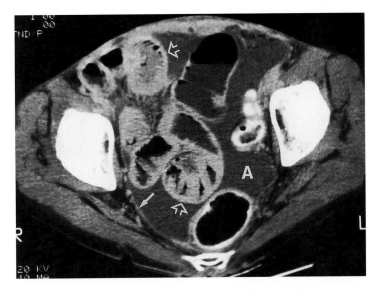

Figure 4-16. Small bowel obstruction following hysterectomy for endometrial carcinoma approximately 1 year ago. There is ascites (A), diffuse thickening of the parietal peritoneum (solid arrow), and thickening of the intestinal wall (open arrows) as a result of tumor implants on the visceral peritoneal surface. Obstruction was due to encasement of pelvic small intestinal segments by the tumor implants.

considered dilated; however, this does not imply that all bowel dilated to this extent is obstructed. The four patients falsely diagnosed with small bowel obstruction in the series by Megibow et al. had bowel dilatation; however, the dilatation in these patients was due to adynamic ileus. In loops of small bowel that are not dilated, are dilated in proportion to the colon, or lack evidence of a transition zone, the findings of air-fluid levels and a fluid-filled appearance are indicative of adynamic ileus rather than mechanical bowel obstruction **(Option (C) is false).**

The imaging method best used to evaluate a patient suspected of having small bowel obstruction depends on the clinical presentation. There have been a few reports of the utility of sonography in the evaluation of patients with small bowel obstruction; however, there is no consensus regarding its use for this indication. Enteroclysis is probably more useful than CT in the evaluation of patients with early, low-grade partial, or intermittent small bowel obstruction. The ability of enteroclysis to localize adhesions accurately is particularly important in view of the increasing use of laparoscopy for the lysis of adhesions. As mentioned above, enteroclysis or small-bowel follow-through examination may be contraindicated in patients in whom cross-sectional imaging is also being

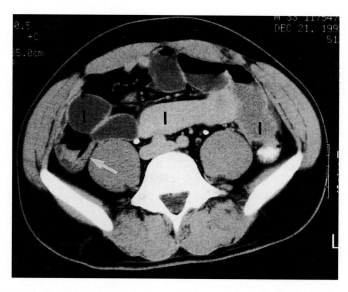

Figure 4-17. Ileal obstruction in a 33-year-old man with acute onset of abdominal pain and no history of prior surgical procedure. A CT scan shows multiple dilated small intestinal loops (I) with collapsed distal ileum (arrow) in the right lower abdominal quadrant. This combination of findings indicates mechanical ileal obstruction, but no cause for the obstruction was seen on CT. At operation, a single adhesive band was found obstructing the distal ileum.

considered, because the high density of the oral barium preparations used in these studies significantly degrades CT image quality.

CT is considered the procedure of choice in the evaluation of patients suspected of having small bowel obstruction in the following settings: (1) patients with radiographic and clinical findings of small bowel obstruction, who have no history of previous surgery and are to undergo nonoperative management (in these patients, CT can show an unsuspected abnormality, such as incarcerated hernia, tumor, or strangulation, that would alter the treatment plan); (2) patients with a history of an abdominal malignancy and clinical symptoms of small bowel obstruction; (3) patients with signs and symptoms of small bowel obstruction and systemic signs of infection or a palpable abdominal or pelvic mass; and (4) patients with signs and symptoms of small bowel obstruction and systemic signs of bowel infarction (a notoriously difficult clinical diagnosis).

Question 13

Concerning CT findings in closed-loop obstruction,

    (A) if strangulation occurs, the wall of the affected bowel loop is stretched thin as it worsens

    (B) the presence of edema and hemorrhage within the affected mesentery suggests strangulation

    (C) a U-shaped loop of bowel is characteristic

    (D) the diagnosis of strangulation is based on the detection of intramural or portal venous gas

    (E) the finding of two collapsed loops adjacent to the site of obstruction suggests the diagnosis

Closed-loop small bowel obstruction, defined as mechanical obstruction caused by occlusion of a segment of bowel at two points along its course, is most commonly due to adhesions or incarcerated hernias (Figure 4-18). The segment of affected bowel can include one or several loops. Closed-loop small bowel obstruction is a surgical emergency because of the propensity for the obstructed bowel to become strangulated and progress to irreversible ischemia, infarction, and perforation.

The strangulation can be caused by vascular compromise from the same mechanism that caused the small bowel obstruction, from volvulus of the obstructed segment, or from increased intraluminal pressure as a result of progressive distension of the obstructed loop. Regardless of the mechanism of strangulation, restriction of the venous outflow from the affected bowel leads to engorgement of the mesenteric vessels supplying the loop; intramural hemorrhage; increased permeability of the bowel wall with weeping of hemorrhagic fluid into the intestinal lumen, surrounding mesentery, and peritoneal space; and, eventually, frank infarction and perforation.

The most important factor affecting the clinical outcome in patients with small bowel obstruction is whether the obstruction has progressed to the point of strangulation. Unfortunately, the diagnosis of strangulation on the basis of clinical and laboratory data is difficult and is missed preoperatively in 50 to 85% of cases. Ischemic injury due to strangulating obstruction can become irreversible before there are any clear clinical manifestations of obstruction. The goal of the radiologist is to identify these patients early in the course of disease, when the bowel ischemia is still reversible.

Abdominal radiography has a limited role in the evaluation of patients suspected of having closed-loop small bowel obstruction. Radiographs often show nonspecific abnormalities or appear normal. They occasionally show a "pseudotumor" due to the fluid-filled closed-loop or to

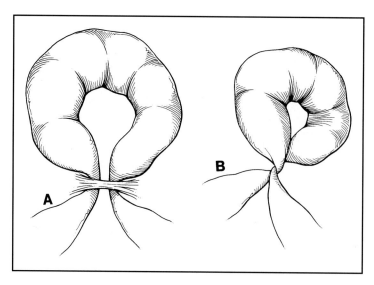

Figure 4-18. Diagram of closed-loop small bowel obstruction. (A) An adhesive band causes obstruction at two points of adjacent segments of bowel. (B) Closed-loop obstruction associated with small bowel volvulus. Twisting of the closed loop (volvulus) is a common but not invariable complication of the incarcerated loop. (Adapted with permission from Balthazar et al. [3].)

the combination of multiple fluid-filled loops and the adjacent congested and hemorrhagic mesentery. Enteroclysis can identify partial closed-loop small bowel obstruction, but its usefulness for documenting complete closed-loop small bowel obstruction and strangulation has not been proven.

The ability of CT to directly visualize the bowel wall, mesenteric vessels, and surrounding mesenteric fat makes it the most promising imaging method currently available for the evaluation of patients suspected of having closed-loop small bowel obstruction and for diagnosing strangulating obstruction. As described by Balthazar et al., the CT findings seen in patients with closed-loop small bowel obstruction include (1) evidence of small bowel obstruction, (2) a U-shaped configuration of a single distended fluid-filled loop of bowel **(Option (C) is true)** or radial distribution of several fluid-filled dilated loops of bowel, (3) mesenteric vessels that converge toward the point of obstruction, and (4) a site of obstruction with a whirl sign, beak sign, triangular loop, or two adjacent collapsed loops (Figure 4-19) **(Option (E) is true).** The appearance of the closed loop on CT depends on whether it is oriented in the transverse or longitudinal plane. If it is oriented transversely, the entire U-shaped loop can be seen on one or two images (Figure 4-20A).

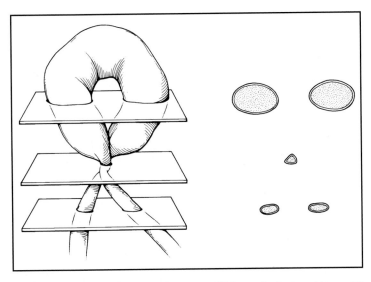

Figure 4-19. Diagram of closed-loop small bowel obstruction with small bowel volvulus. A transverse section of closed loop enables detection of two distended fluid-filled segments of intestine (top right). At the level of the obstruction and volvulus, the loops of bowel are collapsed adjacent to each other or may exhibit a triangular configuration (bottom right). (Adapted with permission from Balthazar et al. [3].)

In addition to the findings described above for closed-loop small bowel obstruction, the CT findings in patients with strangulating obstruction can also include: (1) circumferential thickening, submucosal edema, submucosal hemorrhage (high attenuation), or pneumatosis of the strangulated bowel wall; (2) engorged mesenteric vessels (less than 3 cm in diameter), mesenteric congestion (haziness of the fat and blurring of the margins of the vascular structures), mesenteric hemorrhage adjacent to the affected bowel **(Option (B) is true)**, or portal venous gas; and (3) ascites (Figure 4-20B). In patients with strangulation with mild ischemia and viable bowel, there is mild wall thickening, submucosal edema (as evidenced by a target appearance of the bowel wall), and engorgement of the mesenteric vascular structures. With progression to infarction, the bowel wall thickness and CT attenuation increase as hemorrhage worsens **(Option (A) is false).** Hemorrhage also appears in the mesentery, and there may be intramural pneumatosis and mesenteric or portal venous gas. Pneumatosis and mesenteric and portal venous gas are late findings in bowel ischemia and indicate the presence of bowel wall necrosis **(Option (D) is false).** Pneumatosis has been reported to occur in only 30% of patients with bowel ischemia/infarction; portal

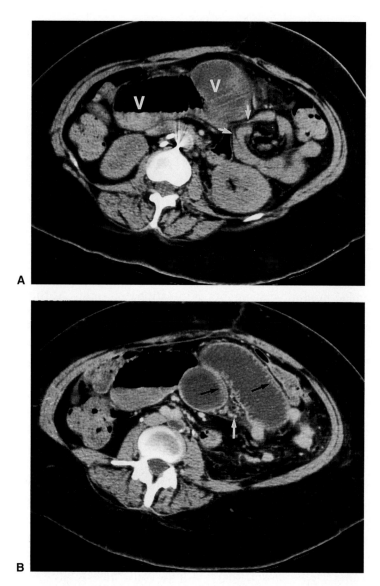

Figure 4-20. Closed-loop small bowel obstruction due to adhesions. (A) A noncontrast CT scan through the level of the obstruction shows a volvulus with the dilated segments of bowel (V) adjacent to two collapsed and undilated loops, which lie in a whirled configuration and appear to come to a point (arrows) as they approach the site of the volvulus. (B) A CT scan at a slightly lower level in the same patient after intravenous contrast administration shows thickening and high attenuation of the wall of the strangulated ileal segment (black arrows). Note venous engorgement and high attenuation consistent with hemorrhage in the attached mesentery (white arrow).

venous or mesenteric gas has been reported to occur in only 13% of patients with bowel ischemia/infarction.

Similar findings can also be seen in patients with entities other than ischemia and infarction. Bowel wall thickening occurs in patients with inflammatory and infectious bowel disease, tumor, or radiation enteritis. Mesenteric or portal venous gas can be seen in patients with abdominal abscess or inflammatory bowel disease or after colonoscopy. Benign causes of pneumatosis (pneumatosis cystoides intestinalis) include obstructive airway disease, ventilator-induced barotrauma, corticosteroid therapy, and collagen vascular disease (especially scleroderma). Furthermore, the absence of any of these findings does not exclude the presence of bowel ischemia. The important point to remember is that in the presence of definitive evidence of small bowel obstruction, the findings described above are strongly suggestive of strangulation and, when communicated to the referring physician, can have a significant impact on the patient's management and clinical outcome.

David S. Memel, M.D.
Robert E. Koehler, M.D.

SUGGESTED READINGS

SMALL BOWEL OBSTRUCTION

1. Balthazar EJ. George W. Holmes Lecture. CT of small-bowel obstruction. AJR 1994; 162:255–261
2. Balthazar EJ, Bauman JS, Megibow AJ. CT diagnosis of closed loop obstruction. J Comput Assist Tomogr 1985; 9:953–955
3. Balthazar EJ, Birnbaum BA, Megibow AJ, Gordon RB, Whelan CA, Hulnick DH. Closed-loop and strangulating intestinal obstruction: CT signs. Radiology 1992; 185:769–775
4. Bessette JR, Maglinte DD, Kelvin FM, Chernish SM. Primary malignant tumors in the small bowel: a comparison of the small-bowel enema and conventional follow-through examination. AJR 1989; 153:741–744
5. Cho KC, Hoffman-Tretin JC, Alterman DD. Closed-loop obstruction of the small bowel: CT and sonographic appearance. J Comput Assist Tomogr 1989; 13:256–258
6. Frager D, Medwid SW, Baer JW, Mollinelli B, Friedman M. CT of small-bowel obstruction: value in establishing the diagnosis and determining the degree and cause. AJR 1994; 162:37–41
7. Fukuya T, Hawes DR, Lu CC, Chang PJ, Barloon TJ. CT diagnosis of small-bowel obstruction: efficacy in 60 patients. AJR 1992; 158:765–769
8. Gazelle GS, Goldberg MA, Wittenberg J, Halpern EF, Pinkney L, Mueller PR. Efficacy of CT in distinguishing small-bowel obstruction from other causes of small-bowel dilatation. AJR 1994; 162:43–47

9. Ha HK, Park CH, Kim SK, et al. CT analysis of intestinal obstruction due to adhesions: early detection of strangulation. J Comput Assist Tomogr 1993; 17:386–389

10. Herlinger H, Maglinte DD. Small bowel obstruction. In: Herlinger H, Maglinte DD (eds), Clinical radiology of the small bowel. Philadelphia: WB Saunders; 1989:479–509

11. Ko YT, Lim JH, Lee DH, Lee HW, Lim JW. Small bowel obstruction: sonographic evaluation. Radiology 1993; 188:649–653

12. Maglinte DD, Gage SN, Harmon BH, et al. Obstruction of the small intestine: accuracy and role of CT in diagnosis. Radiology 1993; 188:61–64

13. Maglinte DD, Herlinger H, Nolan DJ. Radiologic features of closed loop obstruction: analysis of 25 confirmed cases. Radiology 1991; 179:383–387

14. Megibow AJ, Balthazar EJ, Cho KC, Medwid SW, Birnbaum BA, Noz ME. Bowel obstruction: evaluation with CT. Radiology 1991; 180:313–318

15. Mucha P Jr. Small intestinal obstruction. Surg Clin North Am 1987; 67:597–620

16. Rubesin SE, Herlinger H. CT evaluation of bowel obstruction: a landmark article—implications for the future. Radiology 1991; 180:307–308

17. Stewart ET. CT diagnosis of small-bowel obstruction. AJR 1992; 158:771–772

18. Wills JS. Closed-loop and strangulating obstruction of the small intestine: a new twist. Radiology 1992; 185:635–636

ABDOMINAL HERNIAS

19. Balthazar EJ, Subramanyam BR, Megibow A. Spigelian hernia: CT and ultrasonography diagnosis. Gastrointest Radiol 1984; 9:81–84

20. Cubillo E. Obturator hernia diagnosed by computed tomography. AJR 1983; 140:735–736

21. Ghahremani GG, Jimenez MA, Rosenfeld M, Rochester D. CT diagnosis of occult incisional hernias. AJR 1987; 148:139–142

22. Ghahremani GG, Michael AS. Sciatic hernia with incarcerated ileum: CT and radiographic diagnosis. Gastrointest Radiol 1991; 16:120–122

23. Glicklich M, Eliasoph J. Incarcerated obturator hernia: case diagnosed at barium enema fluoroscopy. Radiology 1989; 172:51–52

24. Gray SW, Skandalakis JE, Soria RE, Rowe JS. Strangulated obturator hernia. Surgery 1974; 75:20–27

25. Megibow AJ, Wagner AG. Obturator hernia. J Comput Assist Tomogr 1983; 7:350–352

26. Meziane MA, Fishman EK, Siegelman SS. Computed tomographic diagnosis of obturator foramen hernia. Gastrointest Radiol 1983; 8:375–377

27. Pyatt RS Jr, Alona BR Jr, Daye S, Wenzel DJ, Woods E, Alexieva B. Spigelian hernia. J Comput Assist Tomogr 1982; 6:643–645

28. Santora TA, Roslyn JJ. Incisional hernia. Surg Clin North Am 1993; 73:557–570

29. Wechsler RJ, Kurtz AB, Needleman L, et al. Cross-sectional imaging of abdominal wall hernias. AJR 1989; 153:517–521

30. Williams PL, Warwick R. Myology: IV. The muscles of the abdomen. In: Williams PL, Warwick R (eds), Gray's anatomy, 36th edition. Philadelphia: WB Saunders; 1980:551–559

BOWEL ISCHEMIA AND INFARCTION

31. Alpern MB, Glazer GM, Francis IR. Ischemic or infarcted bowel: CT findings. Radiology 1988; 166:149–152
32. Balthazar EJ, Hulnick D, Megibow AJ, Opulencia JF. Computed tomography of intramural intestinal hemorrhage and bowel ischemia. J Comput Assist Tomogr 1987; 11:67–72
33. Federle MP, Chun G, Jeffrey RB, Rayor R. Computed tomographic findings in bowel infarction. AJR 1984; 142:91–95
34. Lund EC, Han SY, Holley HC, Berland LL. Intestinal ischemia: comparison of plain radiographic and computed tomographic findings. Radio-Graphics 1988; 8:1083–1108
35. Smerud MJ, Johnson CD, Stephens DH. Diagnosis of bowel infarction: a comparison of plain films and CT scans in 23 cases. AJR 1990; 154:99–103

SMALL BOWEL VOLVULUS

36. Fisher JK. Computed tomographic diagnosis of volvulus in intestinal malrotation. Radiology 1981; 140:145–146
37. Jaramillo D, Raval B. CT diagnosis of primary small-bowel volvulus. AJR 1986; 147:941–942

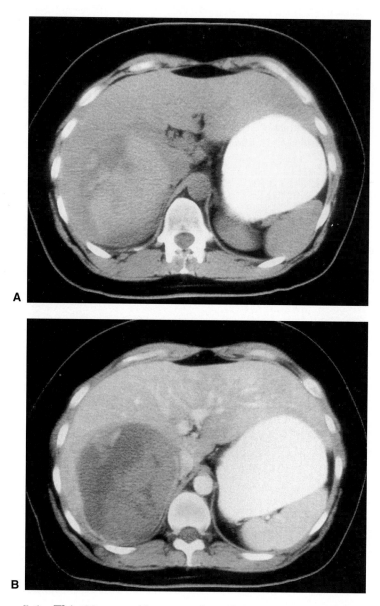

Figure 5-1. This 39-year-old woman has abdominal pain. You are shown precontrast (A) and postcontrast (B) CT scans of the abdomen.

Case 5:   Hepatocellular Adenoma

Question 14

Which *one* of the following is the MOST likely diagnosis?

    (A) Focal nodular hyperplasia
    (B) Cavernous hemangioma
    (C) Hepatocellular adenoma
    (D) Hepatobiliary cystadenoma
    (E) Mesenchymal hamartoma

On the noncontrast test CT scan (Figure 5-1A), a well-defined mass is seen in the right lobe of the liver. The mass is heterogeneous and has a large high-attenuation region, suggesting acute hemorrhage (Figure 5-2A). On the dynamic postcontrast test CT scan (Figure 5-1B), the mass is very sharply defined by an enhancing rim (Figure 5-2B). It is rarely possible to make a histologic diagnosis of the type of hepatic tumor on the basis of the CT appearance alone; however, in this case, the presence of hemorrhage into a liver mass in a young woman should suggest a diagnosis of hepatocellular adenoma **(Option (C) is correct).** Hepatocellular adenoma is a rare benign lesion seen most commonly in young women; the estimated incidence is 3 to 4 per 100,000. Exceedingly rare prior to the widespread use of oral contraceptives, the tumor now characteristically affects women with a history of oral contraceptive use. The exact mechanism by which estrogens induce proliferation of hepatocytes is not known. Regression of lesions after cessation of oral contraceptives has been reported but may take several months.

Pathologically, hepatocellular adenomas are well-circumscribed, often encapsulated lesions. Grossly, resected adenomas frequently demonstrate areas of hemorrhage and infarction. The tumors are composed of neoplastic hepatocytes arranged in cords. Although the tumor hepatocytes histologically resemble normal hepatocytes, the tumors generally do not contain other normal liver constituents (bile ducts, Kupffer cells, etc.).

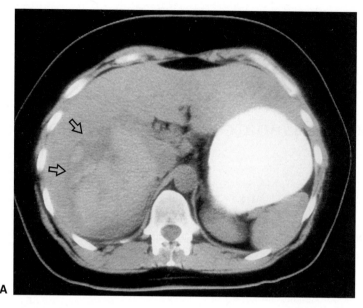

A

Figure 5-2 (Same as Figure 5-1). Hepatocellular adenoma. (A) A noncontrast CT scan of the liver demonstrates a well-circumscribed mass in the right lobe of the liver (arrows). The majority of the lesion is hyperdense, suggesting the presence of acute hemorrhage. (B) After intravenous administration of contrast agent, a CT scan shows an enhancing rim at the periphery of the hemorrhagic lesion (arrows), representing the tumor capsule.

Hepatocellular adenomas are clinically significant because of the high risk of hemorrhage. Hemorrhage can occur within the lesion, as in the test patient, or the tumor can rupture, resulting in hemoperitoneum. Surgical resection of the lesion is recommended in most cases because of the potential for this serious complication as well as a small but significant risk of malignant degeneration. Four cases of hepatocellular carcinoma arising from hepatocellular adenoma have been reported by the Armed Forces Institute of Pathology; the risk is thought to be higher in patients with underlying metabolic disease.

The liver is host to a wide variety of neoplasms. Primary hepatic tumors, both benign and malignant, are derived from hepatocytes, bile duct epithelium, or supporting mesenchymal cells. The liver is also a major site for metastatic neoplasms as well as inflammatory masses. Recognition of the key imaging features of hepatic tumors is important; this is particularly true for those features that allow differentiation of lesions that do not require biopsy or surgical resection (such as focal nodular hyperplasia [FNH] and cavernous hemangioma) from tumors that

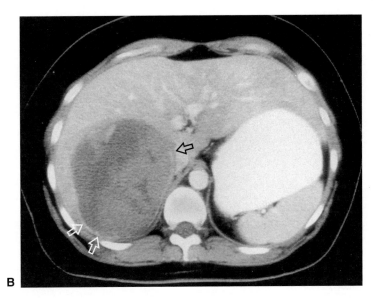

B

require further treatment. Successful differentiation requires a knowledge of typical and atypical features of hepatic tumors on all imaging studies, as well as an understanding of which imaging studies can provide the most valuable information.

FNH (Option (A)) is a benign hepatic lesion that, like hepatocellular adenoma, is found most commonly in young women. Unlike hepatocellular adenoma, however, FNH lesions are usually asymptomatic and are discovered when the liver is imaged for other reasons, although they occasionally present clinically as a palpable right upper quadrant mass. A number of different theories about the pathogenesis of FNH have been proposed, including the speculation that it is a hyperplastic response of normal liver tissue to a localized vascular anomaly. The lesion has no malignant potential and is considered by some to represent a benign "tumor-like condition," rather than a true neoplasm. Presentation of FNH with hemorrhage is extremely rare, making this diagnosis less likely than hepatocellular adenoma in the test case.

Cavernous hemangioma (Option (B)) is another benign hepatic neoplasm that is also more common in women. It is the most common benign non-cystic liver lesion; its prevalence at autopsy has been reported to be up to 20% in one small series, although a larger autopsy series placed the frequency of this tumor at 7.9%. The vast majority of these lesions are asymptomatic. Surgical resection is generally only considered for large, symptomatic lesions. Spontaneous hemorrhage has been reported but is extremely rare. On noncontrast CT, most hemangiomas are less dense

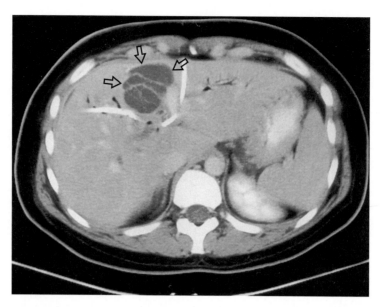

Figure 5-3. Hepatobiliary cystadenoma. A postcontrast CT scan shows a cystic mass with an enhancing rim (arrows) and internal septations occupying the medial segment of the left lobe of the liver in a 32-year-old woman. The mass had resulted in obstruction of the biliary ducts. Biliary drainage catheters and air within the biliary ducts are also seen. This patient subsequently underwent surgical excision of the lesion.

than normal liver. When intravenous contrast agent is administered, hemangiomas demonstrate a characteristic pattern of nodular peripheral enhancement, which is not seen in the test images.

Hepatobiliary cystadenoma (Option (D)), also called biliary cystadenoma, is yet another rare benign hepatic tumor that shows a female predominance. Ishak reported a series of eight patients (all women) with this lesion. Six cases of hepatobiliary cystadenocarcinoma, the malignant counterpart of this lesion, were also reported in four men and two women. As the name implies, cystadenomas are intrahepatic cystic masses, a feature that distinguishes them from the solid mass seen in the test images. CT characteristically demonstrates a low-attenuation mass within the liver, often with internal septations (Figure 5-3). Occasionally, mural nodules are observed. The benign lesions are difficult to distinguish from hepatobiliary cystadenocarcinoma. Total surgical excision of this lesion is usually performed, often with hepatic lobectomy, to prevent local recurrence or malignant degeneration.

Mesenchymal hamartoma (Option (E)) can be dismissed as a possible diagnosis on the basis of the test patient's age alone. Although a few case

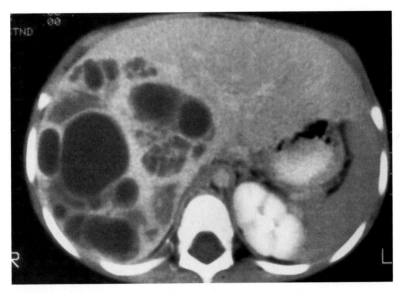

Figure 5-4. Mesenchymal hamartoma. A contrast-enhanced CT scan in a 2-year-old child with a palpable right upper quadrant mass. A well-circumscribed mass is present in the right lobe of the liver, which contains multiple cysts of variable size. (Case courtesy of William Hastrup, M.D., Valley Children's Hospital, Fresno, Calif.)

reports of this tumor occurring in adults have been published, mesenchymal hamartoma is a rare hepatic tumor that occurs predominantly in children, most often boys, with an average age of 15 months. In two large series, this lesion represented 5 to 8% of pediatric liver tumors. Patients usually present with large, solitary hepatic masses, averaging 18 cm in the series published by Lack. The tumor consists of mesenchyme, often with numerous multilocular cysts, and remnants of hepatic parenchyma. CT evaluation most commonly demonstrates a well-circumscribed mass containing cystic areas of various sizes with internal septations (Figure 5-4).

Question 15

Concerning focal nodular hyperplasia,

- (A) most patients have a solitary lesion
- (B) a central scar is specific for this lesion
- (C) a stellate central scar is consistently identified on dynamic contrast-enhanced CT scans
- (D) on T2-weighted MR images, the lesion is typically hypointense relative to normal liver
- (E) on MRI, the lesion does not enhance following gadopentetate dimeglumine injection

FNH is a benign, usually solitary **(Option (A) is true)** liver lesion that characteristically has a central fibrous scar surrounded by nodules of hyperplastic hepatocytes, Kupffer cells, and small bile ductules. There is a female predominance, with a female-to-male ratio of approximately 2 to 1, but FNH is found in both sexes and in all age groups. The central scar consists of dense fibrous tissue that contains abnormal thick-walled blood vessels. It has been proposed that the lesion represents hepatocellular hyperplasia in response to the central vascular malformation. The central scar is not, however, a constant feature pathologically, although it is identified in most lesions larger than 1 cm. Importantly, a central scar is not specific for FNH but can also be seen in patients with fibrolamellar hepatocellular carcinoma and large cavernous hemangiomas **(Option (B) is false).**

Sonographically, FNH has a variable appearance, with some lesions appearing hypoechoic to liver, others appearing isoechoic, and still others appearing hyperechoic. The central scar is seldom demonstrated. The value of color Doppler sonography in the diagnosis of FNH has also been investigated. Golli et al. demonstrated central pulsatile flow in 13 of 19 FNH lesions, not surprising in view of the vascular nature of this lesion. However, since arterial Doppler signals are also seen in malignant hypervascular tumors, particularly hepatocellular carcinoma, the demonstration of intravascular flow has little value in establishing a confident diagnosis of FNH.

On noncontrast CT scans, FNH lesions are usually less dense than liver (Figure 5-5A). On bolus contrast-enhanced CT, these vascular lesions will transiently and diffusely enhance, except for a central stellate area that represents the central scar (Figure 5-5B). Lesions can easily be missed, however, if only contrast-enhanced CT is performed, because they can rapidly become isodense to the rest of the liver. Visualization of the central scar by CT depends to some extent on technical factors but is not a consistent feature **(Option (C) is false).** The capability of spiral CT to obtain thin-section, high-resolution images rapidly during

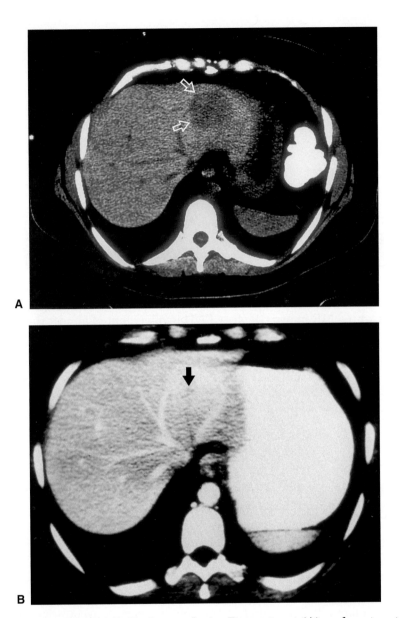

Figure 5-5. Focal nodular hyperplasia. Precontrast (A) and postcontrast (B) CT images of FNH in the left lobe of the liver. On the precontrast image, the lesion is seen as a well-defined region with low attenuation values in the left lobe (arrows in panel A). After bolus intravenous injection of contrast agent, the lesion becomes diffusely hyperdense relative to normal liver, except for a central low-attenuation focus (arrow in panel B), which may represent a central scar.

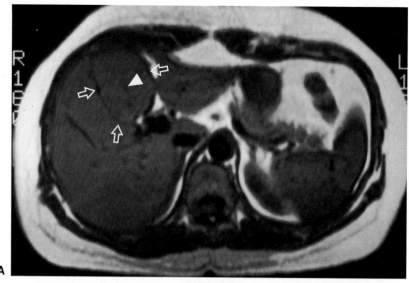

SE 500/20

Figure 5-6. Focal nodular hyperplasia. A T1-weighted MR image (A) and a T2-weighted MR image (B) show FNH involvement of almost the entire medial segment of the left lobe. On the T1-weighted sequence, the lesion (arrows) is isointense to liver, with a focal central low-attenuation region (arrowhead), probably representing the central scar. On the T2-weighted image, the lesion is slightly hyperintense to normal liver, with a focal central hyperintense region (arrowhead) corresponding to the low-intensity region on the T1-weighted image and probably representing the central scar.

a bolus administration of intravenous contrast material can result in increased detection of a visible central scar in these lesions.

Radiocolloid hepatic scintigraphy has been used as a noninvasive technique for identification of FNH and for differentiation of FNH from hepatocellular adenoma. Kupffer cells are present in FNH lesions, so the majority of these lesions take up Tc-99m sulfur colloid. Lubbers et al. report that uptake of Tc-99m sulfur colloid is infrequent in patients with hepatocellular adenomas and is extremely rare in patients with other hepatic tumors, so demonstration of this finding strongly favors the diagnosis of FNH.

On noncontrast MR images, FNH is usually isointense to slightly hyperintense relative to normal liver on all pulse sequences (Figure 5-6A) **(Option (D) is false).** These lesions are usually homogeneous, without evidence of the hemorrhage or necrosis commonly seen in hepatocellular adenoma. However, a wide range of atypical MR appearances

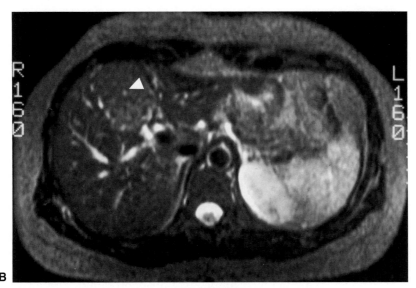

SE 2,500/80

of FNH has been reported, including a heterogeneous appearance and low signal intensity in comparison with the liver on T1-weighted images. The central scar can be visible as a hyperintense area on T2-weighted images (Figure 5-6B). There have been only a few reports of the MR appearance of fibrolamellar hepatocellular carcinoma, but in the two cases reported by Mattison et al., the central scars were of low signal intensity on all pulse sequences; this allowed differentiation from FNH. Characterization of FNH can be improved by combining the noncontrast MR images with images obtained during bolus administration of gadopentetate dimeglumine. Vigorous, early, homogeneous enhancement of the lesion is seen following gadopentetate dimeglumine injection **(Option (E) is false).** Biopsy is warranted in some patients because of atypical features, but the use of Tc-99m sulfur colloid imaging or MRI generally allows a diagnosis to be made noninvasively.

Question 16

Concerning cavernous hemangiomas of the liver,

(A) they are encapsulated
(B) small lesions are typically both hyperechoic and homogeneous sonographically
(C) nodular peripheral enhancement on contrast-enhanced dynamic CT is a characteristic feature
(D) on delayed postcontrast CT images, complete fill-in is essential for establishing the diagnosis
(E) the specificity of SPECT with Tc-99m erythrocytes is less than 50%
(F) the specificity of MRI for diagnosing lesions is about 90%

Hepatic hemangiomas are the most common benign non-cystic tumors in the liver. Histologically, these lesions consist of vascular spaces ranging in size from capillary to cavernous, partly or completely filled with blood, and lined by a single layer of endothelium. These vascular spaces are separated by a scant connective tissue stroma. Especially in larger lesions, areas of fibrosis with obliteration of the vascular spaces, thrombosis, necrosis, or foci of calcification are sometimes seen. The lesion is sharply defined but not encapsulated, and imaging evidence of a tissue capsule excludes the diagnosis of cavernous hemangioma **(Option (A) is false).**

Sonographically, most small lesions are homogeneous and hyperechoic with well-defined margins **(Option (B) is true).** Enhanced through transmission, reflecting the fluid-filled spaces within this lesion, can also be seen (Figure 5-7). Unfortunately, some hemangiomas, particularly the larger ones, do not have this sonographic appearance but, rather, appear as hypoechoic lesions or lesions of mixed echogenicity. Hypoechoic areas may reflect large cystic spaces within the lesion, and complex patterns reflect areas of fibrosis, thrombosis, and necrosis that are often seen pathologically within larger hemangiomas. Lesions can also appear relatively hypoattenuating if present in a liver of increased echogenicity, as seen in fatty infiltration (Figure 5-8).

On CT, most lesions are the same attenuation as flowing blood prior to administration of contrast material; therefore, in most patients they are hypodense compared with liver. After bolus administration of contrast material, CT classically demonstrates early nodular peripheral enhancement, as contrast slowly flows into the numerous vascular channels that make up this lesion **(Option (C) is true)** (Figure 5-9). Progressive opacification toward the lesion center, with complete fill-in between 3 and 60 minutes after initiation of the bolus, completes the classic CT description of this lesion. Freeny and Marks, however, showed that only 55% of hemangiomas fulfill these strict CT criteria for diagnosis. Many

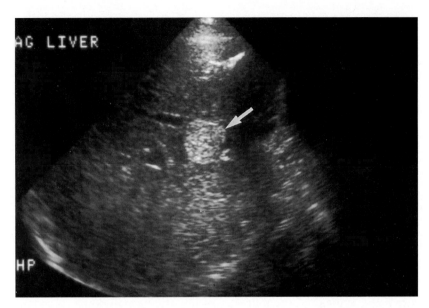

Figure 5-7. Hemangioma. A well-circumscribed hyperechoic lesion is seen in the liver (arrow). The lesion displays no edema ring or tissue capsule, and enhanced through transmission is present. This is the typical sonographic appearance of hemangioma.

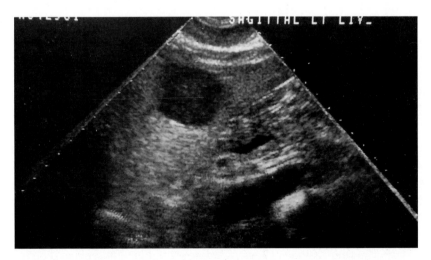

Figure 5-8. Atypical sonographic appearance of hepatic hemangioma. A 4-cm lesion is seen in the left lobe of the liver. The lesion is hypoechoic relative to surrounding parenchyma but does display enhanced through transmission. On CT and SPECT with Tc-99m erythrocytes, the features of this lesion were characteristic of hepatic hemangioma.

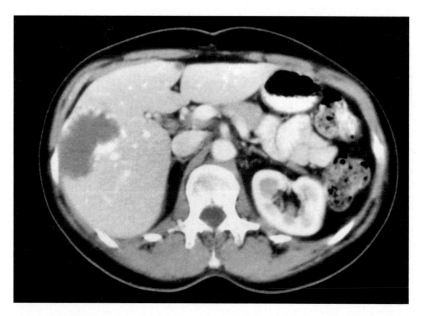

Figure 5-9. Typical CT appearance of hepatic hemangioma. A contrast-enhanced CT scan shows a low-attenuation lesion in the right lobe of the liver with nodular peripheral enhancement of attenuation similar to that seen in the vascular structures.

lesions, particularly larger ones with areas of fibrosis (Figure 5-10), do not demonstrate complete fill-in of the lesion after contrast agent administration **(Option (D) is false).**

On scintigraphy with Tc-99m erythrocytes, a perfusion/blood pool mismatch, with decreased activity on early dynamic images and increased activity on delayed blood pool images, is the classic pattern (Figure 5-11). This pattern allows differentiation of hemangiomas from other vascular neoplasms, both benign and malignant, which generally show early accumulation of labeled erythrocytes and rarely exhibit increased activity relative to surrounding hepatic parenchyma. SPECT with Tc-99m erythrocytes is a very reliable examination for the diagnosis of hemangiomas greater than 2.5 cm in size, with a positive predictive value and specificity near 100% reported by Birnbaum et al. **(Option (E) is false).** Smaller lesions or lesions adjacent to blood vessels can be more difficult to detect because of limitations in spatial resolution.

The ability of MRI to diagnose hemangioma has been extensively reported. Hemangiomas are typically isointense or slightly hypointense on T1-weighted MR images but are markedly hyperintense on T2-weighted images (Figure 5-12). Morphologically, hemangiomas are usually ovoid or

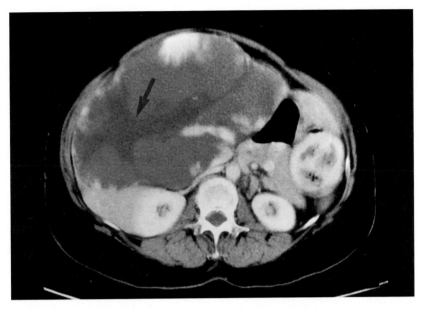

Figure 5-10. Giant cavernous hemangioma. A contrast-enhanced CT scan demonstrates a large lesion with nodular peripheral enhancement characteristic of hemangioma. A large, low-attenuation central scar (arrow) is present in the center of the lesion.

spheroid and homogeneous with well-defined margins but no tissue capsule. With use of both morphologic and signal-intensity characteristics, MRI has been reported to be 90% sensitive and 92% specific for the MR diagnosis of hemangioma **(Option (F) is true).** Given the frequent pathologic finding of fibrosis within lesions larger than 2 cm, it is not surprising that this classic description of MR findings in patients with hemangioma is often not seen with large lesions. Ros et al. reported that hemangiomas frequently have a heterogeneous signal intensity on T2-weighted images, predominantly reflecting areas of central fibrosis seen on pathologic examination. They described other signs that can be helpful in making the diagnosis of hemangioma by MRI, including the findings of sharp margins and a lobulated lesion contour (Figure 5-13A). Injection of gadopentetate dimeglumine can add some specificity to the MR examination by the demonstration of vivid nodular peripheral enhancement, similar to that seen on CT studies (Figure 5-13B).

The high prevalence of hepatic hemangiomas means that the radiologist should be familiar with both the typical and atypical appearances of this lesion on imaging studies in order to avoid unnecessary percutaneous biopsy. Complications following needle biopsy of hemangiomas,

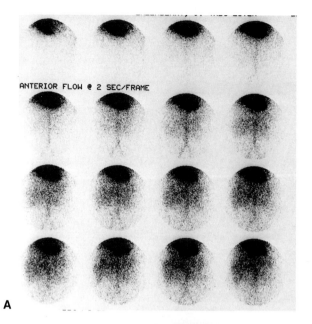

A

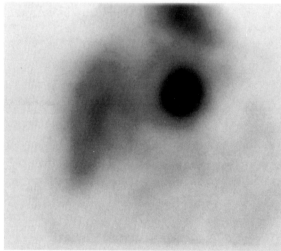

B

Figure 5-11. Same patient as in Figure 5-8. Tc-99m erythrocyte scintigraphy of hemangioma in the left lobe of liver. (A) No increased activity is seen in the left lobe of the liver during the flow phase of the study. (B) A focus of increased blood pool activity compared with normal liver is seen in the left lobe on a delayed coronal SPECT image.

although uncommon, do occur, and most of these lesions can be diagnosed by using a combination of noninvasive imaging studies. The diagnostic evaluation of a suspected hepatic hemangioma will vary depending on the clinical presentation, the patient's history, and the expertise of the radiologist. Most consider that a focal hepatic lesion with a classic appearance for a hemangioma on either ultrasonography, CT, or MRI requires no further evaluation in a patient who is not at increased risk

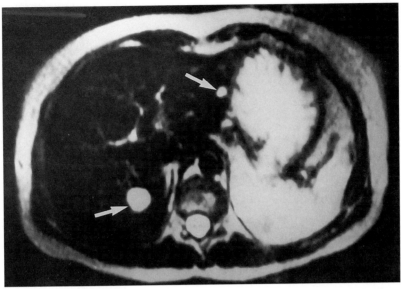

TR 2,000/TE 150

Figure 5-12. Hepatic hemangiomas. Typical T2-weighted MR image shows small hemangiomas. In this patient, two well-circumscribed, homogeneous, high-attenuation lesions are identified, one in the lateral segment of the left hepatic lobe and one in the posterior segment of the right hepatic lobe (arrows).

for primary or metastatic hepatic malignancy. In patients who are at increased risk for hepatic malignancy, the combination of confirmatory findings on two different diagnostic studies is generally necessary to make the diagnosis of hemangioma confidently. If a lesion with an appearance consistent with a cavernous hemangioma is discovered on either CT or ultrasonography, Tc-99m erythrocyte scintigraphy with SPECT is recommended as the confirmatory examination because of the high specificity of this method for assessing lesions larger than 2.5 cm in diameter. For smaller lesions, MRI is recommended for confirmation. If the confirmatory study indicates that the lesion has features consistent with hemangioma, no further evaluation is necessary. If typical features of a hemangioma are not demonstrated, however, percutaneous biopsy can then be performed.

If a lesion suspected to be a hemangioma is initially detected on MRI, Tc-99m erythrocyte scintigraphy is again recommended as the confirmatory test for lesions larger than 2.5 cm. The greater sensitivity of MRI for detecting small lesions, particularly those <1 cm, can lead to a diagnostic dilemma, particularly in a patient at increased risk for hepatic malig-

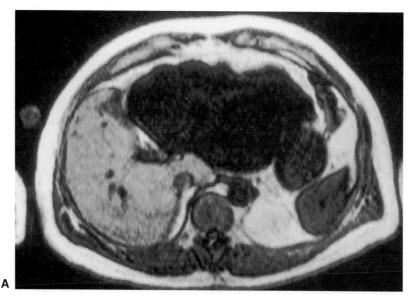

GRE 8/3/25°/760

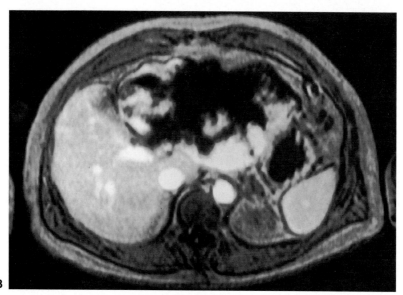

GRE 8/3/25°/760

Figure 5-13. Hepatic hemangiomas. T1-weighted gradient-echo MR images obtained before (A) and after (B) administration of gadolinium DTPA show a large hemangioma occupying almost the entire left lobe of the liver. Prior to injection of contrast agent, the mass has low signal intensity relative to normal hepatic parenchyma. Early in the bolus phase of contrast agent injection, the mass demonstrates peripheral foci of globular enhancement characteristic of hepatic hemangioma and similar to the pattern of contrast enhancement seen on dynamic postcontrast CT.

nancy, since no other imaging modality works well for improving diagnostic specificity in lesions of this size and percutaneous biopsy of such small lesions is difficult. In this situation, follow-up MRI is generally recommended.

Question 17

Concerning hepatocellular adenoma,

(A) use of anabolic steroids is a risk factor
(B) cirrhosis is a risk factor
(C) it does not demonstrate uptake of Tc-99m sulfur colloid
(D) sonographically, the lesion often appears identical to focal nodular hyperplasia
(E) pathologically, it has no distinct surrounding capsule

Most hepatocellular adenomas are associated with oral contraceptive use, but these lesions are also seen in a number of other clinical settings including metabolic diseases (glycogen storage disease type I, galactosemia, and tyrosinemia) and in association with anabolic steroid use **(Option (A) is true)**. Adenomas also arise spontaneously. Unlike hepatocellular carcinoma, no association of hepatocellular adenomas with cirrhosis has been reported **(Option (B) is false)**.

Hepatocellular adenomas consist predominantly of hepatocytes, but careful histologic analysis aslo demonstrates Kupffer cells within the lesions. Most adenomas appear photon deficient on Tc-99m sulfur colloid imaging, but some uptake of Tc-99m sulfur colloid does occur **(Option (C) is false)**. Although this was seen in 25% of lesions in one series, the overall frequency appears to be 10% or less.

Sonographic findings in patients with hepatocellular adenoma are variable, and the lesion is often indistinguishable from FNH or other hepatic lesions, particularly in the absence of hemorrhage **(Option (D) is true)**.

The appearance of hepatocellular adenoma on MRI is not specific; a variety of patterns, particularly on T2-weighted images, has been reported. As frequently seen pathologically, areas of necrosis and hemorrhage within the tumor can result in a complex MR appearance (Figure 5-14A). However, most nonhemorrhagic lesions tend to be isointense to slightly hyperintense to liver on both T1- and T2-weighted spin-echo pulse sequences (Figure 5-14B). A surrounding tissue capsule is sometimes demonstrated **(Option (E) is false)**. An appearance similar to that of a cavernous hemangioma, which has a very high signal intensity

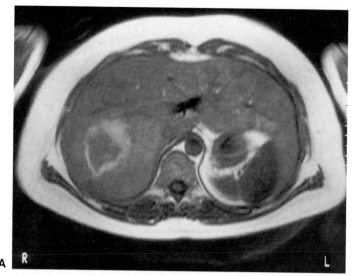

SE 300/15

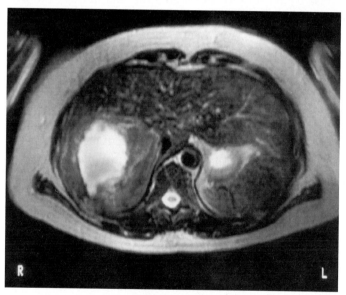

SE 2,000/100

Figure 5-14. Hepatocellular adenoma. T1-weighted (A) and T2-weighted (B) MR images in a patient with a hepatocellular adenoma involving the right lobe of the liver show that the mass itself has slightly higher signal intensity than normal hepatic parenchyma, with areas of high signal intensity on both sequences reflecting the presence of hemorrhage into the lesion.

on T2-weighted images, would not be expected, despite the variability of MR patterns for hepatocellular adenoma.

Judith L. Chezmar, M.D.

SUGGESTED READINGS

HEPATOCELLULAR ADENOMA AND FOCAL NODULAR HYPERPLASIA

1. Golli M, Mathieu D, Anglade MC, Cherqui D, Vasile N, Rahmouni A. Focal nodular hyperplasia of the liver: value of color Doppler US in association with MR imaging. Radiology 1993; 187:113–117
2. Golli M, Van Nhieu JT, Mathieu D, et al. Hepatocellular adenoma: color Doppler US and pathologic correlations. Radiology 1994; 190:741–744
3. Goodman ZD, Mikel UV, Lubbers PR, Ros PR, Langloss JM, Ishak KG. Kupffer cells in hepatocellular adenomas. Am J Surg Pathol 1987; 11:191–196
4. Kerlin P, Davis GL, McGill DB, Weiland LH, Adson MA, Sheedy PF II. Hepatic adenoma and focal nodular hyperplasia: clinical, pathologic, and radiologic features. Gastroenterology 1983; 84:994–1002
5. Learch TJ, Ralls PW, Johnson MB, et al. Hepatic focal nodular hyperplasia: findings with color Doppler sonography. J Ultrasound Med 1993; 12:541–544
6. Lee MJ, Saini S, Hamm B, et al. Focal nodular hyperplasia of the liver: MR findings in 35 proved cases. AJR 1991; 156:317–320
7. Lubbers PR, Ros PR, Goodman ZD, Ishak KG. Accumulation of technetium-99m sulfur colloid by hepatocellular adenoma: scintigraphic-pathologic correlation. AJR 1987; 148:1105–1108
8. Mathieu D, Bruneton JN, Drouillard J, Pointreau CC, Vasile N. Hepatic adenomas and focal nodular hyperplasia: dynamic CT study. Radiology 1986; 160:53–58
9. Mathieu D, Rahmouni A, Anglade MC, et al. Focal nodular hyperplasia of the liver: assessment with contrast-enhanced TurboFLASH MR imaging. Radiology 1991; 180:25–30
10. Mattison GR, Glazer GM, Quint LE, Francis IR, Bree RL, Ensminger WD. MR imaging of hepatic focal nodular hyperplasia: characterization and distinction from primary malignant hepatic tumors. AJR 1987; 148:711–715
11. Paulson EK, McClellan JS, Washington K, Spritzer CE, Meyers WC, Baker ME. Hepatic adenoma: MR characteristics and correlation with pathologic findings. AJR 1994; 163:113–116
12. Vilgrain V, Flejou JF, Arrive L, et al. Focal nodular hyperplasia of the liver: MR imaging and pathologic correlation in 37 patients. Radiology 1992; 184:699–703
13. Wanless IR, Mawdsley C, Adams R. On the pathogenesis of focal nodular hyperplasia of the liver. Hepatology 1985; 5:1194–1200

14. Welch TJ, Sheedy PF II, Johnson CM, et al. Focal nodular hyperplasia and hepatic adenoma: comparison of angiography, CT, US, and scintigraphy. Radiology 1985; 156:593–595

CAVERNOUS HEMANGIOMA

15. Birnbaum BA, Weinreb JC, Megibow AJ, et al. Definitive diagnosis of hepatic hemangiomas: MR imaging versus Tc^{99m}-labeled red blood cell SPECT. Radiology 1990; 176:95–101
16. Freeny PC, Marks WM. Hepatic hemangiomas: dynamic bolus CT. AJR 1986; 147:711–719
17. Gandolfi L, Leo P, Solmi L, Vitelli E, Verros G, Colecchia A. Natural history of hepatic haemangiomas: clinical and ultrasound study. Gut 1991; 32:677–680
18. Nelson RC, Chezmar JL. Diagnostic approach to hepatic hemangiomas. Radiology 1990; 176:11–13
19. Quinn SF, Benjamin GG. Hepatic cavernous hemangiomas: simple diagnostic sign with dynamic bolus CT. Radiology 1992; 182:545–548
20. Ros PR, Lubbers PR, Olmsted WW, Morillo G. Hemangioma of the liver: heterogeneous appearance on T2-weighted images. AJR 1987; 149:1167–1170
21. Stark DD, Felder RC, Wittenberg J, et al. Magnetic resonance imaging of cavernous hemangioma of the liver: tissue-specific characterization. AJR 1985; 145:213–222
22. Tumeh SS, Benson C, Nagel JS, English RJ, Holman BL. Cavernous hemangioma of the liver: detection with single-photon emission computed tomography. Radiology 1987; 164:353–356

HEPATOBILIARY CYSTADENOMA

23. Choi BI, Lim JH, Han MC, et al. Biliary cystadenoma and cystadenocarcinoma: CT and sonographic findings. Radiology 1989; 171:57–61
24. Ishak KG, Willis GW, Cummins SD, Bullock AA. Biliary cystadenoma and cystadenocarcinoma: report of 14 cases and review of the literature. Cancer 1977; 39:322–338
25. Korobkin M, Stephens DH, Lee JK, et al. Biliary cystadenoma and cystadenocarcinoma: CT and sonographic findings. AJR 1989; 153:507–511
26. Stanley J, Vujic I, Schabel SI, Gobien RP, Reines HD. Evaluation of biliary cystadenoma and cystadenocarcinoma. Gastrointest Radiol 1983; 8:245–248

MESENCHYMAL HAMARTOMA

27. DeMaioribus CA, Lally KP, Sim K, Isaacs H, Mahour GH. Mesenchymal hamartoma of the liver. A 35-year review. Arch Surg 1990; 125:598–600
28. Lack EE. Mesenchymal hamartoma of the liver. A clinical and pathologic study of nine cases. Am J Pediatr Hematol Oncol 1986; 8:91–98
29. Ros PR, Goodman ZD, Ishak KG, et al. Mesenchymal hamartoma of the liver: radiologic-pathologic correlation. Radiology 1986; 158:619–624

30. Stocker JT, Ishak KG. Mesenchymal hamartoma of the liver: report of 30 cases and review of the literature. Pediatr Pathol 1983; 1:245–267
31. Wholey MH, Wojno KJ. Pediatric hepatic mesenchymal hamartoma demonstrated on plain film, ultrasound and MRI, and correlated with pathology. Pediatr Radiol 1994; 24:143–144

LIVER TUMORS: GENERAL

32. Craig JR, Peters RL, Edmondson HA. Tumors of the liver and extrahepatic bile ducts: atlas of tumor pathology, 2nd series, fascicle 26. Washington, D.C.: Armed Forces Institute of Pathology; 1989
33. Edmondson HA. Differential diagnosis of tumors and tumor-like lesions of liver in infancy and childhood. Am J Dis Child 1956; 91:168–186
34. Fishman EK, Farmlett E, Kadir S, Siegelman SS. Computed tomography of benign hepatic tumors. J Comput Assist Tomogr 1982; 6:472–481
35. Ishak KG, Rabin L. Benign tumors of the liver. Med Clin North Am 1975; 59:995–1013
36. Karhunen PJ. Incidence of benign liver tumors at autopsy. J Clin Pathol 1986; 39:183–188
37. Powers C, Ros PR, Stoupis C, Johnson WK, Segel KH. Primary liver neoplasms: MR imaging with pathologic correlation. RadioGraphics 1994; 14:459–482
38. Stephens DH, Johnson CD. Benign masses of the liver. In: Silverman PM, Zeman RK (eds), CT and MRI of the liver and biliary tract. New York: Churchill Livingstone; 1990:93–127

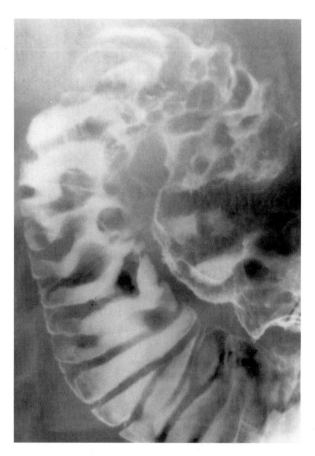

Figure 6-1. This 62-year-old man on chronic hemodialysis has vague abdominal pain. You are shown a spot radiograph of the duodenum from an upper gastrointestinal examination.

Case 6: Duodenitis Secondary to Renal Failure

Question 18

Which *one* of the following is the MOST likely cause of the findings?

- (A) Renal failure
- (B) Pancreatitis
- (C) Ischemia
- (D) Lymphoma
- (E) Crohn's disease

The test image (Figure 6-1) is a double-contrast radiograph of the duodenum showing markedly thickened, lobulated folds in the duodenal bulb and proximal descending duodenum. The diagnosis of duodenitis can be suggested radiographically in patients who have a spastic, irritable duodenal bulb or thickened, nodular folds in the proximal duodenum. For reasons that are unclear, patients with chronic renal failure who are undergoing dialysis often have enlarged duodenal folds to a degree rarely seen in other patients with duodenitis. The cause of this duodenitis is uncertain, but it has been postulated that patients on chronic hemodialysis have increased gastric acid secretion. These individuals can present with epigastric pain, vomiting, or upper gastrointestinal bleeding. The duodenitis has sometimes been found to resolve after renal transplantation. In any case, the test patient is known to be on chronic hemodialysis; therefore, his severe duodenitis is presumably related to his underlying renal failure **(Option (A) is correct).**

In some patients with pancreatitis (Option (B)), an enlarged head of the pancreas can cause widening or compression of the duodenal sweep and/or thickened, spiculated folds, predominantly on the medial aspect of the duodenum. In other patients, pancreatitis can cause circumferential narrowing of the descending duodenum (Figure 6-2), with various degrees of obstruction. In Figure 6-1, however, there is no widening or compression of the duodenal sweep, and fold thickening extends well into the

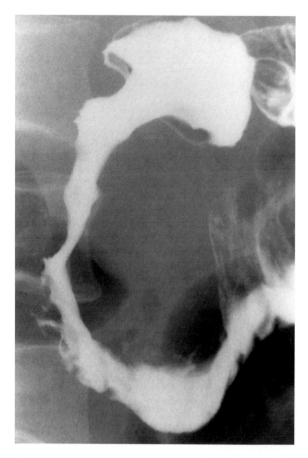

Figure 6-2. Pancreatitis. Widening of the duodenal sweep and circumferential narrowing of the descending duodenum are seen in a patient with underlying pancreatitis.

lateral aspect of the duodenum, so the radiographic findings are not typical of pancreatitis.

Ischemia (Option (C)) of the small bowel is manifested radiographically by thickened, spiculated folds or by large, nodular indentations (i.e., thumbprinting) due to submucosal edema and hemorrhage. Small bowel ischemia can result from atherosclerotic or embolic occlusion of vessels supplying the intestine or from low-flow states due to decreased perfusion of the bowel. However, the small bowel is a less common site of ischemia than the colon, and ischemia of the duodenum is rare.

Duodenal involvement by lymphoma (Option (D)) usually results from contiguous spread of tumor from the distal stomach or proximal jejunum or from encasement of the duodenum by a conglomerate mass of

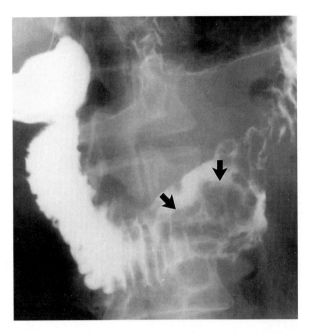

Figure 6-3. Duodenal lymphoma. A barium study shows a bulky mass lesion (arrows) with thickened folds in the third and fourth portions of the duodenum. (Reprinted with permission from Gore et al. [5].)

lymphomatous nodes in the retroperitoneum. There is little lymphoid tissue in the duodenum, and so duodenal lymphoma is a rare lesion, constituting less than 5% of all small bowel lymphomas. Duodenal lymphoma is manifested radiographically by infiltrative, ulcerative, polypoid, or nodular forms (Figure 6-3). Although barium studies may demonstrate thickened duodenal folds, duodenal lymphoma is a much less common condition than duodenitis secondary to renal failure. In patients with duodenal lymphoma, CT can demonstrate nodular masses, cavitated lesions, or long, infiltrated segments with masslike thickening of the duodenum. Occasionally, duodenal or small bowel lymphoma occurs as a complication of long-standing celiac disease.

Most patients with duodenal Crohn's disease (Option (E)) have concomitant Crohn's disease of the small bowel or colon. Aphthous ulcers are the earliest radiographic abnormalities seen in patients with duodenal Crohn's disease. These aphthous ulcers can be indistinguishable from varioliform duodenal erosions. However, erosive duodenitis usually involves the duodenal bulb, whereas the aphthous ulcers of Crohn's disease are located anywhere in the duodenum from the bulb to the ligament of Treitz. With progression of disease, these patients can develop

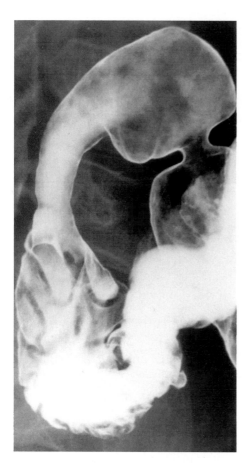

Figure 6-4. Duodenal Crohn's disease. There is smooth, tapered narrowing of the proximal descending duodenum with effacement of mucosal folds. This appearance is characteristic of duodenal involvement by Crohn's disease.

thickened nodular folds, ulcers, or strictures in the proximal duodenum (Figure 6-4). However, in a patient on hemodialysis, thickened duodenal folds are more likely to be caused by renal failure than by Crohn's disease. As in the stomach, suspected duodenal involvement by Crohn's disease should lead to a careful small bowel follow-through or barium enema to rule out Crohn's disease in the small bowel or colon.

Marc S. Levine, M.D.

SUGGESTED READINGS

DUODENITIS SECONDARY TO RENAL FAILURE

1. Wiener SN, Vertes V, Shapiro H. The upper gastrointestinal tract in patients undergoing chronic dialysis. Radiology 1969; 92:110–114

2. Zukerman GR, Mills BA, Koehler RE, Siegel A, Harter HR, DeSchryver-Kecskemeti K. Nodular duodenitis: pathologic and clinical characteristics in patients with end-stage renal disease. Dig Dis Sci 1983; 28:1018–1024

DUODENAL MANIFESTATIONS OF PANCREATITIS

3. Gore RM, Levine MS, Laufer I (eds). Textbook of gastrointestinal radiology. Philadelphia: WB Saunders; 1994:717–741

DUODENAL LYMPHOMA

4. Balikian JP, Nassar NT, Shamma'a MH, Shalid MJ. Primary lymphomas of the small intestine including the duodenum. A roentgen analysis of twenty-nine cases. AJR 1969; 107:131–141
5. Gore RM, Levine MS, Laufer I (eds). Textbook of gastrointestinal radiology. Philadelphia: WB Saunders; 1994:684–716
6. Hricak H, Thoeni RF, Margulis AR, Eyler WR, Francis IR. Extension of gastric lymphoma into the esophagus and duodenum. Radiology 1980; 135:309–312
7. Meyers MA, Katzen B, Alonso DR. Transpyloric extension to duodenal bulb in gastric lymphoma. Radiology 1975; 115:575–580

DUODENAL CROHN'S DISEASE

8. Kelvin FM, Gedgaudas RK. Radiologic diagnosis of Crohn disease (with emphasis on its early manifestations). Crit Rev Diagn Imaging 1981; 16:43–91
9. Legge DA, Carlson HC, Judd ES. Roentgenologic features of regional enteritis of the upper gastrointestinal tract. AJR 1970; 110:355–360
10. Nelson SW. Some interesting and unusual manifestations of Crohn's disease (regional enteritis) of the stomach, duodenum and small intestine. AJR 1969; 107:86–101
11. Thompson WM, Cockrill H Jr, Rice RP. Regional enteritis of the duodenum. AJR 1975; 123:252–262

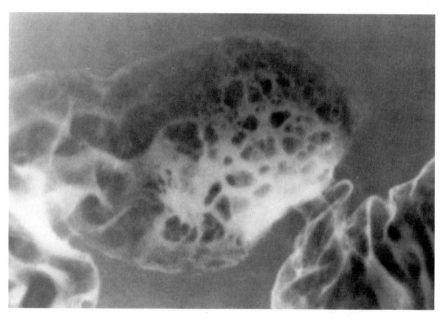

Figure 7-1. This 53-year-old man has epigastric discomfort. You are shown a spot radiograph from an upper gastrointestinal examination.

Case 7:   Heterotopic Gastric Mucosa

Question 19

Which *one* of the following is the MOST likely diagnosis?

(A) Duodenitis
(B) Lymphoid hyperplasia
(C) Brunner's gland hyperplasia
(D) Heterotopic gastric mucosa
(E) Crohn's disease

The test image (Figure 7-1) is a double-contrast radiograph of the duodenum showing multiple discrete, angulated or polygonal defects in the duodenal bulb. This appearance is characteristic of heterotopic gastric mucosa in the bulb **(Option (D) is correct)**, a benign condition of little or no clinical significance. Heterotopic gastric mucosa in the duodenum has such a characteristic appearance that a definitive diagnosis can be made on the basis of barium studies without need for further investigation.

The diagnosis of duodenitis (Option (A)) can be suspected radiographically in patients who have a spastic, irritable duodenal bulb or thickened, nodular folds in the proximal duodenum (Figure 7-2). However, thickened folds and spasm are nonspecific findings, and so the upper gastrointestinal examination generally has not been considered a reliable technique for diagnosing this condition. With the double-contrast technique, however, it is possible to diagnose erosive duodenitis. As in the stomach, varioliform erosions usually appear as punctate barium collections surrounded by radiolucent halos of edematous mucosa (Figure 7-3). In any case, the lesions depicted in the test image do not have the appearance of duodenal erosions.

Lymphoid hyperplasia (Option (B)) is a benign condition manifested radiographically by multiple small, rounded nodules in the duodenal bulb and proximal descending duodenum (Figure 7-4). Thus, hyperplastic lymphoid follicles have a different appearance and location in the duodenum than does heterotopic gastric mucosa. Patients with lymphoid

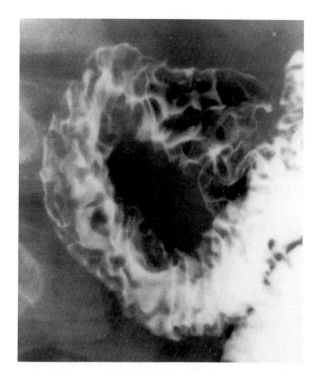

Figure 7-2. Duodenitis with thickened folds. This patient has thickened, nodular folds in the proximal duodenum. Unless the folds are grossly enlarged, however, this is not a reliable sign of duodenitis.

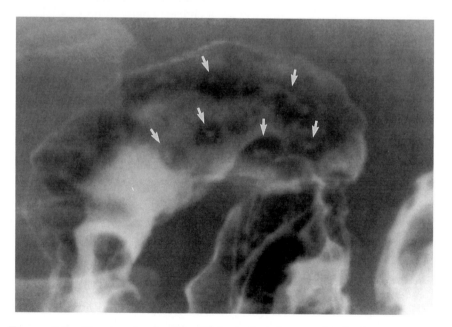

Figure 7-3. Erosive duodenitis. This patient has multiple duodenal erosions, seen as punctate barium collections with surrounding mounds of edema (arrows). (Reprinted with permission from Levine et al. [20].)

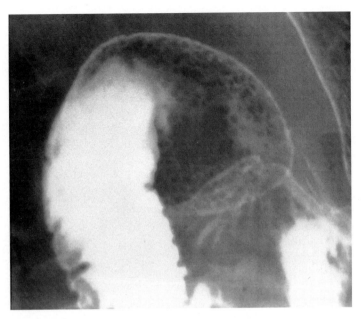

Figure 7-4. Benign lymphoid hyperplasia. Innumerable tiny, rounded nodules are present in the duodenal bulb. (Reprinted with permission from Laufer and Levine [19].)

hyperplasia of the duodenum can also have generalized lymphoid hyperplasia of the small bowel or colon as a result of an underlying immunoglobulin deficiency state.

Brunner's gland hyperplasia (Option (C)), like lymphoid hyperplasia, can be characterized radiographically by multiple small, rounded nodules in the proximal duodenum, producing a "cobblestone" or "Swiss cheese" appearance (Figure 7-5). The nodules are most numerous in the duodenal bulb and less concentrated in the descending duodenum, so that they correspond to the normal anatomic distribution of Brunner's glands. Thus, the lesions of Brunner's gland hyperplasia have a different appearance and location in the duodenum than does heterotopic gastric mucosa.

Duodenal involvement by Crohn's disease (Option (E)) usually occurs in patients who have concomitant antral disease. As elsewhere in the gastrointestinal tract, aphthous ulcers represent the earliest morphologic finding in the duodenum. With progression, duodenal Crohn's disease can be manifested by one or more larger ulcers, thickened nodular folds, cobblestoning, and stricture formation (see Figure 6-4). However, duodenal Crohn's disease is not usually characterized by the discrete, angulated defects seen in the test image.

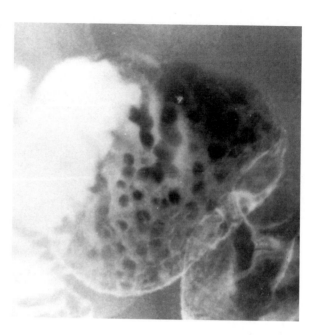

Figure 7-5. Brunner's gland hyperplasia. Multiple small, rounded nodules are present in the duodenal bulb, producing a "Swiss cheese" appearance. Lymphoid hyperplasia of the duodenum could produce similar findings (see Figure 7-4). (Reprinted with permission from Laufer and Levine [19].)

Question 20

Concerning Brunner's gland hyperplasia,

    (A) it occurs in response to increased gastric acid secretion
    (B) it is often associated with duodenitis
    (C) it is confined to the duodenal bulb
    (D) it is a premalignant condition
    (E) lymphoid hyperplasia produces similar radiographic findings

Brunner's glands in the duodenum normally secrete an alkaline mucus, which protects the mucosa from the damaging effects of gastric acid entering the duodenum. As a result, Brunner's gland hyperplasia is thought to occur as a response to hypersecretion of acid in the stomach **(Option (A) is true).** Because of this increased acid secretion, many patients with enlarged Brunner's glands have concomitant duodenitis with thickened, nodular folds in the proximal duodenum **(Option (B) is true).**

The location of Brunner's glands in the duodenal bulb and proximal descending duodenum means that hyperplastic Brunner's glands can be manifested radiographically by multiple small, rounded nodules throughout the proximal duodenum (Figure 7-5) **(Option (C) is false).** Other patients can have massive enlargement of one or more glands,

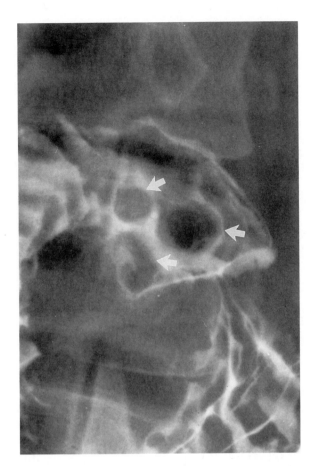

Figure 7-6. Brunner's gland hamartomas. Several submucosal masses (arrows) are seen in the duodenal bulb. (Reprinted with permission from Gore et al. [18].)

resulting in the development of so-called Brunner's gland hamartomas. These hamartomas can appear as one or more submucosal masses, ranging from several millimeters to several centimeters in size (Figure 7-6). Pathologic examination has invariably shown that Brunner's gland hyperplasia, whether characterized by diffuse enlargement of Brunner's glands or by massive enlargement of a single gland, is a benign condition without risk of malignant degeneration **(Option (D) is false).** As indicated above, lymphoid hyperplasia of the duodenum can produce similar radiographic findings **(Option (E) is true).**

Question 21

Concerning heterotopic gastric mucosa in the duodenum,

(A) it is a premalignant condition
(B) it commonly causes epigastric pain
(C) endoscopic biopsies should be performed to confirm the diagnosis when barium studies suggest this condition
(D) it tends to be located near the base of the duodenal bulb
(E) prolapsed gastric mucosa produces similar radiographic findings

Heterotopic gastric mucosa in the duodenum is characterized pathologically by the presence of multiple small foci of ectopic gastric mucosa in the duodenal bulb. It is a benign condition without any known risk of malignant degeneration **(Option (A) is false).** Affected individuals can be symptomatic because of associated inflammatory disease or ulcers, but heterotopic gastric mucosa in the duodenum is not by itself thought to be a cause of epigastric pain or other upper gastrointestinal symptoms **(Option (B) is false).** Indeed, some investigators believe that heterotopic gastric mucosa actually has a protective effect against the development of peptic ulcers. Therefore, it is usually considered to be an incidental radiographic finding with little or no clinical significance, and so endoscopic biopsies are not required to confirm this diagnosis **(Option (C) is false).** The heterotopic mucosa is characterized by angulated or polygonal 1- to 5-mm nodules or plaques that, unlike Brunner's glands or lymphoid follicles, tend to be clustered near the base of the duodenal bulb (Figure 7-1) **(Option (D) is true).** This condition can usually be differentiated from prolapsed gastric mucosa in the duodenal bulb, which is typically manifested by a mushroom-shaped defect at the base of the bulb, often occurring as a transient finding at fluoroscopy (Figure 7-7) **(Option (E) is false).**

Marc S. Levine, M.D.

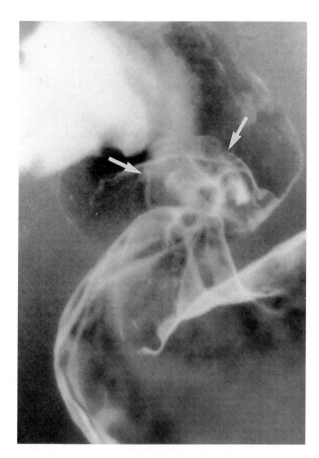

Figure 7-7. Prolapsed gastric mucosa in the duodenal bulb. A mushroom-shaped defect (arrows) is present at the base of the duodenal bulb as a result of prolapsed gastric mucosa. This often occurs as a transient finding at fluoroscopy.

SUGGESTED READINGS

HETEROTOPIC GASTRIC MUCOSA

1. Agha FP, Ghahremani GG, Tsang TK, Victor TA. Heterotopic gastric mucosa in the duodenum: radiographic findings. AJR 1988; 150:291–294
2. Langkemper R, Hoek AC, Dekker W, Op den Orth JO. Elevated lesions in the duodenal bulb caused by heterotopic gastric mucosa. Radiology 1980; 137:621–624
3. Smithuis RH, Vos CG. Heterotopic gastric mucosa in the duodenal bulb: relationship to peptic ulcer. AJR 1989; 152:59–61

DUODENITIS

4. Bova JG, Kamath V, Tio FO, Peters JE Jr, Goldstein HM. The normal mucosal surface pattern of the duodenal bulb: radiologic-histologic correlation. AJR 1985; 145:735–738

5. Gelfand DW, Dale WJ, Ott DJ, et al. Duodenitis: endoscopic-radiologic correlation in 272 patients. Radiology 1985; 157:577–581

6. Levine MS, Turner D, Ekberg O, Rubesin SE, Katzka DA. Duodenitis: a reliable radiologic diagnosis? Gastrointest Radiol 1991; 16:99–103

LYMPHOID HYPERPLASIA

7. Govoni AF. Benign lymphoid hyperplasia of the duodenal bulb. Gastrointest Radiol 1976; 1:267–269

BRUNNER'S GLAND HYPERPLASIA

8. Kaplan EL, Dyson WL, Fitts WT Jr. The relationship of gastric hyperacidity to hyperplasia of Brunner's glands. Arch Surg 1969; 98:636–639

9. Maglinte DD, Mayes SL, Ng AC, Pickett RD. Brunner's gland adenoma: diagnostic considerations. J Clin Gastroenterol 1982; 4:127–131

10. Merine D, Jones B, Ghahremani GG, Hamilton SR, Bayless TM. Hyperplasia of Brunner glands: the spectrum of its radiographic manifestations. Gastrointest Radiol 1991; 16:104–108

11. ReMine WH, Brown PW Jr, Gomes MM, Harrison EG Jr. Polypoid hamartomas of Brunner's glands. Report of six surgical cases. Arch Surg 1970; 100:313–316

12. Weinberg PE, Levin B. Hyperplasia of Brunner's glands. Radiology 1965; 84:259–262

DUODENAL CROHN'S DISEASE

13. Kelvin FM, Gedgaudas RK. Radiologic diagnosis of Crohn disease (with emphasis on its early manifestations). Crit Rev Diagn Imaging 1981; 16:43–91

14. Legge DA, Carlson HC, Judd ES. Roentgenologic features of regional enteritis of the upper gastrointestinal tract. AJR 1970; 110:355–360

15. Levine MS. Crohn's disease of the upper gastrointestinal tract. Radiol Clin North Am 1987; 25:79–91

16. Nelson SW. Some interesting and unusual manifestations of Crohn's disease (regional enteritis) of the stomach, duodenum and small intestine. AJR 1969; 107:86–101

17. Thompson WM, Cockrill H Jr, Rice RP. Regional enteritis of the duodenum. AJR 1975; 123:252–262

DUODENAL LESIONS—GENERAL

18. Gore RM, Levine MS, Laufer I (eds). Textbook of gastrointestinal radiology. Philadelphia: WB Saunders; 1994:628–659

19. Laufer I, Levine MS. Double contrast gastrointestinal radiology, 2nd ed. Philadelphia: WB Saunders; 1992:321–361

20. Levine MS, Rubesin SE, Herlinger H, Laufer I. Double-contrast upper gastrointestinal examination: technique and interpretation. Radiology 1988; 168:593–602

Notes

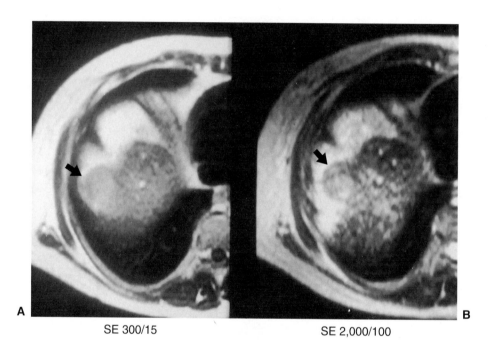

SE 300/15   SE 2,000/100

Figure 8-1. This 60-year-old man with chronic active hepatitis is being evaluated for possible liver transplantation. You are shown T1-weighted (A) and T2-weighted (B) MR images.

Case 8:   Hepatocellular Carcinoma

Question 22

The hepatic lesion (arrow) in the test images MOST probably represents:

    (A) regenerative nodule
    (B) adenomatous hyperplasia (macroregenerative nodule)
    (C) nodular regenerative hyperplasia
    (D) hepatocellular carcinoma
    (E) fibrolamellar hepatocellular carcinoma

A well-circumscribed discrete mass is present in the dome of the liver on the test images (Figure 8-1). The liver is small and is surrounded by ascites, suggesting that cirrhosis is present in this patient with a history of chronic active hepatitis. The lesion exhibits high signal intensity on both T1- and T2-weighted images. The MRI appearance of this lesion, in association with the changes suggesting cirrhosis, makes hepatocellular carcinoma (HCC) the most likely diagnosis **(Option (D) is correct).**

HCC is the most common primary malignant hepatic tumor. It usually occurs in association with chronic hepatic disease, frequently cirrhosis, but can occur in an otherwise normal liver.

Most HCCs exhibit low signal intensity on T1-weighted images and high signal intensity on T2-weighted images, but a significant percentage (ca. 30%) have high signal intensity on T1-weighted images, as seen in the test image (Figure 8-1A). This high signal intensity on T1-weighted images has been found to correlate with steatosis in some lesions. The effect of copper on the signal intensity of these lesions is still controversial. The hyperintense appearance on T1-weighted MR images is not specific for HCC, however, having been reported for rare fat-containing tumors such as hepatic angiomyolipoma (Figure 8-2), as well as for some lesions of metastatic melanoma (Figure 8-3) and hemorrhagic lesions.

Recently, great interest has been focused on the pathologic changes and radiologic detection of small HCCs and associated nodular lesions in the cirrhotic liver. Recent technical advances have improved our ability

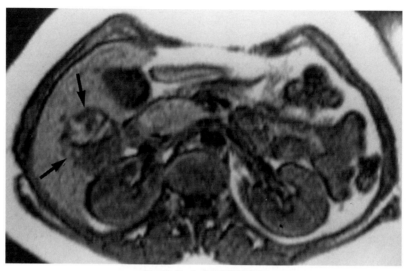

Turboflash 9/3/25°/760

Figure 8-2. Hepatic angiomyolipoma. This rare hepatic lesion (arrows) displays a heterogeneous signal intensity, with regions of high signal intensity due to fat, on this T1-weighted turboflash image.

to diagnose and characterize small lesions. The availability of resected specimens for radiologic-pathologic correlation from patients with cirrhosis who have undergone hepatic resection or liver transplantation has also added enormously to our knowledge of the appearance of these lesions on various imaging studies. Reports of excellent long-term survival after treatment of small HCCs by percutaneous ethanol injection directly into the lesion have also resulted in increased impetus for early diagnosis.

The terminology used for defining these nodular lesions associated with cirrhosis is somewhat controversial, and the histologic distinctions between different types of lesions are not always clear. The importance of these lesions stems from the theory that HCCs evolve within the cirrhotic liver from initially benign lesions, progressing from regenerative nodules to adenomatous hyperplasia to HCC. Regenerative nodules (Option (A)) are formed by replicating hepatocytes, which distort the lobular architecture of the liver. The characteristic appearance of regenerative nodules on MRI is that of multiple small nodules of low signal intensity on T2-weighted images (Figure 8-4) rather than the large nodule of high signal intensity seen on the test image (Figure 8-1B).

Adenomatous hyperplasia, also called macroregenerative nodule (Option (B)), is a distinct nodular lesion that is larger than the surround-

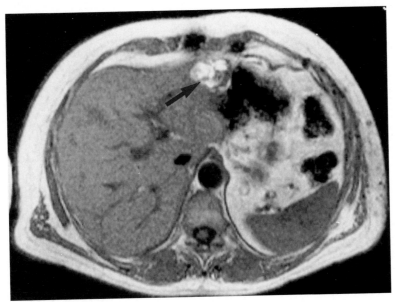

GRE 100/5/80°

Figure 8-3. Hepatic metastasis from melanoma. This lesion in the left lobe of the liver (arrow) displays high signal intensity on a T1-weighted MR image.

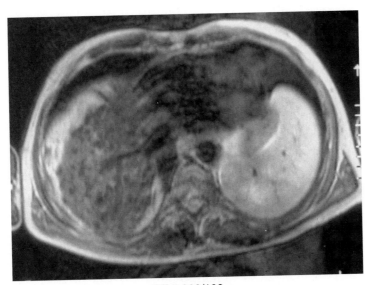

SE 2,000/100

Figure 8-4. Regenerative nodules. A T2-weighted MR image demonstrates multiple nodules of low signal intensity.

ing regenerative nodules in the cirrhotic liver. The lesion is composed of hepatocytes arranged in cords and containing portal areas. Unlike HCC, the typical macroregenerative nodule lacks dysplastic features and does not demonstrate vascular invasion or expansive growth into the adjacent liver. As described by Choi et al., however, some lesions of adenomatous hyperplasia contain atypical hepatocytes and are thought to represent a premalignant condition intermediate between typical adenomatous hyperplasia and early HCC. This belief is supported by the finding of malignant foci within some lesions of adenomatous hyperplasia, as well as by natural history studies (as reported by Caramella et al.) showing progression of these lesions to HCC. Similar to regenerative nodules, adenomatous hyperplasia is frequently not detected on imaging studies. When detected sonographically, adenomatous hyperplasia is typically hypoechoic. On CT, lesions of adenomatous hyperplasia appear as areas of low attenuation relative to hepatic parenchyma. These lesions are supplied by the portal vein, and this difference in blood supply compared with that for malignant lesions (which are supplied by the hepatic artery) can aid in differentiation of these lesions from HCC (Figure 8-5). Matsui et al. described the MRI appearance of adenomatous hyperplasia without atypia as hyperintense on T1-weighted images and hypointense on T2-weighted images (Figure 8-6), allowing its differentiation from HCC. As with regenerative nodules, it is the low signal intensity of these lesions on T2-weighted images that allows differentiation from HCC.

Nodular regenerative hyperplasia (NRH) (Option (C)), also known as nodular transformation, is a rare, distinct clinical and pathologic entity that is not related to the regenerative nodules associated with cirrhosis. NRH is characterized by diffuse nodularity of the liver as a result of multiple regenerative nodules ranging in size from a few millimeters to 1 cm, without fibrous septa between the nodules. This lack of fibrosis is the important feature distinguishing NRH from other nodular lesions of the liver. NRH is associated with portal hypertension in approximately half of all patients and has been reported to occur in patients with a variety of systemic diseases including rheumatoid arthritis and myeloproliferative and lymphoproliferative disorders. Wanless has proposed that NRH is a secondary response of the liver to obliteration of portal veins. Radiologic findings include multiple nodules, large masses, or a normal-appearing liver in patients in whom the nodules are less than 5 mm in size. The nodules are of variable echogenicity and are usually hypoattenuating lesions on postcontrast CT (Figure 8-7). NRH can be associated with hemorrhage due to bleeding varices from portal hypertension or to hemorrhage from the nodules themselves.

Fibrolamellar HCC (Option (E)), considered a tumor distinct from or a subtype of HCC, has epidemiologic and imaging features different from

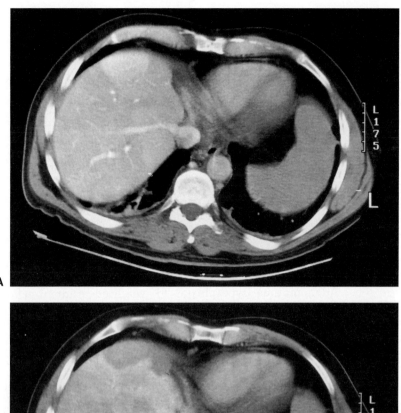

A

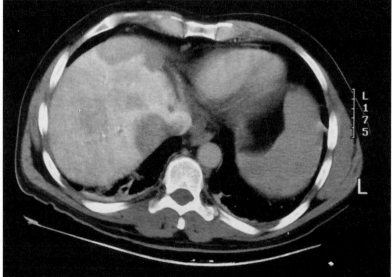

B

Figure 8-5. Macroregenerative nodules. (A) CT performed during contrast injection into a catheter in the superior mesenteric artery demonstrates multiple round lesions in the dome of the liver that enhance to a slightly greater degree than surrounding parenchyma. This demonstrates that these lesions receive their blood supply from the portal vein. (B) CT performed during contrast injection into a catheter in the hepatic artery demonstrates the absence of hepatic arterial supply to these lesions.

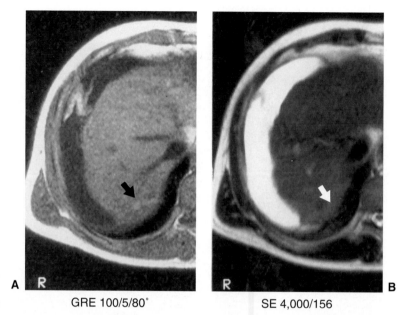

GRE 100/5/80°   SE 4,000/156

Figure 8-6. Adenomatous hyperplasia. T1-weighted gradient-echo (A) and T2-weighted turbo-spin-echo (B) MR images in a patient with cirrhosis. A 1-cm lesion (arrow) with high signal intensity on the T1-weighted image and low signal intensity on the T2-weighted image is identified. These MRI characteristics are consistent with adenomatous hyperplasia.

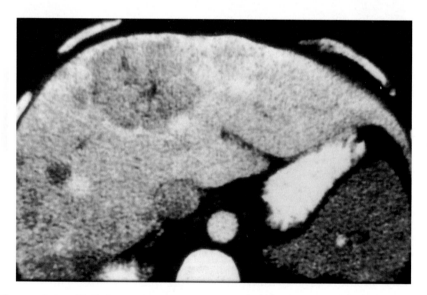

Figure 8-7. Nodular regenerative hyperplasia. Contrast-enhanced CT shows multiple low-density nodules of variable size in the liver parenchyma. Other CT appearances of NRH include a grossly normal liver or a single hepatic mass. (Case courtesy of Abraham Dachman, M.D., University of Chicago Hospital, Chicago, Ill.)

those of other HCCs, making the diagnosis of this rare lesion unlikely (see below).

Question 23

Concerning regenerative nodules,

(A) they are invariably present in the cirrhotic liver
(B) they are composed of hepatocytes surrounded by fibrosis
(C) they are easily identified on contrast-enhanced CT scans
(D) their low signal intensity on T2-weighted MR images is due to iron deposition

Cirrhosis of the liver is defined by the presence of extensive fibrosis and regenerative nodules. These small nodules form as a response to extensive hepatocellular destruction by necrosis or chronic cirrhosis. Radiologic-pathologic correlation in patients undergoing liver transplantation has shown that regenerative nodules are invariably present in the cirrhotic liver but are infrequently seen on imaging studies **(Option (A) is true)**. Regenerative nodules are formed by replicating hepatocytes surrounded by fibrosis **(Option (B) is true)**. Regenerative nodules can be seen on unenhanced CT as multiple small nodules of slightly higher attenuation than the surrounding parenchyma (Figure 8-8); they are less frequently seen after contrast agent administration, which may render them isoattenuating with surrounding parenchyma **(Option (C) is false)**. Regenerative nodules are characteristically small and of low signal intensity on T2-weighted images (Figure 8-4). Iron deposits within regenerative nodules are responsible for this MRI appearance **(Option (D) is true)**.

Question 24

Imaging features suggestive of hepatocellular carcinoma include:

(A) venous invasion
(B) encapsulation
(C) intratumoral septation
(D) intratumoral arterial flow
(E) arterioportal shunting

The radiologic appearance of HCC can simulate that of other hepatic tumors. However, a number of imaging features have been described

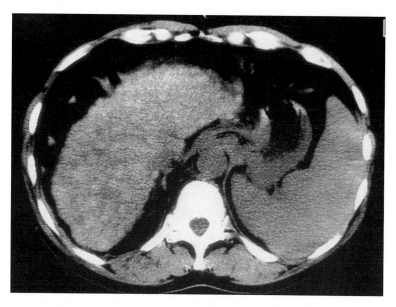

Figure 8-8.   Regenerative nodules. A noncontrast CT scan shows a small liver with a nodular contour and innumerable small round nodules of higher attenuation than surrounding tissue.

that, when present, suggest the diagnosis of HCC. One of the imaging features most strongly suggestive of HCC is its association with concomitant changes of chronic liver disease. Among the numerous conditions associated with HCC are infection with hepatitis virus B or C, cirrhosis of numerous etiologies (including alcoholic cirrhosis), hemochromatosis, and exposure to hepatic toxins including vinyl chloride. HCC can occur in a normal liver, but the strong association with chronic liver disease makes HCC likely when a mass lesion is seen in a cirrhotic liver.

There is considerable variability in the gross pathologic appearance of HCC. Classification has been attempted by numerous authorities. Acuda et al. have proposed a system that classifies lesions of HCC by their growth pattern. The spreading growth pattern is the most common pattern in several large series. In this growth pattern, the tumor margins are indistinct and spread into the cirrhotic nodules in the surrounding liver (Figure 8-9). The expanding pattern is the second most common growth pattern. These tumors compress and displace surrounding hepatic parenchyma and can occur in encapsulated and unencapsulated forms (Figure 8-10). A multifocal or diffuse growth pattern consists of several remote tumor foci without one clear dominant mass.

HCC has a propensity for vascular invasion (Figure 8-11). Invasion of the portal or hepatic veins by an intrahepatic tumor is highly suggestive

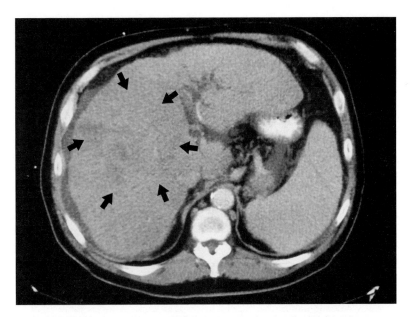

Figure 8-9. Hepatocellular carcinoma, spreading type. A contrast-enhanced CT scan shows a vague hypodense lesion occupying the majority of the right lobe of the liver and the medial segment of the left lobe. The margins between lesion and normal hepatic parenchyma are indistinct (arrows). Normal vascular structures are not seen. Dilated bile ducts are present in the left lobe.

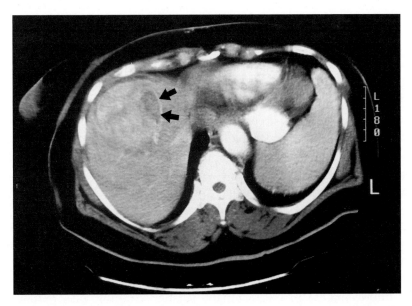

Figure 8-10. Hepatocellular carcinoma, expanding type. A contrast-enhanced CT scan shows a well-circumscribed mass in the dome of the liver, which is predominantly hypervascular but with multiple components of variable enhancement, i.e., a mosaic pattern. A portion of an enhancing tumor capsule (arrows) is seen.

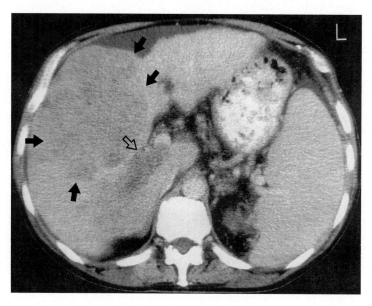

Figure 8-11. Hepatocellular carcinoma with portal vein invasion. A post-contrast CT scan shows a large mass (solid arrows) occupying the anterior segment of the right lobe of the liver and the medial segment of the left lobe. Low-attenuation thrombus is seen filling the right portal vein and extending into the main portal vein (open arrow). Also note the nodular contour of the liver, splenomegaly, and varices, consistent with cirrhosis and portal hypertension.

of HCC; it was recognized on CT in 48% of patients with HCC in the series reported by Freeny et al. and in 33% in a series of 100 patients with HCC reported by Stevens et al. This finding is fairly specific for HCC and is reported to occur in metastases in less than 1% of patients **(Option (A) is true).** Invasion of the biliary tree also can occur.

Encapsulation is another imaging feature suggestive of HCC **(Option (B) is true),** although tumor capsules are also seen in patients with other primary hepatic neoplasms, particularly hepatocellular adenoma. The presence of a capsule is variable and has been reported by Freeny et al. and Ros et al. to occur less frequently in non-Asian patients with HCC than has been reported in Asian patients. Stevens et al., however, found tumor capsules in a higher proportion of patients in their series (31%) than was reported in other non-Asian population studies. It is probable that improvements in CT technique (faster scanning with proportionately more sections obtained during peak enhancement) account for some of the differences. The capsule occurs in the expanding form of the tumor by compression of adjacent hepatic parenchyma and condensation

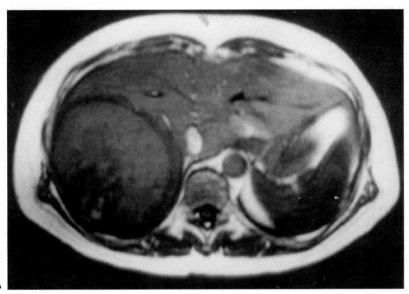

A

SE 300/15

Figure 8-12. Hepatocellular carcinoma. T1-weighted (A) and T2-weighted (B) MR images of the liver demonstrate a capsule surrounding the mass. This capsule has low signal intensity on the T1-weighted sequence and high signal intensity on the T2-weighted sequence. Intratumoral septation, dividing the tumor into multiple compartments, is also demonstrated on the T2-weighted image.

of reticulin fibers along the expanding edge of the mass. It usually appears as a hypodense rim on noncontrast CT and may or may not enhance after intravenous administration of contrast medium (Figure 8-10). On MRI, most tumor capsules appear as hypointense rings on T1-weighted images and as hyperintense bands on T2-weighted images (Figure 8-12); they can appear as double rings on T2-weighted images.

Intratumoral septation is another characteristic imaging feature of HCC **(Option (C) is true).** This feature is best seen on T2-weighted MR images (Figure 8-12) and has been described as a mosaic pattern, with thin fibrous septa dividing the tumor into multiple compartments. The term "mosaic pattern" has been used to describe not only the septated tumors but also those containing multiple nodular components of differing CT attenuation values or MR signal intensities. In the study by Stevens et al., 46 of 100 patients with HCC had a mosaic pattern (usually septations and nodules) on CT; this pattern was always seen best with contrast enhancement. It is more common in larger lesions.

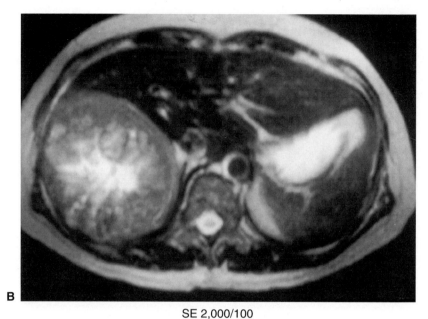

B

SE 2,000/100

Figure 8-12 (Continued)

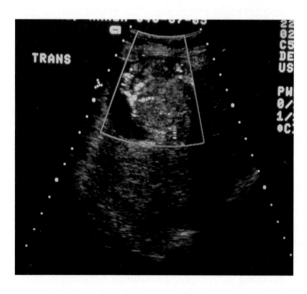

Figure 8-13. Hepato-
cellular carcinoma. A
color Doppler sono-
graphic image shows
marked internal vascu-
larity in this nodular
lesion in a cirrhotic
liver. (Reprinted with
permission from Nino-
Murcia et al. [8].)

Intratumoral arterial flow signal, detectable by pulsed or color Doppler sonography, is another characteristic finding in HCC **(Option (D) is
true)** (Figure 8-13). Nino-Murcia et al. reported that internal vascularity
detectable by Doppler sonography was seen in 75% of lesions of HCC but

in only 33% of metastatic lesions and 15% of hemangiomas. This overlap limits the specificity of the finding in diagnosing a specific type of tumor, but the use of Doppler sonography may increase confidence in the detection of tumor in the cirrhotic liver if it can be shown that a questionable nodule has internal vascularity.

Arterioportal shunting is another common feature of HCC **(Option (E) is true).** It has been demonstrated by angiography in up to 63% of tumors. Postcontrast CT can demonstrate arterioportal shunting by early and prolonged enhancement of the portal vein with irregular intraluminal or periportal vessels. This was an uncommon finding (4% of tumors) in the series reported by Freeny et al., probably because of the difficulty in detecting this feature on an incremental dynamic postcontrast CT examination in comparison with angiography.

Question 25

Concerning fibrolamellar hepatocellular carcinoma,

- (A) it occurs most commonly in elderly patients
- (B) it is associated with cirrhosis
- (C) it is usually multifocal
- (D) central calcification is a characteristic feature
- (E) the prognosis is favorable compared with that for typical hepatocellular carcinoma

Fibrolamellar HCC is a rare, distinctive HCC variant. The tumor is usually a slowly growing neoplasm that arises in a younger age group (adolescents and young adults) than do most HCCs, which have a peak incidence in the fifth to seventh decades **(Option (A) is false).** There is an equal incidence in males and females. The tumor arises in normal liver in at least 75% of patients **(Option (B) is false).** In the remainder, it is associated with cirrhosis or hepatic fibrosis. No specific etiologic agent has been identified.

The tumor has a distinctive microscopic pattern characterized by eosinophilic neoplastic hepatocytes separated into cords by lamellar fibrous strands. The tumor is usually solitary **(Option (C) is false).** Friedman et al. reported that central stellate or nodular calcification is a distinctive radiologic feature **(Option (D) is true)** and appears in a high proportion of these lesions. Teefey et al., however, have reported that calcification can also occur in a significant minority of HCCs of a nonfibrolamellar type. Therefore, the presence of calcification is not specific for this diagnosis. Identification of a central fibrous scar similar to that seen with lesions of focal nodular hyperplasia has been reported; however, most fibrolamellar HCCs do not have this appearance. Prognosis is generally more favorable than with typical HCC, with an average survival of 32 months versus 6 months for typical HCC **(Option (E) is true).**

Discussion

Detection of HCC can be extremely difficult, especially when the tumor occurs in patients with chronic liver disease, the population at greatest risk. The variability of pathologic forms of this tumor, as well as the nodularity and distortion of the normal hepatic architecture that occurs with cirrhosis, often results in poor sensitivity for tumor detection. In order to maximize tumor detection, a number of imaging strategies can be used.

While less sensitive than CT for lesion detection, sonography is often used for evaluation of patients at risk because of its low cost and wide availability. In evaluating a cirrhotic liver with sonography, color Doppler imaging can be a valuable addition to gray-scale imaging. Color Doppler imaging can detect focal hypervascular lesions that are missed with the use of gray-scale imaging alone.

Biphasic spiral CT, in which the liver is scanned first during the arterial phase following intravenous bolus contrast enhancement and then again during the portal venous phase, has been shown to increase detection of hypervascular lesions in the liver by comparison with scanning performed during the portal venous phase alone (Figure 8-14). This technique may find its greatest utility in the detection of HCC.

MRI is also a valuable imaging method for detection and characterization of focal hepatic lesions. However, because of its cost, it is used more often as a problem-solving method than as a screening method.

Regardless of the imaging method used to evaluate the cirrhotic liver, an important principle should be remembered. The incidence of HCC in the cirrhotic liver is high, and the incidence of benign lesions is low; therefore, any focal hepatic lesion must be viewed with a high index of suspicion for HCC.

Judith L. Chezmar, M.D.

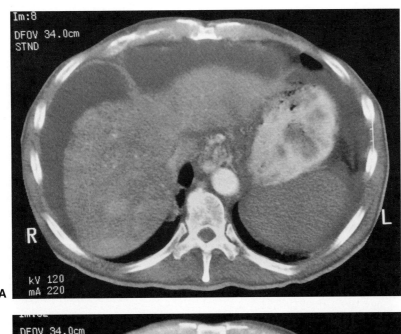

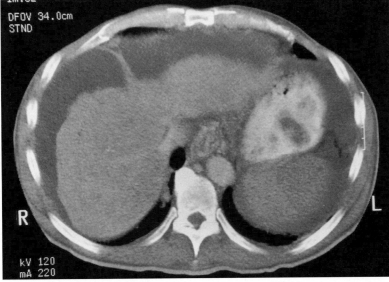

Figure 8-14. Hepatocellular carcinoma, biphasic CT examination. (A) An image obtained during the hepatic arterial phase of bolus intravenous contrast administration demonstrates multiple hypervascular nodules in the cirrhotic liver. These nodules are not detectable on images obtained during the portal venous phase (B).

SUGGESTED READINGS

HEPATOCELLULAR CARCINOMA

1. Choi BI, Takayasu K, Han MC. Small hepatocellular carcinomas and associated nodular lesions of the liver: pathology, pathogenesis, and imaging findings. AJR 1993; 160:1177–1187
2. Ebara M, Ohto M, Watanabe Y, et al. Diagnosis of small hepatocellular carcinoma: correlation of MR imaging and tumor histologic studies. Radiology 1986; 159:371–377
3. Freeny PC, Baron RL, Teefey SA. Hepatocellular carcinoma: reduced frequency of typical findings with dynamic contrast-enhanced CT in a non-Asian population. Radiology 1992; 182:143–148
4. Hollett MD, Jeffrey RB, Nino-Murcia M, Jorgensen MJ, Harris DP. Dual-phase helical CT of the liver: value of arterial phase scans in the detection of small ($\leq$1.5 cm) malignant hepatic neoplasms. AJR 1995; 164:879–884
5. Itoh K, Nishimura K, Togashi K, et al. Hepatocellular carcinoma: MR imaging. Radiology 1987; 164:21–25
6. Kadoya M, Matsui O, Takashima T, Nonomura A. Hepatocellular carcinoma: correlation of MR imaging and histopathologic findings. Radiology 1992; 183:819–825
7. Muramatsu Y, Nawano S, Takayasu K, et al. Early hepatocellular carcinoma: MR imaging. Radiology 1991; 181:209–213
8. Nino-Murcia M, Ralls PW, Jeffrey RB Jr, Johnson M. Color flow Doppler characterization of focal hepatic lesions. AJR 1992; 159:1195–1197
9. Okuda K, Peters RL, Simson IW. Gross anatomic features of hepatocellular carcinoma from three disparate geographic areas. Proposal of new classification. Cancer 1984; 54:2165–2173
10. Ros PR, Murphy BJ, Buck JL, Olmedilla G, Goodman Z. Encapsulated hepatocellular carcinoma: radiologic findings and pathologic correlation. Gastrointest Radiol 1990; 15:233–237
11. Shiina S, Tagawa K, Niwa Y, et al. Percutaneous ethanol injection therapy for hepatocellular carcinoma: results in 146 patients. AJR 1993; 160: 1023–1028
12. Shimamoto K, Sakuma S, Ishigaki T, Ishiguchi T, Itoh S, Fukatsu H. Hepatocellular carcinoma: evaluation with color Doppler US and MR imaging. Radiology 1992; 182:149–153
13. Stevens WR, Johnson CD, Stephens DH, Batts KP. CT findings in hepatocellular carcinoma: correlation of tumor characteristics with causative factors, tumor size, and histologic tumor grade. Radiology 1994; 191: 531–537

REGENERATIVE NODULES AND ADENOMATOUS HYPERPLASIA

14. Caramella D, Pisa I, Lencioni R, Bartolozzi C, Mazzeo S. Natural history of adenomatous hyperplastic nodules in cirrhotic liver: long-term follow-up results. Radiology 1992; 185(P):237

15. Dodd GD III, Oliver JH, Federle MP, et al. Spectrum of imaging findings in hepatic cirrhosis: pathologic correlation in 500 complete hepatectomy specimens. Radiology 1993; 189(P):421

16. Itai Y, Ohnishi S, Ohtomo K, et al. Regenerating nodules of liver cirrhosis: MR imaging. Radiology 1987; 165:419–423

17. Matsui O, Kadoya M, Kameyama T, et al. Adenomatous hyperplastic nodules in the cirrhotic liver: differentiation from hepatocellular carcinoma with MR imaging. Radiology 1991; 173:123–126

18. Matsui O, Kadoya M, Kameyama T, et al. Benign and malignant nodules in cirrhotic livers: distinction based on blood supply. Radiology 1991; 178:493–497

19. Mitchell DG. Focal manifestations of diffuse liver disease at MR imaging. Radiology 1992; 185:1–11

20. Murakami T, Kuroda C, Marukawa T, et al. Regenerating nodules in hepatic cirrhosis: MR findings with pathologic correlation. AJR 1990; 155:1227–1231

21. Ohtomo K, Itai Y, Ohtomo Y, Shiga J, Iio M. Regenerating nodules of liver cirrhosis: MR imaging with pathologic correlation. AJR 1990; 154:505–507

22. Sakamoto M, Hirohashi S, Shimosato Y. Early stages of multistep hepatocarcinogenesis: adenomatous hyperplasia and early hepatocellular carcinoma. Hum Pathol 1991; 22:172–178

NODULAR REGENERATIVE HYPERPLASIA

23. Dachman AH, Ros PR, Goodman ZD, Olmsted WW, Ishak KG. Nodular regenerative hyperplasia of the liver: clinical and radiologic observations. AJR 1987; 148:717–722

24. Steiner PE. Nodular regenerative hyperplasia of liver. Am J Pathol 1959; 35:943–953

25. Stromeyer FW, Ishak KG. Nodular transformation (nodular "regenerative" hyperplasia) of the liver. Hum Pathol 1981; 12:60–71

26. Wanless IR, Godwin TA, Allen F, Feder A. Nodular regenerative hyperplasia of the liver in hematologic disorders: a possible response to obliterative portal venopathy. A morphometric study of nine cases with an hypothesis on the pathogenesis. Medicine 1980; 59:367–379

FIBROLAMELLAR HEPATOCELLULAR CARCINOMA

27. Brandt DJ, Johnson CD, Stephens DH, Weiland LH. Imaging of fibrolamellar hepatocellular carcinoma. AJR 1988; 151:295–299

28. Francis IR, Agha FP, Thompson NW, Keren DF. Fibrolamellar hepatocarcinoma: clinical, radiologic, and pathologic features. Gastrointest Radiol 1986; 11:67–72

29. Friedman AC, Lichtenstein JE, Goodman Z, Fishman EK, Siegelman SS, Dachman AH. Fibrolamellar hepatocellular carcinoma. Radiology 1985; 157:583–587

30. Teefey SA, Stephens DH, Weiland LH. Calcification in hepatocellular carcinoma: not always an indication of fibrolamellar histology. AJR 1987; 149:1173–1174

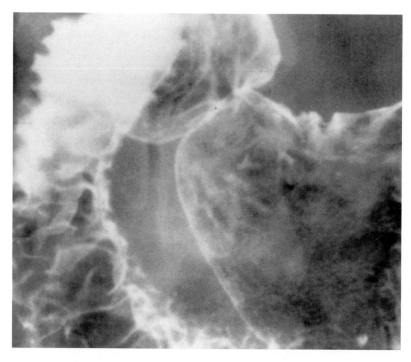

Figure 9-1. This 47-year-old woman has epigastric discomfort and heme-positive stool samples. You are shown a radiograph from an upper gastrointestinal examination.

Case 9: Erosive Gastritis Caused by Nonsteroidal Anti-Inflammatory Drugs

Question 26

Which *one* of the following is the MOST likely cause of the findings?

    (A) *Helicobacter pylori*
    (B) Cytomegalovirus
    (C) Nonsteroidal anti-inflammatory drugs
    (D) Crohn's disease
    (E) Zollinger-Ellison syndrome

The test image (Figure 9-1) demonstrates several small, linear collections of barium in the antrum of the stomach (Figure 9-2). These findings are most consistent with erosive gastritis, an entity that has been diagnosed with increased frequency on double-contrast studies in recent years. Most patients have complete or varioliform erosions that appear radiographically as punctate or slit-like collections of barium surrounded by radiolucent halos of edematous mucosa (Figure 9-3). Varioliform erosions are typically located in the gastric antrum and are often aligned on rugal folds. Major causes of erosive gastritis include aspirin and other nonsteroidal anti-inflammatory drugs (NSAIDs), alcohol, viruses, stress, trauma, and Crohn's disease. However, about 50% of cases are thought to be idiopathic, presumably occurring as a variant of peptic ulcer disease.

Usually, no etiologic significance is attributed to the shape or location of gastric erosions diagnosed on double-contrast studies, but aspirin and other NSAIDs can produce distinctive linear and serpentine erosions in the stomach. The erosions in the test image have this distinctive appearance **(Option (C) is correct).** These erosions are sometimes located in the gastric antrum, as in the test patient. This patient was known to be taking ibuprofen at the time of the barium study. More

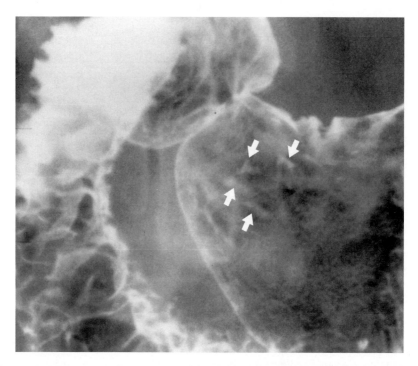

Figure 9-2 (Same as Figure 9-1). Erosive gastritis caused by an NSAID. Multiple linear and serpentine erosions (arrows) are seen in the distal portion of the gastric antrum. This patient was known to be taking ibuprofen at the time of the barium study.

often, however, NSAID-induced erosions are clustered in the body of the stomach, on or near the greater curvature (Figure 9-4). It has been postulated that these erosions result from localized mucosal injury as the dissolving tablets collect by gravity in the most dependent portion of the stomach, burning tiny holes in the adjacent greater curvature. In any case, detection of linear or serpentine erosions in the stomach should lead to careful questioning of the patient about the possibility of NSAID use. If recent ingestion of these drugs is confirmed in symptomatic patients, withdrawal of the offending agent often produces a dramatic clinical response.

Helicobacter pylori (formerly known as *Campylobacter pylori*) (Option (A)) is a gram-negative bacillus that has been cultured from the stomach in 70 to 75% of patients with histologic evidence of gastritis. Furthermore, eradication of the organism by antimicrobial therapy usually results in healing of the gastritis. Such data suggest that *H. pylori* is a cause of chronic gastritis. However, *H. pylori* is frequently present in asymptomatic patients over the age of 60, so that the clinical significance

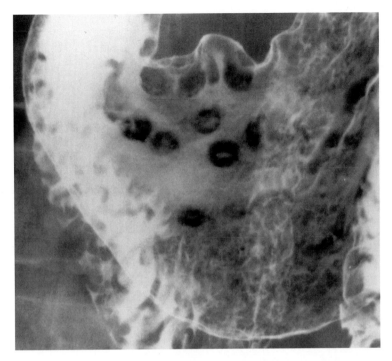

Figure 9-3. Erosive gastritis. Multiple varioliform erosions are seen in the gastric antrum as tiny barium collections surrounded by radiolucent halos of edematous mucosa. (Reprinted with permission from Gore et al. [2].)

of this infection remains uncertain. *H. pylori* gastritis can be manifested radiographically by thickened folds, predominantly in the gastric antrum or body (Figure 9-5). These findings are nonspecific, however, because enlarged folds can result from a variety of inflammatory or neoplastic conditions involving the stomach. In any case, *H. pylori* gastritis has not been described as a cause of linear or serpentine erosions in the stomach.

Cytomegalovirus (CMV) (Option (B)) is a member of the herpesvirus group that has been recognized with increased frequency as an opportunistic invader of the gastrointestinal tract in patients with AIDS. The colon is the most common site of infection, but these patients occasionally develop CMV esophagitis or gastritis. CMV gastritis is manifested radiographically by mucosal nodularity; erosions; shallow or deep ulcers; thickened, nodular folds; and, in advanced disease, antral narrowing (Figure 9-6). Ulceration or narrowing of the stomach should therefore suggest the possibility of CMV gastritis in patients with AIDS. However, the test patient was not known to have AIDS. The appearance of the erosions in Figure 9-1 and the widespread use of NSAIDs in the general

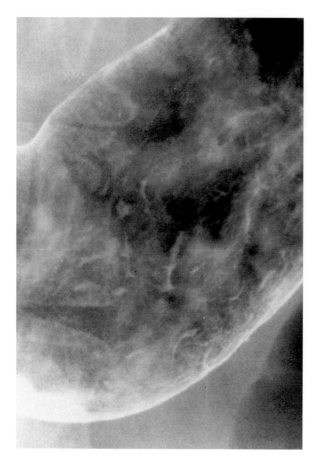

Figure 9-4. Erosive gastritis caused by an NSAID. Distinctive linear and serpentine erosions are seen clustered in the body of the stomach near the greater curvature. This patient was taking indomethacin at the time of the barium study. (Reprinted with permision from Levine et al. [7].)

population make the latter a far more likely cause of the erosive gastritis in the test patient than AIDS-associated CMV infection.

Aphthous ulcers are sometimes seen on double-contrast studies as an early sign of Crohn's disease (Option (D)) involving the stomach (Figure 9-7). Aphthous ulcers can appear as punctate or slit-like collections of barium surrounded by radiolucent mounds of edema, so that they are indistinguishable from gastric erosions. However, patients with aphthous ulcers almost always have associated Crohn's disease involving the small bowel or colon. Again, the absence of a history of inflammatory bowel disease and the high prevalence of NSAID use make Crohn's disease a less likely explanation for the findings in Figure 9-1.

Zollinger-Ellison syndrome (Option (E)) is caused by the uncontrolled release of gastrin from non-beta islet cell tumors known as gastrinomas. About 75% of these tumors are located in the pancreas; most of the rest arise in the duodenal wall. Most gastrinomas are thought to be malig-

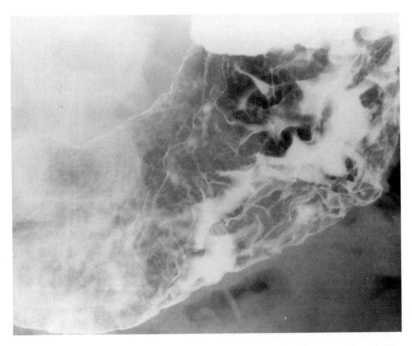

Figure 9-5. *Helicobacter pylori* gastritis. Thickened, irregular folds are seen in the body of the stomach. Gastric brushings and biopsy specimens were positive for *H. pylori* in this patient. However, thickened folds should be recognized as a nonspecific radiographic finding. (Reprinted with permission from Gore et al. [2].)

nant, because metastases are present at the time of diagnosis in 30 to 50% of patients. Because of the high gastrin levels in these patients, marked hypersecretion of gastric acid can result in the development of gastric, duodenal, or even jejunal ulcers. Barium studies can reveal characteristic findings. Hypersecretion of acid often results in a large volume of fluid in the stomach, duodenum, and proximal jejunum that dilutes the barium and compromises mucosal coating. Many patients have markedly thickened gastric and duodenal folds as a result of edema, inflammation, and increased acid secretion (Figure 9-8). Thickened folds can be caused by a variety of conditions; however, the combination of thickened folds and excessive fluid in the stomach, duodenum, and proximal jejunum should suggest the possibility of Zollinger-Ellison syndrome.

The hallmark of Zollinger-Ellison syndrome is ulceration. About 75% of the ulcers are located in the stomach or duodenal bulb, but the remaining 25% are located in the postbulbar duodenum or proximal jejunum. Peptic ulcers rarely occur distal to the papilla of Vater, so the

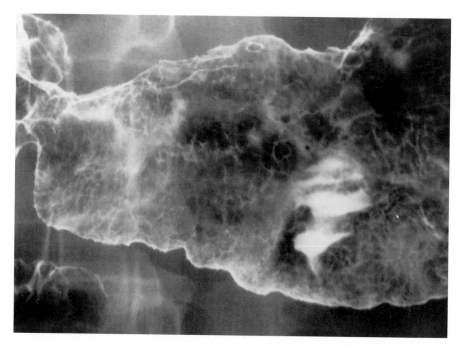

Figure 9-6. Cytomegalovirus gastritis. Mucosal nodularity and tiny ulcerations are seen in the gastric antrum, which has an irregular contour. This patient has AIDS. (Reprinted with permission from Gore et al. [2].)

presence of one or more ulcers in the third or fourth portion of the duodenum or in the proximal jejunum should be highly suggestive of Zollinger-Ellison syndrome. It should be noted that the test figure shows no evidence of increased secretions or thickened folds in the stomach or duodenum. The findings in the test patient are therefore not suggestive of Zollinger-Ellison syndrome.

Marc S. Levine, M.D.

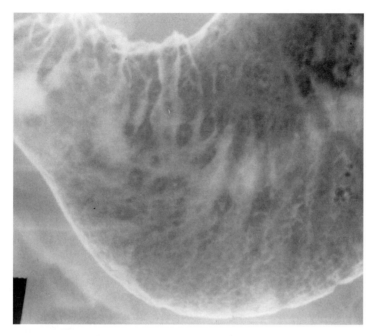

Figure 9-7. Early Crohn's disease with multiple aphthous ulcers. These lesions are indistinguishable from varioliform erosions in the stomach. However, this patient has advanced changes of Crohn's disease in the small bowel. (Reprinted with permission from Levine [21].)

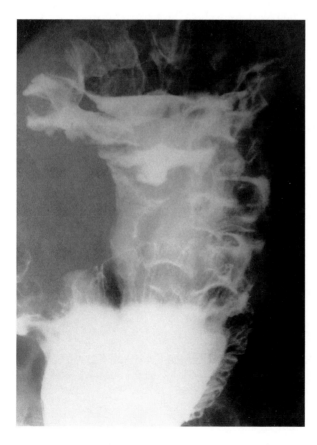

Figure 9-8 (left). Zollinger-Ellison syndrome. Markedly thickened folds are present in the gastric fundus and body. Also note how the barium is diluted by excessive fluid in the stomach. (Reprinted with permission from Gore et al. [24].)

EROSIVE GASTRITIS AND NONSTEROIDAL ANTI-INFLAMMATORY DRUGS

1. Catalano D, Pagliari U. Gastroduodenal erosions: radiological findings. Gastrointest Radiol 1982; 7:235–240

2. Gore RM, Levine MS, Laufer I (eds). Textbook of gastrointestinal radiology. Philadelphia: WB Saunders; 1994:598–627

3. Lanza F, Royer G, Nelson R. An endoscopic evaluation of the effects of nonsteroidal anti-inflammatory drugs on the gastric mucosa. Gastrointest Endosc 1975; 21:103–105

4. Lanza FL, Nelson RS, Rack MF. A controlled endoscopic study comparing the toxic effects of sulindac, naproxen, aspirin, and placebo on the gastric mucosa of healthy volunteers. J Clin Pharmacol 1984; 24:89–95

5. Laufer I, Hamilton J, Mullens JE. Demonstration of superficial gastric erosions by double contrast radiography. Gastroenterology 1975; 68:387–391

6. Levine MS. Stomach. In: Levine MS, Laufer I (eds), Double contrast gastrointestinal radiology, 2nd ed. Philadelphia: WB Saunders; 1992:191–248

7. Levine MS, Verstandig A, Laufer I. Serpiginous gastric erosions caused by aspirin and other nonsteroidal antiinflammatory drugs. AJR 1986; 146:31–34

8. Poplack W, Paul RE, Goldsmith M, Matsue H, Moore JP, Norton R. Demonstration of erosive gastritis by the double-contrast technique. Radiology 1975; 117:519–521

HELICOBACTER PYLORI GASTRITIS

9. Chaloupka JC, Gay BB, Caplan D. *Campylobacter* gastritis simulating Menetrier's disease by upper gastrointestinal radiography. Pediatr Radiol 1990; 20:200–201

10. Chamberlain CE, Peura DA. *Campylobacter (Helicobacter) pylori*. Is peptic disease a bacterial infection? Arch Intern Med 1990; 150:951–955

11. Dooley CP, Cohen H, Fitzgibbons PL, et al. Prevalence of *Helicobacter pylori* infection and histologic gastritis in asymptomatic persons. N Engl J Med 1989; 321:1562–1566

12. Morrison S, Dahms BB, Hoffenberg E, Czinn SJ. Enlarged gastric folds in association with *Campylobacter pylori* gastritis. Radiology 1989; 171:819–821

13. Urban BA, Fishman EK, Hruban RH. *Helicobacter pylori* gastritis mimicking gastric carcinoma at CT evaluation. Radiology 1991; 179:689–691

CYTOMEGALOVIRUS GASTRITIS

14. Falcone S, Murphy BJ, Weinfeld A. Gastric manifestations of AIDS: radiographic findings on upper gastrointestinal examination. Gastrointest Radiol 1991; 16:95–98

15. Farman J, Lerner ME, Ng C, et al. Cytomegalovirus gastritis: protean radiologic manifestations. Gastrointest Radiol 1992; 17:202–206
16. Megibow AJ, Balthazar EJ, Hulnick DH. Radiology of nonneoplastic gastrointestinal disorders in acquired immune deficiency syndrome. Semin Roentgenol 1987; 22:31–41
17. Teixidor HS, Honig CL, Norsoph E, Albert S, Mouradian JA, Whalen JP. Cytomegalovirus infection of the alimentary canal: radiologic findings with pathologic correlation. Radiology 1987; 163:317–323

GASTRIC CROHN'S DISEASE

18. Ariyama J, Wehlin L, Lindstrom CG, Wenkert A, Roberts GM. Gastroduodenal erosions in Crohn's disease. Gastrointest Radiol 1980; 5:121–125
19. Kelvin FM, Gedgaudas RK. Radiologic diagnosis of Crohn disease (with emphasis on its early manifestations). Crit Rev Diagn Imaging 1981; 16:43–91
20. Laufer I, Trueman T. Multiple superficial gastric erosions due to Crohn's disease of the stomach. Radiologic and endoscopic diagnosis. Br J Radiol 1976; 49:726–728
21. Levine MS. Crohn's disease of the upper gastrointestinal tract. Radiol Clin North Am 1987; 25:79–91

ZOLLINGER-ELLISON SYNDROME

22. Amberg JR, Ellison EH, Wilson SD, et al. Roentgenographic observations in the Zollinger-Ellison syndrome. JAMA 1964; 190:185–187
23. Ellison EH, Wilson SD. The Zollinger-Ellison syndrome: reappraisal and evaluation of 260 registered cases. Ann Surg 1964; 160:514–530
24. Gore RM, Levine MS, Laufer I (eds). Textbook of gastrointestinal radiology. Philadelphia: WB Saunders; 1994:562–597
25. Missakian MM, Carlson HC, Huzenga KA. Roentgenographic findings in Zollinger-Ellison syndrome. AJR 1965; 94:429–437
26. Nelson SW, Christoforidis AJ. Roentgenologic features of the Zollinger-Ellison syndrome: ulcerogenic tumor of the pancreas. Semin Roentgenol 1968; 3:254–266
27. Zboralske FF, Amberg JR. Detection of the Zollinger-Ellison syndrome: the radiologist's responsibility. AJR 1968; 104:529–543

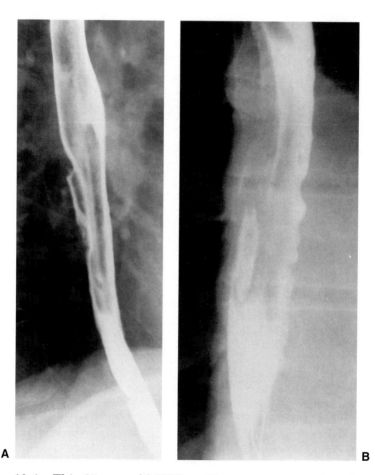

Figure 10-1. This 35-year-old HIV-positive man presented with odyno-phagia. You are shown double-contrast (A) and single-contrast (B) radio-graphs from an esophagram.

Case 10: HIV Esophagitis

Question 27

Which *one* of the following is the MOST likely diagnosis?

    (A) *Candida* esophagitis
    (B) Herpes esophagitis
    (C) HIV esophagitis
    (D) Lymphoma
    (E) Kaposi's sarcoma

Two radiographs (Figure 10-1) from a biphasic esophagram show a giant (diameter, 5 cm), relatively flat midesophageal ulcer both in profile (Figure 10-2A) and *en face* (Figure 10-2B). Cytomegalovirus (CMV) and HIV esophagitis are by far the most common causes of giant esophageal ulcers in HIV-positive patients with odynophagia. However, CMV esophagitis is not listed as an option, so HIV esophagitis is the most likely diagnosis **(Option (C) is correct).**

CMV, a member of the herpesvirus group, has been recognized as a cause of opportunistic esophagitis in patients with AIDS. Affected individuals usually present with severe odynophagia. CMV esophagitis can be manifested radiographically by discrete, superficial ulcers that are indistinguishable from those of herpes esophagitis. However, other patients can have one or more giant, relatively flat esophageal ulcers that are 2 cm or more in length (Figure 10-3). A diagnosis of CMV esophagitis can be made on the basis of endoscopic cultures or endoscopic brushings and biopsy specimens when characteristic intranuclear inclusions are detected in endothelial cells or fibroblasts at or near the base of the ulcers. The treatment for CMV esophagitis includes relatively toxic antiviral agents, such as ganciclovir, that are associated with bone marrow suppression. Thus, endoscopic brushings, biopsy specimens, or cultures are required to confirm the presence of CMV infection prior to initiating treatment.

HIV infection itself has been recognized with increasing frequency as another cause of giant esophageal ulcers in HIV-positive patients with

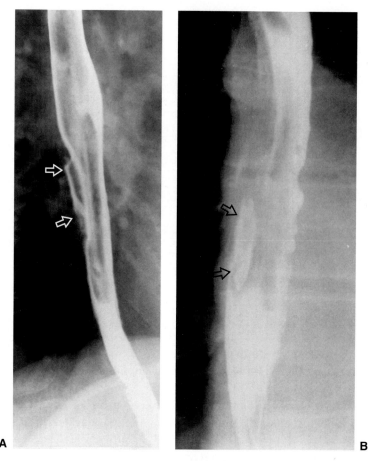

Figure 10-2 (Same as Figure 10-1). HIV esophagitis. A giant, relatively flat ulcer (arrows) is seen in the midesophagus both in profile on the double-contrast radiograph (A) and *en face* on the single-contrast radiograph (B). CMV esophagitis can produce identical findings in HIV-positive patients with odynophagia.

odynophagia. HIV esophagitis is usually manifested on esophagography by one or more giant, relatively flat esophageal ulcers that are indistinguishable from those caused by CMV esophagitis. Endoscopy is therefore required to differentiate these conditions.

Candida esophagitis (Option (A)) is the most common opportunistic infection in the esophagus. When ulceration is present in patients with candidiasis, however, it almost always occurs against a background of diffuse plaque formation (Figure 10-4). Furthermore, giant ulcers are almost never seen in patients with *Candida* esophagitis.

Figure 10-3 (right). CMV esophagitis. This patient with AIDS has a giant, flat ulcer (arrows) in the distal esophagus that is indistinguishable from the HIV ulcer in Figure 10-1. Endoscopic brushings, biopsy specimens, or cultures are therefore required to differentiate these infections. (Reprinted with permission from Gore et al. [13].)

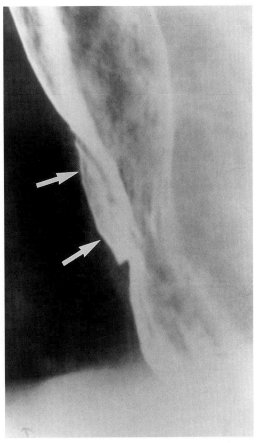

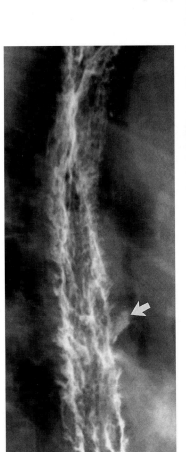

Figure 10-4 (left). Advanced *Candida* esophagitis. The esophagus has a grossly irregular or "shaggy" contour due to trapping of barium between innumerable plaques and pseudomembranes. There is also a deep ulcer (arrow) superimposed on a background of plaque formation.

Herpes simplex virus is also a relatively common cause of esophagitis in HIV-positive patients. Herpes esophagitis (Option (B)) is usually mani-

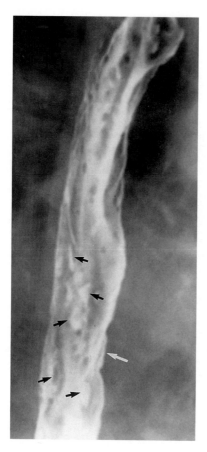

Figure 10-5. Herpes esophagitis. Multiple small, discrete ulcers are seen both *en face* (black arrows) and in profile (white arrow) in the midesophagus. These findings should be highly suggestive of herpes esophagitis in an immunocompromised patient with odynophagia.

fested radiographically by multiple discrete, superficial ulcers in the upper esophagus or midesophagus (Figure 10-5). However, herpetic ulcers rarely become as large as the ulcer in the test images, so CMV esophagitis and HIV esophagitis are much more likely diagnoses.

Lymphoma (Option (D)) and Kaposi's sarcoma (Option (E)) are malignant tumors that occur with increased frequency in the gastrointestinal tract of HIV-positive patients. When these tumors involve the esophagus, they are usually manifested radiographically by submucosal nodules (Figure 10-6), enlarged folds, polypoid or ulcerated masses, or strictures. Thus, neither of these tumors would be likely in the test patient.

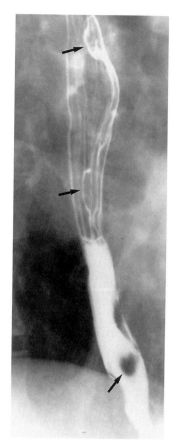

Figure 10-6. Kaposi's sarcoma involving the esophagus. This patient has multiple submucosal masses (arrows) in the esophagus. (Case courtesy of Robert Goren, M.D., Philadelphia, Pa.)

Question 28

Concerning *Candida* esophagitis,

    (A) it is the most common type of opportunistic esophagitis

    (B) about 90% of patients have associated oropharyngeal candidiasis

    (C) plaques are seen on double-contrast esophagrams in about 90% of endoscopically proven cases

    (D) a shaggy esophageal contour is characteristic of early candidiasis

    (E) an infiltrating esophageal carcinoma produces similar radiographic findings

Candidiasis is by far the most common cause of opportunistic esophagitis **(Option (A) is true).** Patients can be immunocompromised by underlying malignancy; debilitating illness; diabetes; treatment with radiation, steroids, or other cytotoxic agents; or AIDS, a severe disorder of cellular immunity.

Most patients with *Candida* esophagitis have acute onset of odynophagia, characterized by intense substernal pain during swallowing. Other patients can develop dysphagia. The presence of oropharyngeal candidiasis (i.e., thrush) should suggest the correct diagnosis, but about 50% of patients with *Candida* esophagitis do not have active infection of the oropharynx **(Option (B) is false).** Patients with oropharyngeal candidiasis can also have herpes or CMV esophagitis, so the presence of fungal infection in the oropharynx does not preclude the possibility of viral infection in the esophagus. Thus, it can be difficult or impossible to differentiate fungal and viral esophagitis on clinical grounds.

The radiologic diagnosis of *Candida* esophagitis has been limited by the fact that it tends to be a superficial disease with mucosal abnormalities that are difficult to detect on single-contrast barium studies. However, double-contrast esophagography has a reported sensitivity of about 90% in diagnosing *Candida* esophagitis, primarily because of its ability to demonstrate mucosal plaques that cannot easily be seen on single-contrast studies **(Option (C) is true).** These lesions typically appear as discrete plaquelike defects that have a linear configuration and are separated by segments of normal mucosa (Figure 10-7). Pathologically, the plaques consist of heaped-up areas of necrotic epithelial debris and actual colonies of *Candida albicans* on the esophageal mucosa.

In severe *Candida* esophagitis, the esophagus eventually can have a grossly irregular or "shaggy" contour caused by coalescent plaque and pseudomembrane formation with barium trapped between these plaques and pseudomembranes (Figure 10-4). Thus, a shaggy esophagus clearly is not a sign of early candidiasis **(Option (D) is false)** but instead indicates advanced disease. This fulminant form of candidiasis occurs primarily in patients with AIDS.

A diffusely infiltrating esophageal carcinoma can also produce an irregular esophageal contour. However, such lesions are usually associated with various degrees of luminal narrowing and almost always have relatively abrupt, shelf-like proximal and distal borders (Figure 10-8). Thus, an infiltrating esophageal carcinoma can almost always be differentiated from the shaggy esophagus of candidiasis **(Option (E) is false).**

Figure 10-7 (right). Candida esophagitis. Multiple discrete plaquelike lesions are seen in the midesophagus. The plaques have a linear configuration and are separated by segments of normal mucosa. These findings are characteristic of *Candida* esophagitis.

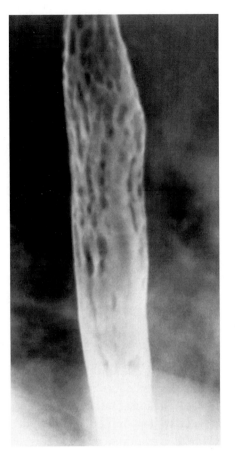

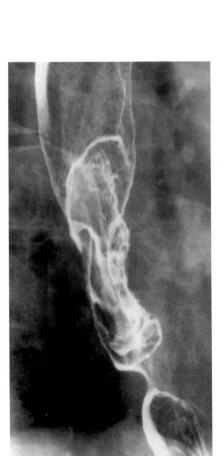

Figure 10-8 (left). Infiltrating esophageal carcinoma. The lesion is manifested by irregular luminal narrowing with abrupt, shelf-like borders. These findings are characteristic of advanced esophageal carcinoma.

Question 29

Concerning herpes esophagitis,

    (A) it is characterized by discrete, superficial ulcers
    (B) it occasionally occurs as an acute, self-limited syndrome in otherwise healthy patients
    (C) eosinophilic intranuclear inclusions are characteristic
    (D) it often leads to the formation of esophageal strictures
    (E) drug-induced esophagitis produces similar radiographic findings

Esophagitis due to herpes simplex virus type 1 is usually manifested radiographically by discrete, superficial ulcers in the midesophagus without evidence of plaques **(Option (A) is true).** The ulcers can have a punctate, linear, or stellate configuration and are often surrounded by radiolucent halos of edematous mucosa (Figure 10-5). In contrast, ulceration in patients with candidiasis almost always occurs on a background of diffuse plaque formation (see Figure 10-4). Therefore, discrete ulcers on an otherwise normal mucosa should be highly suggestive of herpes esophagitis in immunocompromised patients with odynophagia.

Herpes esophagitis is usually seen in immunocompromised patients, but it occasionally occurs as an acute, self-limited illness in otherwise healthy individuals who have no underlying immunologic problems **(Option (B) is true).** These immunocompetent patients are typically young men who have a history of recent exposure to sexual partners with herpetic lesions on the lips or buccal mucosa. Most of these patients have a 3- to 10-day influenzalike prodrome with fever, headache, or myalgias prior to the sudden onset of intense odynophagia. Despite the severity of symptoms, these patients almost always have self-limited disease, with symptoms resolving within 3 to 14 days after presentation. Double-contrast esophagography can reveal multiple tiny ulcers that are clustered in the midesophagus near the level of the left main bronchus (Figure 10-9). Thus, in otherwise healthy patients, the diagnosis of herpes esophagitis can usually be suggested on the basis of the clinical and radiographic findings without need for endoscopy.

In patients with herpes esophagitis, the histologic or cytologic findings on biopsy specimens or brushings from the esophagus are relatively specific for the herpesvirus group. The classic finding of Cowdry type A intranuclear inclusions in intact epithelial cells adjacent to ulcers is virtually pathognomonic of herpetic infection **(Option (C) is true).** The diagnosis of herpes esophagitis can also be confirmed by obtaining positive viral cultures from the esophagus or by direct immunofluorescent staining for the herpes simplex antigen.

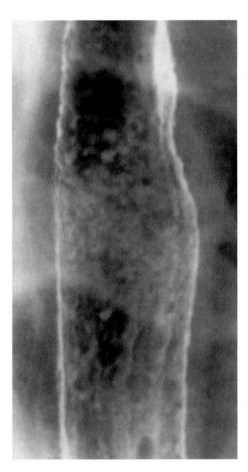

Figure 10-9. Herpes esophagitis in an otherwise healthy patient. Multiple punctate areas of ulceration are seen clustered in the midesophagus below the level of the left main bronchus. The diagnosis of herpes esophagitis can be suggested on the basis of the clinical and radiographic findings without need for endoscopy. (Reprinted with permission from Shortsleeve and Levine [22].)

Even in immunocompromised patients, herpes esophagitis is usually a self-limited disease, and most cases resolve without sequelae. As a result, these patients almost never develop esophageal strictures **(Option (D) is false)**.

Certain oral medications, e.g., tetracycline and doxycycline, can cause a focal contact esophagitis, manifested on double-contrast esophagography by the development of shallow ulcers indistinguishable from those of herpes esophagitis (see Case 2, Figure 2-1) **(Option (E) is true)**. However, a temporal relationship between ingestion of the offending medication and the onset of esophagitis should suggest the correct diagnosis. Reflux esophagitis is a more common cause of ulceration, but it tends to involve the distal esophagus and is usually associated with a hiatal hernia or gastroesophageal reflux. Other causes of ulceration, such as radiation esophagitis, caustic esophagitis, and Crohn's disease, can usually be differentiated from herpes esophagitis by the clinical history and presentation.

Question 30

Concerning HIV esophagitis,

(A) not all affected individuals have AIDS at the time of presentation
(B) it can be associated with a maculopapular rash on the upper half of the body
(C) cytomegalovirus esophagitis produces similar radiographic findings
(D) treatment with oral steroids is recommended

A new clinical syndrome of odynophagia and giant esophageal ulcers has been recognized in patients with HIV infection. Although most patients have known AIDS at the time of presentation, some have recently become HIV positive, so that HIV esophagitis can occur at about the time of seroconversion **(Option (A) is true).** Thus, giant esophageal ulcers can be a manifestation of acute or chronic HIV infection.

Patients with HIV esophagitis can have associated ulcers on the hard palate or a distinctive maculopapular rash involving the face, trunk, and upper extremities **(Option (B) is true).** The possibility of HIV esophagitis should therefore be suspected in HIV-positive patients with the characteristic maculopapular rash who develop odynophagia at about the time of seroconversion.

CMV esophagitis can also be manifested radiographically by the development of one or more giant, flat ulcers in the esophagus (Figure 10-3) **(Option (C) is true),** so endoscopy is required to differentiate it from HIV esophagitis. Although it is not possible to make a definitive diagnosis of HIV esophagitis at endoscopy, HIV ulcers should be suspected if endoscopic brushings, biopsy specimens, and cultures are all negative for CMV or other opportunistic organisms. HIV ulcers can heal spontaneously or can respond dramatically to treatment with oral steroids **(Option (D) is true),** but they do not require treatment with other antiviral agents such as ganciclovir. Thus, endoscopy should be performed on HIV-positive patients with giant esophageal ulcers to differentiate HIV from CMV infection in the esophagus.

In summary, double-contrast esophagography is a useful technique for evaluating patients with AIDS who present clinically with odynophagia or dysphagia. When opportunistic infection is present, most such patients are found to have *Candida* esophagitis, manifested radiographically by discrete plaquelike lesions in the esophagus. A smaller number of patients are found to have herpes esophagitis, as demonstrated by the presence of superficial ulcers without plaques. Fungal and viral esophagitis can therefore usually be differentiated on double-contrast studies, eliminating the need for endoscopy in most of these patients. However, endoscopy is required if the radiographic findings are equivocal or if appropriate treatment with antifungal or antiviral agents fails to produce an adequate clinical response. Finally, esophagography can demonstrate one or more giant, relatively flat ulcers due to CMV or HIV esophagitis. In such cases, endoscopy is also required for a definitive diagnosis, since these disorders are treated differently.

Marc S. Levine, M.D.

SUGGESTED READINGS

HIV ESOPHAGITIS

1. Bach MC, Howell DA, Valenti AJ, Smith TJ, Winslow DL. Aphthous ulceration of the gastrointestinal tract in patients with the acquired immunodeficiency syndrome (AIDS). Ann Intern Med 1990; 112:465–467
2. Bach MC, Valenti AJ, Howell DA, Smith TJ. Odynophagia from aphthous ulcers of the pharynx and esophagus in the acquired immunodeficiency syndrome (AIDS). Ann Intern Med 1988; 109:338–339
3. Dretler RH, Rausher DB. Giant esophageal ulcer healed with steroid therapy in an AIDS patient. Rev Infect Dis 1989; 11:768–769
4. Kumar A, Posner G, Colby S, Nicholas A. Giant esophageal ulcers in AIDS-related complex. Gastrointest Endosc 1988; 34:153–154
5. Levine MS, Loercher G, Katzka DA, Herlinger H, Rubesin SE, Laufer I. Giant, human immunodeficiency virus-related ulcers in the esophagus. Radiology 1991; 180:323–326
6. Rabeneck L, Popovic M, Gartner S, et al. Acute HIV infection presenting with painful swallowing and esophageal ulcers. JAMA 1990; 263:2318–2322
7. Sor S, Levine MS, Kowalski TE, et al. Giant ulcers of the esophagus in patients with human immunodeficiency virus: clinical, radiographic, and pathologic findings. Radiology 1995; 194:447–451

CANDIDA ESOPHAGITIS

8. Athey PA, Goldstein HM, Dodd GD. Radiologic spectrum of opportunistic infections of the upper gastrointestinal tract. AJR 1977; 129:419–424
9. Hartong WA, Moeller DD, Laing RR. Esophageal moniliasis. Radiographic, endoscopic, and pathologic criteria for diagnosis. J Kans Med Soc 1972; 73:470–474
10. Laufer I. Radiology of esophagitis. Radiol Clin North Am 1982; 20:687–699
11. Levine MS, Macones AJ Jr, Laufer I. *Candida* esophagitis: accuracy of radiographic diagnosis. Radiology 1985; 154:581–587

12. Levine MS, Woldenberg R, Herlinger H, Laufer I. Opportunistic esophagitis in AIDS: radiographic diagnosis. Radiology 1987; 165:815–820

13. Gore RM, Levine MS, Laufer I (eds). Textbook of gastrointestinal radiology. Philadelphia: WB Saunders; 1994:385–402

14. Vahey TN, Maglinte DD, Chernish AM. State-of-the-art barium examination in opportunistic esophagitis. Dig Dis Sci 1986; 31:1192–1195

HERPES ESOPHAGITIS

15. Agha FP, Lee HH, Nostrant TT. Herpetic esophagitis: a diagnostic challenge in immunocompromised patients. Am J Gastroenterol 1986; 81:246–253

16. DeGaeta L, Levine MS, Guglielmi GE, Raffensperger EC, Laufer I. Herpes esophagitis in an otherwise healthy patient. AJR 1985; 144:1205–1206

17. Levine MS, Laufer I, Kressel HY, Friedman HM. Herpes esophagitis. AJR 1981; 136:863–866

18. Levine MS, Loevner LA, Saul SH, Rubesin SE, Herlinger H, Laufer I. Herpes esophagitis: sensitivity of double-contrast esophagography. AJR 1988; 151:57–62

19. Lightdale CJ, Wolf DJ, Marcucci RA, Salyer WR. Herpetic esophagitis in patients with cancer: ante mortem diagnosis by brush cytology. Cancer 1977; 39:223–226

20. Nash G, Ross JS. Herpetic esophagitis. A common cause of esophageal ulceration. Hum Pathol 1974; 5:339–345

21. Shortsleeve MJ, Gauvin GP, Gardner RC, Greenberg MS. Herpetic esophagitis. Radiology 1981; 141:611–617

22. Shortsleeve MJ, Levine MS. Herpes esophagitis in otherwise healthy patients: clinical and radiographic findings. Radiology 1992; 182:859–861

LYMPHOMA

23. Carnovale RL, Goldstein HM, Zornoza J, Dodd GD. Radiologic manifestations of esophageal lymphoma. AJR 1977; 128:751–754

24. Caruso RD, Berk RN. Lymphoma of the esophagus. Radiology 1970; 95:381–382

25. Gedgaudas-McClees RK, Maglinte DD. Lymphomatous esophageal nodules: the difficulty in radiological differential diagnosis. Am J Gastroenterol 1985; 80:529–530

26. Levine MS, Sunshine AG, Reynolds JC, Saul SH. Diffuse nodularity in esophageal lymphoma. AJR 1985; 145:1218–1220

27. Zornoza J, Dodd GD. Lymphoma of the gastrointestinal tract. Semin Roentgenol 1980; 15:272–287

KAPOSI'S SARCOMA

28. Friedman SL, Wright TL, Altman DF. Gastrointestinal Kaposi's sarcoma in patients with acquired immunodeficiency syndrome. Endoscopic and autopsy findings. Gastroenterology 1985; 89:102–108

29. Rose HS, Balthazar EJ, Megibow AJ, Horowitz L, Laubenstein LJ. Alimentary tract involvement in Kaposi sarcoma: radiographic and endoscopic findings in 25 homosexual men. AJR 1982; 139:661–666

30. Wall SD, Friedman SL, Margulis AR. Gastrointestinal Kaposi's sarcoma in AIDS: radiographic manifestations. J Clin Gastroenterol 1984; 6:165–171

CYTOMEGALOVIRUS ESOPHAGITIS

31. Balthazar EJ, Megibow AJ, Hulnick D, Cho KC, Berenbaum E. Cytomegalovirus esophagitis in AIDS: radiographic features in 16 patients. AJR 1987; 149:919–923

32. Balthazar EJ, Megibow AJ, Hulnick DH. Cytomegalovirus esophagitis and gastritis in AIDS. AJR 1985; 144:1201–1204

33. Frager DH, Frager JD, Brandt LJ, et al. Gastrointestinal complications of AIDS: radiologic features. Radiology 1986; 158:597–603

34. Teixidor HS, Honig CL, Norsoph E, Albert S, Mouradian JA, Whalen JP. Cytomegalovirus infection of the alimentary canal: radiologic findings with pathologic correlation. Radiology 1987; 163:317–323

35. Wilcox CM, Diehl DL, Cello JP, Margaretten W, Jacobson MA. Cytomegalovirus esophagitis in patients with AIDS. A clinical, endoscopic, and pathologic correlation. Ann Intern Med 1990; 113:589–593

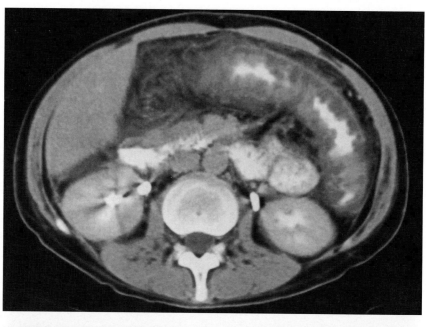

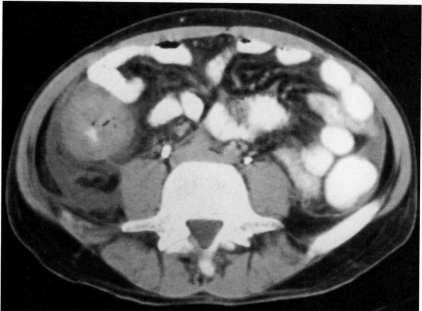

Figure 11-1. This 22-year-old man with AIDS has fever, leukocytosis, right lower quadrant pain, and bloody diarrhea. You are shown two images from an abdominal CT scan.

Case 11: Cytomegalovirus Colitis

Question 31

Which *one* of the following is the MOST likely diagnosis?

    (A) Lymphoma
    (B) Cytomegalovirus colitis
    (C) Herpes simplex colitis
    (D) Pseudomembranous colitis
    (E) Gonococcal colitis

Figure 11-1 demonstrates marked thickening of the wall of the colon, with severe involvement of the ascending and transverse colon and relative sparing of the descending colon (Figure 11-2). The bowel wall has low attenuation due to submucosal edema, suggesting an inflammatory or infectious process rather than a colonic neoplasm. Pericolonic inflammatory changes are evident, manifested by soft tissue stranding in the fat adjacent to the colon. Minimal ascites is also seen. The radiographic findings are consistent with colitis, which, in a patient with AIDS, can be due to any one or a combination of several different pathogens, including viral, fungal, bacterial, and protozoal organisms. Of the options presented, the most likely cause of colitis in the test patient is cytomegalovirus (CMV) infection of the colon, and the CT findings are characteristic of those described for CMV colitis **(Option (B) is correct).** This diagnosis was confirmed by mucosal biopsy.

CMV is one of the most common gastrointestinal pathogens in patients with AIDS, and colitis is the most common manifestation of enteric CMV infection, although CMV esophagitis, gastritis, small intestinal enteritis, and biliary infection are also prevalent. The clinical course of CMV colitis varies, but it is characterized by diarrhea (100% of patients) and frequently by fever (80%), hematochezia (74 to 80%), and abdominal pain (82%). Severe involvement can result in bowel ischemia and, in some cases, perforation. Pathologic findings are variable and include focal or diffuse inflammation, hemorrhagic plaques, and superficial or deep ulceration.

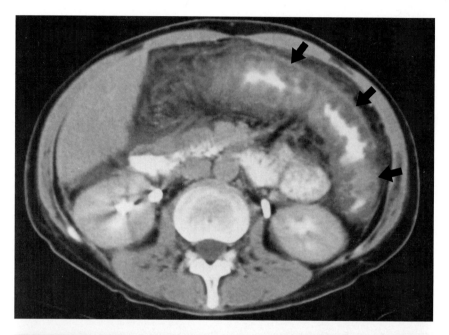

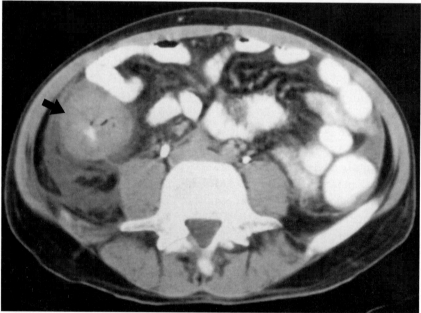

Figure 11-2 (Same as Figure 11-1). Cytomegalovirus colitis in association with AIDS. Marked thickening of the wall of the right and transverse colon as a result of submucosal edema is evident (arrows). Soft tissue stranding in the fat adjacent to the colon and minimal ascites in the right paracolic gutter are also seen.

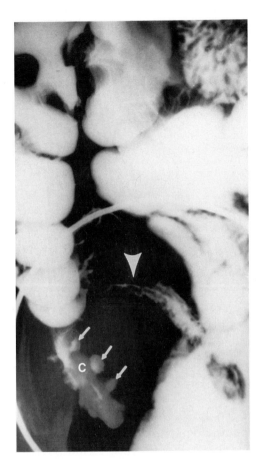

Figure 11-3. CMV colitis in a 29-year-old man with AIDS. This film was obtained during a barium examination of the small intestine and shows a markedly contracted cecum (C). Multiple discrete ulcerations (arrows) with surrounding edema are present. The distal ileum (arrowhead) is displaced superiorly by the thickened cecal wall, but it is radiographically normal.

Reported findings on barium enema reflect this variability in pathologic findings. Balthazar et al. reported the results of barium enema examinations in 10 patients with CMV colitis; a variety of abnormalities, including diffuse mucosal granularity, aphthous ulcers, thickened folds, and spasticity, were noted. In two patients in this series, the barium enema was normal. In this and other reported series, the abnormalities were diffuse in some patients and segmental or focal in others. When the abnormalities are segmental or focal, there is a predilection for the cecum and right colon. Large discrete ulcers on barium studies have also been reported in association with CMV colitis (Figure 11-3).

At most institutions, barium enema is seldom used to diagnose colitis in patients with AIDS. Many patients do, however, undergo CT scanning to evaluate the abdomen for malignancy or evidence of infection and are found to have evidence of severe colitis on this examination. Thickening

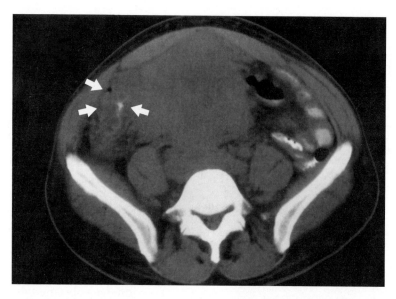

Figure 11-4. Non-Hodgkin's lymphoma associated with AIDS. Marked thickening of the wall of the right colon (arrows) is seen in association with a bulky nodal mass.

of the wall of the colon, with low attenuation of the wall reflecting submucosal edema, is the most common finding, as seen in the test patient. The differential diagnosis of colitis associated with AIDS includes adenovirus infection; infection with bacterial agents, including *Shigella flexneri, Campylobacter jejuni, Clostridium difficile,* and *Mycobacterium avium-intracellulare* (MAI); and protozoan infestations, particularly by *Cryptosporidium* species. The specific diagnosis of CMV colitis is established by biopsy, with histopathologic findings including identification of the characteristic "owl eye" appearance of intranuclear or cytoplasmic CMV inclusions. Treatment is with antiviral agents (ganciclovir).

Diffuse thickening of the wall of the colon is one of the CT findings associated with AIDS-related lymphoma (Option (A)) (Figure 11-4); however, the low attenuation of the colonic wall seen in the test images, reflecting submucosal edema and increased density of the pericolonic fat, suggests an inflammatory rather than a neoplastic condition. Although the absence of associated findings such as enlarged lymph nodes does not exclude lymphoma from consideration, there is no support for this diagnosis. The patient's presentation with fever, abdominal pain, and diarrhea also favors infection over neoplasm.

Herpes simplex virus (Option (C)) has been identified as a cause of bowel infection associated with HIV infection, but it typically produces perianal lesions and proctitis rather than colitis. Diarrhea associated with herpes simplex virus infection has not been described. The diagnosis is made by sigmoidoscopy, with barium enema examination usually not indicated. Lesions begin as small vesicles, which may progress to ulceration. Symptoms of herpes simplex virus proctitis include severe anorectal pain and tenesmus. The absence of severe anorectal pain and the presence of pancolitis in the test patient make herpes simplex colitis an unlikely option.

With the exception of *Clostridium difficile* toxin-induced colitis (pseudomembranous colitis [Option (D)]), no characteristic radiographic findings have yet been described for infections with the other organisms that frequently cause colitis in this population. The CT appearance of pseudomembranous colitis, a well-known complication of antibiotic therapy in immunocompetent individuals, has been described and can be similar to CMV colitis, with diffuse or segmental colon wall thickening (Figure 11-5). The radiologic appearance of pseudomembranous colitis is the same in immunocompetent and immunocompromised patients. Adjacent pericolonic inflammatory changes are usually absent or less striking in patients with pseudomembranous colitis; this and the lack of a history of antibiotic use make pseudomembranous colitis a less likely diagnosis in the test patient. *Neisseria gonorrhoeae* is a common sexually transmitted organism but has not been implicated as a cause of AIDS-related colitis. Hence, gonococcal colitis (Option (E)) is unlikely.

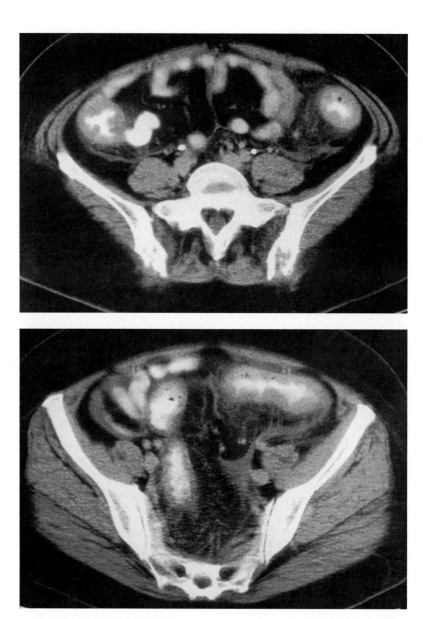

Figure 11-5. Pseudomembranous colitis. These images from a CT scan in a middle-aged woman on antibiotic therapy show diffuse thickening of the entire colon, with minimal pericolonic inflammatory changes and minimal intraperitoneal fluid. Endoscopic evaluation demonstrated confluent pseudomembranes consisting of necrotic debris and ulcerated colonic mucosa.

Question 32

Concerning gastrointestinal infections in patients with AIDS,

(A) symptomatic infection occurs in most patients with AIDS
(B) a specific pathogen is identified in fewer than 50% of patients with diarrhea
(C) there is little geographic variation in causative pathogens
(D) mucosal biopsy is usually necessary to establish a diagnosis of viral infection
(E) infections of the small bowel usually have nonspecific radiologic findings

Symptomatic gastrointestinal infections, predominantly manifested by diarrhea, affect most patients with AIDS worldwide **(Option (A) is true)** and are a significant cause of morbidity and mortality. Gastrointestinal symptoms, predominantly diarrhea, have been reported to affect 30 to 50% of North Americans and Europeans with AIDS and approximately 90% of persons with AIDS in developing countries. A wide variety of pathogens, including viral, fungal, bacterial, and protozoal organisms, can infect the bowel in this population. Identification of the specific etiologic agent has been stressed by many investigators, because specific and very different therapies are available for treatment of bowel infection and such therapies can significantly improve the quality of life in these patients. The toxicity of many agents used to treat these infections also dictates that an accurate and specific diagnosis be obtained when possible. With a thorough diagnostic evaluation, the specific pathogen(s) can be identified in the vast majority of patients (65 to 85%) with diarrhea **(Option (B) is false).**

Recognition that there is a geographic variation in the causes of diarrhea in patients with AIDS is important in helping to determine which pathogens are most likely to be the causative agent of illness in a particular patient **(Option (C) is false).** For example, rotavirus is frequently associated with diarrhea in patients with AIDS in Australia but not in the United States. There are also reported regional differences in the organisms causing gastrointestinal infection within the United States.

Examination of the stool for parasites and culture of stool samples for *Salmonella* species and *Shigella flexneri* are often the first steps in the diagnostic evaluation of patients with AIDS-associated diarrhea. Endoscopic evaluation is performed if further diagnostic evaluation is necessary; it includes mucosal biopsy, which is necessary for the diagnosis of viral pathogens **(Options (D) is true),** and the evaluation for protozoan organisms in the biopsy specimen or fluid. Viral agents, such as CMV, can also be detected by culture, but a positive culture does not differentiate between the presence of CMV and infection by the virus. This full evaluation has been stressed by some investigators; however, others

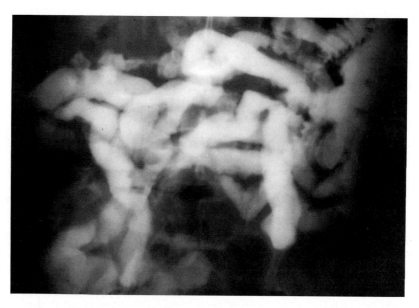

Figure 11-6. Cryptosporidiosis. Sloughing of the mucosa has resulted in a "toothpaste" appearance of the small bowel. (Reprinted with permission from Johanson and Sonnenberg [4].)

believe that a minimal initial evaluation involving only stool culture and symptomatic treatment, with full evaluation reserved for nonresponders, is a more cost-effective and equally efficacious approach. Empirical antibiotic therapy is not recommended because of the wide variety of potential pathogens and the availability of specific treatment and particularly because drug intolerance and drug incompatibility are common in these patients.

Most small bowel infections associated with AIDS do not have specific radiographic findings, and radiology often does not have a definitive role in the evaluation of these patients **(Option (E) is true).** This lack of specific radiographic findings in most patients with small bowel infection is similar to the situation with infection of the colon, as discussed above.

Gastrointestinal pathogens commonly infecting the small bowel include protozoa (*Cryptosporidium* species, *Isospora belli*, and *Enterocytozoon bieneusi* [*Microsporidium*]), bacteria (MAI, *Salmonella* species), and viruses, particularly CMV. Radiologic features of cryptosporidiosis include prominence of mucosal folds and dilatation of the small bowel, affecting the jejunum preferentially or the entire small bowel. Mucosal sloughing, resulting in a "toothpaste" appearance of the small bowel, has also been described in severe cases (Figure 11-6). Characteristic radiologic findings in patients with MAI infection have included findings similar to those seen in patients with Whipple's disease: villous hypertrophy resulting in a prominent fine nodular fold pattern of the small bowel. On CT examination MAI is frequently associated with bulky retroperitoneal or mesenteric adenopathy, which may have low attenuation. Recognition of these patterns is useful, but findings are usually nonspecific and insufficient case material has been accumulated for a number of the causes of infection to allow for definitive radiologic diagnosis.

Unfortunately, many AIDS-associated infections resulting in diarrhea recur after cessation of therapy. Emergence of drug resistance is also a problem. Resistance to *Shigella* and *Campylobacter* species, CMV, and herpes simplex virus has been reported. Nevertheless, thorough diagnostic evaluation and appropriate therapy can significantly reduce morbidity and mortality in this group of patients.

Question 33

Concerning gastrointestinal tumors in patients with AIDS,

    (A) lymphoma arises more commonly in the stomach than in the duodenum
    (B) bowel involvement with lymphoma is infrequent in the absence of nodal disease
    (C) most patients with Kaposi's sarcoma involving the bowel have skin lesions
    (D) submucosal nodules are the characteristic radiologic finding in patients with gastrointestinal Kaposi's sarcoma
    (E) there is a high incidence of anal cancer

Non-Hodgkin's lymphoma and Kaposi's sarcoma are the two most common neoplasms to involve the gastrointestinal tract in patients with AIDS. AIDS-related lymphoma can involve any abdominal organ but most commonly affects the gastrointestinal tract, lymph nodes, liver, kidneys, and adrenal glands. In the series reported by Radin et al. of patients with AIDS-related lymphoma who underwent CT evaluation, the gastrointestinal tract was the most frequent site of extranodal involvement; in this study, gastrointestinal tract involvement occurred in 54% of patients with intra-abdominal lymphoma.

AIDS-related lymphoma involving the bowel can have a variety of appearances, as can lymphoma not associated with AIDS. Infiltrating tumor masses with focal or diffuse bowel wall thickening (Figure 11-4) and masses containing ulceration or central excavation, the so-called cavitary or endoexoenteric forms of lymphoma, are the most common appearances (Figure 11-7). Multiple tumor nodules or discrete polypoid lesions simulating adenocarcinoma have also been reported. The disease commonly involves the stomach, as does non-Hodgkin's lymphoma not

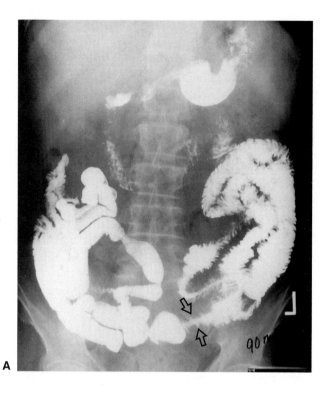

Figure 11-7. Gastrointestinal lymphoma in a patient with AIDS. (A) A radiograph from a small bowel examination demonstrates tumor infiltration of a segment of jejunum, causing irregular fold thickening and segmental narrowing. (B and C) CT scans show the large soft tissue mass involving the affected jejunal segment, with marked luminal irregularity, ulceration, and luminal narrowing.

A

associated with AIDS, but duodenal, small bowel, and colonic involvement are also frequent. In Radin's series, the sites of alimentary tract involvement by lymphoma were distributed as follows: stomach, 15; duodenum, 4; small intestine, 14; colon, 2; rectum, 10; perianal, 7 **(Option (A) is true).** Perianal lymphoma is almost exclusively associated with AIDS (Figure 11-8).

Gastrointestinal involvement with AIDS-related lymphoma can occur in the absence of nodal disease, and the absence of enlarged lymph nodes in association with gastrointestinal masses or focal or diffuse bowel wall thickening should not exclude lymphoma from the differential diagnosis **(Option (B) is false).** As reported by Radin, 51% of patients with gastrointestinal involvement by lymphoma did not have enlarged abdominal lymph nodes.

Kaposi's sarcoma was one of the first unusual neoplasms described as a manifestation of AIDS. It was initially described by Moritz Kaposi in 1872 and was generally seen in men over 50 years of age, often of Jewish or Italian descent; it was clinically manifested as violaceous flat or nodular lesions often limited to the lower extremities, with occasional widespread dissemination. In the early 1980s descriptions of a fulminant

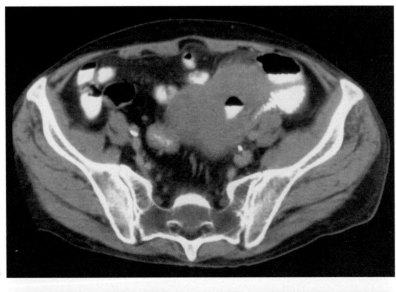

B

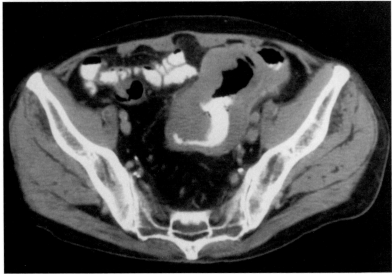

C

form of the disease in homosexual or bisexual young men in New York and California began to appear and helped to define AIDS, now recognized to be caused by infection with HIV, isolated in 1983.

The incidence of Kaposi's sarcoma is significantly higher in homosexual men than among other populations of patients with AIDS, such as drug abusers. Epidemiologic studies suggest a sexually transmitted agent, as yet unidentified, in combination with immunosuppression as a cause of the disease. The incidence of Kaposi's sarcoma is declining, pos-

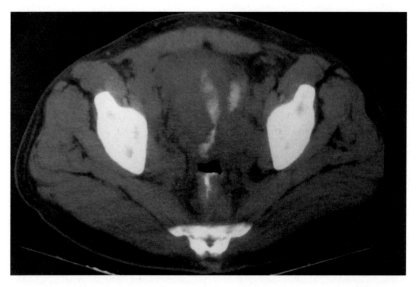

Figure 11-8. Non-Hodgkin's lymphoma associated with AIDS. A bulky tumor mass involves the sigmoid colon and rectum. Perianal and iliac lymphadenopathy are also seen.

sibly as a result of modifications in high-risk sexual behavior in the group at highest risk.

Kaposi's sarcoma can involve almost any organ but most commonly involves the skin, mucous membranes, lymph nodes, and gastrointestinal tract. Most patients (approximately 95%) have skin lesions when gastrointestinal involvement is diagnosed **(Option (C) is true).** Gastrointestinal involvement is seen in approximately 40% of patients with skin lesions of Kaposi's sarcoma, but many affected patients have no symptoms. When present, symptoms are often nonspecific and include rectal pain, diarrhea, bleeding or signs of occult blood loss, and rectal mass. Occasional massive gastrointestinal hemorrhage has been reported. Kaposi's sarcoma is rarely a cause of death in patients with AIDS, however, even when it involves multiple organs.

Lesions of Kaposi's sarcoma can involve the esophagus, but the stomach and small bowel are the most commonly affected sites. The lesions are predominantly submucosal, with later involvement of the mucosa or muscular layers of the bowel. Endoscopically, lesions have been described as vascular-appearing umbilicated nodules, pigmented papules, or telangiectasias of variable size.

The characteristic radiologic findings in patients with Kaposi's sarcoma are discrete submucosal nodules of different sizes but usually less

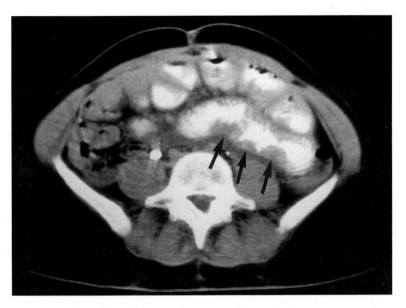

Figure 11-9. Kaposi's sarcoma of the small bowel in a patient with AIDS. A CT scan of the abdomen demonstrates multiple soft tissue nodules (arrows) in the small bowel.

than 2 cm in diameter **(Option (D) is true)** (Figure 11-9). Isolated or confluent mucosal masses with focal areas of submucosal infiltration appearing as plaquelike lesions have been found in the colon.

Lymphoma and Kaposi's sarcoma involving the gastrointestinal tract are common and are the best-documented AIDS-related tumors, but new tumors continue to be described in association with this disease. Multiple tumors of smooth muscle origin involving the lungs, gastrointestinal tract, or both have recently been reported. In addition, patients with AIDS have a documented increased risk of epidermoid anal cancer **(Option (E) is true).** Comparing observed with expected cases of this neoplasm, Melbye et al. reported a relative risk of anal cancer of 84:1 among homosexual patients and 37:7 among non-homosexual patients. Anal epithelial abnormalities have also been described in association with human papillomavirus in homosexual men, with the frequency of anal epithelial dysplasia and atypia higher in men with both HIV and human papillomavirus than in men with either virus alone.

Judith L. Chezmar, M.D.

SUGGESTED READINGS

GASTROINTESTINAL INFECTIONS IN PATIENTS WITH AIDS

1. Balthazar EJ, Megibow AJ, Fazzini E, Opulencia JF, Engel I. Cytomegalovirus colitis in AIDS: radiographic findings in 11 patients. Radiology 1985; 155:585–589
2. Berk RN, Wall SD, McArdle CB, et al. Cryptosporidiosis of the stomach and small intestine in patients with AIDS. AJR 1984; 143:549–554
3. Frager DH, Frager JD, Wolfe EL, et al. Cytomegalovirus colitis in acquired immune deficiency syndrome: radiologic spectrum. Gastrointest Radiol 1986; 11:241–246
4. Johanson JF, Sonnenberg A. Efficient management of diarrhea in the acquired immunodeficiency syndrome (AIDS). A medical decision analysis. Ann Intern Med 1990; 112:942–948
5. Megibow AJ, Wall SD, Balthazar EJ, et al. Gastrointestinal radiology in AIDS patients. In: Federle M, Megibow A, Naidich DP (eds), Radiology of acquired immune deficiency syndrome. New York: Raven Press; 1988:77–105
6. Rene E, Marche C, Chevalier T, et al. Cytomegalovirus colitis in patients with acquired immunodeficiency syndrome. Dig Dis Sci 1988; 33:741–750
7. Smith PD, Quinn TC, Strober W, Janoff EN, Masur H. NIH conference. Gastrointestinal infections in AIDS. Ann Intern Med 1992; 116:63–77
8. Vincent ME, Robbins AH. Mycobacterium avium-intracellulare complex enteritis: pseudo-Whipple disease in AIDS. AJR 1985; 144:921–922
9. Wall SD, Jones B. Gastrointestinal tract in the immunocompromised host: opportunistic infections and other complications. Radiology 1992; 185:327–335
10. Wall SD, Ominsky S, Altman DF, et al. Multifocal abnormalities of the gastrointestinal tract in AIDS. AJR 1986; 146:1–5

AIDS-RELATED NEOPLASMS

11. Buchbinder A, Friedman-Kien AE. Clinical aspects of epidemic Kaposi's sarcoma. Cancer Surv 1991; 10:39–52
12. Melbye M, Cote TR, Kessler L, Gail M, Biggar RJ. High incidence of anal cancer among AIDS patients. The AIDS/Cancer Working Group. Lancet 1994; 343:636–639
13. Nyberg DA, Jeffrey RB Jr, Federle MP, Bottles K, Abrams DI. AIDS-related lymphomas: evaluation by abdominal CT. Radiology 1986; 159:59–63
14. Radin DR, Esplin JA, Levine AM, Ralls PW. AIDS-related non-Hodgkin's lymphoma: abdominal CT findings in 112 patients. AJR 1993; 160:1133–1139
15. Radin DR, Kiyabu M. Multiple smooth-muscle tumors of the colon and adrenal gland in an adult with AIDS. AJR 1992; 159:545–546
16. Rose HS, Balthazar EJ, Megibow AJ, Horowitz L, Laubenstein LJ. Alimentary tract involvement in Kaposi sarcoma: radiographic and endoscopic findings in 25 homosexual men. AJR 1982; 139:661–666

Notes

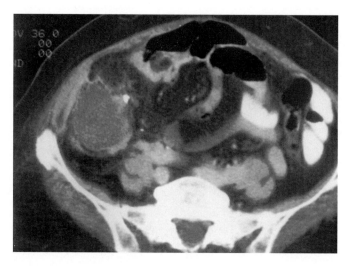

Figure 12-1. This 47-year-old man has fever and right lower quadrant pain. You are shown a postcontrast CT scan of the lower abdomen.

Case 12: Periappendiceal Abscess

Question 34

Which *one* of the following is the MOST likely diagnosis?

(A) Ruptured cecal carcinoma
(B) Ruptured cecal diverticulum
(C) Periappendiceal phlegmon
(D) Periappendiceal abscess
(E) Mucocele of the appendix

The primary abnormality demonstrated in the test image (Figure 12-1) is a well-defined fluid-density mass in the right iliac fossa, which is associated with a punctate calcification (Figure 12-2). Given the patient's history of fever and right lower quadrant pain, an inflammatory process seems the most likely explanation. The low attenuation of the lesion and its mass effect are consistent with an abscess. A large number of pathologic processes (e.g., Crohn's disease, tuberculosis, and diverticulitis) can result in right lower quadrant abscesses; however, the presence of an associated punctate calcification (appendicolith) is virtually diagnostic of a periappendiceal abscess **(Option (D) is correct).** In the absence of an appendicolith, a specific diagnosis often cannot be made for many right lower quadrant inflammatory lesions. Further evaluation with a barium enema or colonoscopy is often required to establish the diagnosis in such patients.

A ruptured cecal carcinoma (Option (A)) (Figure 12-3) or ruptured diverticulum of the right colon (Option (B)) (Figure 12-4) can result in CT findings similar to those associated with a perforated appendix (focal bowel wall thickening and surrounding inflammatory changes). However, the visualization of an appendicolith in the test image establishes the diagnosis of appendicitis and makes these other entities much less likely. Narrow (5-mm) collimated scans through the iliac fossa can aid in the visualization of a small appendicolith (Figure 12-5). In the absence of an appendicolith, the location of the inflammatory process can aid in the differential diagnosis. Phlegmons or abscesses immediately adjacent to

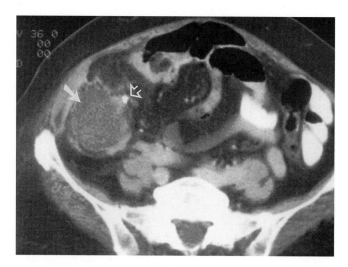

Figure 12-2 (Same as Figure 12-1). A contrast-enhanced CT scan demonstrates a well-defined low-density mass in the right iliac fossa (solid arrow). Note the adjacent punctate calcification (open arrow) representing an appendicolith. This combination of findings strongly suggests the diagnosis of a periappendiceal abscess.

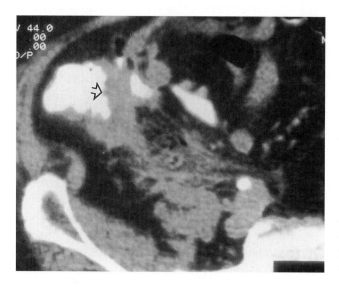

Figure 12-3. Ruptured cecal carcinoma. Note the focal wall thickening of the medial aspect of the cecum (arrow) with surrounding edema of pericecal fat.

the cecal tip are commonly related to appendicitis. Phlegmons (Option (C)) are solid inflammatory masses of the omentum and mesentery (Figure 12-6). They are of soft tissue density (>30 HU) rather than fluid density on CT. The low-density mass in the test patient (Figure 12-1) is most

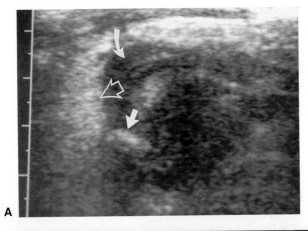

A

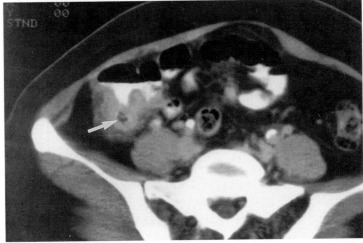

B

Figure 12-4. Ruptured cecal diverticulum. (A) A transverse sonogram of the cecum demonstrates an echogenic cecal diverticulum (straight arrow) within a thickened cecal wall (curved arrow). Note the edematous, echogenic pericecal fat (open arrow). (B) A CT scan reveals gas-forming infection within the cecal diverticulum (arrow). Note the thickened cecal wall and edema of adjacent fat.

consistent with a liquefied abscess rather than a phlegmon. However, when no appendicolith is identified, a contrast enema is routinely performed to distinguish other lesions (cecal diverticulitis, carcinoma, Crohn's disease, etc.) from appendicitis. The contrast enema does not have to be performed urgently and can be deferred until the acute inflammatory process has begun to resolve 24 to 48 hours later.

Patients with mucocele of the appendix (Option (E)) often have mild, generally chronic right lower quadrant pain. They rarely present with

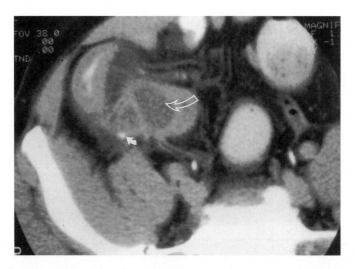

Figure 12-5. Small appendicolith identified by 5-mm collimated CT scanning. Note the low-density abscess (open arrow) and adjacent tiny appendicolith (solid arrow). The abscess cavity was less than 3 cm in diameter. The patient responded to antibiotic therapy alone and did not require surgery or percutaneous drainage.

acute symptoms. On CT and sonography, mucoceles typically appear as rounded or tubular cystic masses at the base of the cecum (Figures 12-7 and 12-8). Mucoceles of the appendix can demonstrate curvilinear mural calcification (Figure 12-7), but they are not associated with the typical punctate or lamellated calcification of an appendicolith.

The imaging workup of a patient with suspected appendicitis has been a topic of controversy in the last decade. Many patients, particularly young males, with classic signs and symptoms of acute appendicitis (i.e., midepigastric pain migrating to the right lower quadrant, fever, and leukocytosis) require no preoperative imaging. However, imaging is indicated in any patient in whom the clinical diagnosis is in doubt; this includes patients with unusual patterns of abdominal pain, patients without fever, or patients with normal or equivocal laboratory test results. Imaging should also be considered for female patients in their reproductive years. Clinical experience indicates that these patients frequently exhibit signs and symptoms mimicking those of appendicitis that are due to other pathologic processes, often of gynecologic origin.

Once it has been decided to perform further imaging, three major radiologic examinations should be considered: graded-compression sonography, CT, and contrast enema.

Sonography with graded compression is an accurate means of diagnosing appendicitis; several series report sensitivity and specificity val-

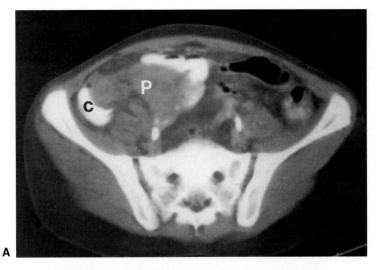

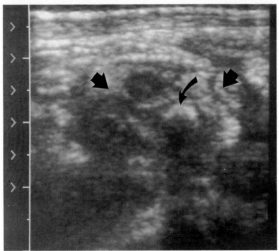

Figure 12-6. Periappendiceal phlegmon in two different patients. (A) A contrast-enhanced CT scan demonstrates an inflammatory mass of soft tissue density adjacent to the cecum (c), representing a periappendiceal phlegmon (P). The inflammatory mass is isodense with adjacent muscle and shows no areas of liquefied pus. (B) A transverse sonogram of the right lower quadrant in another patient demonstrates a poorly defined mass (straight arrows) of mixed echogenicity. Echogenic components represent inflamed fat. Note the appendicoliths within the phlegmon (curved arrow).

ues greater than 90%. Advantages specific to sonography are its ability to (1) define all layers of the bowel wall, (2) provide real-time observation of peristalsis and bowel compressibility, (3) rapidly evaluate both the abdo-

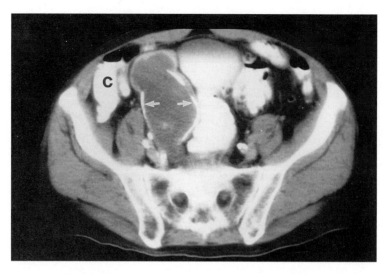

Figure 12-7. Mucocele of the appendix. Note the tubular low-density mass near the base of the cecum (c). Curvilinear calcification is present in the walls of the mucocele (arrows).

men and pelvis using both transabdominal and endovaginal techniques, and (4) provide direct correlation of imaging abnormalities with the site of pain. As pointed out in the study of Gaensler et al., sonography has considerable potential to establish an alternative diagnosis when the clinical suspicion of appendicitis is not borne out. However, sonography has several drawbacks as well. The sensitivity and specificity values reported above are only applicable in centers where there is considerable experience with the method. Moreover, in obese patients, it is difficult to perform adequate graded compression and it can be impossible to define the cecum and appendix. When abscesses are present, sonography is poor in defining their precise location and extent, particularly if the abscesses have a significant retroperitoneal component or contain gas. Practice guidelines differ at various institutions; however, sonography is ideally suited for thin to average-sized patients who are not clinically suspected of having appendiceal perforation.

CT has a number of potential advantages. The ability of CT to display abdominal and pelvic anatomy is relatively uninfluenced by patient size, the presence of gas overlying areas of interest, or the technical skill of the operator. Its contrast sensitivity allows observation of relatively subtle soft tissue stranding within inflamed mesenteric or pericolic fat, a finding that may be difficult to perceive sonographically. The full extent of fluid collections is optimally displayed by CT. Its drawbacks include (1)

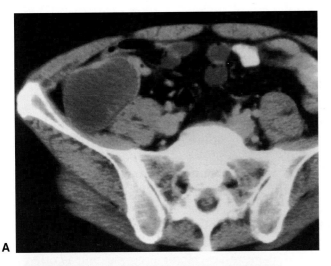

A

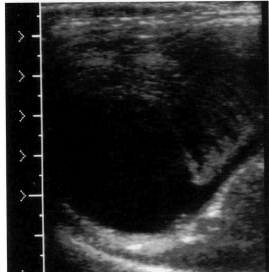

B

Figure 12-8. Mucocele of the appendix. A CT scan of the right lower quadrant (A) and a transverse sonogram (B) demonstrate a rounded cystic mass at the base of the cecum.

ionizing radiation exposure, a factor of some concern in any young patient and particularly in young women of reproductive age; (2) reduced accessibility in the emergency room situation; and (3) relatively poor specificity in making gynecologic diagnoses. Patients most likely to profit from CT examinations include those with signs and symptoms of abscess clinically amenable to percutaneous drainage and those with a confusing clinical picture unlikely to be related to gynecologic pathology. CT is more often the imaging method of choice in obese patients or if perforation is likely. Patients with appendiceal perforation often have a clinical history of right lower quadrant pain and fever lasting longer than 48 hours. It should be noted, however, that fever and leukocytosis can be minimal or absent in immunocompromised patients with appendicitis or periappendiceal abscess.

Contrast-enhanced CT can differentiate a liquefied abscess from a phlegmon more readily than can sonography. Unlike phlegmons, lique-fied abscesses demonstrate little or no enhancement with intravenous administration of contrast agent. CT can also define the extraperitoneal extension of a periappendiceal abscess better than can sonography.

The importance of the contrast enema in the evaluation of suspected appendicitis has diminished in recent years, since sonography and CT have become clinically accepted. The major advantage of the contrast enema is that complete filling of the appendix absolutely excludes the diagnosis of appendicitis. When appendicitis is not present, the contrast enema provides information about other colonic processes but is other-wise not helpful in establishing an alternative diagnosis. Other draw-backs include lack of information about pericolonic tissues, so that the presence and extent of an abscess can only be based on inferential evi-dence. Moreover, retained contrast material within the colon after the performance of the enema can prevent subsequent CT examination. The major role for the contrast enema is in those relatively infrequent cir-cumstances in which a colonic disease other than appendicitis is clini-cally suspected.

Question 35

Concerning periappendiceal inflammatory masses,

(A) percutaneous drainage of periappendiceal phlegmons is contraindicated

(B) small (1- to 2-cm) periappendiceal abscesses can be treated successfully with broad-spectrum intravenous antibiotics

(C) percutaneous drainage of periappendiceal abscesses has a complication rate of less than 10%

(D) fistulas to the cecum or base of the appendix are commonly demonstrated on immediate post-drainage abscess sinograms

(E) fistulas to the cecum or base of the appendix rarely close without operative intervention

Percutaneous drainage of periappendiceal abscesses is a safe and ef-fective alternative to surgery. Contrast-enhanced CT is often essential for patient selection because of its accuracy in defining the nature and extent of the inflammatory process. CT is also helpful in identifying an appropriate access route for percutaneous catheter insertion (Figure

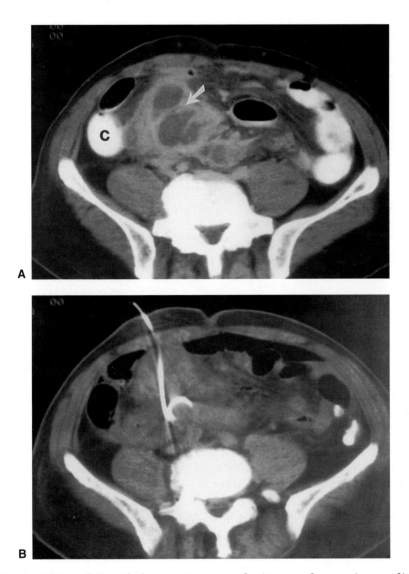

Figure 12-9. CT-guided percutaneous drainage of a periappendiceal abscess. (A) A CT scan demonstrates an abscess (arrow) adjacent to the cecum (c). (B) Note that the percutaneous catheter (arrow) has been inserted into the abscess cavity without traversing the bowel. The abscess has been completely evacuated.

12-9). By definition, periappendiceal phlegmons (Figure 12-6) do not contain liquefied pus, so patients with phlegmons are not candidates for percutaneous catheter drainage **(Option (A) is true).** Patients with phlegmons often respond to intravenous therapy with broad-spectrum antibiotics. Similarly, most patients with small periappendiceal ab-

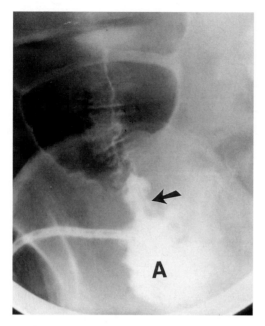

Figure 12-10. Cecal fistula following percutaneous drainage of a periappendiceal abscess. Contrast injected via a percutaneous drainage catheter 3 days after the initial drainage procedure fills the abscess cavity (A). The abscess communicates with the cecum through the base of the appendix (arrow). The fistula closed spontaneously with a combination of intravenous antibiotics and percutaneous drainage.

scesses (1 to 2 cm) do well with intravenous antibiotic therapy alone (Figure 12-5) **(Option (B) is true).** In our series, 28 of 32 small abscesses were managed successfully with antibiotic therapy alone. A trial of intravenous antibiotic therapy should continue for at least 72 hours, since even patients who are responding may not defervesce immediately. Complications of percutaneous drainage of periappendiceal abscesses are infrequent; they include post-procedural bacteremia, hemorrhage, inadvertent bowel perforation, and delayed abscess recurrence. In general, complications occur in fewer than 10% of patients **(Option (C) is true).**

Immediately after percutaneous drainage, injection of a small amount of contrast material into the abscess via the catheter frequently fails to demonstrate an underlying communication to the appendix or cecum **(Option (D) is false).** In fact, high-pressure catheter injections performed immediately after insertion of a drainage catheter are contraindicated, because there is some likelihood of inducing sepsis. The track often does not fill during a low-volume, low-pressure injection because of the inflammatory debris and edema in the vicinity of the fistula. However, abscess sinography repeated 3 to 4 days after the initial drainage shows that approximately 45% of patients have an underlying appendiceal or cecal fistula (Figure 12-10). These fistulas generally have low output (≤50 mL/day) and close spontaneously within 10 days when treated with a combination of percutaneous drainage and antibiotic therapy **(Option (E) is false).** The catheter must be left in place, however, until fistula closure is documented by follow-up abscess sinography. Recurrence of periappendiceal abscess can be due to an unrecognized fistula and premature catheter withdrawal. Patients with higher-output fistulas typically require prolonged catheter drainage and are better managed with operative repair.

Question 36

Concerning mucoceles of the appendix,

    (A) they are found in approximately 5% of all appendectomy specimens
    (B) the most common CT appearance is a tubular low-density mass
    (C) they are a cause of enteroenteric intussusception
    (D) they are associated with pseudomyxoma peritonei

Pathologically, a mucocele of the appendix represents a dilated appendiceal lumen filled with mucus. The diameter of the mucocele is generally 3 to 6 cm. Obstruction of the base of the appendix is the etiology of mucocele in most patients. An appendicolith or postinflammatory scarring from appendicitis is the most common cause. Other obstructing lesions such as a cecal carcinoma, an appendiceal carcinoma, or an appendiceal polyp can result in a mucocele. Appendiceal cystadenomas or cystadenocarcinomas are occasionally associated with a dilated mucus-filled appendix. It is uncertain whether a cystadenoma or cystadenocarcinoma first develops and then obstructs the lumen of the appendix or whether the mucosal lining of an obstructed appendix undergoes neoplastic degeneration and evolves into a cystadenoma or cystadenocarcinoma. Radiographically visible calcification in the wall of a mucocele is not uncommon (Figure 12-7).

Mucoceles are rare, occurring in only 0.2 to 0.3% of all appendectomy specimens **(Option (A) is false).** A preoperative diagnosis of an appendiceal mucocele can be established on the basis of typical CT and sonographic findings. On CT, a mucocele is a tubular low-density mass at the cecal tip **(Option (B) is true).** On sonography, mucoceles are complex cystic masses. Echogenic mucoid material is present within a tubular mass with well-defined walls. Mucoceles occasionally serve as the lead point for intussusception **(Option (C) is true).** If a cystic mass is identified by CT or sonography in a patient with an intussusception of the right or transverse colon, a mucocele of the appendix should be a strong candidate as the etiology (Figure 12-11).

An important complication of appendiceal mucoceles is peritoneal rupture. This results in pseudomyxoma peritonei, which is an accumula-

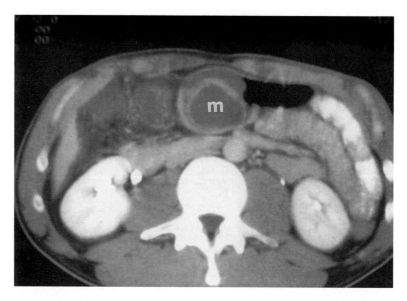

Figure 12-11. Mucocele of the appendix causing intussusception. Note the cystic mass (m) within the lumen of the transverse colon, representing an intussuscepting mucocele.

tion of gelatinous material throughout the peritoneal cavity (Figure 12-12) **(Option (D) is true).** Both benign and malignant mucoceles can cause pseudomyxoma peritonei. Cystic peritoneal implants from pseudomyxoma peritonei often cause subtle mass effect with scalloping of the contour of the liver or spleen. Small bowel obstruction is often a recurrent problem in patients with malignant peritoneal implants.

R. Brooke Jeffrey, M.D.

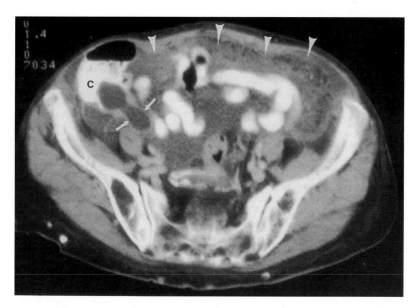

Figure 12-12.   Pseudomyxoma peritonei due to mucinous carcinoma of the appendix. CT section at the level of the pelvic brim in an elderly woman with complaints of increasing abdominal girth shows a low-attenuation flask-shaped collection (arrows) originating from the posteromedial aspect of the cecum (C). Amorphous soft tissue attenuation material is present throughout the peritoneal space (arrowheads).

SUGGESTED READINGS

APPENDICITIS AND PERIAPPENDICEAL ABSCESS

1. Balthazar EJ, Birnbaum BA, Yee J, Megibow AJ, Roshkow J, Gray C. Acute appendicitis: CT and US correlation in 100 patients. Radiology 1994; 190:31–35

2. Balthazar EJ, Megibow AJ, Siegel SE, Birnbaum BA. Appendicitis: prospective evaluation with high-resolution CT. Radiology 1991; 180:21–24

3. Brown JJ. Acute appendicitis: the radiologist's role. Radiology 1991; 180:13–14

4. Gaensler EH, Jeffrey RB Jr, Laing FC, Townsend RR. Sonography in patients with suspected acute appendicitis: value in establishing alternative diagnoses. AJR 1989; 152:49–51

5. Jeffrey RB Jr. Management of the periappendiceal inflammatory mass. Semin US CT MR 1989; 10:341–347

6. Jeffrey RB Jr, Laing FC, Lewis FR. Acute appendicitis: high-resolution real-time US findings. Radiology 1987; 163:11–14

7. Malone AJ Jr, Wolf CR, Malmed AS, Melliere BF. Diagnosis of acute appendicitis: value of unenhanced CT. AJR 1993; 160:763–766

8. Puylaert JB. Acute appendicitis: US evaluation using graded compression. Radiology 1986; 158:355–360

9. vanSonnenberg E, Wittich GR, Casola G, et al. Periappendiceal abscesses: percutaneous drainage. Radiology 1987; 163:23–26

10. Wong CH, Trinh TM, Robbins AN, Rowen SJ, Cohen AJ. Diagnosis of appendicitis: imaging findings in patients with atypical clinical features. AJR 1993; 161:1199–1203

APPENDICEAL MUCOCELE

11. Dachman AH, Lichtenstein JE, Friedman AC. Mucocele of the appendix and pseudomyxoma peritonei. AJR 1985; 144:923–929

12. Madwed D, Mindelzun R, Jeffrey RB Jr. Mucocele of the appendix: imaging findings. AJR 1992; 159:69–72

Notes

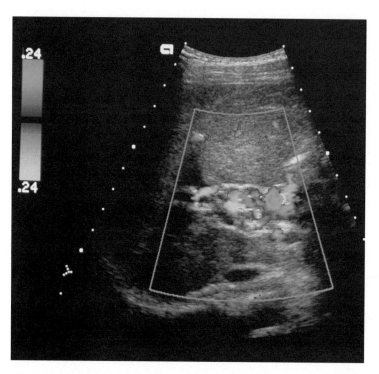

Figure 13-1. This 64-year-old alcoholic man has abnormal liver function tests. You are shown an oblique color Doppler sonogram of the porta hepatis.

Case 13: Cavernous Transformation of the Portal Vein

Question 37

Which *one* of the following is the MOST likely diagnosis?

  (A) Cavernous transformation of the portal vein
  (B) Acute portal vein thrombosis
  (C) Hepatic artery aneurysm
  (D) Pylephlebitis
  (E) Periportal adenopathy

The color Doppler sonogram in the test patient (Figure 13-1) demonstrates numerous color-coded vessels in the porta hepatis and no main extrahepatic portal vein. These findings (Figure 13-2) are typical of cavernous transformation of the portal vein **(Option (A) is correct).** In patients with cavernous transformation, the main extrahepatic portal vein is thrombosed and is often not identifiable as a discrete structure. Numerous collateral veins are present in the hepatoduodenal ligament and porta hepatis. Color Doppler sonography can rapidly determine the patency and direction of flow within abdominal blood vessels. In the test image, the varices have different color coding due to their different flow directions. In normal patients, the hepatic artery and portal vein have similar flow direction and will be color coded the same.

Gray-scale sonographic findings in acute portal vein thrombosis (Option (B)) include demonstration of an echogenic intraluminal mass and enlargement of the thrombosed segment of the vein; color flow Doppler imaging or spectral waveform analysis shows absence of flow in cases of complete venous obstruction (Figure 13-3). Pitfalls of gray-scale sonography include the presence of artifactual echoes mimicking a thrombus as well as slow flow (common in patients with portal hypertension) that is below the threshold for observation by Doppler sonographic methods. Early in the evolution of acute portal vein thrombosis, extensive collateral vessels would not be an expected finding.

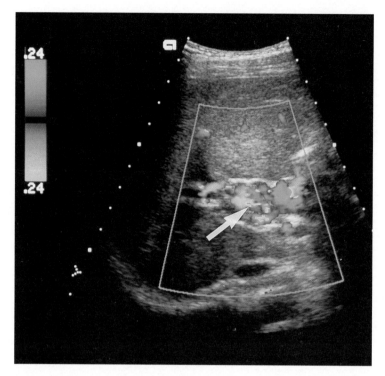

Figure 13-2 (Same as Figure 13-1). Cavernous transformation of the portal vein. An oblique color Doppler sonogram demonstrates numerous color-coded varices in the porta hepatis (arrow) without a normal extrahepatic portal vein. These findings are diagnostic of cavernous transformation.

An aneurysm of the hepatic artery (Option (C)) would not be associated with the extensive collateral vasculature demonstrated on the test image and would be identified as a rounded cystic mass adjacent to a normal extrahepatic portal vein. Spectral Doppler tracings obtained from within the cystic mass would demonstrate an arterial waveform (Figure 13-4). True aneurysms of the hepatic artery are rare; etiologies include atherosclerotic disease and vasculitis (particularly polyarteritis nodosa). Hepatic artery pseudoaneurysms are far more common in clinical practice. The most common etiologies include pancreatitis, penetrating trauma, and percutaneous interventional procedures such as percutaneous biliary drainage. Treatment of these pseudoaneurysms should be performed by angiographic embolization whenever feasible.

Pylephlebitis (Option (D)) from portal venous bacteremia can result in septic thrombosis of the portal vein (Figure 13-5). The radiologic (CT, sonographic, or MR) findings are similar to those in patients with acute

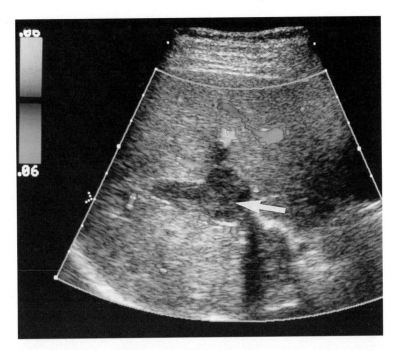

Figure 13-3. Acute thrombosis of the portal vein. An oblique color Doppler sonogram demonstrates low-level echoes within the portal vein (arrow) without evidence of color Doppler flow. The patient had progressively abnormal liver function tests following splenectomy.

portal vein thrombosis due to other etiologies (Figures 13-3 and 13-6). If the infected thrombus does not lyse, pylephlebitis can ultimately result in cavernous transformation.

Periportal adenopathy (Option (E)) can be readily excluded in the test patient, because all of the structures in the porta hepatis are vessels, as evidenced by their color Doppler flow signals. On noncontrast CT, periportal vessels can mimic lymphadenopathy; therefore, use of intravenous contrast enhancement to establish the CT diagnosis of cavernous transformation is essential.

Portal vein thrombosis is most typically seen in conditions with chronically reduced portal blood flow (such as cirrhosis), with acute inflammation (pancreatitis or pyelonephritis), or with clotting disorders. When there is occlusion to flow within the main portal vein, collateral vessels within the hepatoduodenal ligament are recruited to re-establish blood flow to the liver. These collaterals enlarge with time and eventually replace the ligamentous portion of the portal vein. This tangle of collateral vessels that lies along the course of the portal vein has been termed "cavernous transformation" or portal cavernoma. The time sequence over

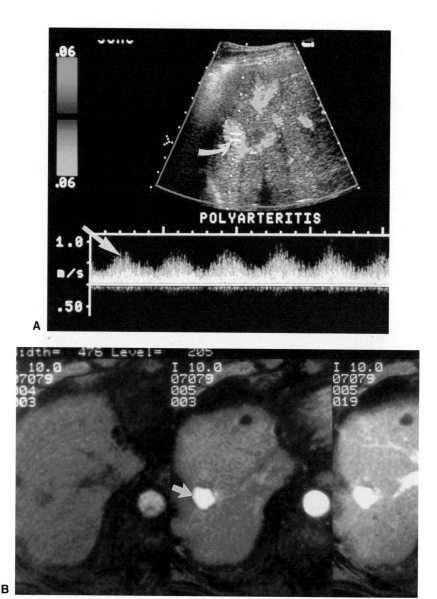

Figure 13-4. Hepatic artery aneurysm associated with vasculitis. (A) A color Doppler sonogram reveals an arterial waveform (straight arrow) within the peripheral hepatic artery aneurysm (curved arrow). (B) A dynamic postcontrast MR scan demonstrates intense enhancement of the aneurysm (arrow) during the arterial phase of the injection.

which cavernous transformation develops is not completely known; however, cases of acute portal vein thrombosis suggest that small collateral veins can be identified within the hepatoduodenal ligament or in the

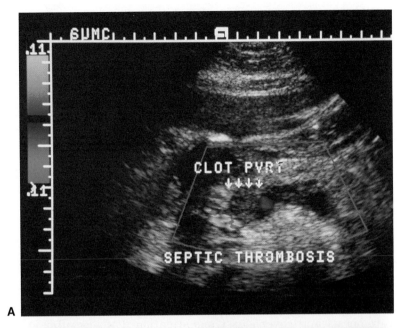

A

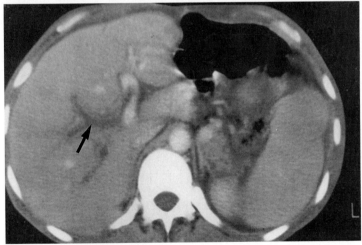

B

Figure 13-5. Pylephlebitis (septic thrombosis of the portal vein) in two patients. (A) A color Doppler sonogram of the splenic-portal venous confluence demonstrates an echogenic clot (arrows) involving the extra-hepatic portal vein and the splenic vein. (B) A postcontrast CT scan in another patient demonstrates low-density thrombosis. The thrombus extends throughout the right portal venous system into the ascending left portal vein (arrow). The thrombosis in the patient in panel A did not resolve with antibiotic therapy, and the process progressed to cavernous transformation. The patient in panel B responded well to antibiotic therapy, and the follow-up studies showed that thrombus had completely lysed.

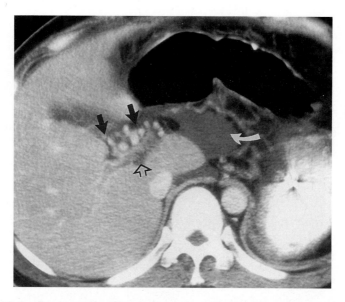

Figure 13-6. Periportal collaterals in a patient with cavernous transformation of acute portal vein thrombosis. The patient developed portal vein thrombosis and cavernous transformation 3 weeks after splenectomy. A postcontrast CT scan demonstrates numerous periportal collaterals (black arrows). Note the thrombosed main and right portal veins with low-density thrombus (open arrow). Fluid is also evident in the lesser sac (curved white arrow).

gallbladder fossa within 3 to 4 days. CT findings include the absence of a definitive portal vein and the presence of numerous blood-density structures within the porta hepatis. Findings within the hepatic parenchyma depend on the extent of intraportal clot (Figure 13-7). When a lobar branch of the portal system is involved along with the main portal vein, that lobe will exhibit hyperdense enhancement during the arterial phase of hepatic imaging. If both lobar branches are involved, imaging during the arterial phase demonstrates peripheral hepatic hyperdensity (see Case 26). MRI is similarly capable of demonstrating the characteristic serpentine vessels that are diagnostic of this entity (Figure 13-8).

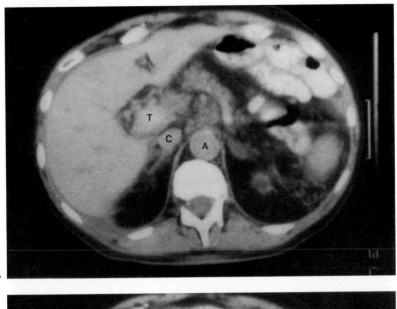

A

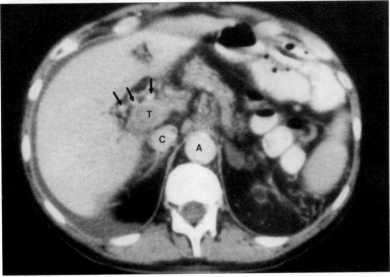

B

Figure 13-7. Acute portal vein thrombosis. (A) A CT section at the level of the porta hepatis, obtained prior to the administration of intravenous contrast agent, shows portal venous thrombus. Its attenuation is higher than that of the flowing blood within the aorta and inferior vena cava. (B) A CT section at the same level after administration of intravenous contrast agent shows no change in the attenuation of the portal venous thrombus (T), but it does show the expected rise in attenuation of the flowing blood in the aorta (A) and inferior vena cava (C). Note the enhancement of multiple small collateral vessels (arrows) within the hepatoduodenal ligament. T = portal venous thrombus; A = aorta; C= inferior vena cava.

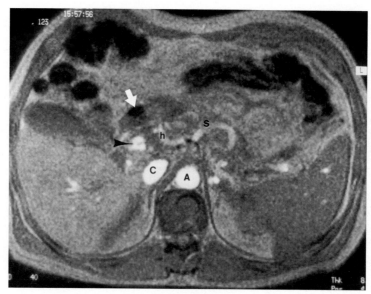

GRE 50/8/40°

Figure 13-8. Cavernous transformation of the portal vein. An MR section obtained during a single breath-hold (flow-sensitive image) obtained through the inferior aspect of the hepatoduodenal ligament shows absence of signal (arrow) in the expected position of the portal vein. Flow is observed within multiple small collateral vessels (arrowhead), which comprise the cavernous transformation. A = aorta; C = inferior vena cava; h = hepatic artery; s = splenic artery.

Question 38

Concerning portal vein thrombosis,

(A) septic thrombosis is associated with *Bacteroides fragilis* septicemia
(B) signal within the portal vein on spin-echo MR images is diagnostic for thrombosis
(C) duplex sonography demonstrating arterial flow within a portal vein thrombus suggests tumor thrombosis
(D) its high intensity on T2-weighted spin-echo MR images is due to extracellular methemoglobin
(E) on noncontrast CT, acute thrombus in the portal vein has an attenuation lower than flowing blood

The clinical diagnosis of portal vein thrombosis is often imprecise. There are often no obvious signs or symptoms. Portal vein thrombosis can be suspected on the basis of increasing ascites due to extrahepatic portal hypertension. There can be clinical evidence of a hypercoagulable state such as polycythemia. It is not uncommon, however, for the diagnosis to be established first by CT or sonography. Thrombosis of the portal vein is associated with a wide variety of disorders including pancreatitis, hypercoagulable states, neoplastic invasion, and pylephlebitis. It can occur after splenectomy as a result of thrombocytosis. Pylephlebitis results from portal venous bacteremia typically associated with appendicitis or diverticulitis. *Bacteroides fragilis* and *Escherichia coli* are the most common organisms associated with septic thrombosis of the portal vein **(Option (A) is true)**. *Bacteroides* species can promote clot formation by elaborating enzymes that are potent coagulants.

Color Doppler sonography and MRI are both accurate techniques for diagnosis of portal vein thrombosis. On spin-echo MR images, however, the presence of signal within the portal vein is not diagnostic for portal vein thrombosis **(Option (B) is false)**. Slowly flowing blood in the portal vein can cause intraluminal signal (Figure 13-9A). Other causes of intraluminal vascular signal not related to thrombosis include entry-slice flow-related enhancement and even-echo rephasing. Confirmation of suspected portal vein thrombosis on spin-echo imaging is often best performed with either gradient-recalled sequences or imaging after intravenous administration of gadolinium, similar to contrast-enhanced CT (Figure 13-9B). On gradient-recalled images, areas of normal portal flow, even if relatively slow, appear as bright signal. Similarly, with gadolinium enhancement the portal vessels will demonstrate a uniform increase in signal compared with nonenhanced scans. Thrombus will appear as an intraluminal filling defect within the enhancing portal vein (Figure 13-10). Neoplasms invading the portal vein can demonstrate enhancement of tumor thrombus on postcontrast MRI. Tumor thrombus can also be diagnosed if arterial flow is identified within a thrombus by duplex sonography **(Option (C) is true)**.

The appearance of blood on CT images depends on its physical state. Acute hemorrhage has the same composition as flowing blood and therefore exhibits the same attenuation value. However, as the blood forms a clot (or thrombus), the serous elements within the plasma are squeezed out; since the attenuation of the elements thus removed is low (on the order of 20 to 30 HU), this process has the effect of increasing the attenuation of the clot. Hence, an acute portal vein thrombus is more dense than flowing blood on a noncontrast CT scan **(Option (E) is false)**. This effect continues until the clot is lysed, a process that may take place quickly, in a vessel (such as the portal vein) or in a mesothelium-lined space such as the pleura or peritoneum, or slowly, within a confined space (such as the musculature of the abdominal wall). Whatever the

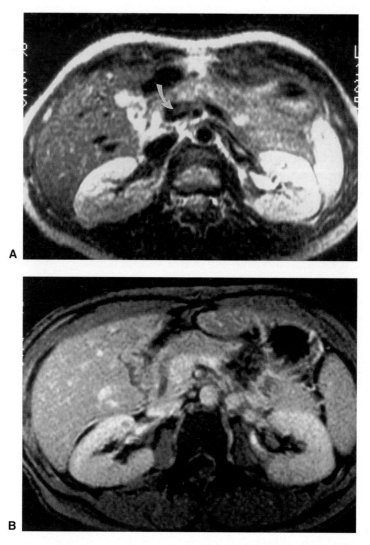

Figure 13-9. Slowly flowing blood in the portal vein. (A) A T2-weighted spin-echo image demonstrates intravascular signal within the portal vein (arrow) as a result of slow flow. (B) A postcontrast dynamic MR scan demonstrates no evidence of thrombus in the portal vein.

rate of lysis, the process steadily decreases the average attenuation values within the clot or thrombus.

The appearance of blood on MR images is more complex; it depends both on the physical state and the chemical composition of the blood components. Specifically, the T1 and T2 signal intensity characteristics depend on the chemical structure of the hemoglobin molecule and the

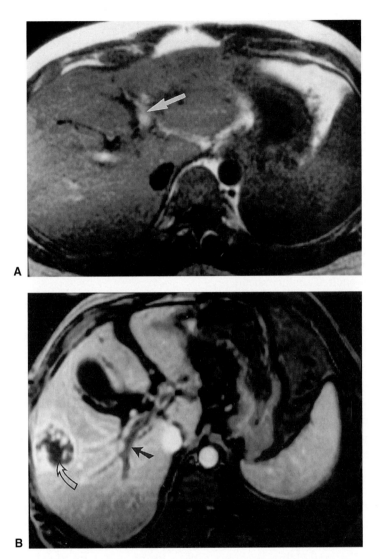

Figure 13-10. Subacute portal vein thrombosis in two patients. (A) A T1-weighted MR image demonstrates high-intensity thrombus within the ascending left portal vein (arrow). (B) In another patient, a multiplanar spoiled-GRASS MR image obtained after administration of gadolinium DTPA demonstrates low-intensity thrombus within the posterior branch of the right portal vein (solid arrow). The patient had septic thrombosis. Note the adjacent liver abscess (curved open arrow).

rate at which its degradation products develop. Although the time course of these chemical transformations is well documented for the central nervous system, it has yet to be established for extracerebral sites. The

Table 13-1: MR appearance of blood breakdown products

Blood component	MR appearance
Oxyhemoglobin	No magnetic effect
Deoxyhemoglobin	T1 dark
Intracellular methemoglobin	T1 bright, T2 dark
Extracellular methemoglobin	T1 bright, T2 bright
Hemosiderin	T2 dark (superparamagnetic effect)

description that follows therefore does not attempt to specify the precise timing of each transformation.

After blood exits the vascular compartment, the oxyhemoglobin molecules within the erythrocytes begin to lose oxygen to the surrounding tissues and are transformed into deoxyhemoglobin. Deoxyhemoglobin is a paramagnetic substance; however, its geometric configuration inhibits the close interaction of surrounding water molecules with the iron and, accordingly, T1 shortening does not occur. Within a few days, the ferrous ion in hemoglobin is oxidized to ferric ion and the molecule becomes methemoglobin. This structural change is accompanied by the loss of the hydrophobic effect described above. The magnetic effect of methemoglobin depends on whether it is bound within the erythrocyte or free within the extracellular space. Intracellular methemoglobin produces a marked degree of T1 shortening, resulting in hyperintensity on T1-weighted images. Because they are distributed inhomogeneously, they exert local magnetic field effects that result in shortening of T2. This translates to reduced signal on T2-weighted images. With time, the erythrocytes lyse and the methemoglobin becomes extracellular. Since its distribution in the extracellular fluid is homogeneous, it no longer produces local field effects and therefore does not shorten the T2 of water protons. Accordingly, T2-weighted images obtained when methemoglobin is extracellular show hyperintensity **(Option (D) is true)**. A summary of the chemical forms of hemoglobin and of blood breakdown products and their MR effects is given in Table 13-1.

R. Brooke Jeffrey, M.D.

SUGGESTED READINGS

1. Levy HM, Newhouse JH. MR imaging of portal vein thrombosis. AJR 1988; 151:283–286
2. Lim GM, Jeffrey RB Jr, Ralls PW, Marn CS. Septic thrombosis of the portal vein: CT and clinical observations. J Comput Assist Tomogr 1989; 13:656–658
3. Marn CS, Francis IR. CT of portal venous occlusion. AJR 1992; 159:717–726
4. Martin K, Balfe DM, Lee JK. Computed tomography of portal vein thrombosis: unusual appearances and pitfalls in diagnosis. J Comput Assist Tomogr 1989; 13:811–816
5. Martinoli C, Cittadini G, Pastorino C, et al. Gradient echo MRI of portal vein thrombosis. J Comput Assist Tomogr 1992; 16:226–234
6. Mathieu D, Vasile N, Dibie C, Grenier P. Portal cavernoma: dynamic CT features and transient differences in hepatic attenuation. Radiology 1985; 154:743–748
7. Miller VE, Berland LL. Pulsed Doppler duplex sonography and CT of portal vein thrombosis. AJR 1985; 145:73–76
8. Mori H, Hayashi K, Uetani M, Matsuoka Y, Iwao M, Maeda H. High-attenuation recent thrombus of the portal vein: CT demonstration and clinical significance. Radiology 1987; 163:353–356
9. Parvey HR, Raval B, Sandler CM. Portal vein thrombosis: imaging findings. AJR 1994; 162:77–81
10. Ralls PW. Color Doppler sonography of the hepatic artery and portal venous system. AJR 1990; 155:517–525
11. Silverman PM, Patt RH, Garra BS, et al. MR imaging of the portal venous system: value of gradient-echo imaging as an adjunct to spin-echo imaging. AJR 1991; 157:297–302
12. Zirinsky K, Markisz JA, Rubenstein WA, et al. MR imaging of portal venous thrombosis: correlation with CT and sonography. AJR 1988; 150:283–288

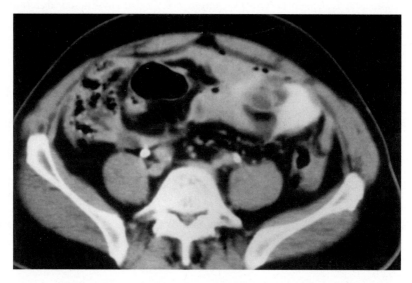

Figure 14-1. This 27-year-old man sustained blunt abdominal trauma in a motor vehicle accident. You are shown a CT scan obtained after both oral and intravenous administration of contrast medium.

Case 14: Traumatic Small Bowel Perforation

Question 39

Which *one* of the following is the MOST likely diagnosis?

    (A) Intraperitoneal hemorrhage
    (B) Mesenteric hematoma
    (C) Small bowel obstruction
    (D) Colonic hematoma
    (E) Jejunal perforation

The primary abnormalities visible in the test image (Figure 14-1) are the roughly triangular collections of high-attenuation fluid adjacent to a loop of bowel. Their position and configuration strongly suggest that they are extraluminal in location, and the very high attenuation of one of the loops is evidence that it represents contrast material (Figure 14-2). A further clue to the origin of the collections is the presence of gas bubbles on the nondependent surface of two of them, clear evidence of pneumoperitoneum. The bowel loop with which these collections are associated is located in the left mid-abdomen and is well anterior to the descending colon; therefore, it almost certainly represents a loop of jejunum. Taken together, in a patient with blunt abdominal trauma, the findings are highly suggestive of jejunal perforation **(Option (E) is correct).**

An intraperitoneal hemorrhage (Option (A)) would be expected to occupy a location similar to that shown in the test image, and, if the hemorrhage were recent, the blood could have a relatively high attenuation value. However, the attenuation of the most lateral collection is far too high to be related to anything other than contrast material, and extraluminal gas bubbles would not be present within an intraperitoneal hemorrhage. The discussion in Question 40 elaborates on the clinical and radiographic findings in patients with hemoperitoneum.

Mesenteric hematomas (Option (B)) also have the attenuation of fresh blood and could not achieve the density of the most lateral collec-

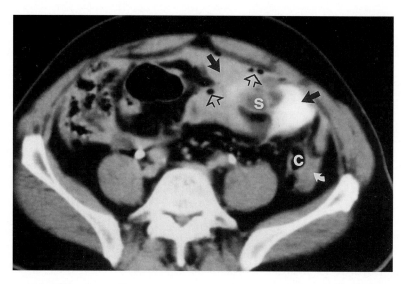

Figure 14-2 (Same as Figure 14-1). Traumatic small bowel perforation. A postcontrast CT scan demonstrates two roughly triangular collections of extraluminal oral contrast agent (solid black arrows) adjacent to a loop of small bowel (S). The most lateral part of the collection has the greatest attenuation value; it represents undiluted contrast material adjacent to the site of leakage. Note the multiple tiny bubbles (open arrows) indicative of pneumoperitoneum. Some high-density fluid (curved white arrow) has extended into the left paracolic gutter adjacent to the colon (c). This may represent either blood or dilute oral contrast agent. These findings are diagnostic of small bowel perforation.

tion in the test image. Moreover, mesenteric collections surround the intramesenteric vessels and infiltrate the mesenteric fat. Since they are confined within the mesenteric loop, they do not take on the triangular appearance illustrated in the test case.

In patients with small bowel obstruction (Option (C)), CT images show dilated loops of bowel proximal to the obstruction site, and collapsed loops distal to it. Administered oral contrast material typically becomes dilute as it passes through the fluid-filled bowel, and often there is no identifiable contrast material present near the site of obstruction. There are no distended, fluid-filled loops of small intestine shown in the test image. The CT findings in small bowel obstruction are discussed in Case 4.

Intramural hematomas of the small bowel or colon (Option (D)) occur frequently in patients sustaining abdominal trauma. They produce focal bowel wall thickening, which can be relatively high in attenuation value (see the discussion in Question 40). In the test image, segments of both ascending and descending colon are shown; although there is fluid adjacent to the descending colon, within the paracolic gutter, there is no evidence for intrinsic colonic wall thickening.

CT is the imaging method of choice to evaluate hemodynamically stable patients with significant blunt abdominal trauma. Sonography and peritoneal lavage are sensitive for demonstration of free intraperitoneal fluid, but they have significant limitations in demonstrating extraperitoneal injuries. In addition, the mere demonstration of hemoperitoneum is not sufficient information to determine the need for surgery. A high percentage of patients with small hepatic and mesenteric lacerations have associated hemoperitoneum. Surgical repair of these lacerations is often not required if these patients remain hemodynamically stable.

Blunt trauma to the bowel and mesentery occurs in approximately 5% of patients with abdominal trauma. The mortality from undiagnosed injuries to the bowel is significant. Delayed diagnosis of perforation of the duodenum is associated with a mortality rate of up to 65%. Observation of extraluminal contrast material directly confirms the presence of alimentary tract disruption, as illustrated by the test case. The presence of intraluminal contrast material also makes the diagnosis of intramural hemorrhage somewhat easier; a blood-thickened intestinal wall can mimic a collapsed loop, and the administered contrast agent distends the loop and identifies the luminal contour.

There is some controversy, however, as to whether oral contrast material should be given in every case of blunt trauma to the abdomen. Foley points out that many traumatized patients will require general anesthesia soon after the CT scan, so that the presence of intragastric contrast material presents a risk of aspiration. Withdrawal of gastric contents through a nasogastric tube is a reasonable solution to this problem. On balance, oral contrast material should be administered unless it is clearly risky to do so.

Because of the possibility of extraluminal leakage of the administered contrast agent, a water-soluble material should be chosen. Patients who are alert and cooperative can generally drink the few hundred milliliters required to opacify the stomach, duodenum, and upper small bowel; in obtunded or uncooperative patients, the contrast agent should be administered through a nasogastric tube. The tube should be withdrawn into the esophagus while the patient is being examined, so that streak artifacts are minimized in the upper abdomen. After the examination is completed, the tube can be reinserted and, if necessary, residual contrast material can be withdrawn from the stomach. Generally, only the stomach, duodenum, and proximal jejunum are opacified with the oral contrast material. No attempt is made to opacify the distal small bowel or colon. In the setting of acute abdominal trauma, it is unnecessary and potentially hazardous to delay the examination until the contrast material reaches the colon.

In some cases, it is either impossible or imprudent to administer oral contrast material prior to scanning the abdomen. In that setting, it is critically important to search the images for evidence of interloop fluid, which can be the only sign of intestinal perforation (see the discussion in Question 40).

Question 40

Concerning CT of blunt abdominal trauma,

  (A) the most common site of gastrointestinal injury is the jejunum
  (B) free air is nearly always noted if the jejunum is perforated
  (C) interloop blood is a common finding in patients with splenic lacerations
  (D) focal bowel wall thickening is a sign of intramural hematoma
  (E) water-density interloop fluid is a sign of small bowel perforation

Blunt injuries to the bowel typically occur at anatomic sites of relative fixation of the gastrointestinal tract. The most common injuries involve the proximal jejunum (just beyond its fixation at the ligament of Treitz) and the duodenum (because of its retroperitoneal attachments) **(Option (A) is true).** Abdominal radiographs are of limited value in the diagnosis of complications from blunt injury to the bowel, although they can demonstrate pneumoperitoneum in cases of bowel perforation. However, CT is more sensitive in demonstrating tiny extraluminal gas bubbles that are present in patients with laceration of the gastrointestinal tract. Experience with plain films of the abdomen in normal individuals suggests that there is little or no gas present in jejunal segments—this portion of the bowel is usually collapsed or filled with fluid only. Accordingly, perforation of the jejunum is frequently unassociated with significant pneumoperitoneum **(Option (B) is false).** In the series of Rizzo et al., free intraperitoneal air was observed in only 9 of 16 surgically confirmed bowel lacerations.

Interloop blood is an extremely important CT sign of bowel or mesenteric injury. Interloop fluid collections are triangular in configuration because of the reflections of the mesenteric folds. With most hepatic and splenic injuries, hemoperitoneum extends from the upper abdomen to the pelvis via the paracolic gutters. Blood in the interloop compartments in patients with hepatic or splenic injuries is infrequently observed **(Option (C) is false);** therefore, interloop blood strongly suggests bowel or mesenteric injury.

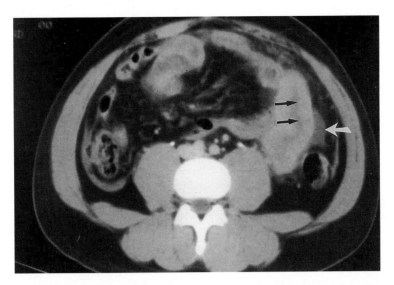

Figure 14-3. Intramural hematoma of the jejunum associated with small bowel perforation. A CT scan performed after intravenous contrast administration demonstrates mural thickening of the proximal jejunum just distal to the ligament of Treitz (black arrows). Adjacent to this thickened loop is a small amount of water-density fluid (white arrow). This proved at surgery to represent leakage of small bowel contents due to a 1-cm laceration of the jejunum. Note the absence of pneumoperitoneum.

Focal bowel wall thickening on CT in the setting of trauma is typically due to an intramural hematoma **(Option (D) is true)** (Figure 14-3). This is best appreciated when the lumen is distended with oral contrast medium. Following intravenous administration of iodinated contrast medium, there may be intense enhancement of the bowel wall in patients with mesenteric or intramural hematomas. This is due to delayed transit of contrast agent through the bowel wall as a result of partial venous outflow obstruction. Perforation of the small bowel can result in leakage of small bowel fluid, which is a mixture of bile, gastric juice, pancreatic secretions, and succus entericus. Small bowel contents are of water density on CT and can be misconstrued as simple ascites. Simple ascites is more often noted adjacent to the liver, in the paracolic gutters, and in the pelvis. It is uncommon to identify isolated interloop fluid in patients with simple ascites. Isolated interloop water-density fluid in traumatized patients is a worrisome finding that suggests bowel perforation (Figure 14-3) **(Option (E) is true)**. Other secondary signs of bowel injury should be carefully sought in these patients.

Question 41

Concerning intra-abdominal hemorrhage on CT scans of blunt abdominal trauma,

(A) the fluid attenuation value with acute hemoperitoneum is typically greater than 30 HU

(B) the fluid attenuation value with acute hemoperitoneum is lower in patients with severe anemia than in patients who are not anemic

(C) clotted blood has a higher attenuation value than free lysed blood does

(D) the "sentinel clot" sign refers to the observation that blood has higher attenuation values closer to the site of injury

(E) on precontrast studies, areas of active arterial extravasation are often isodense with adjacent major arterial structures

The accurate diagnosis of hemoperitoneum is one of the major contributions of CT to the evaluation of abdominal trauma. In patients without underlying anemia, the attenuation value of the blood in patients with acute hemoperitoneum is generally greater than 30 HU **(Option (A) is true).** However, in patients with anemia, the attenuation value of blood can be substantially lower **(Option (B) is true).** The factors determining the attenuation value of blood on CT are the concentration of hemoglobin and the physiologic state of the blood. Clotted blood typically has attenuation values of 45 to 60 HU, significantly higher than that of free lysed blood in the peritoneal cavity **(Option (C) is true).**

One of the major problems encountered in interpreting abdominal CT in patients with abdominal trauma is determining the precise site of injury when a large quantity of blood is present in the abdominal cavity. Orwig and Federle observed that the attenuation value of intraperitoneal blood adjacent to the site of visceral injury tended to be higher than that of blood elsewhere in the peritoneal space (Figure 14-4) **(Option (D) is true).** This "sentinel clot" sign proved to be of value in determining the site of visceral injury in 84% of cases studied. The rationale for this sign depends on the fact that free lysed blood is present in areas remote from the injury; as mentioned above, the attenuation value of lysed blood is considerably lower than that of freshly extravasated blood or clot.

In patients undergoing dynamic bolus CT, active arterial extravasation is also a critically important observation. Most patients with relatively minor blunt visceral injuries can be managed nonoperatively; however, the CT diagnosis of active arterial extravasation requires urgent intervention (Figure 14-5). The diagnosis of active arterial extravasation is facilitated by the use of intravenous contrast material; in these cases, contrast-rich blood is seen central to a mass composed of unopacified fresh blood. However, it can be more difficult to identify active extravasation on noncontrast CT scans. Typically, those areas of active bleeding

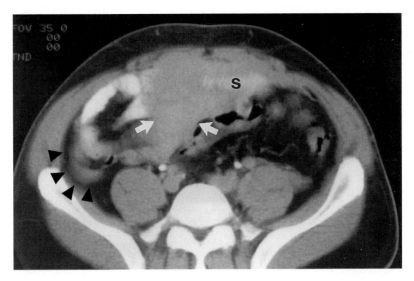

Figure 14-4. "Sentinel clot" sign of mesenteric injury. A CT scan obtained after administration of oral and intravenous contrast material demonstrates a triangular collection of high-density interloop hematoma (arrows) adjacent to the distal small bowel (S). At surgery, a large interloop hematoma was noted in association with an intramural hematoma of the small bowel. There was no perforation of the bowel. Note the lower attenuation of the lysed blood in the right paracolic gutter (arrowheads).

are isodense with the flowing blood within adjacent arterial structures **(Option (E) is true).**

When active extravasation is observed on CT, the findings aid in determining the appropriate form of urgent intervention; surgical exploration is indicated in patients with active intraperitoneal arterial extravasation because there is a high likelihood of other intraperitoneal injuries. However, in patients with active extraperitoneal arterial extravasation (e.g., from a lumbar artery), angiographic embolization is the treatment of choice. The precise site of retroperitoneal bleeding is very difficult to identify at the time of surgical exploration; moreover, radiologic methods have proved highly successful in nonoperatively managing patients with retroperitoneal arterial bleeding.

Midstream aortic angiography can sometimes identify the site of lumbar artery hemorrhage; selective catheterization of the vessel is then performed (Figure 14-6A and B). Even if no extravasation is seen on aortography, selective lumbar arteriography is warranted if there is sufficient suspicion of an injury to these vessels. Injured lumbar arteries can opacify slowly and incompletely on a nonselective angiogram.

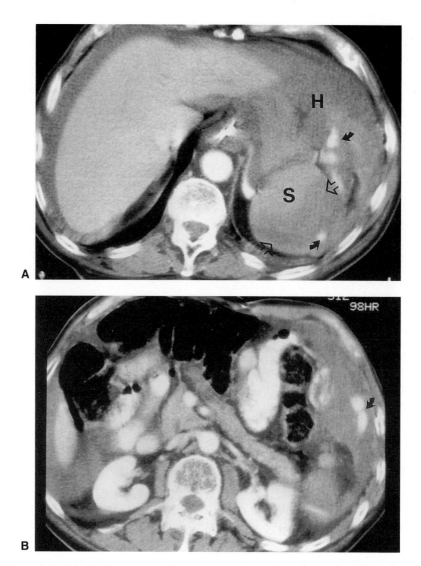

Figure 14-5. Active arterial extravasation from splenic trauma. (A) A CT scan obtained after oral contrast agent administration and during intravenous contrast agent infusion demonstrates a large perisplenic hematoma (H). Note the compression of the splenic parenchyma (S) by the subcapsular hematoma (open arrows). Adjacent to the spleen are several foci (solid arrows) with extremely high attenuation fluid (120 HU) isodense with the adjacent aorta. These represent areas of active arterial extravasation. (B) A more inferior CT section demonstrates active arterial extravasation extending into the left paracolic gutter (curved arrow).

Typically, digital subtraction angiography is performed after selective catheterization of the target lumbar artery. The subsequent images

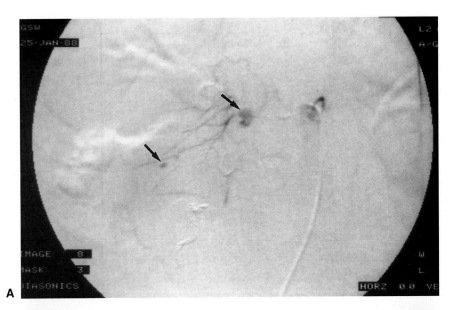

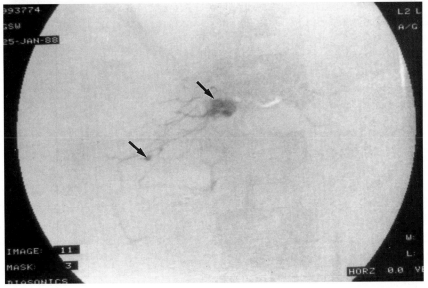

Figure 14-6. Selective catheter embolization of lumbar artery extravasation. (A and B) Subtraction images from a selective lumbar arteriogram reveal extravasation of contrast agent (arrows) following blunt trauma.

should be searched for confirmation of active extravasation and for possible communication with spinal artery branches. If a spinal artery is identified, the catheter must be passed beyond the origin of this branch before embolization is undertaken.

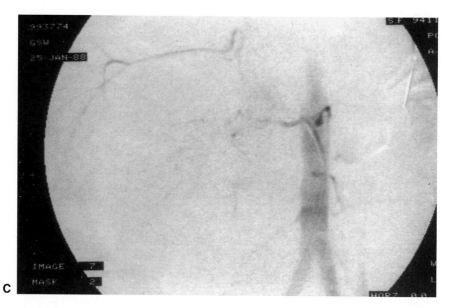

C

Figure 14-6 (Continued). Selective catheter embolization of lumbar artery extravasation. (C) After embolization with Gelfoam pledgets, repeat arteriography shows that the lumbar artery is occluded. No hemorrhage is evident. The patient became hemodynamically stable after the embolization procedure.

The embolization procedure can be performed using Gelfoam pledgets or small coils (Figure 14-6C). The embolic agent used depends on the size and location of the vessel injury. Gelfoam pledgets can be injected and flow-directed to occlude a peripheral injury to the lumbar artery, whereas injury to the main lumbar trunk might be easier to occlude with coils. Lumbar arteries adjacent to the target vessel should be studied after embolization to ensure that there is not continued extravasation due to collateral blood flow.

R. Brooke Jeffrey, M.D.

SUGGESTED READINGS

1. Donohue JH, Federle MP, Griffiths BG, Trunkey DD. Computed tomography in the diagnosis of blunt intestinal and mesenteric injuries. J Trauma 1987; 27:11–17
2. Foley WD. Imaging in abdominal trauma. In: Freeny PC, Stevenson GW (eds), Margulis and Buchenne's alimentary tract radiology, 5th ed. St. Louis: Mosby-Year Book; 1993:2120–2142.

3. Hara H, Babyn PS, Bourgeois D. Significance of bowel wall enhancement on CT following blunt abdominal trauma in childhood. J Comput Assist Tomogr 1992; 16:94–98

4. Hofer GA, Cohen AJ. CT signs of duodenal perforation secondary to blunt abdominal trauma. J Comput Assist Tomogr 1989; 13:430–432

5. Jeffrey RB Jr, Cardoza JD, Olcott EW. Detection of active intraabdominal arterial hemorrhage: value of dynamic contrast-enhanced CT. AJR 1991; 156:725–729

6. Nghiem HV, Jeffrey RB Jr, Mindelzun RE. CT of blunt trauma to the bowel and mesentery. AJR 1993; 160:53–58

7. Orwig D, Federle MP. Localized clotted blood as evidence of visceral trauma on CT: the sentinel clot sign. AJR 1989; 153:747–749

8. Rizzo MJ, Federle MP, Griffiths BG. Bowel and mesenteric injury following blunt abdominal trauma: evaluation with CT. Radiology 1989; 173:143–148

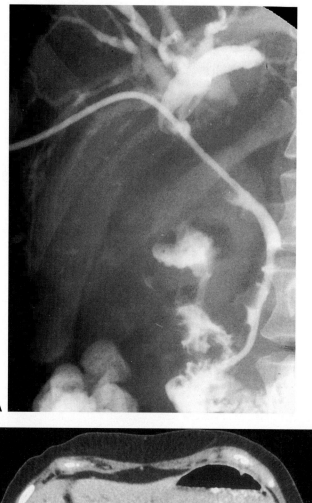

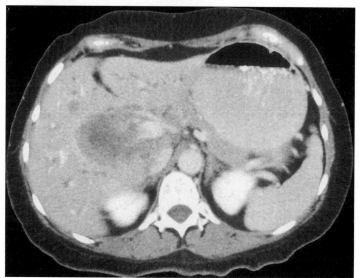

Figure 15-1

Case 15: Suprapancreatic Biliary Obstruction

Questions 42 through 45

Four patients referred for evaluation of obstructive jaundice underwent cholangiography and CT studies (Figures 15-1 through 15-4). For each numbered set of images listed below (Questions 42 through 45), select the *one* lettered diagnosis (A, B, C, D, or E) that is MOST closely associated with it. Each lettered diagnosis may be used once, more than once, or not at all.

42. Figure 15-1
43. Figure 15-2
44. Figure 15-3
45. Figure 15-4

    (A) Carcinoma of the bile duct
    (B) AIDS cholangiopathy
    (C) Nodal metastases to the porta hepatis
    (D) Carcinoma of the gallbladder
    (E) Mirizzi's syndrome

    The cholangiogram of the first patient (Figure 15-1A) shows intrahepatic biliary obstruction; the obstructing lesion is located at the level of the origin of the hepatic duct, and the proximal 3 cm of the duct is narrowed (Figure 15-5A). There is also marked displacement of the extrahepatic duct from right to left, providing inferential evidence that a mass is present, centered about the level of the porta hepatis. The cystic duct and gallbladder are not filled with contrast material.

    The CT image (Figure 15-1B) shows a large, predominantly low-attenuation mass located lateral and posterior to the portal vein and hepatic artery, i.e., within the intrahepatic portion of the hepatoduodenal ligament (Figure 15-5B). There is associated peripheral biliary dilatation. A bulky mass lateral to the expected course of the common bile duct is quite characteristic of gallbladder carcinoma **(Option (D) is the correct answer to Question 42).** Other diagnostic considerations would

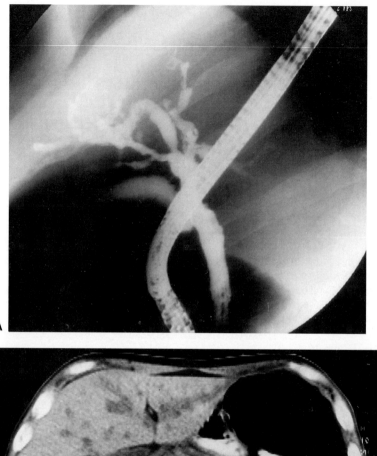

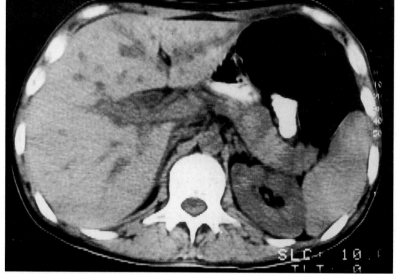

Figure 15-2

include lymphoma and hepatocellular carcinoma, but they were not listed as options.

Carcinoma of the bile duct is another form of a tumor with the same histologic characteristics, cholangiocarcinoma, but arises from bile duct

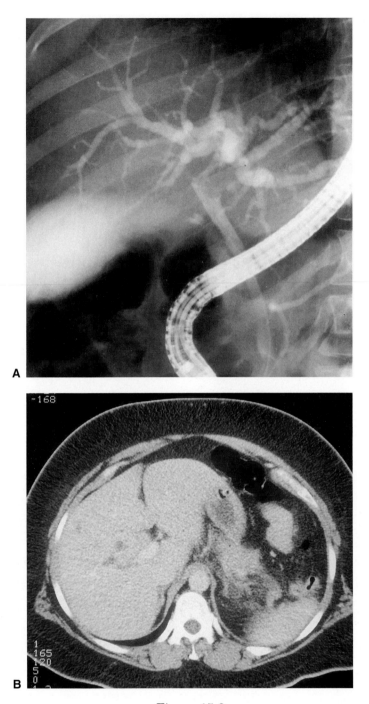

Figure 15-3

epithelium and is therefore centered along the course of the intrahepatic, common hepatic, or common bile duct. Also, most bile duct cholangiocar-

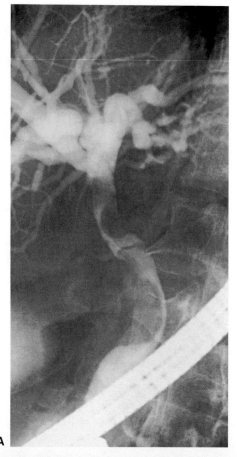

A

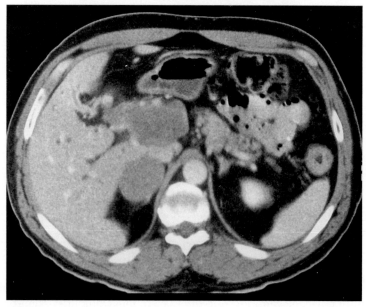

B

Figure 15-4

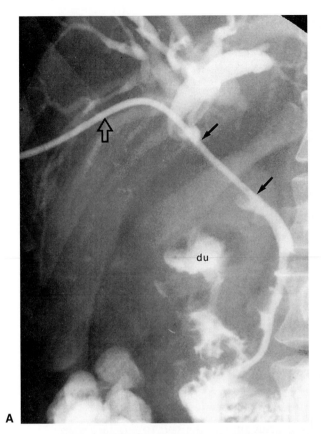

Figure 15-5 (Same as Figure 15-1). Gallbladder carcinoma: "massive" form. (A) A cholangiogram performed via a percutaneous catheter (open arrow) shows luminal narrowing involving the proximal 3 cm of the common hepatic duct (solid arrows). There is marked leftward displacement of the extrahepatic ducts. du = duodenal bulb. (B) A CT section through the porta hepatis shows a large heterogeneous mass (M) lateral to the portal vein (pv) and hepatic artery (open arrow) within the lateral portion of the hepatoduodenal ligament. Note the biliary dilatation in the periphery of the liver.

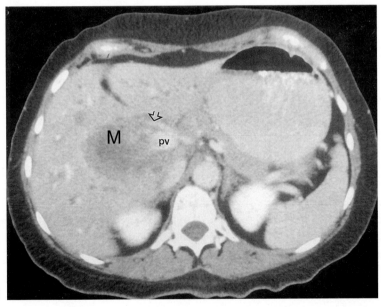

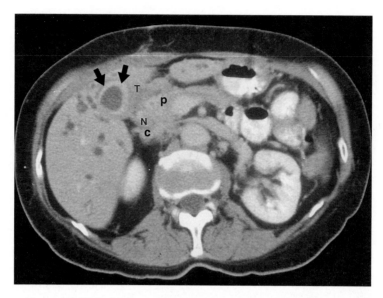

Figure 15-6. Gallbladder carcinoma: "thick-wall" form. A CT section through the gallbladder displays marked wall thickening (arrows) with striking contrast enhancement. Tumor (T) has extended into the fat around the periphery of the gallbladder fossa, and there is an enlarged node (N) in the pancreaticoduodenal chain. p = pancreas; c = inferior vena cava.

cinomas are relatively small, not bulky like the tumor in Figure 15-1. AIDS cholangiopathy is a fibrotic process unassociated with a mass. Nodal metastases to the porta hepatis can be quite bulky but are almost always centered between the portal vein and the inferior vena cava, in what has been termed the portacaval space. Also, nodal metastases are more commonly multiple masses rather than large, solitary lesions. Mirizzi's syndrome (obstruction of the common duct by inflammation from a stone in the cystic duct) can be associated with an inflammatory mass but would not produce smooth displacement of the common hepatic and common bile duct.

Carcinoma of the gallbladder is not a common tumor, and the prognosis of patients with this condition is extremely poor. This is very probably a reflection of the advanced stage at which most patients present. It is probable that gallbladder cancers arise in patients with long-standing chronic cholecystitis; 70 to 80% of cases are associated with gallstones.

Itai et al. described three recognizable CT patterns: "massive" (the most common pattern, seen in 60 to 70% of tumors in most series and the type illustrated in Figure 15-1), "thickened wall" (Figure 15-6), and "intraluminal" (Figure 15-7). The gallbladder lies adjacent to the hepa-

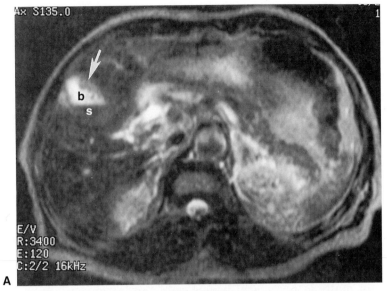

SE 3,400/120

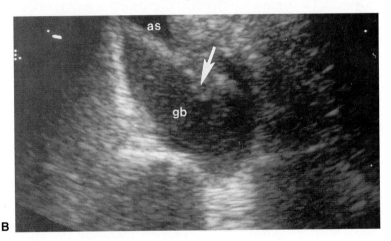

Figure 15-7. Gallbladder carcinoma: "intraluminal" polypoid form. (A) An MR section through the gallbladder fossa was obtained with strong T2 weighting. Bile (b) and small stones (s) are present within the gallbladder lumen. An irregular polypoid mass (arrow) is observed on the anteromedial surface. (B) A sonogram in the same patient shows the hyperechoic polyp (arrow) arising from the wall of the gallbladder (gb). A small amount of ascites (as) is also present.

toduodenal ligament, and so it is very common for gallbladder cancers to infiltrate into the porta hepatis, producing encasement of the common hepatic duct, portal vein, and hepatic artery. This infiltration is typically observed lateral to the portal vein. Inferiorly, tumor within the ligament extends into the retroperitoneum on the posterolateral surface of the pancreas and frequently produces bile duct obstruction in the pancreatic segment. The surface of the gallbladder is covered almost entirely by peritoneum, and another common mode of spread is peritoneal dissemination. In these cases, CT may depict ascites or peritoneal masses. In one series, 45% of patients had surgically proven peritoneal dissemination at the time they presented. Metastatic adenopathy to the nodal chain that accompanies the hepatic artery and continues along the retroperitoneal portion of the bile duct is also present in up to 70% of patients.

Cholangiography is usually performed in patients with biliary obstruction (and hence advanced disease). Encasement of the common hepatic duct within the porta hepatis and displacement of the extrahepatic ducts by a mass are the most common findings. It is rare for the cystic duct or gallbladder to be directly opacified during cholangiography in this condition.

The cholangiogram of the second patient (Figure 15-2A) shows narrowing of multiple segmental branches of the intrahepatic biliary tree (Figure 15-8A). The right posterior duct narrowing is well profiled. There are also numerous intraluminal filling defects within the contrast column, in both the intra- and extrahepatic segments. There is minimal dilatation within the bile ducts.

The CT scan (Figure 15-2B) was obtained without intravenous contrast agent administration (because of the patient's severely compromised clinical condition). The wall of the right hepatic and common hepatic duct is shown to be symmetrically thickened (Figure 15-8B). Also, there is water-density infiltration surrounding the portal triads and minimal dilatation of the intrahepatic ducts. Primary sclerosing cholangitis would be a viable diagnosis but is not among the options listed. The radiographic appearance is also quite consistent with AIDS cholangiopathy and should be considered diagnostic in conjunction with a history of HIV infection (withheld in this patient) **(Option (B) is the correct answer to Question 43).**

Cholangiocarcinoma, nodal metastases, and carcinoma of the gallbladder would be expected to have an associated mass and evidence of biliary obstruction, but these are not present in Figure 15-2. Mirizzi's syndrome is unlikely since obstruction is not present. Moreover, the striking changes of cholangitis would not be expected in patients with Mirizzi's syndrome.

Acalculous inflammation of both the gallbladder and the biliary tract is a known complication of AIDS. Its exact prevalance is unknown, because a large number of affected patients are asymptomatic or their biliary symptoms are overshadowed by other complications of the disease. When symptoms do occur, they are often nonspecific, e.g., fever and ab-

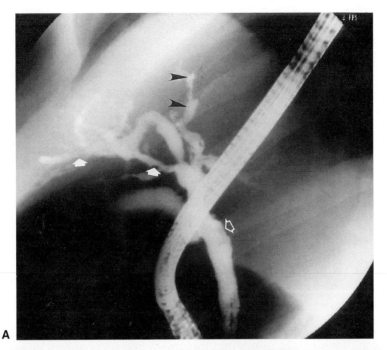

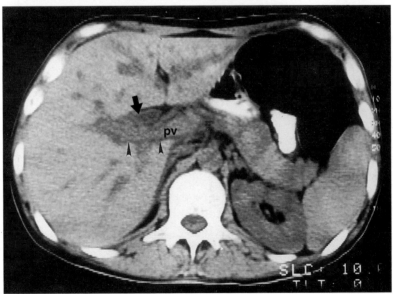

Figure 15-8 (Same as Figure 15-2). AIDS cholangiopathy. (A) An endo-scopic cholangiogram shows markedly irregular narrowing of the left (arrowheads) and right (white arrows) intrahepatic ducts. At least one filling defect (open arrow) is present within the proximal common bile duct. (B) A CT section through the porta hepatis shows slight thickening of the wall of the bile duct (arrow). A rim of edema (arrowheads) is present and is best detected posterior to the portal vein (pv).

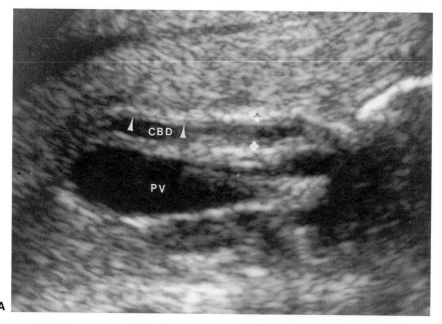

A

Figure 15-9. AIDS cholangiography. (A) Sonographic examination of a young man with right upper quadrant pain and fever shows no evidence of ductal dilatation. However, there is thickening of the wall (arrowheads) of the common bile duct (CBD). This sonographic finding is common in AIDS cholangiopathy. PV = portal vein. (B) A CT section obtained in another patient with AIDS cholangiopathy shows marked contrast enhancement within the thick-walled common bile duct (arrow).

dominal pain. The organisms most commonly implicated include cytomegalovirus, *Cryptosporidium* species, and *Enterocytozoon bieneusi* (microsporidiosis).

Ultrasonography of the gallbladder in patients with AIDS frequently shows a thick wall, often with accompanying pericholecystic fluid. In many cases the bile ducts are thickened as well, and there is usually modest biliary dilatation (Figure 15-9A). CT findings similarly reflect biliary dilatation and thickening of the bile duct wall. When intravenous contrast is administered, there is usually moderate to marked enhancement of the thickened duct wall (Figure 15-9B).

Direct cholangiography has been reported to show findings characteristic for AIDS cholangiopathy. Most patients have a smooth stenosis in the region of the papilla. Intrahepatic strictures with proximal dilated areas, resembling the pattern seen in patients with sclerosing cholangitis, are a frequent observation. Less common are intraluminal filling defects, such as those shown in Figure 15-2. The cause of these plaque-like areas has not been determined.

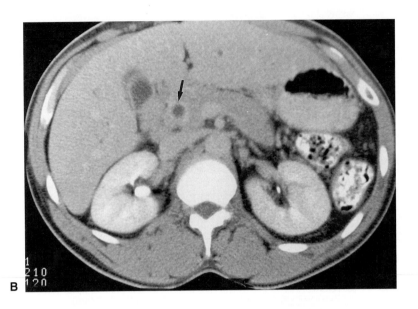

B

The cholangiogram of the third patient (Figure 15-3A) shows dilatation of both left and right intrahepatic ducts. The confluence of the two major ducts is not opacified, and there is a smooth, convex filling defect within the contrast column within the proximal common hepatic duct (Figure 15-10A).

The CT scan (Figure 15-3B) shows intrahepatic duct dilatation. The dilated ducts can be traced to a soft tissue mass, within the periportal fat, that replaces both the right and left hepatic ducts (Figure 15-10B). These radiographic findings are diagnostic of a primary cholangiocarcinoma **(Option (A) is the correct answer to Question 44).**

AIDS cholangiopathy is not associated with a focal mass or duct obstruction. Nodal metastasis is a possible diagnosis in this patient, but extension of tumor into both left and right intrahepatic ducts is very rare. Carcinoma of the gallbladder is highly unlikely; the gallbladder fills readily during the cholangiogram and has a normal appearance. Mirizzi's syndrome is also excluded, because the cystic duct is clearly patent. Also, the site of obstruction in patients with Mirizzi's syndrome is in the distal duct, not at the origin of the common hepatic duct.

Cholangiocarcinoma is a relatively rare tumor, making up only 0.5% of all malignancies. It is known to be associated with inflammatory bowel disease, probably because of the sclerosing cholangitis that frequently attends ulcerative colitis and Crohn's disease. Choledochal cysts are also known to predispose to development of cholangiocarcinoma (Figure 15-11).

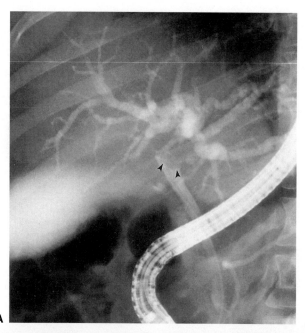

A

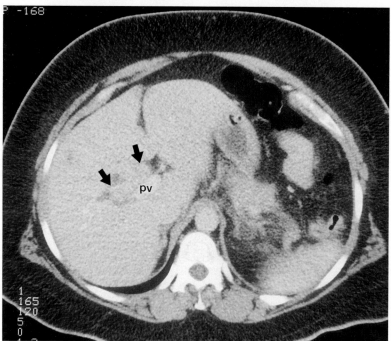

B

Figure 15-10 (Same as Figure 15-3). Cholangiocarcinoma: polypoid form. (A) An endoscopic cholangiogram shows a polypoid lesion (arrowheads) at the origin of the common hepatic duct. The polyp extends into the distal left and right hepatic ducts. (B) A CT section through the porta hepatis shows soft tissue density filling the distal left and right hepatic ducts (arrows) anterior to the portal vein (pv).

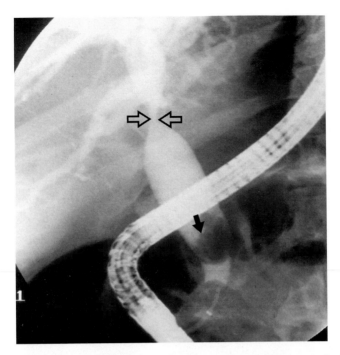

Figure 15-11. Two cholangiocarcinomas arising within a choledochal cyst. An endoscopic cholangiogram shows moderate fusiform dilatation of the extrahepatic common duct. A polypoid mass (solid arrow) is present near the papilla of Vater, and a circumferential stricture (open arrows) is observed at the original of the common hepatic duct. Both were cholangiocarcinomas, and there was diffuse dysplasia of the intervening duct epithelium.

Histologically, most cholangiocarcinomas are mucin-secreting epithelial adenocarcinomas. They exhibit three morphologic types: infiltrative (or scirrhous), exophytic, and polypoid. The infiltrative form is the most common in the hilar lesions. The biological behavior of these cancers depends chiefly on their location; intrahepatic tumors are often asymptomatic until they are quite advanced, since the normal function of the unaffected hepatic lobes prevents jaundice from developing. Long-term stenosis or occlusion of an intrahepatic duct system leads to segmental or lobar atrophy of the involved liver parenchyma, with compensatory hypertrophy of the spared areas. This condition is not specific for cholangiocarcinoma, since it can be observed in any condition characterized by chronic segmental biliary obstruction.

Biliary carcinomas can be located anywhere from the peripheral ducts in the liver to the papilla of Vater. Precise statistics regarding sites of occurrence are difficult to obtain, since most series reflect referral

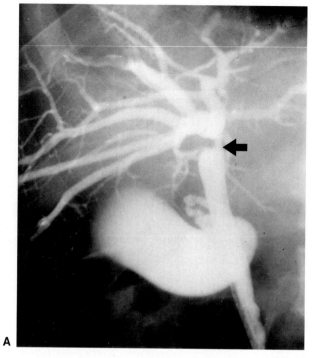

A

Figure 15-12. Cholangiocarcinoma: fibrotic form. (A) A cholangiogram shows a very short, slightly eccentric stricture (arrow) involving the proximal common hepatic duct. (B) A CT section through the stricture shows eccentric thickening of the duct wall (arrowhead), with no evidence of an associated mass.

bias. Most large series give frequencies of 10% for intrahepatic tumors, 25% for hilar cholangiocarcinomas, 5% for cystic duct cancers, 10% for common hepatic duct tumors, and 50% for cancers of the common bile duct. Specialized cancer centers tend to report higher frequencies for more proximal tumors, since those tumors are more difficult to treat and are therefore referred.

Direct cholangiography is frequently performed to diagnose cholangiocarcinoma. In patients with the polypoid form (represented by the test patient in this question), a discrete rounded intraluminal filling defect is observed. The more frequent scirrhous form has the appearance of a smooth stricture involving relatively short segments of the ductal system, commonly involving the distal left and right intrahepatic segments, and the proximal common hepatic duct (Figure 15-12A). In 1965, Klatskin described a series of 13 patients who had a peculiar scarlike form of cholangiocarcinoma characterized by small size, low potential for

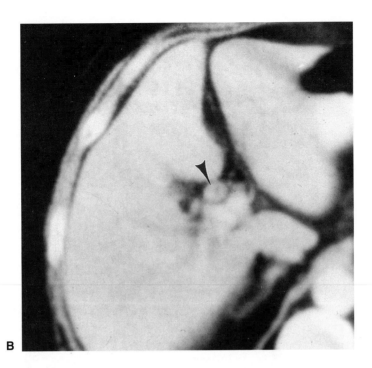

B

widespread metastasis, and accordingly longer survival time, even when palliative procedures were the only therapy. Histopathologic specimens showed relatively well-differentiated adenocarcinoma cells embedded in a dense connective tissue stroma. All of the tumors in this series arose in the liver hilus and involved the distal portions of the right and left hepatic ducts and the proximal portion of the common hepatic duct. Subsequent to this description, the name "Klatskin tumor" has been applied to all cholangiocarcinomas arising at this anatomic site, regardless of histology. Although most hilar tumors fit Klatskin's description, some cholangiocarcinomas at this site are moderately or poorly differentiated and can be associated with appreciable size and widespread metastases. The major impact of cholangiography in staging these tumors is in demonstrating epithelial intraductal spread of tumor; this form of spread cannot be detected by other radiologic methods. For cases that are clearly inoperable, direct endoscopic or transhepatic cholangiography is also of use in providing long-term therapy by placement of indwelling stents.

CT scans of scirrhous cholangiocarcinoma often show only duct wall thickening (Figure 15-12B). More-extensive tumors exhibit ill-defined periductal stranding into the portal fat. One peculiar feature of the fibrous tumors is their propensity to demonstrate marked contrast

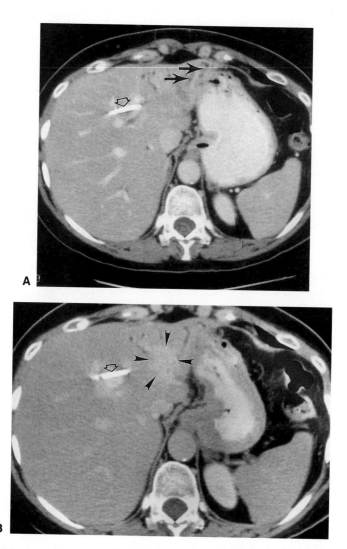

Figure 15-13. Cholangiocarcinoma demonstrating delayed tumor enhancement. (A) A CT section through the upper abdomen shows focal dilatation of segmental bile ducts in the lateral segment of the left hepatic lobe (arrows). No obvious mass is present at the site of duct termination. (B) CT section obtained several minutes after panel A at the same anatomic region. A mass (arrowheads) is now recognized because its attenuation is increased with respect to the surrounding liver. This phenomenon can occur in any tumor with a large extracellular fluid space but is most commonly observed in cholangiocarcinomas. Open arrow = biliary drainage catheter. (Case courtesy of Richard L. Baron, M.D., University of Pittsburgh, Pittsburgh, Penn.)

enhancement on delayed images (obtained in the equilibrium phase, 5 to 10 minutes after contrast administration) (Figure 15-13).

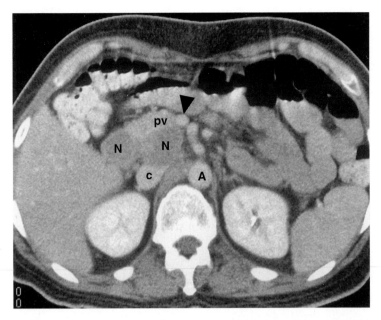

Figure 15-14. Nodal metastases from cholangiocarcinoma. A CT section through the superior mesenteric artery shows two discrete masses (N) within the pancreaticoduodenal nodal chain, lying between the portal vein (pv) and the inferior vena cava (c). A = aorta. The arrowhead indicates the superior mesenteric vein.

Metastatic deposits within the biliary lymphatics are commonly observed in patients with cholangiocarcinoma; the nodes most commonly involved are within the hepatic, gastroduodenal, and pancreaticoduodenal systems (Figure 15-14). The frequency of lymph node metastases at the time of presentation also varies from series to series. In general, distal tumors have a slightly lower likelihood of lymphatic spread. In one series, 73% of proximal cancers had surgically proven lymph node metastases, compared with 33% of distal or diffuse cholangiocarcinomas.

Direct invasion or encasement of surrounding structures is also a feature of cholangiocarcinoma. When the site of involvement is the liver hilus or intrahepatic ducts, the portal vein may be encased; this occurs in about 20% of proximal cancers. It should be stressed that the observation of an atrophic lobe or segment is not reliable evidence of portal vein invasion; portal flow is diverted merely because of the presence of biliary obstruction, and lobar atrophy will result.

Peritoneal metastases are present in a relatively small percentage of patients and are usually a relatively late occurrence. About 25% of patients with cholangiocarcinoma ultimately develop peritoneal spread.

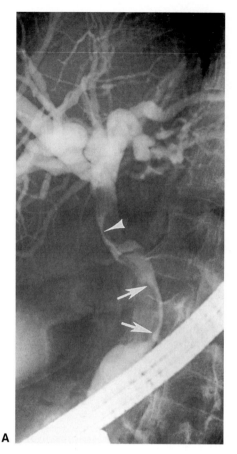

A

Figure 15-15 (Same as Figure 15-4). Biliary obstruction by large pancreaticoduodenal nodes as a result of metastatic malignant melanoma. (A) A cholangiogram shows small proximal (arrowhead) and larger distal (arrows) smooth filling defects that both narrow and alter the axis of the extrahepatic duct. (B) A CT section just below the porta hepatis (through the larger of the two masses) shows a low-attenuation nodal metastasis (N) displacing the portal vein (open arrow) and hepatic artery (solid arrow), producing biliary obstruction (note the peripheral ductal dilatation within the liver). Note also the large mass replacing the right adrenal gland (ad).

Several diseases are known to predispose to the development of cholangiocarcinoma. The most important in the United States are sclerosing cholangitis and choledochal cyst (Figure 15-11). Infestation with liver flukes, such as *Clonorchis sinensis*, is strongly associated with cholangiocarcinoma in Asia.

The cholangiogram of the fourth patient (Figure 15-4A) shows two large, smooth, eccentrically placed filling defects in the contrast column, the larger measuring approximately 4 cm (Figure 15-15A). Moderate intrahepatic duct dilatation is also present. The cystic duct is patent, and there is contrast within the gallbladder (Figure 15-15A).

The CT scan (Figure 15-4B) shows a 5-cm mass arising anterior to the inferior vena cava, just inferior to the porta hepatis (Figure 15-15B). There is also a large mass replacing the right adrenal gland. These two findings strongly suggest the diagnosis of metastatic disease; therefore, the most likely diagnosis among those listed is metastatic adenopathy

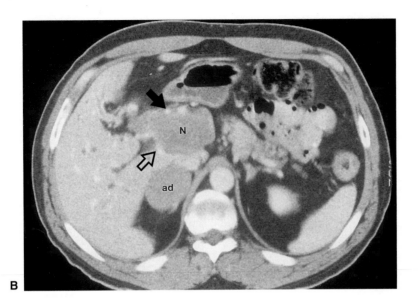

B

within the hepatoduodenal ligament **(Option (C) is the correct answer to Question 45).** This diagnosis is even more compelling when the patient's history of previous melanoma is disclosed.

Cholangiocarcinoma would be very unlikely to produce two discrete lesions, as seen on the cholangiogram. It is also very unlikely to cause metastases to the adrenal gland. AIDS cholangiopathy and Mirizzi's syndrome are not associated with large masses. Carcinoma of the gallbladder is not impossible, but there is evidence of contrast filling the gallbladder on the cholangiogram, which virtually excludes the diagnosis.

The major chain of lymph nodes within the hepatoduodenal ligament is the hepatic chain, which relates to branches of the hepatic artery. These nodes drain the liver and biliary tree directly and are also part of the celiac chain, which may be involved in cancers of the stomach, pancreas, and transverse colon. Metastases from other primary sites also involve the celiac or hepatic chain; those from breast carcinoma and renal cell carcinoma are most common. Systemic lymphomas, particularly non-Hodgkin cell types, also commonly enlarge the portal nodes.

Contrast cholangiography demonstrates hepatoduodenal ligament nodes as smooth indentations into the contrast column. The nodes sometimes have the appearance of intramural lesions, because the ligament is an enclosed space. Multiple nodes are frequently present and give rise to the characteristic sinuous appearance of the common hepatic duct, illustrated in Figure 15-4A.

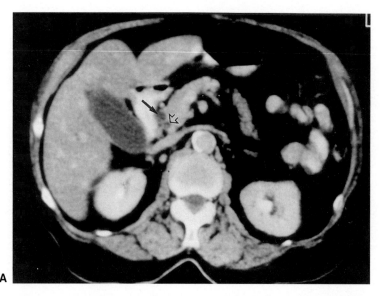

Figure 15-16. Mirizzi's syndrome. (A) A CT section obtained near the papilla of Vater in a 40-year-old woman with known cholelithiasis and intermittent episodes of jaundice. The common hepatic duct (solid arrow) is slightly dilated. Immediately posterior to it lies the cystic duct (open arrow), within which a high-density calculus can be faintly seen. (B) A percutaneous cholangiogram obtained in lateral projection shows the calculus (arrowheads), chiefly within the posterior cystic duct (CYD), with a portion protruding into the common bile duct immediately proximal to the papilla of Vater. CHD = common hepatic duct.

CT provides the means for direct observation of the lymph node chains that characteristically accompany the major arterial branches. The observation of discrete masses along the course of the hepatic artery, gastroduodenal artery, or pancreaticoduodenal arcade should prompt the consideration of lymph node metastases.

Mirizzi's syndrome involves obstruction of the common hepatic duct by a calculus (and surrounding inflammation) in the cystic duct. Frequently, there exists a long common channel in which the cystic duct travels posterior to the common hepatic duct before joining it above the sphincter of Oddi. Inflammation arising in the cystic duct can readily affect the common hepatic duct in this anatomic situation.

Cholangiography in patients with Mirizzi's syndrome frequently demonstrates only an extrinsic mass impinging on the common hepatic duct; filling of the cystic duct is not always easily accomplished, and in these patients it is not obvious that the mass is really a stone within the cystic duct. Cross-sectional imaging by CT or sonography will demon-

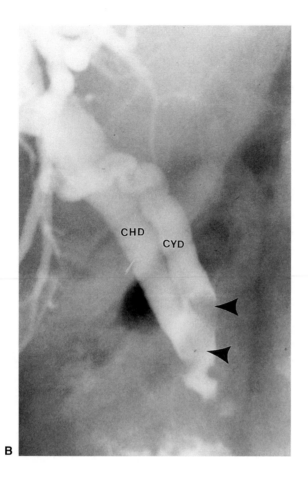

CHD CYD

B

strate both tubular structures (when there is a common channel, the cystic duct is characteristically posterior to the common hepatic duct) and may also show the obstructing stone (Figure 15-16).

In some patients the obstructing stone is within the neck of the gallbladder or proximal cystic duct, in which case the obstruction is closer to the liver hilus. Imaging in these patients frequently shows a thickened gallbladder wall, with an inflammatory mass extending to the proximal common hepatic duct.

Approach to the patient with biliary obstruction. Evaluation of a patient with jaundice is a frequent clinical problem. Clinical skill and problem-solving intuition are more valuable than a strict algorithmic approach, but there are certain valid generalizations regarding the appropriate work-up of these patients.

History, physical examination, and liver function tests usually suffice to determine whether the jaundice is likely to be due to mechanical obstruction (or cholestasis) or hepatocellular disease. When the issue is in doubt, sonography is a simple and reliable means of detecting the duct dilatation that almost always accompanies mechanical obstruction.

Sonography has other strengths as well; it is far better than CT in detecting stones in the gallbladder and at least equivalent to CT in detecting calculi within the common duct. (Study results vary, but both imaging methods are on the order of 70 to 80% sensitive to common duct calculi.) Also, subtle pancreatic lesions are occasionally easier to identify by sonography than by CT since the alteration in echotexture may be more pronounced than the alteration in density in a small cancer. However, sonography has the limitation that some anatomic regions are virtually inaccessible to examination (because of loops of gas-filled bowel). Much of the retroperitoneum falls into this category.

CT displays abdominal anatomy quite well and is most useful when clinical management depends on extrahepatic information. This is quite often the case when malignant biliary obstruction is known or suspected and the choice between curative and palliative intervention depends on precise staging information. CT excels in evaluating abdominal vessels, retroperitoneal and mesenteric nodes, and the walls of hollow viscera. It is approximately equivalent to MRI in evaluating the liver for metastases.

MRI has recently been considered as a means of evaluating biliary obstruction; among its assets is the ability to collect and render information in nonaxial planes of section. This is particularly valuable in assessing anatomic structures that curve in and out of transverse sections—the diaphragm is a typical example. MR images can noninvasively display the entire pancreatic and biliary system. Whether MRI will prove to be clinically useful in evaluating jaundice is still under investigation.

Many patients with jaundice present urgently, with sepsis, shock, or severe abdominal pain. In this setting, diagnostic procedures should properly take a back seat to therapeutic interventions. Direct cholangiography via endoscopic catheterization has emerged as the method of choice; not only can the nature of the obstruction be characterized, but therapeutic drainage can also be performed at the same sitting. For patients in whom endoscopic catheterization cannot be carried out, percutaneous biliary drainage (discussed in Question 46) is an excellent alternative. The choice between these procedures often depends on regional expertise; other situations favoring percutaneous drainage include unusual anatomy (prior gastric surgery or periampullary duodenal diverticulum preventing cannulation) and hilar obstruction (often difficult to navigate from below).

Gathering all the clinical data while performing the fewest imaging procedures is a daunting task; success depends on clear communication between the clinical team and the radiologist.

Question 46

Concerning percutaneous biliary drainage,

- (A) direct drainage of the left hepatic duct is contraindicated
- (B) it is important to attempt placement of an internal (duodenal) drainage catheter during the initial procedure
- (C) in patients with multiple obstructed segments, all hepatic segments should be drained
- (D) in patients with distal obstruction, endoscopic drainage is preferable
- (E) in patients undergoing catheter drainage who develop hemobilia, a cholangiogram is the first radiologic examination that should be performed

Percutaneous transhepatic biliary drainage (PTBD) is a well-accepted treatment for biliary obstructions of all kinds. It represents a logical extension of the diagnostic procedure transhepatic cholangiography. Once the biliary tree is opacified, access to the intrahepatic radicles is readily available, allowing catheter-based intervention to be performed. Depending on the clinical problem to be addressed, percutaneous puncture can be performed through either left or right hepatic segments **(Option (A) is false).** When the obstructing lesion is within the common hepatic or common bile duct, there may be some advantages to performing the procedure via the left hepatic duct; the pathway from skin to biliary radicle is shorter, and the normal course of the left lateral segmental hepatic duct is somewhat straighter from peripheral to central than the course of the right posterior segmental duct. The major disadvantage of puncturing the left hepatic duct is that manipulation of the catheter places the operator's hands in the center of the X-ray beam. However, most interventional suites are equipped with C-arm fluoroscopic units, allowing the operator to work without undue exposure.

The major immediate benefit of PTBD occurs when the biliary obstruction is relieved; this will begin to ameliorate the hepatic dysfunction that attends biliary obstruction and will provide drainage of infected bile. In the long term, it is optimal to reestablish continuity between the intrahepatic flow of bile and the duodenum, but this is not an important goal during the initial drainage procedure. In fact, extended initial manipulation can result in sepsis **(Option (B) is false).**

The major goal of PTBD is to restore hepatic function; therefore, it is acceptable to leave segments undrained if they are unlikely to contribute significantly to overall hepatic function **(Option (C) is false).** Segments with long-standing biliary obstruction frequently undergo atrophy, and catheter placement within these segments is generally performed only if the bile is infected.

PTBD is not without risk, and an alternative method that offers comparable success, endoscopic catheterization and drainage, has become widely available. In a 1986 study, Stanley et al. compared the complications, mortality, and survival of 34 patients who underwent PTBD with 24 patients who had endoscopic decompression. Patients in this series had comparable complication and survival rates, but the 30-day mortality rate for PTBD was 32% compared with 4% for endoscopic intervention. Without question, patient selection bias exerted an important effect on these results. However, there is also no question that, in the vast majority of centers, most patients are managed with endoscopic therapy, with PTBD reserved for the few cases that are problematic for the endoscopist. Obstructing lesions near the papilla of Vater are technically less difficult to approach endoscopically than are more-proximal lesions; accordingly, in this setting, endoscopic therapy is preferred **(Option (D) is true).**

Hemobilia is an important complication of PTBD and has a number of possible etiologies. By far the most common, however, is the placement of a catheter side-hole next to an intrahepatic vessel. This diagnosis can be made quickly and definitively by a catheter cholangiogram, and this procedure is the first test to perform **(Option (E) is true).** If bleeding is brisk and arterial, a hepatic artery aneurysm may be the cause, and angiography is then indicated.

Dennis M. Balfe, M.D.

SUGGESTED READINGS

GALLBLADDER CARCINOMA

1. Itai Y, Araki T, Yoshikawa K, Furui S, Yashiro N, Tasaka A. Computed tomography of gallbladder carcinoma. Radiology 1980; 137:713–718
2. Rooholamini SA, Tehrani NS, Razavi MK, et al. Imaging of gallbladder carcinoma. RadioGraphics 1994; 14:291–306
3. Sagoh T, Itoh K, Togashi K, et al. Gallbladder carcinoma: evaluation with MR imaging. Radiology 1990; 174:131–136

AIDS CHOLANGIOPATHY

4. Da Silva F, Boudghene F, Lecomte I, Delage Y, Grange J-D, Bigot J-M. Sonography in AIDS-related cholangitis: prevalence and cause of an

echogenic nodule in the distal end of the common bile duct. AJR 1993; 160:1205–1207

5. Dolmatch BL, Laing FC, Federle MP, Jeffrey RB, Cello J. AIDS-related cholangitis: radiographic findings in nine patients. Radiology 1987; 163: 313–316

6. Romano AJ, vanSonnenberg E, Casola G, et al. Gallbladder and bile duct abnormalities in AIDS: sonographic findings in eight patients. AJR 1988; 150:123–127

7. Teixidor HS, Godwin TA, Ramirez EA. Cryptosporidiosis of the biliary tract in AIDS. Radiology 1991; 180:51–56

CHOLANGIOCARCINOMA

8. Carr DH, Hadjis NS, Banks LM, Hemingway AP, Blumgart LH. Computed tomography of hilar cholangiocarcinoma: a new sign. AJR 1985; 145:53–56

9. Choi BI, Lee JH, Han MC, Kim SH, Yi JG, Kim CW. Hilar cholangiocarcinoma: comparative study with sonography and CT. Radiology 1989; 172:689–692

10. Dooms GC, Kerlan RK Jr, Hricak H, Wall SD, Margulis AR. Cholangiocarcinoma: imaging by MR. Radiology 1986; 159:89–94

11. Engels JT, Balfe DM, Lee JK. Biliary carcinoma: CT evaluation of extrahepatic spread. Radiology 1989; 172:35–40

12. Honda H, Onitsuka H, Yasumori K, et al. Intrahepatic peripheral cholangiocarcinoma: two-phase dynamic incremental CT and pathologic correlation. J Comput Assist Tomogr 1993; 17:397–402

13. Klatskin G. Adenocarcinoma of the hepatic duct at its bifurcation within the porta hepatis. An unusual tumor with distinctive clinical and pathologic features. Am J Med 1965; 38:241–256

14. Nesbit GM, Johnson CD, James EM, MacCarty RL, Nagorney DM, Bender CE. Cholangiocarcinoma: diagnosis and evaluation of resectability by CT and sonography as procedures complementary to cholangiography. AJR 1988; 151:933–938

15. Takayasu K, Ikeya S, Mukai K, Muramatsu Y, Makuuchi M, Hasegawa H. CT of hilar cholangiocarcinoma: late contrast enhancement in six patients. AJR 1990; 154:1203–1206

16. Takayasu K, Muramatsu Y, Shima Y, Moriyama N, Yamada T, Makuuchi M. Hepatic lobar atrophy following obstruction of the ipsilateral portal vein from hilar cholangiocarcinoma. Radiology 1986; 160:389–393

17. Thorsen MK, Quiroz F, Lawson TL, Smith DF, Foley WD, Stewart ET. Primary biliary carcinoma: CT evaluation. Radiology 1984; 152:479–483

NODES IN THE PORTA HEPATIS

18. Baker ME, Silverman PM, Halvorsen RA Jr, Cohan RH. Computed tomography of masses in periportal/hepatoduodenal ligament. J Comput Assist Tomogr 1987; 11:258–263

19. Weinstein JB, Heiken JP, Lee JK, et al. High resolution CT of the porta hepatis and hepatoduodenal ligament. RadioGraphics 1986; 6:55–74

20. Zirinsky K, Auh YH, Rubenstein WA, Kneeland JB, Whalen JP, Kazam E. The portacaval space: CT with MR correlation. Radiology 1985; 156: 453–460

MIRIZZI'S SYNDROME

21. Cruz FO, Barriga P, Tocornal J, Burhenne HJ. Radiology of the Mirizzi syndrome: diagnostic importance of the transhepatic cholangiogram. Gastrointest Radiol 1983; 8:249–253

EVALUATION OF BILIARY OBSTRUCTION BY CT

22. Barakos JA, Ralls PW, Lapin SA, et al. Cholelithiasis: evaluation with CT. Radiology 1987; 162:415–418
23. Gulliver DJ, Baker ME, Cheng CA, Meyers WC, Pappas TN. Malignant biliary obstruction: efficacy of thin-section dynamic CT in determining resectability. AJR 1992; 159:503–507
24. Reiman TH, Balfe DM, Weyman PJ. Suprapancreatic biliary obstruction: CT evaluation. Radiology 1987; 163:49–56

EVALUATION OF BILIARY OBSTRUCTION BY MRI

25. Dooms GC, Fisher MR, Higgins CB, Hricak H, Goldberg HI, Margulis AR. MR imaging of the dilated biliary tract. Radiology 1986; 158:337–341
26. Low RN, Sigeti JS, Francis IR, et al. Evaluation of malignant biliary obstruction: efficacy of fast multiplanar spoiled gradient-recalled MR imaging vs. spin-echo MR imaging, CT, and cholangiography. AJR 1994; 162:315–323

EVALUATION OF BILIARY OBSTRUCTION BY SONOGRAPHY

27. Laing FC, Jeffrey RB, Wing VW. Improved visualization of choledocholithiasis by sonography. AJR 1984; 143:949–952
28. Laing FC, Jeffrey RB Jr, Wing VW, Nyberg DA. Biliary dilatation: defining the level and cause by real-time US. Radiology 1986; 160:39–42

COMPARATIVE STUDIES

29. Baron RL, Stanley RJ, Lee JKT, et al. A prospective comparison of the evaluation of biliary obstruction using computed tomography and ultrasonography. Radiology 1982; 145:91–98
30. Gibson RN, Yeung E, Thompson JN, et al. Bile duct obstruction: radiologic evaluation of level, cause, and tumor resectability. Radiology 1986; 160: 43–47

31. Hamlin JA, Friedman M, Stein MG, Bray JF. Percutaneous biliary drainage: complications of 118 consecutive catheterizations. Radiology 1986; 158:199–202

32. Lee MJ, Dawson SL, Mueller PR, et al. Percutaneous management of hilar biliary malignancies with metallic endoprostheses: results, technical problems, and causes of failure. RadioGraphics 1993; 13:1249–1263

33. Mueller PR, vanSonnenberg E, Ferrucci JT. Percutaneous biliary drainage: technical and catheter-related problems in 200 procedures. AJR 1982; 138:17–23

34. Stanley J, Gobien RP, Cunningham J, Andriole J. Biliary decompression: an institutional comparison of percutaneous and endoscopic methods. Radiology 1986; 158:195–197

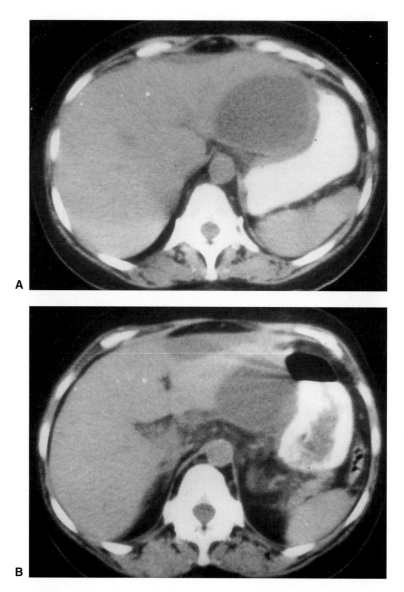

Figure 16-1. This 50-year-old woman has fever, right upper quadrant abdominal pain, and pleuritic left chest pain. You are shown two images from an abdominal CT scan.

Case 16: Abscess in the Greater Peritoneal Cavity

Question 47

Which *one* of the following is the MOST likely diagnosis?

(A) Pyogenic liver abscess
(B) Amebic liver abscess
(C) Echinococcosis
(D) Abscess in the greater peritoneal sac
(E) Abscess in the lesser peritoneal sac

Figure 16-1A shows a large, homogeneous fluid density collection posterior to the left hepatic lobe, displacing the contour of the contrast-filled stomach (Figure 16-2A). The posterior surface of the collection is anterior to the fat within the fissure for the ligamentum venosum. There is a small lenticular collection with similar attenuation lying on the anterior surface of the left lobe; its boundaries are difficult to define on this section. Figure 16-1B, obtained 16 mm caudal to the section in Figure 16-1A, shows that the small lenticular collection is bounded on its right side by the falciform ligament (Figure 16-2B). The contour of the lateral segment of the left hepatic lobe is distorted by the fluid collections.

The clinical findings of fever and pain, combined with these radiographic findings, strongly support the diagnosis of an abscess in the peritoneal space surrounding the left hepatic lobe; this space is part of the greater peritoneal sac **(Option (D) is correct).**

A peritoneal abscess forms when infected fluid enters the peritoneal cavity or when preexisting fluid collections are secondarily infected. The abscess forms as a result of the intense neutrophilic inflammatory reaction produced by the vascular mesothelium. Most abscesses become walled off by deposition of fibrinous material at the periphery of the collection or by adherence of the fluid to adjacent bowel loops or omentum.

Large infected fluid collections can, however, extend into adjacent peritoneal spaces. In the test patient, the abscess extended from the left anterior perihepatic space into the left anterior subphrenic space (Figure

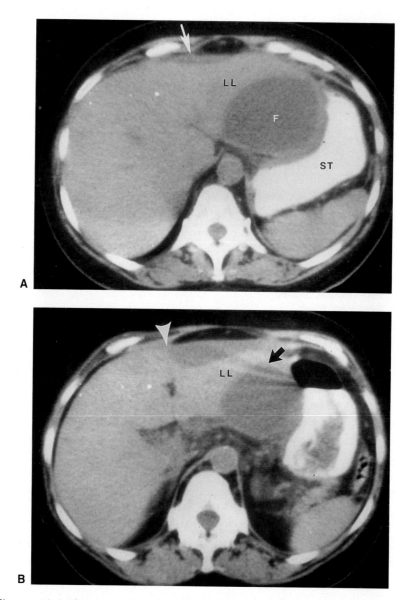

Figure 16-2 (Same as Figure 16-1). Abscess in the left posterior perihepatic space. (A) A CT section obtained at the level of the gastroesophageal junction shows a round, well-circumscribed, low-density fluid
collection (F) distorting the contour of the left hepatic lobe (LL) and the
lesser curve of the stomach (ST). A small lenticular collection (arrow) is
present anterior to the left hepatic lobe. (B) A CT section obtained 16 mm
inferior to panel A shows that the anterior collection is delimited on the
right by the falciform ligament (arrowhead). The anterior and posterior
portions of this fluid collection connect lateral to the left lateral segment
(arrow).

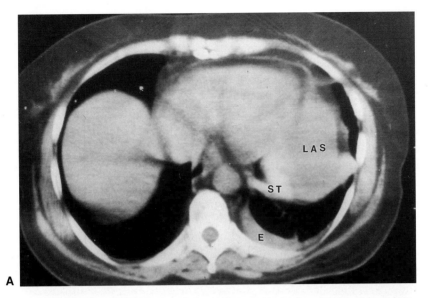

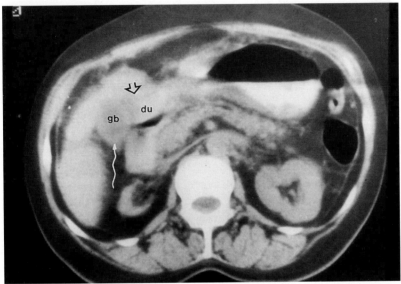

Figure 16-3. Same patient as in Figures 16-1 and 16-2. Abscess in the left posterior perihepatic space. (A) A CT section obtained 16 mm superior to that in Figure 16-2A shows a fluid collection (LAS) in the left anterior subphrenic space, displacing the gastric fundus (ST) and giving rise to a sympathetic pleural effusion (E). (B) A CT section through the gallbladder (gb) shows the inferior extent of the posterior collection noted in Figure 16-2 (open arrow). The gallbladder wall (wavy arrow) is markedly thickened by acute cholecystitis. du = duodenum.

16-3A), where the diaphragmatic irritation induced by the purulent material gave rise to her pleuritic symptoms.

Common causes of abscess in the peritoneal spaces of the upper abdomen include trauma, gastric or duodenal perforation, cholecystitis, and seeding from an adjacent intravisceral abscess in the liver, spleen, or pancreas. Cholecystitis was the underlying cause in the test patient, explaining her right upper quadrant pain (Figure 16-3B).

The history of fever and right upper quadrant pain also suggests a diagnosis of pyogenic liver abscess (Option (A)). However, an abscess within the hepatic parenchyma would be expected to bulge the liver contour outward and would not be sharply confined by the falciform ligament.

Most pyogenic liver abscesses are etiologically related either to biliary infections or to seeding of the portal vein from diverticulitis or appendicitis. Trauma with superinfection of an intrahepatic hematoma is another common cause. Almost half of the abscesses reported in the 1984 series of Halvorsen et al. were polymicrobial; typical organisms include *Streptococcus* species, *Escherichia coli*, and, in children, *Staphylococcus aureus*. Not infrequently, clinical findings are masked by administration of broad-spectrum antibiotics, so that patients frequently present with low-grade fever and relatively mild systemic symptoms.

Mature solitary abscesses have an avascular, liquid center that is separated from liver by a rim of granulation tissue of variable thickness. CT images would therefore be expected to display a spherical mass of near-water attenuation, surrounded by a thin region that undergoes contrast enhancement. In practice, however, abscesses have a variety of appearances; in the 1984 series of Halvorsen et al., septations were visible in 19% of patients and multiple cavities were apparent in 34%. In 69%, the liquid center was heterogeneous and had higher attenuation than water. In 1988, Jeffrey et al. reported a variation that was observed in 14% of pyogenic abscesses in their series: a "cluster" of multiple small (<2-cm) discrete fluid collections in a single segment or lobe (Figure 16-4A). It has been speculated that abscesses that form as the result of biliary infection have a tendency to be multiple. The presence of gas in a pyogenic abscess cavity is relatively uncommon, occurring in only 19% of the patients in the series of Halvorsen et al. (Figure 16-4B).

An amebic liver abscess (Option (B)) will develop in roughly 10% of patients who have invasive amebiasis; it is likely that the parasite reaches the liver by way of the portal vein during the colitic phase of the disease. The clinical presentation can mimic that of a pyogenic abscess, except that most patients will have had an episode of amebic dysentery during the year preceding presentation. The diagnosis is excluded in the test patient because the fluid collection is entirely extrahepatic.

The CT appearance of amebic abscesses is as variable as that of pyogenic abscesses. In the series of 23 patients with amebic liver abscesses

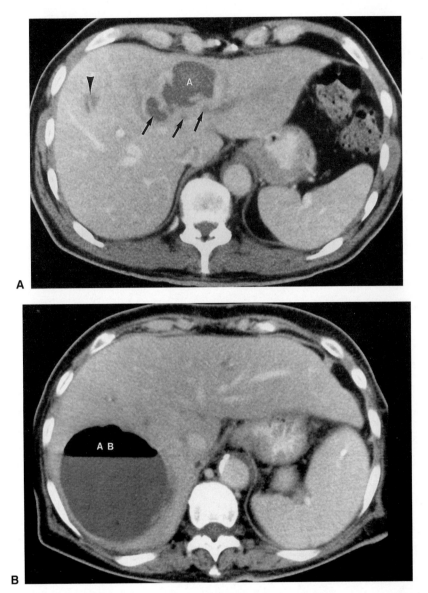

Figure 16-4. Pyogenic liver abscesses. (A) A CT section in a middle-aged man recently treated for acute cholecystitis shows a large, irregular abscess cavity (A) with a thick, enhancing wall in the medial segment of the left hepatic lobe. Multiple smaller abscesses are clustered about it (arrows), and there is a separate small abscess (arrowhead) in the right anterior hepatic segment. (B) A CT section in a 30-year-old man with abdominal trauma. A large gas-containing fluid collection (AB) occupies the dome of the liver.

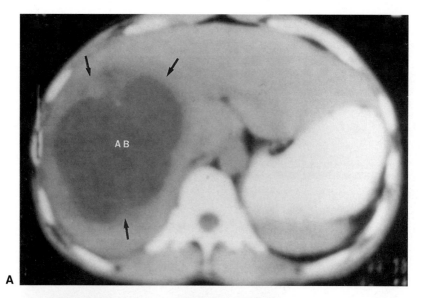

A

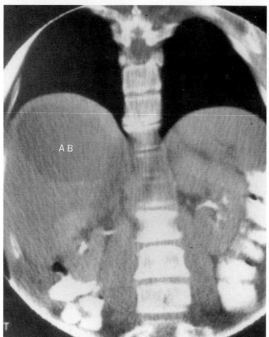

B

Figure 16-5. Amebic abscess. (A) An axial CT section in a 30-year-old male immigrant shows a large cavity with a liquid center (AB) and thick, irregular walls (arrows) in the right posterior hepatic segment near the diaphragm. (B) A direct coronal CT section shows the characteristic relationship of the large solitary cavity (AB) to the diaphragm.

reported by Radin et al., the most common features were a solitary cavity and location within the right lobe (both of these features were present in 74% of patients) (Figure 16-5). Enhancement of the abscess wall was characteristic, and the wall was nodular in 37% of patients. One possibly distinctive feature of amebic abscesses is their potential to spread to extrahepatic locations via the retroperitoneum or diaphragm, an unusual occurrence for pyogenic abscesses.

Echinococcosis (Option (C)) or hydatid disease occurs when an intermediate host (e.g., a sheep or a human) ingests the eggs of the helminthic parasite *Echinococcus* (most often *E. granulosus*). The wall of the ingested eggs is destroyed by upper gastrointestinal digestion; the motile organism then enters the portal vein and becomes encysted within the hepatic parenchyma. The inner wall of the cyst is a germinal layer, and secondary (daughter) cysts are frequently observed. Acute clinical symptoms are uncommon unless the cyst becomes secondarily infected. The extrahepatic location and the absence of daughter cysts exclude this diagnosis in the test patient.

Imaging findings in patients with echinococcosis depend on the status of the organism and on the host response. When the germinal layer is viable, multiple internal daughter cysts form along the periphery and project toward the center of the large hydatid cyst. Death of the parasite leads to separation of the germinal layer from the rest of the wall. Peripheral calcification within the pericyst occurs later (Figure 16-6).

The liver can also be affected by *E. multilocularis*, an entity that differs both clinically and radiologically from the more common hydatid disease. *E. multilocularis* produces numerous small (1- to 10-mm) cysts that form a large conglomerate mass; unlike *E. granulosus*, no well-defined membrane separates the process from the surrounding liver. The disease process almost always extends into the porta hepatis, producing jaundice, venous thrombosis, and portal hypertension. In contrast to the clinical silence of *E. granulosus*, patients with *E. multilocularis* are nearly always symptomatic; jaundice, septicemia (from superinfection of necrotic portions of the process), and variceal bleeding are common modes of presentation.

CT examination in patients with *E. multilocularis* shows a heterogeneous low-attenuation mass with poorly defined boundaries and no discernible enhancement after administration of intravenous contrast material. When calcification occurs, it is punctate rather than arcuate; biliary dilatation is a common feature. It can be difficult to differentiate between hepatocellular carcinoma and *E. multilocularis*.

Abscesses in the lesser peritoneal sac (Option (E)) form under the same conditions as greater peritoneal collections and cannot be clinically distinguished from them. However, the lesser sac lies posterior to the gastrohepatic ligament and does not contact the falciform ligament.

Abscesses in the inferior recess of the lesser sac typically lie between the pancreas and the stomach. Abscesses are generally spherical, and lesser sac abscesses frequently cause marked distortion of the posterior gastric wall because the pancreas is relatively immobile (Figure 16-7).

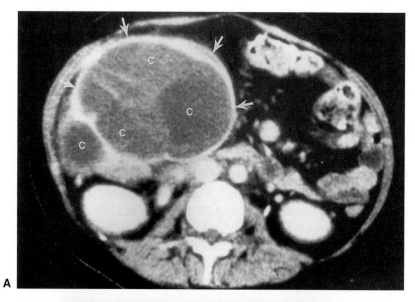

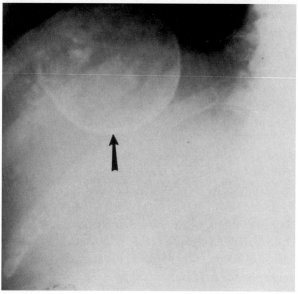

Figure 16-6. Echinococcal cyst. (A) A CT section in an asymptomatic middle-aged patient shows a large, chiefly cystic mass (arrows) with a high-attenuation periphery. There are several smaller (daughter) cysts (C) within the larger mass. (B) An anteroposterior view of the chest shows a peripherally calcified hydatid cyst (arrow) in the dome of the liver.

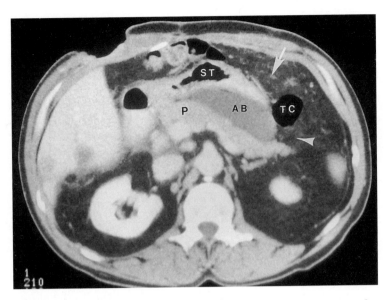

Figure 16-7. Lesser sac abscess. A CT section in a patient undergoing chemotherapy for widespread peritoneal metastases shows a fluid collection (AB) in the inferior recess of the lesser sac, bounded by the pancreas (P) posteriorly and distorting the greater curvature of the stomach (ST) anteriorly. The left side of the collection is bounded by the greater omentum (arrow) and transverse mesocolon (arrowhead). TC = transverse colon.

Question 48

Concerning the lesser peritoneal sac,

- (A) a needle can be placed into a collection in the inferior recess without traversing any structure except properitoneal fat
- (B) collections in the inferior recess occasionally extend into the greater omentum
- (C) in draining collections in the superior recess, a catheter traversing the left lobe of the liver is acceptable
- (D) part of the anterior border of the inferior recess is formed by the lesser omentum
- (E) abscesses within the superior recess usually extend into the hepatorenal recess (Morison's pouch)

The peritoneal spaces of the upper abdomen are divided into two unequal parts, left and right, by the abdominal mesenteries. The ventral mesentery suspends the developing foregut from the anterior abdominal

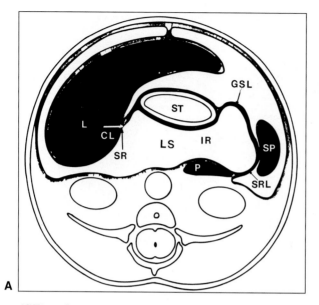

Figure 16-8. Anatomy of peritoneal spaces (A) Embryologically the lesser sac (LS) is a part of the right peritoneal space that is displaced from its original site by the liver (L), which rotates into it as it grows. The superior recess of the lesser sac (SR) lies behind the gastrohepatic ligament (white arrow) and surrounds the caudate lobe (CL). The inferior recess (IR) lies posterior to the stomach (ST) and anterior to the pancreas (P) and is surrounded on the left by the gastrosplenic ligament (GSL) and splenorenal ligament (SRL). The splenorenal ligament eventually fuses to the posterior abdominal wall; the gastrosplenic ligament becomes redundant and ultimately forms the greater omentum and part of the transverse mesocolon. SP = spleen. (B) Adult anatomy of the peritoneal spaces. Left peritoneal spaces: the lateral segment of the left lobe of the liver (LL) divides the anterior (LAP) from the posterior (LPP) left perihepatic space. These spaces are continuous with the left anterior subphrenic space (LAS) just anterior to the stomach (ST). The LAS, in turn, communicates with the left posterior subphrenic space (LPS) (perisplenic space) surrounding the surface of the spleen (S). Right peritoneal spaces: the right subphrenic space (RS) extends from the falciform ligament (bold arrow) to cover the smooth interface between the liver and diaphragm. Posteriorly, it is delimited by the bare area (BA). Caudal to the section drawn here, the posterior part of the space follows the liver surface medially and anteriorly, passing between the liver and the right kidney to form the hepatorenal fossa (Morison's pouch). This communicates through the foramen of Winslow to the upper recess of the lesser sac (SR), which, in turn, empties into the inferior recess of the lesser sac (IR). LK = left kidney.

wall. The liver develops within the ventral mesentery, and the umbilical vein passes through it. As the liver grows, it bulges into the left peritoneal space, deforming its contour and producing compartments anterior and posterior to the liver surface. These compartments, in turn, communicate with the peritoneal surfaces that lie between the left hemidiaphragm and the stomach (anterior subphrenic space) and the spleen (posterior subphrenic or perisplenic space).

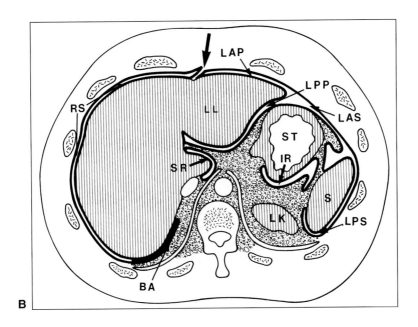

B

At the same time, the liver also rotates into the right peritoneal cavity, so that the left sides of both the ventral mesentery and stomach become anterior in position and their right surfaces become posterior. Therefore, the left peritoneal spaces lie anterior to the lesser omentum (which is the remnant of the ventral mesentery in adults).

In a similar manner, the right-sided peritoneal spaces are subdivided by the growth and rotation of the right lobe of the liver. The right subphrenic space is the smooth, broad surface between the right lobe and the right hemidiaphragm. Below the bare area of the liver, this compartment is continuous with the peritoneal space anterior to the right kidney (the hepatorenal fossa, or Morison's pouch). The right surface of the ventral mesentery (lesser omentum) becomes posterior in location because of the mesenteric rotation described above. The peritoneal space adjacent to this surface is an extension of the right peritoneal space behind the lesser omentum and the stomach and is termed the lesser sac (Figure 16-8A).

The lesser sac is thus formed during embryologic development of the upper abdomen, when the right peritoneal space, displaced by the rotation of the liver, extends behind the lesser omentum and stomach. The gastrosplenic ligament stretches markedly at the same time, so that the right peritoneal space comes to lie between the leaves of the redundant gastrosplenic mesentery to form the omental bursa. As the fetus grows, the anterior and posterior leaves of the gastrosplenic ligament fuse to form the gastrocolic ligament, or greater omentum. As a result, in adults

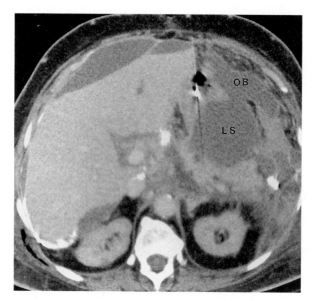

Figure 16-9. Extension of a lesser sac abscess. CT shows that the large lesser sac fluid collection (LS) has extended between the leaves of the greater omentum into the "omental bursa" (OB).

the inferior recess of the lesser sac is surrounded on all sides by visceral structures (Figure 16-8B) and small collections are accordingly technically difficult to drain with a catheter; a needle placed into such a collection must therefore traverse the greater omentum, the stomach, or the lesser omentum before entering the lesser sac **(Option (A) is false).**

In some patients, the embryologic fusion between the anterior and posterior leaves of the greater omentum is incomplete and effusions within the lesser sac can continue into the greater omentum **(Option (B) is true).** When this occurs, the collection often lies anterior to the transverse colon immediately beneath the anterior abdominal wall and so is much easier to drain than most lesser sac abscesses (Figure 16-9).

Loculated fluid collections within the superior recess of the lesser sac usually follow the contour of the caudate lobe. They are bounded by the lesser omentum anteriorly, the caudate lobe on the right, and the retroperitoneal portion of the left gastric artery on the left. Inferiorly, the superior recess empties into the inferior recess and, by way of the foramen of Winslow, into the remainder of the right peritoneal space.

Collections within the superior recess (Figure 16-10) are often very close to the inferior vena cava on the right and the aorta posteriorly on the left. Catheter drainage of such collections usually traverses the left lobe of the liver, because no safer access route is feasible **(Option (C) is true).**

The inferior recess of the lesser sac is bounded anteriorly by the lesser omentum **(Option (D) is true)** and the body of the stomach, later-

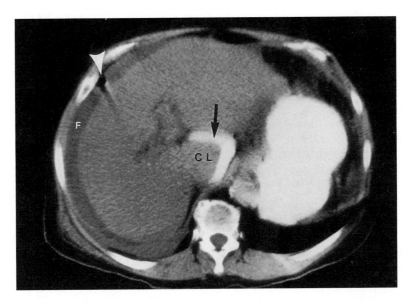

Figure 16-10. Collection within the superior recess of the lesser sac. Contrast agent leaking from a penetrating gastric ulcer (not shown) has entered the superior recess of the lesser sac (arrow), surrounding the leftward surface of the caudate lobe (CL). Note gas (arrowhead) and fluid (F) in the right subphrenic space.

ally by the greater omentum, and posteroinferiorly by the transverse mesocolon.

Fluid collections, chiefly abscesses and pseudocysts, that form in one compartment of the lesser sac typically become walled off quickly, so that they do not communicate with adjacent portions of the peritoneal space. It is particularly uncommon for a lesser sac abscess within the superior recess to extend through the foramen of Winslow into the hepatorenal recess of the greater peritoneal space, even though the two spaces are anatomically continuous **(Option (E) is false).**

Question 49

Concerning intrahepatic infectious lesions,

(A) pyogenic abscesses are solitary in over 95% of patients
(B) in immunocompetent patients, most abscesses result from seeding of the portal vein from appendicitis
(C) in immunocompromised patients, multiple small (<2-cm) collections are most likely to be caused by *Candida albicans*
(D) hydatid cysts can be successfully treated by percutaneous aspiration
(E) peripheral calcification is a characteristic of hydatid cysts

The liver receives its portal blood supply from the veins draining both the small intestine and the colon. Accordingly, infections or infestations arising in the alimentary tract are frequently seeded to the hepatic parenchyma. Also, inflammation of the biliary system can spread directly to the liver surrounding it.

Pyogenic liver abscesses are usually the result of portal contamination by diverticulitis or appendicitis, or from cholecystitis or cholangitis. Less common causes include trauma and inflammation of nearby organs (such as duodenal ulcer disease or pancreatitis). Abscesses that originate in the bile ducts are typically multiple, and those seeded by the portal vein are multifocal in up to one-fourth of patients **(Option (A) is false)**.

Before the antibiotic era, most liver abscesses were the result of portal vein pylephlebitis. Today, in patients who are not immunocompromised, the biliary tree accounts for the vast majority of pyogenic abscesses within the liver parenchyma **(Option (B) is false)**. Gram-negative bacilli (most frequently *E. coli*) are the most common organisms cultured from these collections.

Immunocompromised patients have a different spectrum of focal liver abscesses than do immunocompetent patients. Patients undergoing treatment for hematologic malignancies are at particular risk of developing fungal abscesses. The typical CT appearance of fungal liver abscesses is that of multiple low-density, well-circumscribed lesions scattered throughout the liver parenchyma. Rarely do individual lesions exceed 2 cm in diameter. The vast majority of abscesses with this CT appearance are caused by *Candida albicans* **(Option (C) is true)**. As reported by Shirkhoda et al., the spleen and kidneys may have similar lesions (Figure 16-11A). Sonography has been reported to show several different patterns of candidal abscesses. An echogenic center surrounded by a hypoechoic rim ("bull's-eye" pattern) is the most characteristic (Figure 16-11B) but is not as commonly observed as the uniformly hypoechoic lesion. The differential diagnosis of this appearance includes infections caused by other fungi (*Aspergillus* spp. are common), granulomatous dis-

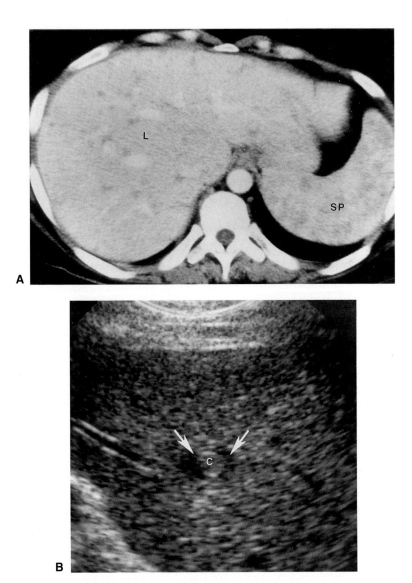

Figure 16-11. Abscesses due to *Candida albicans.* (A) A CT scan in an immunosuppressed patient with fever and abdominal pain shows multiple focal low-attenuation areas throughout both the liver (L) and spleen (SP). Aspiration and culture showed invasive *Candida* organisms. (B) A sonogram in another immunocompromised patient shows a characteristic "target" appearance, consisting of a highly echogenic center (C) surrounded by an annular hypoechoic zone (arrows).

eases such as sarcoidosis, *Yersinia enterocolitica* infection, non-Hodgkin's lymphoma, and chemical injury (such as tetracycline intoxication).

Percutaneous therapy of pyogenic liver abscesses has been accepted for more than a decade, but aspiration of hydatid cysts has been discouraged because of the potential risk of lethal complications (typically due to anaphylactic shock). However, Acunas et al. reported their experience with 12 patients with purely cystic hydatid disease. Percutaneous aspiration combined with injection of hypertonic saline was successful in all cases **(Option (D) is true).**

Imaging features of echinococcal liver cysts depend on the stage of the disease. Internal septations are frequently present. When daughter cysts form, their walls sometimes can be seen within the larger "mother" cyst. Ring-shaped or crescentic calcifications are present within the pericyst in up to 60% of patients **(Option (E) is true)** and are associated with the death of the parasite (Figure 16-6B).

Question 50

Contraindications to percutaneous abscess drainage include:

(A) multiple loculations
(B) ascites
(C) lack of a safe access route
(D) bleeding diathesis
(E) infected pseudoaneurysms

Few radiologic procedures have been received as enthusiastically by primary care physicians as percutaneous abscess drainage. In the early development of this technique, radiologists were selective in identifying candidates appropriate for the drainage procedure. Included were patients with unilocular cavities, those in whom an access track to the abscess cavity did not pass through unaffected solid viscera, and those with cavities that were unassociated with fistulas or sinus tracts. All other patients were considered inappropriate candidates for percutaneous drainage. However, the gratifying success of the percutaneous approach led radiologists to expand these restrictive criteria. Multiple loculations can be successfully approached with multiple catheters **(Option (A) is false).** In patients in whom complex fluid collections are being drained, it is important that post-drainage imaging be performed to assess the completeness of the drainage procedure and that additional catheters be placed as necessary to achieve complete resolution.

Placing catheters into an abscess cavity through a pocket of ascitic fluid often leads to some catheter care problems, since ascites frequently tracks along the tube, causing persistent leakage onto the skin. This

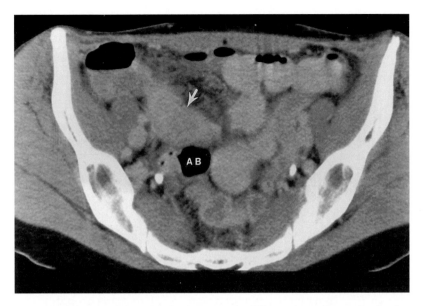

Figure 16-12. "Undrainable" abscess. A CT section through the lower abdomen in a 25-year-old patient with known Crohn's disease shows a thick-walled loop of distal ileum (arrow), which had perforated posteriorly into a small gas-containing abscess cavity (AB). Percutaneous drainage was not performed, because of the lack of a safe access route to this small collection.

problem may be aggravating, but it is not a contraindication to performing abscess drainage **(Option (B) is false).**

Fluid collections are occasionally surrounded on all sides by structures that are unsafe to traverse. Deep pelvic abscesses sometimes fall into this category, being shielded by the ilium and sacrum on the posterior and lateral sides and by loops of sigmoid colon or ileum anteriorly (Figure 16-12) **(Option (C) is true).** It must be remembered, however, that the word "safety" has no consistent definition, and, in the context of a critically ill patient, a risky drainage procedure sometimes must be undertaken because it is the only choice. Individual decisions depend less on absolute rules than on clinical judgment and procedural innovation.

Many patients with abscesses have underlying deficits in their clotting mechanism, either because of an underlying condition or because of consumptive coagulopathy produced by the infection. In general, these conditions can be temporarily corrected by administration of fresh-frozen plasma or platelets and should not prevent the performance of a successful drainage procedure **(Option (D) is false).**

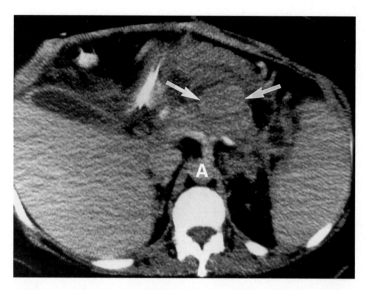

Figure 16-13. Infected pseudoaneurysm. A CT section through the celiac axis in a patient with recurrent severe pancreatitis, fever, and abdominal pain shows a rounded fluid collection (arrows) which demonstrates contrast enhancement to the same degree as the aorta (A). Direct percutaneous embolization was successfully performed.

One potential pitfall in the path of the interventional radiologist is the pseudoaneurysm. Pseudoaneurysms are most commonly observed in patients who have had necrotizing pancreatitis (Figure 16-13). Enzymatic dissolution of the adventitia of small to medium-sized peripancreatic vessels produces a weakened wall, leading to pseudoaneurysm formation. The appropriate nonsurgical therapy for these lesions is transcatheter (or, occasionally, percutaneous) embolization; drainage catheter insertion is not appropriate, even if the pseudoaneurysms are infected **(Option (E) is true).**

Question 51

Concerning percutaneous abscess drainage,

(A) successful drainage of a pleural space collection requires a larger-diameter catheter than does drainage of an abdominal abscess
(B) routine irrigation of the abscess cavity with an antibiotic solution is beneficial
(C) an enteric fistula is a cause of therapeutic failure
(D) complete distension of the abscess cavity is potentially hazardous

Selection of catheter size, and the size and number of side holes within the catheter, is a function of the abscess contents; the fluid material within a mature pyogenic collection can be drained with a 12F to 14F catheter, independent of the geometry or location of the cavity **(Option (A) is false).** Collections due to pancreatitis are frequently semisolid (Figure 16-14), and larger catheters are helpful in allowing the solid components to pass through the tube without clogging it.

The major benefit of percutaneous catheter drainage of abscesses occurs when the purulent material is removed, and the widespread acceptance of the procedure stems from the fact that this simple maneuver alone is highly successful. Accordingly, additional procedures, such as injection of antibiotics or mucolytic agents into the cavity, should be reserved for cases in which a problem occurs and should not be performed routinely **(Option (B) is false).** Antibiotic therapy should be directed to the systemic rather than the local effects of the abscess.

The success rate of percutaneous drainage procedures is quite high but is not 100%. There are some situations in which catheter drainage has a higher likelihood of failure as a curative procedure. These include drainage of an infected tumor, attempted drainage of an inflammatory process with a large semisolid component, and abscess cavities associated with enteric fistulas (Figure 16-15) **(Option (C) is true).** It is important to recognize that the presence of a fistula does not mandate that the drainage will be a failure; however, there is a higher likelihood that catheter drainage times will be prolonged or that complications requiring repositioning or additional catheters will occur.

It is important to document that all of the purulent material in the body cavity has been successfully drained; however, reinjection of the catheter immediately after intubation of the cavity is not effective in making that assessment, and reinflation of the cavity can cause the remaining abscess contents to be driven into the periphery of the abscess, where bacteria will be introduced into the venous system. This results in sepsis **(Option (D) is true).**

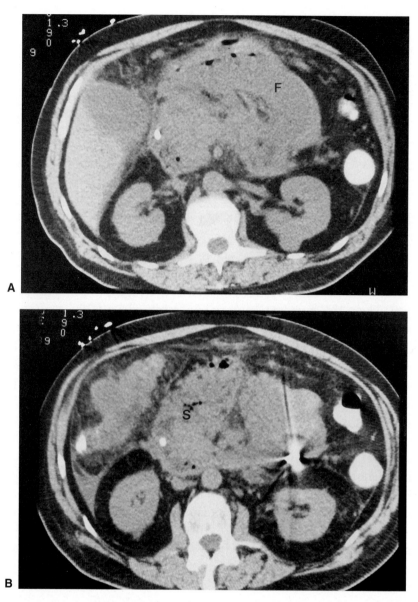

Figure 16-14. Pancreatitis with solid component. (A) A CT section through the upper portion of the pancreas shows a homogeneous high-attenuation fluid collection (F) that was successfully drained with a percutaneous catheter. (B) A CT section 16 mm inferior to that in panel A shows a complex mixed-attenuation portion of the collection (S), containing gas bubbles. This area was chiefly solid, and a catheter positioned in this collection initially drained scant fluid.

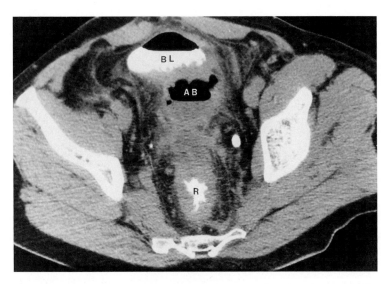

Figure 16-15. Abscess due to diverticulitis with persistent sigmoid fistula. A CT section through the pelvis in an elderly man with clinical evidence of diverticulitis shows an abscess cavity (AB) that communicated to the sigmoid colon (shown on a higher section). There is inflammatory thickening of the base of the bladder (BL); gas in the bladder is due to communication of the abscess with the bladder lumen. There is also marked thickening of the rectum (R) as a result of the surrounding inflammation, but no fistula was present. Percutaneous catheter drainage was performed, with continued drainage for 6 weeks, despite bowel rest.

Question 52

Concerning injection of contrast agent into an abscess cavity (abscess sinography),

- (A) it is indicated when CT, ultrasonography, or clinical evaluation suggests the presence of a residual cavity
- (B) it is essential before removal of the drainage catheter
- (C) it is helpful in evaluating patients with persistent or increasing drainage
- (D) in conjunction with CT, it is useful in detecting residual pockets not drained by the abscess catheter

Catheter care and follow-up is at least as important to the success of percutaneous abscess drainage as the technical success of catheter introduction. In uncomplicated cases, in which the purulent material has been successfully withdrawn during the initial drainage procedure, the patient's clinical status has improved, and the output of the drainage

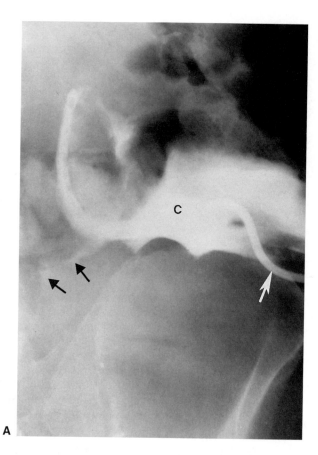

Figure 16-16. Catheter repositioning for adequate drainage. The patient had an iliac fossa abscess drained 5 days previously and now has recurrent fever and left psoas muscle irritation. (A) Abscess sinography through the indwelling catheter (white arrow) shows almost total collapse of the initial abscess cavity (C). Contrast is noted to track inferiorly (black arrows) from a portion of the cavity.

catheter ceases, the catheter can be removed without any additional imaging **(Option (B) is false).** However, when the clinical evolution is not straightforward, it can be very helpful to perform catheter injections in specific circumstances. Probably the most common situation is that in which persistent or increasing drainage through the catheter prompts a follow-up CT or sonogram that shows a residual cavity **(Option (C) is true).** In that situation, the most efficient maneuver is to determine whether simple repositioning of the indwelling catheter will solve the problem, and catheter injection will demonstrate whether the new collection can be filled via the existing catheter (Figure 16-16) **(Option (A) is true).** Conversely, if the contrast injection shows no connection to the second abscess, a second drainage catheter is mandated.

Occasionally, it is unclear whether the cavity filled by injection of contrast agent corresponds to the extent of the fluid collection demonstrated by CT. In these cases, the simplest maneuver is to inject dilute

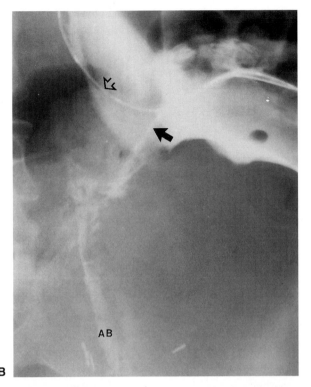

B

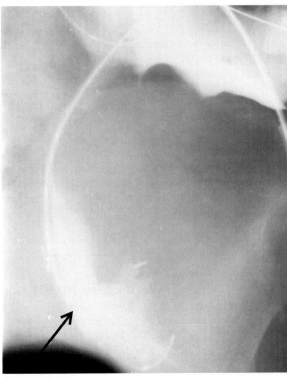

C

Figure 16-16 (Continued). Catheter repositioning for adequate drainage. (B) A safety wire (open arrow) has been placed. A 5F catheter (solid arrow) has been manipulated into the inferior track; water-soluble contrast agent (injected through the catheter) fills a long fusiform abscess (AB) corresponding to the distribution of the left psoas muscle. (C) A guidewire (arrow) has been inserted into the second collection, which was subsequently successfully drained with a second catheter.

contrast material (1 to 2% iodine) into the drainage catheter and repeat the CT scan **(Option (D) is true).** Undrained collections can be readily differentiated from portions of a complex cavity.

Dennis M. Balfe, M.D.

SUGGESTED READINGS

PERITONEAL ABSCESS

1. Crass JR, Maile CW, Frick MP. Catheter drainage of the left posterior subphrenic space: a reliable percutaneous approach. Gastrointest Radiol 1985; 10:397–398
2. Goldman R, Hunter TB, Haber K. The silent abdominal abscess: role of the radiologist. AJR 1983; 141:21–25
3. Jaques P, Mauro M, Safrit H, Yankaskas B, Piggott B. CT features of intra-abdominal abscesses: prediction of successful percutaneous drainage. AJR 1986; 146:1041–1045

PYOGENIC LIVER ABSCESS

4. Halvorsen RA, Korobkin M, Foster WL, Silverman PM, Thompson WM. The variable CT appearance of hepatic abscesses. AJR 1984; 141:941–946
5. Jeffrey RB Jr, Tolentino CS, Chang FC, Federle MP. CT of small pyogenic hepatic abscesses: the cluster sign. AJR 1988; 151:487–489
6. Mendez RJ, Schiebler ML, Outwater EK, Kressel HY. Hepatic abscesses: MR imaging findings. Radiology 1994; 190:431–436

AMEBIC LIVER ABSCESS

7. Elizondo G, Weissleder R, Stark DD, et al. Amebic liver abscess: diagnosis and treatment evaluation with MR imaging. Radiology 1987; 165:795–800
8. Radin DR, Ralls PW, Colletti PM, Halls JM. CT of amebic liver abscess. AJR 1988; 150:1297–1301
9. Ralls PW, Henley DS, Colletti PM, et al. Amebic liver abscess: MR imaging. Radiology 1987; 165:801–804

HYDATID DISEASE

10. Bezzi M, Teggi A, De Rosa F, et al. Abdominal hydatid disease: US findings during medical treatment. Radiology 1987; 162:91–95
11. Didier D, Weiler S, Rohmer P, et al. Hepatic alveolar echinococcosis: correlative US and CT study. Radiology 1985; 154:179–186
12. Lewall DB, McCorkell SJ. Hepatic echinococcal cysts: sonographic appearance and classification. Radiology 1985; 155:773–775

13. Taourel P, Marty-Ane B, Charasset S, Mattei M, Devred P, Bruel JM. Hydatid cyst of the liver: comparison of CT and MRI. J Comput Assist Tomogr 1993; 17:80–85

PERITONEAL ANATOMY

14. Dodds WJ, Foley WD, Lawson TL, Stewart ET, Taylor A. Anatomy and imaging of the lesser peritoneal sac. AJR 1985; 144:567–575
15. Halvorsen RA, Jones MA, Rice RP, Thompson WM. Anterior left subphrenic abscess: characteristic plain film and CT appearance. AJR 1982; 139:283–289
16. Jeffrey RB, Federle MP, Goodman PC. Computed tomography of the lesser peritoneal sac. Radiology 1981; 141:117–122
17. Min P-Q, Yang Z-G, Lei Q-F, et al. Peritoneal reflections of left perihepatic region: radiologic-anatomic study. Radiology 1992; 182:553–557
18. Rubenstein WA, Auh YH, Whalen JP, Kazam E. The perihepatic spaces: computed tomographic and ultrasound imaging. Radiology 1983; 149:231–239
19. Rubenstein WA, Auh YH, Zirinsky K, Kneeland JB, Whalen JP, Kazam E. Posterior peritoneal recesses: assessment using CT. Radiology 1985; 156:461–468
20. Vincent LM, Mauro MA, Mittelstaedt CA. The lesser sac and gastrohepatic recess: sonographic appearance and differentiation of fluid collections. Radiology 1984; 150:515–519

CANDIDA LIVER ABSCESSES

21. Pastakia B, Shawker TH, Thaler M, O'Leary T, Pizzo PA. Hepatosplenic candidiasis: wheels within wheels. Radiology 1988; 166:417–421
22. Shirkhoda A, Lopez-Berestein G, Holbert JM, Luna MA. Hepatosplenic fungal infection: CT and pathologic evaluation after treatment with liposomal amphotericin B. Radiology 1986; 159:349–353

PERCUTANEOUS ABSCESS DRAINAGE

23. Casola G, vanSonnenberg E, Neff CC, Saba RM, Withers C, Emarine CW. Abscesses in Crohn disease: percutaneous drainage. Radiology 1987; 163:19–22
24. Gerzof SG, Johnson WC, Robbins AH, Nabseth DC. Expanded criteria for percutaneous abscess drainage. Arch Surg 1985; 120:227–232
25. Haaga JR, Weinstein AJ. CT-guided percutaneous aspiration and drainage of abscesses. AJR 1980; 135:1187–1194
26. Lambiase RE, Cronan JJ, Dorfman GS, Paolella LP, Haas RA. Percutaneous drainage of abscesses in patients with Crohn disease. AJR 1988; 150:1043–1045
27. Lambiase RE, Deyoe L, Cronan JJ, Dorfman GS. Percutaneous drainage of 335 consecutive abscesses: results of primary drainage with 1-year follow-up. Radiology 1992; 184:167–179

28. Lang EK, Springer RM, Glorioso LW III, Cammarata CA. Abdominal abscess drainage under radiologic guidance: causes of failure. Radiology 1986; 159:329–336

29. Mueller PR, Ferrucci JT Jr, Simeone JF, et al. Lesser sac abscesses and fluid collections: drainage by transhepatic approach. Radiology 1985; 155:615–618

30. Neff CC, vanSonnenberg E, Casola G, et al. Diverticular abscesses: percutaneous drainage. Radiology 1987; 163:15–18

31. vanSonnenberg E, D'Agostino HB, Casola G, Halasz NA, Sanchez RB, Goodacre BW. Percutaneous abscess drainage: current concepts. Radiology 1991; 181:617–626

32. vanSonnenberg E, Wing VW, Casola G, et al. Temporizing effect of percutaneous drainage of complicated abscesses in critically ill pateints. AJR 1984; 142:821–826

PERCUTANEOUS ABSCESS DRAINAGE OF HYDATID DISEASE

33. Acunas B, Rozanes I, Celik L, et al. Purely cystic hydatid disease of the liver: treatment with percutaneous aspiration and injection of hypertonic saline. Radiology 1992; 182:541–543

34. Giorgio A, Tarantino L, Francica G, et al. Unilocular hydatid liver cysts: treatment with US-guided, double percutaneous aspiration and alcohol injection. Radiology 1992; 184:705–710

Notes

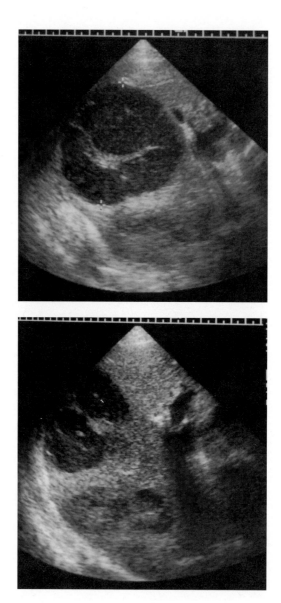

Figure 17-1. This 32-year-old HIV-positive man has vague right upper quadrant pain. You are shown transverse sonograms of the liver.

Case 17: AIDS-Related Lymphoma

Question 53

Which *one* of the following is the MOST likely diagnosis?

(A) Pyogenic abscess
(B) Lymphoma
(C) Kaposi's sarcoma
(D) Mycobacterial infection
(E) *Pneumocystis carinii* infection

The test images (Figure 17-1) demonstrate multiple large hypoechoic masses within the liver in the HIV-positive test patient. The masses are well defined, have internal septations, and exhibit slightly enhanced through transmission (Figure 17-2). These features can be observed either in a complex fluid collection, such as pyogenic abscess, or in a solid mass with relatively homogeneous internal structure, such as lymphoma. HIV-positive patients are not more susceptible to pyogenic liver abscesses than the general population, but they are quite likely to develop lymphoma, either as their AIDS-defining illness or later in the course of the disease. Moreover, up to 45% of patients with AIDS-related abdominal lymphomas develop hepatic involvement. For this reason, of the choices listed, AIDS-related lymphoma is the most likely explanation for the sonographic findings **(Option (B) is correct).**

Patients with a pyogenic abscess (Option (A)) involving the liver can have a variety of underlying etiologies and clinical presentations. Although severe systemic symptoms with chills, hectic fevers, and focal right upper quadrant pain are still common modes of presentation, many patients have low-grade fever, mild or absent local pain, and no overt systemic symptoms. In part, this may reflect the increased use of broad-spectrum antibiotics, which are often administered during the early phase of the illness (when some other diagnosis is suspected) and thus modify its evolution. The vague right upper quadrant pain described in the history of the test patient does not, by itself, exclude the diagnosis of pyogenic abscess.

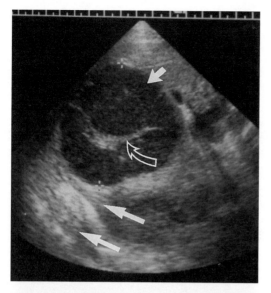

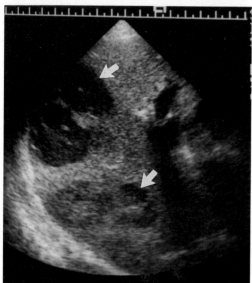

Figure 17-2 (Same as Figure 17-1). AIDS-related hepatic lymphoma. Transverse sonograms of the right lobe of the liver demonstrate multiple hypoechoic masses (short white arrows). Note the internal septation within the lesion in panel A (curved open arrow). Slight enhancement of through transmission is also noted (long white arrows). Percutaneous biopsy revealed non-Hodgkin's lymphoma.

The sonographic appearance of pyogenic abscesses is quite variable. Many are focal hypoechoic lesions. If the abscess contains gas, acoustic shadowing with a characteristic "comet-tail" appearance can be seen emerging from multiple sites within the collection. Unlike amebic abscesses, which tend to be round or oval, most pyogenic abscesses have irregular margins (Figure 17-3). The lobular margin is probably a reflection of the tendency of pyogenic abscesses to cluster within an affected

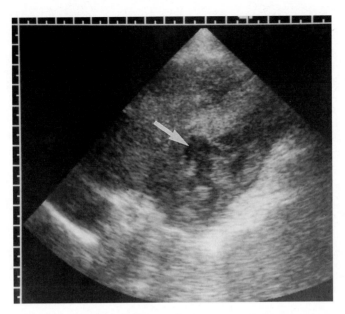

Figure 17-3. Pyogenic liver abscess. A transverse sonogram of the left lobe of the liver demonstrates a poorly defined hypoechoic lesion with irregular margins (arrow). Culture of a needle aspirate was positive for *Escherichia coli.*

lobe or segment (Figure 17-4). The individual pockets within the cluster have variably thick fibrinous walls, producing the sonographic appearance of multiple septations. However, despite their multilocular appearance, single-catheter percutaneous drainage is almost always successful; the components of the cavity typically interconnect (Figure 17-5).

Hepatic involvement in patients with AIDS-related Kaposi's sarcoma (Option (C)) is a common autopsy finding. However, it is rarely symptomatic and often goes clinically undetected. Not infrequently, hepatic lesions due to AIDS-related Kaposi's sarcoma are microscopic and cannot be detected by CT or sonography. Hepatic Kaposi's sarcoma has a predilection for periportal involvement. Periportal tumor infiltration can manifest as delayed enhancement on postcontrast CT. In addition to periportal involvement, peripheral parenchymal nodules can be detected by CT and sonography (Figure 17-6). Peripheral nodules of hepatic Kaposi's sarcoma typically are echogenic on sonography and have low attenuation on CT. The differential diagnosis of multiple echogenic hepatic lesions in a patient with AIDS includes Kaposi's sarcoma, fungal microabscesses, metastatic carcinoma, and multiple hemangiomas. Fine-needle aspiration biopsy is a safe and effective technique to confirm hepatic involve-

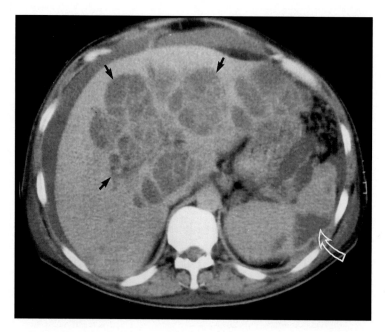

Figure 17-4. Cluster sign of pyogenic liver abscess. A contrast-enhanced CT scan of a large pyogenic abscess demonstrates a multiseptated appearance (black arrows). A splenic abscess was also noted (curved open arrow). Cultures grew anaerobic streptococci.

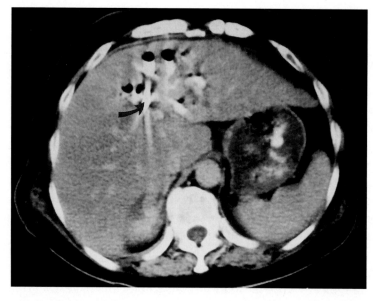

Figure 17-5. Successful percutaneous drainage of a multiseptated pyogenic abscess. Following catheter drainage of the left-lobe liver abscess, dilute water-soluble contrast was injected into the abscess via the percutaneous catheter (arrow). Note that all of the various components of the abscess intercommunicate. The abscess resolved with single-catheter drainage.

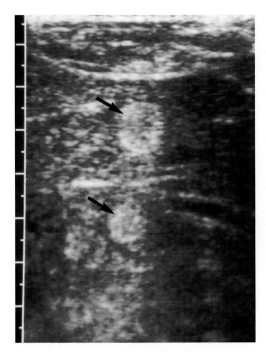

Figure 17-6. Hepatic involvement with AIDS-related Kaposi's sarcoma. A transverse sonogram of the left lobe of the liver demonstrates multiple echogenic nodules (arrows). A percutaneous biopsy revealed Kaposi's sarcoma. The differential diagnosis includes fungal abscesses, hemangiomas, and metastasis.

ment by Kaposi's sarcoma. Clusters of pleomorphic spindle cells are characteristic cytologic features of Kaposi's sarcoma (Figure 17-7).

Mycobacterial infection of the liver (Option (D)) is a well-known complication of AIDS. Organisms include both *Mycobacterium tuberculosis* and *Mycobacterium avium-intracellulare* complex. Most mycobacterial lesions in the liver are microscopic and are not detected by imaging studies. When visible, they are typically less than 1 to 2 cm in size, not bulky as in the test images. In a 1991 report, Radin retrospectively analyzed the abdominal CT scans of 27 patients with *M. tuberculosis* infection and compared them with those of 44 patients with *M. avium-intracellulare* complex infection. Of these patients, 11% had hepatic involvement by *M. tuberculosis* and 9% had hepatic involvement by *M. avium-intracellulare* complex. Marked hepatomegaly was noted in 20% of patients with *M. avium-intracellulare* infection. Low-attenuation lymphadenopathy was found with both *M. tuberculosis* and *M. avium-intracellulare* complex infections (Figure 17-8) but was more common in the former. Fine-needle aspiration biopsy may be extremely valuable in diagnosing mycobacterial infections in patients with AIDS. Smears demonstrate enlarged histiocytes that contain acid-fast organisms on specialized stains.

Extrapulmonary involvement by *P. carinii* (Option (E)) is being recognized with increasing frequency in patients with AIDS who receive

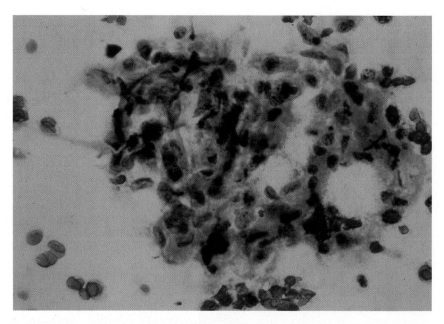

Figure 17-7. Fine-needle aspiration cytology of Kaposi's sarcoma. A sample obtained during percutaneous biopsy of a retroperitoneal lymph node contains typical cytologic features of Kaposi's sarcoma. Note the adherent clusters of pleomorphic spindle cells with hyperchromatic nuclei.

aerosolized pentamidine prophylaxis. Widespread involvement of the liver, spleen, kidneys, and bone marrow can occur. Hepatic involvement by *P. carinii* typically results in multiple punctate calcifications. Calcifications can also occur in the spleen, kidneys, adrenal glands, and lymph nodes. Sonographically, hepatic lesions appear as tiny punctate echogenic foci that are diffusely scattered throughout the entire liver, unlike the lesions in the test images.

Recent observations suggest that *P. carinii* infections can produce focal masses, both in the pulmonary parenchyma and in the abdomen (Figure 17-9). However, tumefactive involvement of the hepatic parenchyma has not been reported.

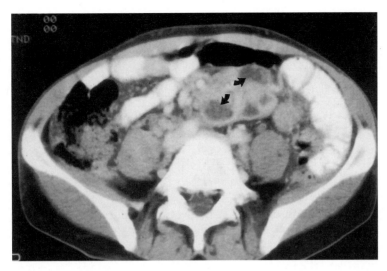

Figure 17-8. Low-density mesenteric lymph nodes as a result of *M. avium-intracellulare* complex infection. Note the multiple areas of necrosis within the enlarged mesenteric lymph nodes (arrows). Biopsy and cultures revealed *M. avium-intracellulare* complex.

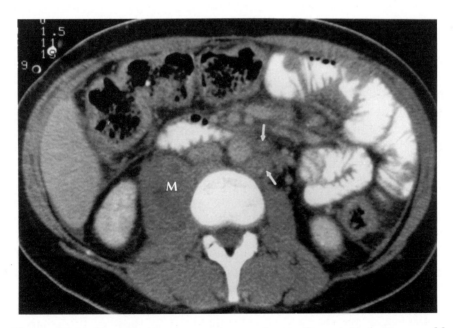

Figure 17-9. Tumefactive psoas abscess due to *P. carinii.* A 41-year-old man underwent prophylactic therapy with aerosolized pentamidine. The CT section demonstrates a mixed-attenuation mass (M) producing enlargement and contour deformity of the right psoas muscle. Note the enlarged left para-aortic nodes (arrows), a common but nonspecific finding in patients with AIDS.

Question 54

Concerning lymphadenopathy in patients with HIV infection,

(A) mild enlargement of retroperitoneal lymph nodes (less than 1.5 cm) is often due to reactive hyperplasia

(B) Kaposi's sarcoma is a cause of bulky retroperitoneal lymphadenopathy

(C) on postcontrast CT, low-attenuation areas within the lymph nodes are typically due to Kaposi's sarcoma

(D) percutaneous fine-needle aspiration biopsy of enlarged lymph nodes often yields a specific diagnosis

Lymphadenopathy is one of the primary abdominal abnormalities in patients with HIV infection and is a common feature of several diseases that occur in patients with AIDS. The differential diagnosis of lymphadenopathy in an HIV-infected patient is broad and includes reactive hyperplasia, AIDS-related lymphoma, Kaposi's sarcoma, and mycobacterial infection. Rare etiologies include extrapulmonary *P. carinii* and bacillary angiomatosis (vascular proliferation caused by a rickettsial organism). Reactive lymphoid hyperplasia (often associated with mild splenomegaly) is commonly observed on cross-sectional images of patients with HIV infection, well before they develop an AIDS-defining illness. These reactive nodes occur in the usual abdominal nodal distribution, typically para-aortic and mesenteric, and rarely exceed 1.5 cm in greatest dimension. Common pathologic processes that involve these nodal groups in patients with HIV infection include non-Hodgkin's lymphoma, Kaposi's sarcoma, and mycobacterial infection. Each of these entities (particularly lymphoma) typically produces bulky lymphadenopathy, with maximum nodal diameters well in excess of 1.5 cm. Accordingly, the commonest cause for the CT finding of multiple, well-defined, minimally enlarged lymph nodes is reactive hyperplasia **(Option (A) is true).**

The manifestations of Kaposi's sarcoma in the abdomen are protean. An infiltrative form can occur within the portal structures in the liver, as mentioned in the discussion of Question 53; however, an adenopathic form that produces moderate nodal enlargement also exists **(Option (B) is true).** Because Kaposi's sarcoma is a vascular neoplasm, there is typically visible enhancement of the lymph node masses after intravenous administration of contrast material. The attenuation values of involved lymph nodes are characteristically higher than those of the adjacent abdominal musculature (Figure 17-10). In a retrospective analysis of patients with abdominal and pelvic lymphadenopathy due to AIDS, Herts et al. noted that 26 of 38 patients with widespread Kaposi's sarcoma had lymph node attenuation values higher than that of the iliopsoas muscle. The positive predictive value for this observation in diag-

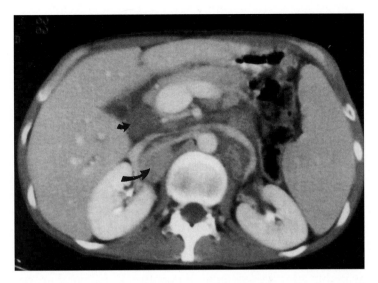

Figure 17-10. Hyperattenuating retroperitoneal lymphadenopathy from AIDS-related Kaposi's sarcoma. A postcontrast CT scan demonstrates a large renal hilus lymph node (large arrow) with attenuation values significantly greater than those of the adjacent abdominal musculature. Fine-needle aspiration biopsy revealed Kaposi's sarcoma. The patient experienced persistent fever, so a biopsy of an enlarged periportal lymph node was performed. Note the low-attenuation lymph node adjacent to the splenic-portal venous confluence (small arrow). Percutaneous needle biopsy and subsequent cultures of periportal lymph node revealed *M. avium-intracellulare* complex.

nosing nodal Kaposi's sarcoma was 79%. Only one patient in this series had Kaposi's sarcoma producing low-attenuation adenopathy **(Option (C) is false).**

Mycobacterial infections also involve retroperitoneal and mesenteric lymph nodes and likewise produce enlargement of these nodes in excess of 1.5 cm. Low-density areas, presumably reflecting the caseating necrosis that occurs late in the course of the disease, are frequently observed in the central portion of the node (Figure 17-8). On scans enhanced by intravenous contrast material, a hyperattenuating rim can be observed.

Non-Hodgkin's lymphoma is decidedly common in patients with HIV infection. As discussed previously, the lymphoma frequently involves the hepatic parenchyma but also characteristically causes massive enlargement of retroperitoneal and mesenteric nodes. These nodes usually have attenuation values equal to that of adjacent abdominal musculature; they can have lower attenuation values if they contain areas of central necrosis (see the discussion of Question 55).

Bacillary angiomatosis is a recently described infectious disorder (caused by the rickettsial organism *Rochalimaea henselae*) that occurs predominantly in patients with AIDS. Cutaneous lesions are quite common and can mimic the clinical appearance of Kaposi's sarcoma or pyogenic granuloma. Massive visceral lymphadenopathy can occur in patients with this entity. Biopsy of skin lesions can be quite valuable for establishing the diagnosis. The lesions are readily treatable with antibiotic therapy, so this entity should be considered when massive visceral lymphadenopathy is noted in patients with characteristic skin lesions.

Fine-needle aspiration cytology is often quite valuable in diagnosing a variety of causes of lymphadenopathy in patients with AIDS **(Option (D) is true)**. Mycobacterial infection, Kaposi's sarcoma, and non-Hodgkin's lymphoma have very distinctive cytologic features that can be readily demonstrated by the fine-needle aspiration technique. Treatment options for Kaposi's sarcoma are quite limited because there is no currently available effective systemic chemotherapy. Chemotherapy for non-Hodgkin's lymphoma can result in short-term remission. The long-term prognosis is poor in patients with AIDS, however, since the disease is frequently advanced at the time of presentation. Mycobacterial infections such as *M. tuberculosis* and *M. avium-intracellulare* complex infections respond variably to chemotherapy depending on the extent of pulmonary, visceral, and systemic involvement. The prognosis is generally poor when these diseases are detected in debilitated patients.

Question 55

Concerning AIDS-related lymphomas,

    (A) they are aggressive histologic subtypes of non-Hodgkin's lymphoma
    (B) most patients present with advanced disease
    (C) there is a predilection for extranodal sites of involvement
    (D) the liver is a commonly involved extranodal site

Lymphoma is sometimes the initial clinical presentation of AIDS. AIDS-related lymphomas are aggressive forms of non-Hodgkin's B-cell lymphoma **(Option (A) is true)**. The most common histologic subtypes include small cell noncleaved lymphoma (either Burkitt's or non-Burkitt's), large cell lymphoma, and immunoblastic lymphoma. Patients typically present with stage III or IV disease **(Option (B) is true)**. AIDS-related lymphomas have a strong predilection for extranodal sites of involvement **(Option (C) is true)**. Virtually any abdominal organ can be involved with lymphoma in patients with AIDS. In a 1993 clinical review of 112 patients with AIDS-related lymphomas, Radin et al. noted extra-

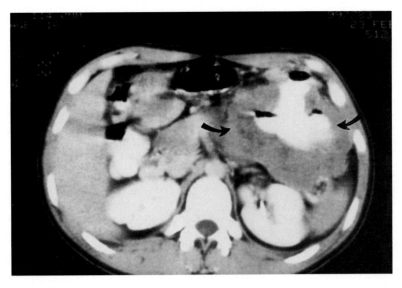

Figure 17-11. Gastric lymphoma in a patient with AIDS. A CT scan demonstrates diffuse mural thickening of the stomach (arrows). Endoscopic biopsy revealed non-Hodgkin's lymphoma.

nodal disease in 86% of patients. The gastrointestinal tract was involved in 54% of patients (Figure 17-11), the liver was involved in 29%, the kidney was involved in 11%, and the adrenal gland was involved in 11%. Other authors also report a significant percentage of patients with hepatic involvement in AIDS. Townsend, in a review of 38 patients with abdominal lymphoma, noted liver involvement in 17 (45%) **(Option (D) is true).** There are two distinct morphologic patterns of hepatic involvement by AIDS-related lymphoma: (1) small scattered nodules that are difficult to distinguish from microabscesses (Figure 17-12), and (2) large conglomerate masses (as in the test patient [Figure 17-1]). Hepatic lymphoma typically is hypoechoic on sonography and has low attenuation on contrast-enhanced CT. Lymphoma can produce a solid mass in virtually any abdominal organ. Diffuse peritoneal involvement occurs occasionally, and its CT appearance mimics carcinomatosis (Figure 17-13). Some patients with AIDS-related lymphomas respond to conventional chemotherapy in the short term. It is therefore of some importance to differentiate lymphoma (for which treatment is available) from other causes of lymphadenopathy. Ultimately, however, patients succumb to disseminated AIDS lymphoma as a result of either tumor recurrence or complications such as overwhelming opportunistic infection.

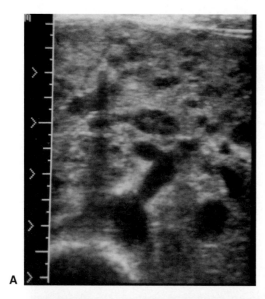

Figure 17-12. AIDS-related hepatic lymphoma. (A) A sonogram demonstrates innumerable hypoechoic nodules scattered throughout the liver. (B) A sonogram in another patient demonstrates two discrete hypoechoic nodules in the right lobe (arrows). (C) Fine-needle aspiration biopsy from liver lesions in the patient in panel A reveals typical cytologic features of non-Hodgkin's lymphoma. Note the monotonous sheet of abnormal lymphocytes with hyperchromatic nuclei.

A

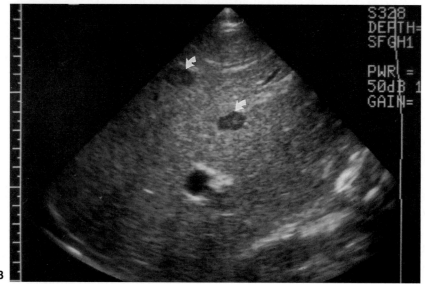

B

Fine-needle aspiration biopsy of AIDS-related lymphomas is adequate for subtyping. Core biopsy is rarely required for definitive diagnosis.

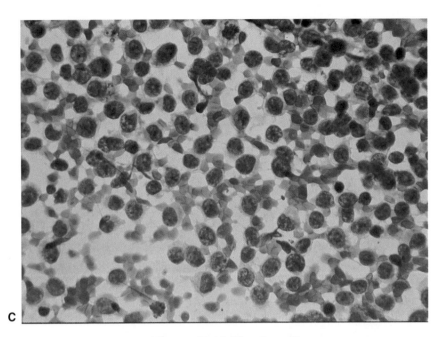

C

Figure 17-12 (Continued)

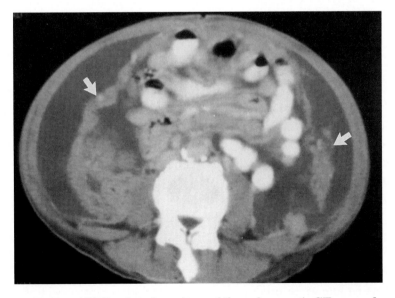

Figure 17-13. AIDS-related peritoneal lymphoma. A CT scan demonstrates marked ascites and omental masses (arrows). These findings mimic carcinomatosis. Laparoscopic biopsy of the omentum revealed non-Hodgkin's lymphoma.

Question 56

Features of extrapulmonary *Pneumocystis carinii* infection in patients with AIDS include:

(A) punctate calcifications in the liver and spleen
(B) generalized renal hypoechogenicity
(C) splenic abscesses
(D) biliary obstruction
(E) association with prophylactic pentamidine inhalation therapy

The use of pentamidine aerosol inhalers for prophylactic control of pulmonary infection by *P. carinii* in patients with AIDS has led to the development of extrapulmonary sites of involvement by this organism **(Option (E) is true).** Extrapulmonary *P. carinii* infection can result in diffuse microcalcifications throughout the liver, spleen, kidneys, adrenal glands, and lymph nodes **(Option (A) is true).** On CT, low-attenuation abscesses can be present in these organs, particularly the spleen (Figure 17-14) **(Option (C) is true).** On sonography, tiny microechogenic foci are noted in the involved visceral organs (Figure 17-15). It should be noted that microcalcifications of the liver, spleen, and kidneys can be due to other opportunistic infections in patients with AIDS; there are recent reports of these findings in patients with AIDS who have cytomegalovirus infection or *M. avium-intracellulare* complex infection.

Diffuse renal hyperechogenicity is not a feature of extrapulmonary *P. carinii* infection **(Option (B) is false).** However, renal involvement in patients with AIDS (AIDS-related nephropathy) causes nephromegaly and a diffuse increase in renal echogenicity. The increased cortical echogenicity correlates histologically with focal and segmental glomerulosclerosis and dilated renal tubules. These findings indicate irreversible renal disease. Renal biopsy is therefore generally unrewarding, because no treatment is available.

AIDS-related cholangitis is a cause of biliary obstruction. Radiographic findings in patients with this entity include diffuse intrahepatic strictures resembling those seen in sclerosing cholangitis and slight thickening of the wall of the bile ducts. Strictures of the papilla of Vater are also frequently reported. Rarely, acalculous cholecystitis can occur. Pathogens known to produce this entity include cryptosporidium, cytomegalovirus, and microsporidiosis. However, *P. carinii* has not been reported to cause AIDS-related cholangitis **(Option (D) is false).**

R. Brooke Jeffrey, M.D.

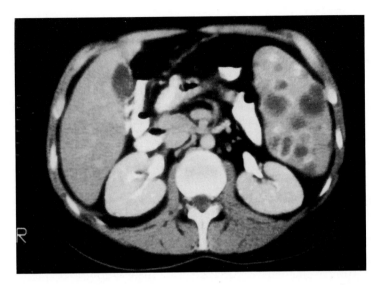

Figure 17-14. Splenic abscesses caused by *P. carinii*. A contrast-enhanced CT scan demonstrates numerous low-density splenic abscesses. Biopsy revealed *P. carinii*.

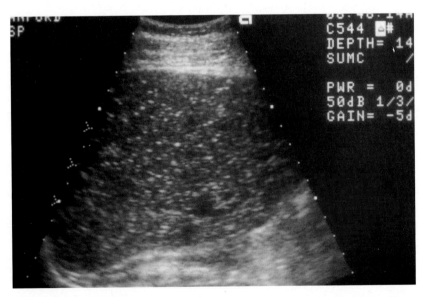

Figure 17-15. Hepatic involvement by *P. carinii*. A sagittal sonogram of the right lobe of the liver demonstrates innumerable tiny echogenic foci. A core biopsy revealed *P. carinii*.

SUGGESTED READINGS

AIDS-RELATED LYMPHOMA

1. Bottles K, McPhaul LW, Volberding P. Fine-needle aspiration biopsy of patients with acquired immunodeficiency syndrome (AIDS): experience in an outpatient clinic. Ann Intern Med 1988; 108:42–45

2. Haskal ZJ, Lindan CE, Goodman PC. Lymphoma in the immunocompromised patient. Radiol Clin North Am 1990; 28:885–899

3. Jeffrey RB Jr. Abdominal imaging in the immunocompromised patient. Radiol Clin North Am 1992; 30:579–596

4. Nyberg DA, Jeffrey RB Jr, Federle MP, Bottles K, Abrams DI. AIDS-related lymphomas: evaluation by abdominal CT. Radiology 1986; 159:59–63

5. Radin DR, Esplin JA, Levin AM, Ralls PW. AIDS-related non-Hodgkin's lymphoma: abdominal CT findings in 112 patients. AJR 1993; 160:1133–1139

6. Townsend RR. CT of AIDS-related lymphoma. AJR 1991; 156:969–974

7. Townsend RR, Laing FC, Jeffrey RB Jr, Bottles K. Abdominal lymphoma in AIDS: evaluation with US. Radiology 1989; 171:719–724

PYOGENIC LIVER ABSCESS

8. Bernardino ME, Berkman WA, Plemmons M, Sones PJ Jr, Price RB, Casarella WJ. Percutaneous drainage of multiseptated hepatic abscess. J Comput Assist Tomogr 1984; 8:38–41

9. Jeffrey RB Jr, Tolentino CS, Chang FC, Federle MP. CT of small pyogenic hepatic abscesses: the cluster sign. AJR 1988; 151:487–489

10. Johnson RD, Mueller PR, Ferrucci JT Jr, et al. Percutaneous drainage of pyogenic liver abscesses. AJR 1985; 144:463–467

11. Kuligowska E, Connors SK, Shapiro JH. Liver abscess: sonography in diagnosis and treatment. AJR 1982; 138:253–257

12. McDonald AP, Howard RJ. Pyogenic liver abscess. World J Surg 1980; 4:369–380

KAPOSI'S SARCOMA

13. Hammerman AM, Kotner LM Jr, Doyle TB. Periportal contrast enhancement on CT scans of the liver. AJR 1991; 156:313–315

14. Herts BR, Megibow AJ, Birnbaum BA, Kanzer GK, Noz ME. High-attenuation lymphadenopathy in AIDS patients: significance of findings at CT. Radiology 1992; 185:777–781

15. Luburich P, Bru C, Ayuso MC, Azon A, Condom E. Hepatic Kaposi sarcoma in AIDS: US and CT finding. Radiology 1990; 175:172–174

16. Moon KL Jr, Federle MP, Abrams DI, Volberding P, Lewis BJ. Kaposi sarcoma and lymphadenopathy syndrome: limitations of abdominal CT in acquired immunodeficiency syndrome. Radiology 1984; 15:479–483

17. Safai B, Johnson KG, Myskowski PL, et al. The natural history of Kaposi's sarcoma in the acquired immunodeficiency syndrome. Ann Intern Med 1985; 103:744–750

18. Schneiderman DJ, Arenson DM, Cello JP, Margaretten W, Weber TE. Hepatic disease in patients with acquired immunodeficiency syndrome (AIDS). Hepatology 1987; 7:925–930

19. Valls C, Cañas C, Turell LG, Pruna X. Hepatosplenic AIDS-related Kaposi's sarcoma. Gastrointest Radiol 1991; 16:342–344

MYCOBACTERIAL INFECTIONS

20. Radin DR. Intraabdominal *Mycobacterium tuberculosis* vs *Mycobacterium avium-intracellulare* infections in patients with AIDS: distinction based on CT findings. AJR 1991; 156:487–491

PNEUMOCYSTIS CARINII INFECTION

21. Feuerstein IM, Francis P, Raffeld M, Pluda J. Widespread visceral calcifications in disseminated *Pneumocystis carinii* infection: CT characteristics. J Comput Assist Tomogr 1990; 141:149–151

22. Radin DR, Baker EL, Klatt EC, et al. Visceral and nodal calcification in patients with AIDS-related *Pneumocystis carinii* infection. AJR 1990; 154:27–31

23. Spouge AR, Wilson S, Gopinath N, Sherman M, Blendis LM. Extrapulmonary *Pneumocystis carinii* in patient with AIDS: sonographic findings. AJR 1990; 155:76–78

24. Telzak EE, Cote RJ, Gold JW, Campbell SW, Armstrong D. Extrapulmonary *Pneumocystis carinii* infections. Rev Infect Dis 1990; 12:380–386

25. Towers MJ, Withers CE, Hamilton PA, Kolin A, Walmsley S. Visceral calcification in patients with AIDS may not always be due to *Pneumocystis carinii*. AJR 1991; 156:745–747

BACILLARY ANGIOMATOSIS

26. Haught WH, Steinbach J, Zander DS, Wingo CS. Case report: bacillary angiomatosis with massive visceral lymphadenopathy. Am J Med Sci 1993; 306:236–240

27. Kunberger LE, Montalvo BM. Bacillary angiomatosis in the abdomen: Doppler and CT features. J Comput Assist Tomogr 1994; 18:308–309

28. Wyatt SH, Fishman EK. Hepatic bacillary angiomatosis in a patient with AIDS. Abdom Imaging 1993; 18:336–338

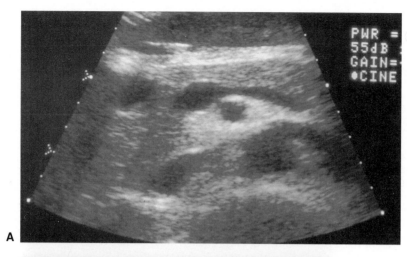

A

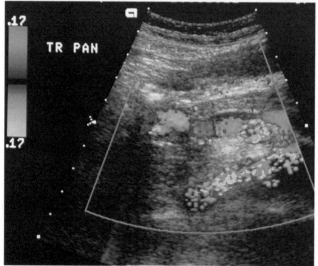

B

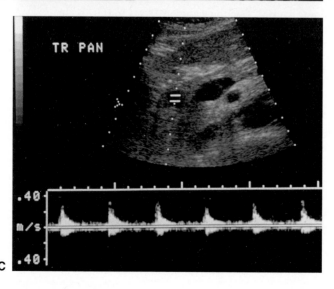

C

Figure 18-1.
This 52-year-old
man has vague
abdominal dis-
comfort 6 months
after an episode
of pancreatitis.
You are shown
a transverse sono-
gram of the up-
per abdomen
(A), a corres-
ponding color
Doppler sono-
gram (B), and
a spectral Dop-
pler waveform
tracing at the
same level (C).

298

Case 18: Pseudoaneurysm of the Gastroduodenal Artery

Question 57

Which *one* of the following is the MOST likely diagnosis?

(A) Arteriovenous malformation
(B) Pseudocyst
(C) Neuroendocrine tumor
(D) Pseudoaneurysm
(E) Varix

The transverse sonogram (Figure 18-1A) at the level of the splenic-portal confluence demonstrates a cystic structure just anterolateral to the head of the pancreas (Figure 18-2A). The color Doppler sonogram (Figure 18-1B) clearly shows that there is blood flow filling the lumen of the cystic mass (Figure 18-2B), and the spectral Doppler waveform tracing (Figure 18-1C) shows the typical pattern of arterial pulsation (Figure 18-2C). The site of the cystic mass is characteristic of the expected position of the gastroduodenal artery, but the structure is clearly much larger than a normal gastroduodenal artery. The sonographic findings are classic for a pseudoaneurysm arising from the gastroduodenal artery, a diagnosis made even more secure when taking into account the history of pancreatitis **(Option (D) is correct).** The diagnosis was confirmed by MRI and selective visceral angiography (Figure 18-3).

An arteriovenous malformation (Option (A)) would be expected to display intraluminal signal on a color flow Doppler examination. However, on gray-scale imaging, arteriovenous malformations are characterized by a tangle of vessels with multiple feeding arteries and draining veins; they do not demonstrate a single large cystic structure, as is seen in the test images. Moreover, spectral Doppler analysis of arteriovenous malformations demonstrates markedly chaotic, turbulent flow. The abnormal direct artery-to-vein communications that define this entity are associated with high peak velocities and prominent diastolic flow; blood

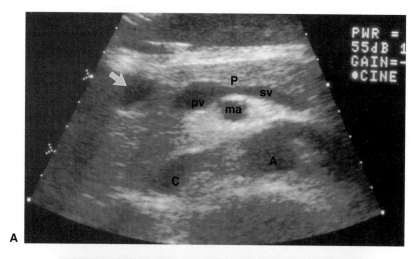

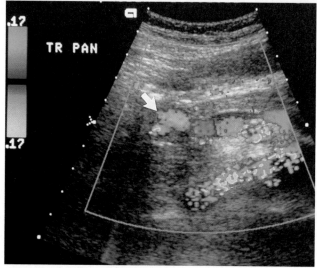

Figure 18-2 (Same as Figure 18-1).   Pseudoaneurysm of the gastroduod-enal artery. (A) A transverse gray-scale sonogram of the pancreas at the level of the splenic-portal venous confluence demonstrates a cystic mass (arrow) in the expected location of the gastroduodenal artery. (B) A corre-sponding color Doppler sonogram demonstrates flow within the cystic mass (arrow), indicative of a blood vessel. (C) A spectral Doppler tracing demonstrates a typical arterial waveform. These findings suggest the diagnosis of a pseudoaneurysm of the gastroduodenal artery. pv = portal vein; sv = splenic vein; A = aorta; C = inferior vena cava; ma = superior mesenteric artery; P = pancreas.

flow through the malformation is essentially continuous throughout the cardiac cycle due to markedly lowered resistance. Tracings obtained in a

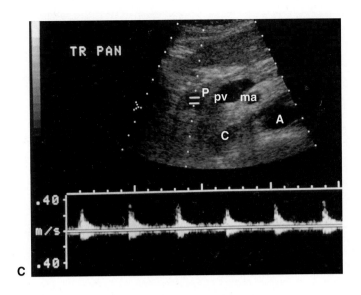

C

vein draining an arteriovenous malformation accordingly show arterial waveforms.

Arteriovenous malformations are rare in the abdomen; etiologies include penetrating trauma and interventional procedures such as percutaneous biopsies. Renal biopsies are particularly likely to give rise to this complication, because of the close juxtaposition of the arcuate arteries and veins in the area targeted for biopsy. Patients with Osler-Weber-Rendu disease can also develop arteriovenous malformations. The enlarged vascular channels branch in a way that mimics dilated intrahepatic ducts on gray-scale sonography (Figure 18-4A). Color Doppler imaging, aided by spectral waveform analysis, can clearly demonstrate the vascular nature of the phenomenon (Figure 18-4B).

A pancreatic pseudocyst (Option (B)) could develop in the location shown in the test images, particularly in a patient with a well-documented episode of pancreatitis. However, arterial flow would not be evident within a pseudocyst on color or spectral Doppler examination. The sonographic appearance of pancreatic pseudocysts is variable depending on the presence of hemorrhage or infection. Acute hemorrhage within a pancreatic pseudocyst can be quite echogenic (Figure 18-5A). If hemorrhage is suspected either clinically or on the basis of sonographic findings, a noncontrast CT scan should be obtained to confirm the presence of blood; high attenuation (e.g., >30 HU) is characteristic (Figure 18-5B).

Infected pancreatic pseudocysts often demonstrate medium- or low-level echoes (representing pus and debris), fluid-debris levels, and inter-

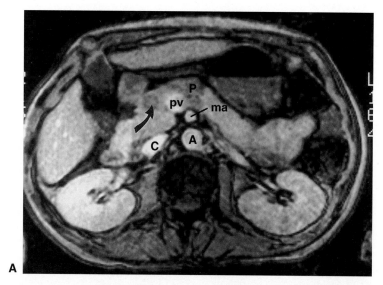

A

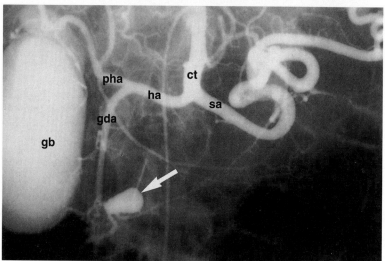

B

Figure 18-3. Same patient as in Figures 18-1 and 18-2. Pseudoaneurysm of the gastroduodenal artery. (A) A T1-weighted gadolinium-enhanced dynamic MR scan obtained by the gradient-echo technique demonstrates slight enhancement (arrow) due to a pseudoaneurysm. (B) A celiac arteriogram demonstrates a large pseudoaneurysm (arrow) arising from the anterior inferior pancreaticoduodenal branch of the gastroduodenal artery. This was successfully embolized with multiple steel coils. Note the contrast agent filling the gallbladder owing to a recent direct cholangiogram. (C) A postembolization arteriogram (open arrows denote the embolic coils) demonstrates complete occlusion (arrowhead) of the distal gastroduodenal artery, as well as the pseudoaneurysm. A = aorta; C = inferior vena cava; ct = celiac trunk; ha = common hepatic artery; gb = gallbladder; gda = gastroduodenal artery; ma = superior mesenteric artery; P = pancreas; pha = proper hepatic artery; pv = portal vein; sa = splenic artery.

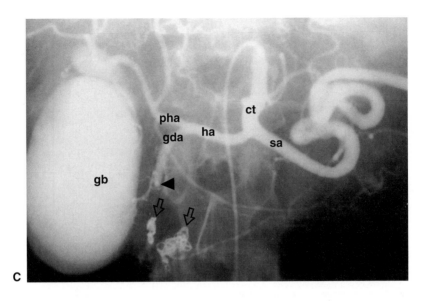

C

nal septations on sonography (Figure 18-6). These features are often difficult to appreciate on CT scans. Imaging-guided diagnostic needle aspiration is a valuable technique to differentiate an infected from a non-infected pseudocyst (Figure 18-7). Pancreatic pseudocysts are readily amenable to guided percutaneous drainage because they are, by definition, encapsulated (Figure 18-8).

Neuroendocrine tumors of the pancreas (Option (C)) have a broad range of imaging findings, depending on their underlying pathologic subtype. In general, they are solid tumors, although rare cystic islet cell neoplasms have been described. Although these tumors are richly supplied with arterial blood, the presence of uniform arterial signal throughout the mass is not compatible with the diagnosis of neuroendocrine tumor. Neuroendocrine tumors include functioning (e.g., hormonally active) and nonfunctioning islet cell tumors. Typically, hormonally active tumors (particularly insulinomas) produce clinical symptoms even when they are quite small, so that functioning tumors tend to be considerably smaller than nonfunctioning tumors at the time they are discovered. All neuroendocrine tumors tend to be malignant (insulinoma is an exception) and can be multiple. Nonfunctioning islet cell tumors do, in fact, elaborate hormones, but they do not produce clinical symptoms; when patients eventually develop symptoms, they are typically related to mass effect. Most islet cell tumors are intrinsic lesions of the pancreas, but gastrinomas, in particular, can be ectopic in location and can arise in adjacent tissues such as the wall of the duodenum.

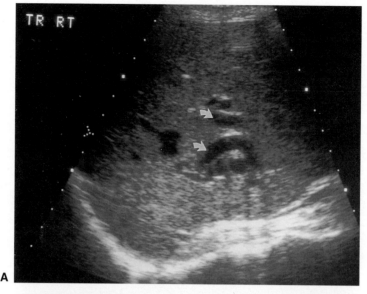

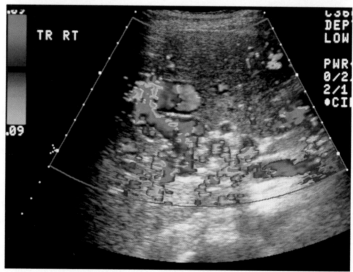

Figure 18-4. Hepatic arteriovenous malformation in a patient with Osler-Weber-Rendu disease. (A) A transverse sonogram of the right lobe of the liver demonstrates numerous dilated tubular structures (arrows). This appearance could mimic dilated intrahepatic bile ducts. (B) A color Doppler sonogram of the right lobe of the liver reveals multiple dilated intrahepatic vascular channels from arteriovenous malformation due to Osler-Weber-Rendu disease.

For therapeutic purposes, it is important to localize the precise anatomic site of these tumors (since they are often difficult to detect during

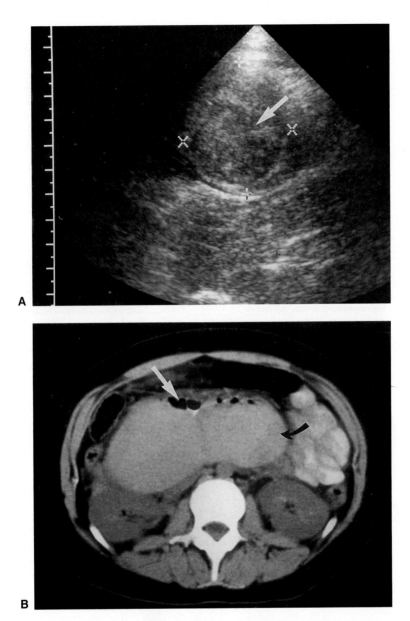

Figure 18-5. Hemorrhagic pancreatic pseudocyst. (A) A sagittal sonogram in the region of the duodenum demonstrates an echogenic mass (arrow). (B) A noncontrast CT scan demonstrates a large hemorrhagic intramural pseudocyst of the duodenum (black arrow). Gas is apparent within the transverse duodenum (white arrow).

surgical exploration) and to determine whether liver metastases are present. Several invasive and noninvasive imaging techniques have been

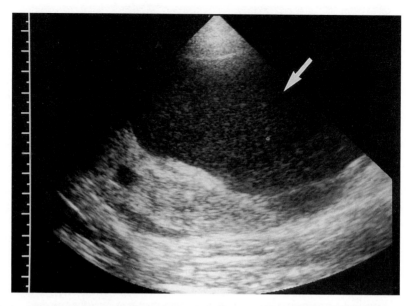

Figure 18-6. Infected pancreatic pseudocyst. A sagittal sonogram of the left upper quadrant demonstrates a large, complex fluid collection with diffuse low-level echoes (arrow). Percutaneous catheter drainage confirmed the presence of an infected pancreatic pseudocyst.

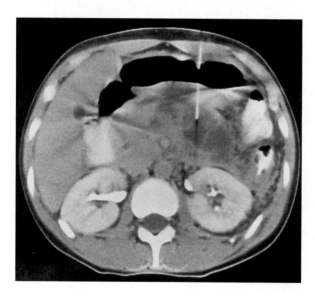

Figure 18-7. Diagnostic needle aspiration of an infected pancreatic pseudocyst. A contrast-enhanced CT scan demonstrates transgastric needle aspiration of an infected pseudocyst in the tail of the pancreas.

used in the preoperative localization of functioning islet cell tumors. Transabdominal sonography depends on identifying an echotexture difference between the hyperechoic normal pancreatic tissue and the hypo-

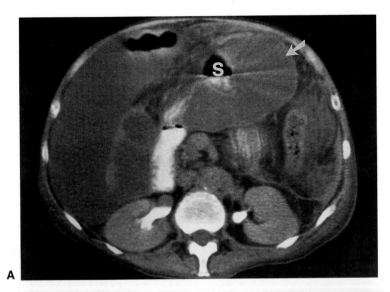

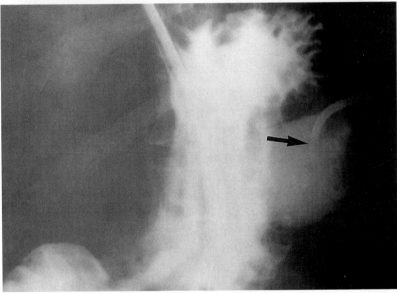

Figure 18-8. Percutaneous drainage of infected lesser sac pseudocyst. (A) A contrast-enhanced CT scan demonstrates a large infected pseudocyst (arrow) in the lesser sac. S = stomach. (B) Following percutaneous catheter drainage, the fluid collection was successfully drained without complications. The arrow indicates the pigtail drainage catheter.

echoic tumor. Small tumors, localized to the pancreatic tail, are very difficult to detect sonographically. Intraoperative sonography, however, has been of considerable use when the surgeon is unable to localize the

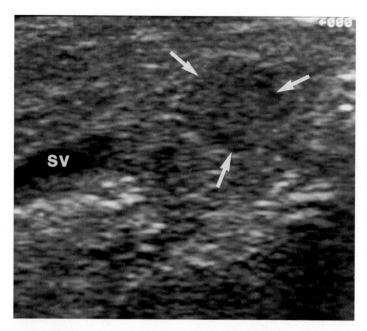

Figure 18-9. Pancreatic insulinoma localized by intraoperative sonography. An intraoperative scan of the pancreas demonstrates a 1-cm hypoechoic lesion (arrows) within the tail of the pancreas. The lesion was not clinically palpable. SV = splenic vein.

tumor site during exploration (Fgure 18-9). Identification of the tumor by CT requires rapid administration of intravenous contrast material and imaging of the entire pancreas during the arterial phase of enhancement. Its success depends on the fact that the tumors are highly vascular and achieve considerably higher attenuation during peak enhancement than does the normal pancreatic parenchyma. However, small tumors can masquerade as normal splenic vessels and can be impossible to resolve when they are less than 1 cm in greatest dimension. MRI has similar drawbacks; its advantage in contrast resolution is balanced by its reduced spatial resolution. Selective angiography depends on detecting the characteristic arterial tumor staining and is likewise insensitive to small lesions.

Imaging methods that rely on the functional properties of islet cell tumors have met with some success. Selective venography of the splenic vein maps the concentration of elaborated hormone along the course of the venous drainage of the pancreas. This technique is tedious and requires percutaneous liver puncture to obtain access to the portal venous system. A recently developed scintigraphic method exploits the fact that

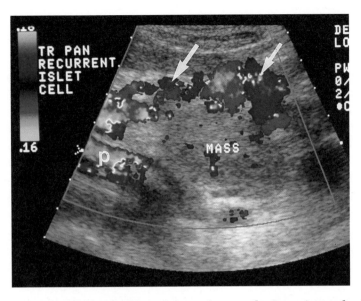

Figure 18-10. Gastroepiploic varices from splenic vein occlusion. A transverse color Doppler sonogram of the pancreas demonstrates a large mass in the pancreatic bed, representing a recurrent islet cell tumor. There is lack of visualization of the splenic vein posterior to the mass. The sonogram demonstrates large gastroepiploic varices (arrows) due to splenic vein occlusion. P = portal vein.

most islet cell tumors express a membrane receptor for the naturally occurring inhibitory hormone, somatostatin. Imaging with In-111 pentetreotide, an In-111-labeled somatostatin analog, allows identification of both primary and secondary islet cell tumors. In the extensive review of this agent by Krenning et al., 45 (80%) of 56 islet cell tumors were successfully imaged with this method. Its success depends on the tumor's expression of a somatostatin receptor in sufficient concentration that accumulation of the radiopharmaceutical can be detected.

Upper abdominal varices (Option (E)) are most often due to portal hypertension or thrombosis of the splenic-portal venous system. They can appear as large cystic masses on gray-scale sonography, but the spectral Doppler waveform analysis would not show arterial pulsations, as were exhibited in the test case. Flow within varices is typically very slow and is relatively constant throughout the cardiac cycle.

The distribution of the varices can be an important clue to identifying the underlying abnormality. A recanalized paraumbilical vein and enlarged coronary (left gastric) vein are typical features of portal hypertension. The presence of short gastric and gastroepiploic varices (Figure 18-10) suggests splenic vein occlusion with collateral venous drainage.

Discussion

Pseudoaneurysm formation is a well-documented complication of pancreatitis and can cause massive hemorrhage. Proteolytic enzymes produced during pancreatitis directly weaken the arterial walls of adjacent blood vessels, resulting in a contained perforation or pseudoaneurysm. Clinical presentation generally results from bleeding. Hemorrhage into the alimentary tract, biliary tree, or pancreatic duct causes symptoms related to the specific site of bleeding and is generally associated with hematemesis or hematochezia. Bleeding into a pseudocyst can cause local pain and hypotension. Pseudoaneurysms associated with pancreatitis can occur anywhere in the visceral arterial circulation but typically occur in the splenic, hepatic, or gastroduodenal arteries. They can arise from the main trunk of these vessels or from smaller side branches. They can also occur within the walls of a pancreatic pseudocyst. Pseudoaneurysms can be asymptomatic; however, life-threatening hemorrhage is possible. Pseudoaneurysms can cause gastrointestinal hemorrhage by erosion into either the pancreatic duct or the biliary tree. Angiographic embolization is the treatment of choice for most visceral artery pseudoaneurysms. These lesions are challenging to treat surgically. The surgical dissection is often made difficult by extensive peripancreatic inflammation.

Patients selected for angiographic treatment should undergo selective arteriography of the target vessel. Aneurysms that arise from major vascular trunks or in regions with dual blood supply (such as the pancreaticoduodenal arcade) will require interruption of flow to both sides of the aneurysm. Occlusion of only one side will allow back-filling of the aneurysm via collateral vessels, with continued risk of arterial hemorrhage. The test patient underwent successful angiographic embolization of the pseudoaneurysm with steel coils (Figure 18-3C). Gelfoam particles can also be used for embolization of small peripancreatic pseudoaneurysms (Figure 18-11). They are probably less desirable than coils, since the pancreatitis that produces the pseudoaneurysm is often of prolonged duration; Gelfoam allows recanalization of the occluded vessel within a few days of embolic therapy. If the inflammatory changes have not subsided, there is some risk of rebleeding.

R. Brooke Jeffrey, M.D.

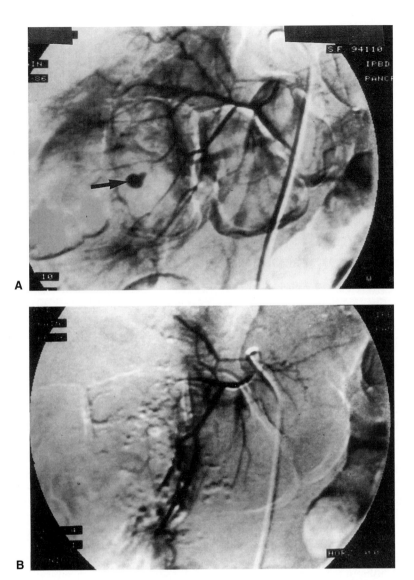

Figure 18-11.   Gelfoam embolization of peripancreatic pseudoaneurysm.
(A) A selective arteriogram of the inferior pancreaticoduodenal artery
demonstrates a small pseudoaneurysm (arrow). (B) Following Gelfoam
embolization, the pseudoaneurysm has been occluded.

SUGGESTED READINGS

PSEUDOANEURYSMS

1. Boudghéne F, L'Hermine C, Bigot JM. Arterial complications of pancreati-

tis: diagnostic and therapeutic aspects in 104 cases. J Vasc Interv Radiol 1993; 4:551–558

2. Burke JW, Erickson SJ, Kellum CD, Tegtmeyer CJ, Williamson BR, Hansen MF. Pseudoaneurysms complicating pancreatitis: detection by CT. Radiology 1986; 161:445–450

3. Falkoff GE, Taylor KJ, Morse S. Hepatic artery pseudoaneurysm: diagnosis with real-time and pulsed Doppler US. Radiology 1986; 158:55–56

4. Isikoff MB, Hill MC, Silverstein W, Barkin J. The clinical significance of acute pancreatic hemorrhage. AJR 1981; 136:679–684

5. Mandel SR, Jaques PJ, Sanofsky S, Mauro MA. Nonoperative management of peripancreatic arterial aneurysms. A 10-year experience. Ann Surg 1987; 205:126–128

6. Yoshikai T, Murakami J, Nishihara H, Oshiumi Y. Hemosuccus pancreaticus: CT manifestations. J Comput Assist Tomogr 1986; 10:510–512

ARTERIOVENOUS MALFORMATIONS

7. Hubsch PJ, Mostbeck G, Barton PP, et al. Evaluation of arteriovenous fistulas and pseudoaneurysms in renal allografts following percutaneous needle biopsy. Color-coded Doppler sonography versus duplex Doppler sonography. J Ultrasound Med 1990; 9:95–100

8. Peery WH. Clinical spectrum of hereditary hemorrhagic telangiectasia (Osler-Weber-Rendu disease). Amer J Med 1987; 82:989–997

PSEUDOCYSTS

9. Gerzof SG, Johnson WC, Robbins AH, Spechler SJ, Nabseth DC. Percutaneous drainage of infected pancreatic pseudocysts. Arch Surg 1984; 119:888–893

10. Hashimoto BE, Laing FC, Jeffrey RB Jr, Federle MP. Hemorrhagic pancreatic fluid collections examined by ultrasound. Radiology 1984; 150:803–808

11. Matzinger FR, Ho CS, Yee AC, Gray RR. Pancreatic pseudocysts drained through a percutaneous transgastric approach: further experience. Radiology 1988; 167:431–434

12. vanSonnenberg E, Wittich GR, Casola G, et al. Complicated pancreatic inflammatory disease: diagnostic and therapeutic role of interventional radiology. Radiology 1985; 155:335–340

NEUROENDOCRINE TUMORS

13. Eelkema EA, Stephens DH, Ward EM, Sheedy PF II. CT features of nonfunctioning islet cell carcinoma. AJR 1984; 143:943–948

14. Frucht H, Doppman JL, Nortan JA, et al. Gastrinomas: comparison of MR imaging with CT, angiography, and US. Radiology 1989; 171:713–717

15. Gunther RW, Klose KJ, Ruckert K, Beyer J, Kuhn FP, Klotter HJ. Localization of small islet-cell tumors. Preoperative and intraoperative ultrasound, computed tomography, arteriography, digital subtraction angiography, and pancreatic venous sampling. Gastrointest Radiol 1985; 10:145–152

16. Kraus BB, Ros PR. Insulinoma: diagnosis with fat-suppressed MR imaging. AJR 1994; 162:69–70
17. Krenning EP, Kwekkeboom DJ, Bakker WH, et al. Somatostatin receptor scintigraphy with [^{111}In-DTPA-D-Phe1]- and [^{123}I-Tyr3]-octreotide: the Rotterdam experience with more than 1000 patients. Eur J Nucl Med 1993; 20:716–731
18. Pogany AC, Kerlan RK Jr, Karam JH, Le Quesne LP, Ring EJ. Cystic insulinoma. AJR 1984; 142:951–952
19. Smith TR, Koenigsberg M. Low-density insulinoma on dynamic CT. AJR 1990; 155:995–996

VARICES

20. Balthazar EJ, Megibow A, Naidich D, LeFleur RS. Computed tomographic recognition of gastric varices. AJR 1984; 142:1121–1125
21. Marn CS, Glazer GM, William DM, Francis IR. CT-angiographic correlation of collateral venous pathways in isolated splenic vein occlusions: new observations. Radiology 1990; 175:375–380

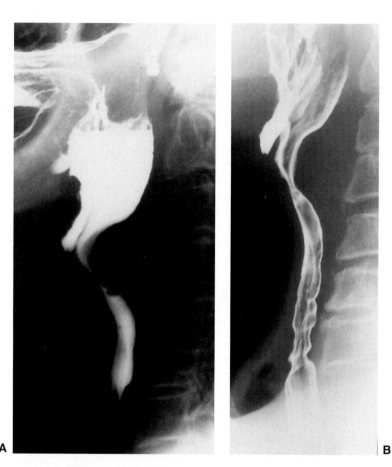

Figure 19-1. This 64-year-old man underwent total laryngectomy 13 months ago for a large epiglottic carcinoma. He now complains of slowly progressive dysphagia for solid food. You are shown solid-column (A) and air-contrast (B) lateral radiographs of the pharynx.

Case 19: Benign Stricture after Total Laryngectomy

Question 58

Which *one* of the following is the MOST likely diagnosis?

    (A) Ulceration of the neopharynx
    (B) Recurrent carcinoma of the posterior pharyngeal mucosa
    (C) Expected postoperative appearance of the pharynx after total laryngectomy
    (D) Benign stricture of the neopharynx
    (E) Abscess within the soft tissues at the base of the neck

The lateral solid-column radiograph (Figure 19-1A) shows moderate retention of the contrast agent in the oropharynx, with the height of the air-barium level at the floor of the mouth (indicating that the pressure within the pharynx is higher than normal) (Figure 19-2A). Also, there is barium coating the floor of the nasopharynx, a reliable sign of nasopharyngeal reflux. There is smooth narrowing of the pharynx immediately below the base of the tongue, but the air-contrast radiograph (Figure 19-1B) shows no evidence of mucosal destruction (Figure 19-2B).

All of the radiologic findings, as well as the clinical history of slowly progressive dysphagia, are most compatible with the diagnosis of benign postoperative stricture **(Option (D) is correct).**

Ulceration of the mucosal surface of the surgically reconstructed pharynx ("neopharynx") (Option (A)) occurs as a late complication in patients who develop postoperative recurrent carcinoma; less commonly, it is seen as an early complication (in the immediate postoperative period) and is probably due to mucosal ischemia. These patients have often had extensive radiotherapy prior to laryngectomy. In patients with either condition, the crater would be irregular (Figure 19-3) and its contours would not change during the course of the examination. There is a collection of barium anterior to the oropharynx in the region of the tongue base in the test patient (Figure 19-1A), but its margins are smooth and it clearly changes in both size and position relative to the oropharynx. Its

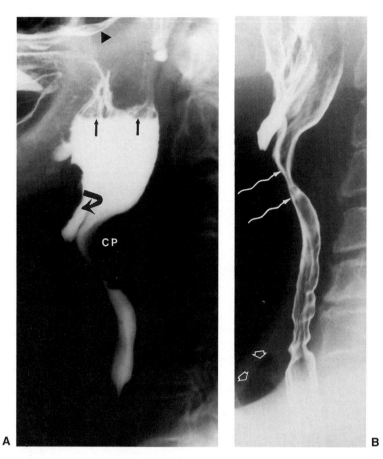

Figure 19-2 (Same as Figure 19-1).   Benign stricture. (A) A lateral radiograph from a solid-column pharyngogram demonstrates an air-barium
level (straight arrows) posterior to the tongue base. Barium has refluxed
into the nasopharynx (arrowhead). A large, smooth posterior indentation
(CP) is present; it represents the cricopharyngeus muscle. A small pseudodiverticulum (curved arrow) is also noted. (B) A lateral radiograph
from an air-contrast pharyngogram performed the same day demonstrates the smooth neopharyngeal narrowing (wavy arrows) at the time
of maximal distension. An air collection (open arrows) is observed anterior to the cervical esophagus; it represents a portion of the trachea,
curving forward toward the stoma in the suprasternal region.

location, at the upper margin of the surgical suture line, is also characteristic of a pseudodiverticulum. These pseudodiverticula develop because the powerful tongue muscles put almost constant strain on the
surgical suture line. This produces an anterior weak area, through which
pharyngeal mucosa protrudes. This is observed to some degree in most
patients who have undergone total laryngectomy. The pseudodiverticula

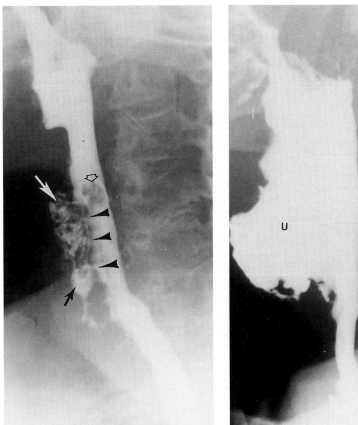

A B

Figure 19-3. Neopharyngeal ulceration. (A) This patient developed swelling in the neck 7 months after total laryngectomy for an extensive transglottic tumor. An oblique pharyngogram demonstrates extensive ulceration of the anterior neopharynx (arrowheads), with contrast material filling an irregular cavity (black and white arrows) within the soft tissues of the neck. A nodular mass (open arrow) is present within the neopharyngeal lumen. At biopsy, extensive recurrent epidermoid carcinoma was found. (B) This patient underwent total laryngectomy for recurrence after full-course radiation therapy and developed extensive neck swelling, pain, and tenderness 14 days after the surgery. A lateral radiograph from a water-soluble contrast study demonstrates a large irregular ulcer cavity (U) filling the anterior neck. Laryngoscopy revealed necrosis of the entire anterior wall of the neopharynx.

are asymptomatic in most individuals but can cause dysphagia if they become large enough to trap food (Figure 19-4).

Recurrent mucosal carcinoma (Option (B)) appears radiographically as an irregular intraluminal mass and is usually associated with ulceration (Figure 19-5). A mass is present in the posterior portion of the

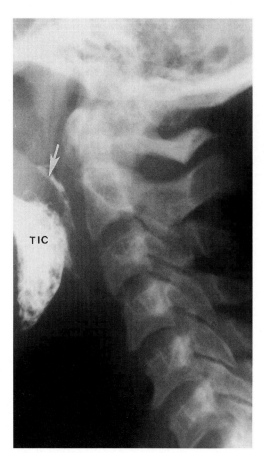

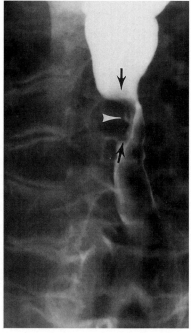

Figure 19-4 (left). Pseudo-diverticulum in a patient who complained of food sticking in the pharynx 1 year after total laryngectomy. A lateral view from a pharyngogram demonstrates barium and food particles retained within a large pseudodiverticulum (TIC) arising at the upper margin of the neopharynx. There is a small amount of nasopharyngeal regurgitation (arrow).

Figure 19-5 (right). Recurrent epidermoid carcinoma. An anteroposterior view from a pharyngogram obtained in a patient 10 months after total laryngectomy demonstrates a smooth mass (arrows) narrowing the distal neopharynx. There is a tiny central ulcer (arrowhead). At biopsy, local recurrence was found.

oropharynx in the test image (Figure 19-1A), but there is no radiologic evidence of mucosal abnormality. Also, the location of the mass in the test image is characteristic for a postlaryngectomy cricopharyngeus muscle indentation. After the surgeon removes the thyroid cartilage to which the anterior portion of the cricopharyngeus muscle is attached, the muscle retracts into a posterior location, where it produces a smooth bulge of variable size on the posterior aspect of the pharynx.

Many of the radiologic features in the test images are normally expected to be present after total laryngectomy (Option (C)); however, the presence of oropharyngeal dilatation and nasopharyngeal reflux and the smooth mid-pharyngeal narrowing are not normal features. In normal postoperative patients, a barium pharyngogram should show only modest tapering of the neopharyngeal walls (Figure 19-6).

Abscess (Option (E)) (Figure 19-7) occurs most commonly in the early postoperative period and is often associated with a sinus tract leading from the pharynx to the abscess cavity. The findings on physical examination of local mass, tenderness, or crepitation of the soft tissues in a febrile patient are highly suggestive of this complication. A collection of gas is present at the base of the neck in the test image (Figure 19-1B), but its shape and position are characteristic; it represents the proximal portion of the trachea, which has been surgically directed toward the chest wall to form the tracheal stoma.

Total laryngectomy is a radical method of treating carcinomas of the laryngopharynx; it destroys the natural voice, so it is usually reserved for patients with large tumors. However, voice-conserving surgical procedures are associated with a higher frequency of complications, and rehabilitation is more difficult because of the risk of aspiration. Accordingly, many patients with smaller tumors but severe underlying medical problems (who may not survive the rehabilitation period) are also selected to undergo total laryngectomy. Medical morbidity is substantial even in patients undergoing total laryngectomy, however; in one series, 6.3% of patients had significant postoperative medical problems, the most prevalent being respiratory failure. This relatively high morbidity probably reflects the older population, as well as the common risk factor of tobacco abuse leading to pulmonary compromise. Considering that most patients selected for total laryngectomy have relatively advanced-stage disease, the 5-year survival rates of 50 to 60% are acceptable.

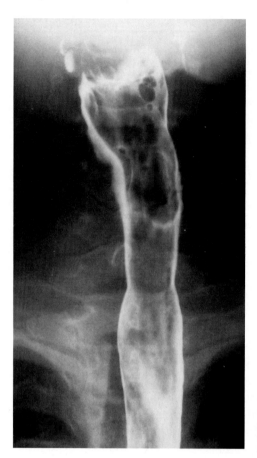

Figure 19-6 (left). Expected appearance after total laryngectomy. An anteroposterior radiograph of an asymptomatic volunteer 5 years after total laryngectomy demonstrates smoothly tapered lateral borders of the neopharynx with gradual widening at the level of the proximal cervical esophagus.

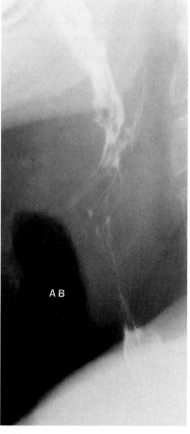

Figure 19-7 (right). Postoperative abscess. A lateral view from a water-soluble contrast pharyngogram performed 7 days after total laryngectomy in a patient with fever, neck pain, and tenderness demonstrates a large gas-containing abscess (AB) in the soft tissues of the anterior neck. No sinus tract was observed.

Question 59

Concerning the complications of total laryngectomy,

(A) pharyngeal ulceration is a common early postoperative complication
(B) fistulas and sinus tracts originate most often from the lower margin of the surgical suture line
(C) preoperative radiation therapy increases the frequency of fistulas and sinus tracts
(D) recurrent carcinoma occurs more commonly in the soft tissues of the neck than in the remaining pharyngeal mucosa
(E) about 15% of patients will develop dysphagia

Total laryngectomy is radical surgery performed for T3 or T4 carcinomas of the pharynx and larynx. It can also be performed for less-extensive carcinomas in patients with a severe underlying medical disorder that would make it hazardous to attempt voice-conserving subtotal procedures. Diabetes, emphysema, and dementia are examples of such conditions. Patients who develop recurrent or persistent disease after full-course radiation therapy or subtotal surgery are candidates for salvage by total laryngectomy.

The operation entails removal of the entire laryngeal skeleton, extending inferiorly to include the first tracheal ring (Figure 19-8). The trachea is then brought anteriorly to form a stoma in the neck just above the manubrium. The operation creates a large defect in the anterior portion of the pharynx extending from the base of the tongue to the cricopharyngeus muscle. Portions of the cricopharyngeus muscle and thyroid perichondrium are used to strengthen the closure. The most vulnerable point of the closure line is the attachment of the pharynx to the tongue base, since the powerful muscles of the tongue put considerable tension on this suture line.

Complications of total laryngectomy fall into two general categories: early, which are usually observed within the first 2 weeks after the procedure; and late, which can occur months to years later.

The most common early complication of total laryngectomy is the formation of a sinus tract (which is termed a fistula if it extends to another mucosal surface, generally the skin of the anterior neck) (Figure 19-9). The mean time to occurrence of these tracts is 7 days after the operation. Numerous studies have documented that the most common pharyngeal site of origin for sinus tracts is at the upper margin of the suture line, where the neopharynx is joined to the tongue base **(Option (B) is false).** Patients who have undergone radiation therapy prior to total laryngectomy are at substantially higher risk for developing this complication **(Option (C) is true).** In a study of 357 patients, McCombe and Jones found that the prevalence of fistula was 39% in the irradiated group com-

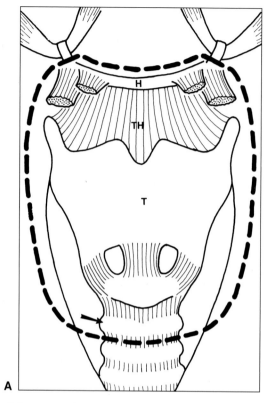

Figure 19-8. Schematic diagrams of total laryngectomy: surgical procedure. (A) Laryngeal cartilages in frontal projection show the margin of surgical resection (dashed line). Structures removed include the thyroid cartilage (T), the thyrohyoid membrane (TH), the hyoid bone (H), and the first tracheal ring (arrow). (B) Laryngeal cartilages in lateral projection show the margin of surgical resection (dashed line). The epiglottis (E) is removed along with the thyroid cartilage (T), thyrohyoid membrane (TH), and hyoid bone (H). Note that the insertion of the anterior part of the cricopharyngeus muscle (CP) is severed. (C) Surgical reconstruction of the nasopharynx. The trachea (TR) is brought anteriorly to form a stoma in the neck. The pharyngeal defect is sutured anteriorly. A nasogastric tube (arrowhead) is present within the lumen of the nasopharynx.

pared with 4% in the nonirradiated group and that the median time to fistula closure was four times longer (112 days versus 28 days) in the irradiated group. Postoperative abscesses (Figure 19-7) are part of this spectrum, since most are observed in conjunction with a sinus tract to the soft tissues of the neck.

Pharyngeal necrosis with ulceration is not a common complication **(Option (A) is false);** it is not specifically mentioned in review articles

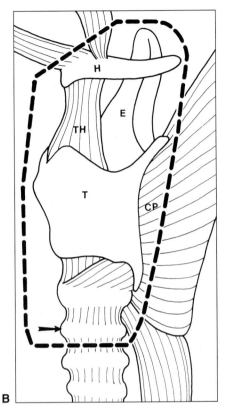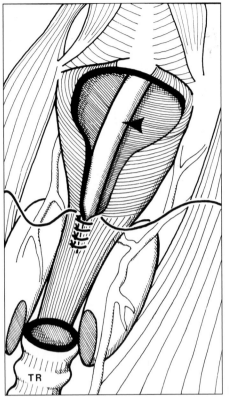

B

C

of postoperative complications. We have observed only a few examples (Figure 19-3), and these usually occurred in patients who had undergone full-course radiation therapy, developed persistent or recurrent cancer, and then had total laryngectomy for salvage.

Late complications include both benign and malignant conditions. Most patients with complications in the late postoperative period experience dysphagia. It has been estimated that approximately 15% of all patients undergoing total laryngectomy will develop dysphagia (**Option (E) is true**).

Stenosis of some portion of the surgically reconstructed pharynx is observed in a number of patients with dysphagia and was the cause of the clinical symptoms in the test patient. In the series of 47 patients undergoing cineradiography observed by Muller-Miny et al., some degree of stenosis was present in 24 patients. The prevalence of stenosis is considerably higher in patients with primary tumors originating in the piriform sinuses or posterior hypopharynx. Kaplan reported a 73% steno-

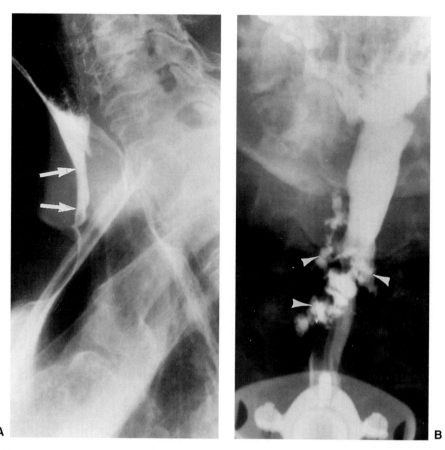

Figure 19-9. Pharyngocutaneous fistula. (A) An oblique view from a pharyngogram obtained in a patient 7 days after total laryngectomy demonstrates a fistula (arrows) arising near the proximal part of the suture line and extending anteriorly to the skin. (B) A radiograph in another patient who had undergone extensive neck irradiation after total laryngectomy demonstrates formation of a large irregular sinus tract (arrowheads) from the anterior aspect of the lower suture margin.

sis rate for tumors at this site (Figure 19-10). Functional evaluation is important in these patients, since many have apparent areas of narrowing without clinical complaints. Administration of various thicknesses of barium, puree, and solid material will frequently elicit symptoms and aids in identifying the narrowing as the basis for clinical complaints.

As mentioned previously, the consistent traction of the powerful tongue muscles on the superior margin of the suture line frequently creates a weakened area on the anterior margin of the neopharynx (the

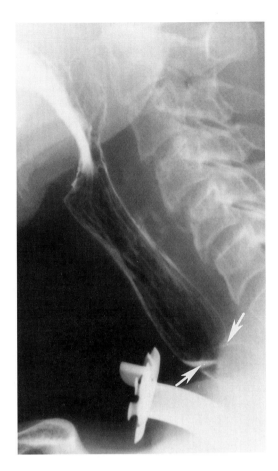

Figure 19-10. Proximal cervical esophageal stenosis (arrows) 2 months after total laryngectomy. The stenosis recurred despite multiple attempts at dilation.

mechanism is the same as that for producing postoperative sinus tracts at this site). Pouches, or pseudodiverticula, are frequently observed in this region as pharyngeal mucosa protrudes through the weakened area. In most patients they are of no clinical consequence, but large diverticula can trap food particles and thereby produce mechanical impingement on swallowing (Figure 19-4). Pouches can also develop elsewhere in the neopharynx and are due to protrusion of mucosa through a muscular defect at the suture line (Figure 19-11).

The surgical procedure results in removal of the anterior attachment of the cricopharyngeus muscle, which retracts to form a posterior bulge on the neopharynx. During normal swallowing the cricopharyngeus relaxes, producing a negative pressure in this pharyngeal segment that helps pass the swallowed bolus into the proximal esophagus. In the post-laryngectomy patient, this negative pressure response is blunted and the

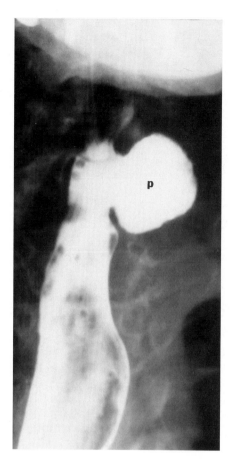

Figure 19-11. Unusual lateral cervical esophageal pouch (p) at the lower left suture margin. Food trapped in this pouch was the genesis of the patient's clinical dysphagia.

bulk of the retracted muscle can act as a mechanical impediment to swallowing (Figure 19-12).

Total laryngectomy is a well-accepted method for treating primary cancers; however, recurrence rates in large surgical series vary from 25 to 50%. The higher end of this spectrum comes from institutions in which surgery is reserved for large, advanced-stage tumors or for patients who have recurrence after radiation therapy. The patterns of recurrence are similar for all reported series; the most common site is in the soft tissues of the neck **(Option (D) is true),** either within unresected cervical lymph nodes or within the neck musculature. Another important site of recurrence is the parastomal region; recurrence in this region occurs in about 10% of operated patients and is associated with a very poor prognosis. The mechanism for tumor recurrence at this site is not certain, but it may be related to seeding of the parastomal tissues during the opera-

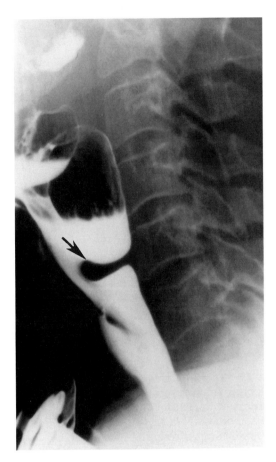

Figure 19-12. Mechanical obstruction. Large cricopharyngeus muscle (arrow) extends nearly all the way across the neopharynx, producing relative mechanical obstruction to the passage of a food bolus.

tive procedure. Mucosal persistence or recurrence is relatively rare in all surgical series.

The risk factors associated with epidermoid carcinoma of the neck are tobacco and alcohol abuse; since these are the same risk factors for the development of epidermoid carcinomas elsewhere, it is not surprising that second-primary cancers arise in 10 to 15% of patients undergoing total laryngectomy. Postoperative evaluation of dysphagia in laryngectomy patients should therefore include a thorough study of the esophagus for both second-primary malignancy (Figure 19-13) and benign esophageal dysmotility that may likewise produce pharyngeal swallowing symptoms.

As indicated by the preceding discussion, barium pharyngography and cross-sectional imaging studies are complementary in evaluating patients with dysphagia after total laryngectomy. Motility disturbances, mechanical problems (strictures, diverticula, fistulas, etc.), and esoph-

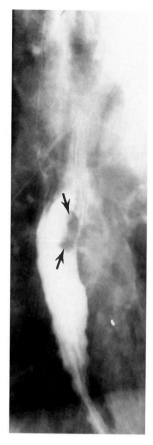

Figure 19-13. Epidermoid carcinoma in a patient examined several years after total laryngectomy. A radiograph shows a nodular mass (arrows) arising from the midesophagus. At biopsy, epidermoid carcinoma was found.

ageal second-primary cancers are best diagnosed by luminal studies; CT and MRI are better for establishing the presence of neck or peristomal recurrences.

Dennis M. Balfe, M.D.

SUGGESTED READINGS

MEDICAL COMPLICATIONS OF TOTAL LARYNGECTOMY

1. Arriaga MA, Kanel KT, Johnson JT, Myers EN. Medical complications in total laryngectomy: incidence and risk factors. Ann Otol Rhinol Laryngol 1990; 99:611–615

SUCCESS RATES AND PATTERNS OF FAILURE IN TOTAL LARYNGECTOMY

2. Esteban F, Moreno JA, Delgado-Rodriguez M, Mochon A. Risk factors involved in stomal recurrence following laryngectomy. J Laryngol Otol 1993; 107:527–531
3. Foote RL, Buskirk SJ, Stanley RJ, et al. Patterns of failure after total laryngectomy for glottic carcinoma. Cancer 1989; 64:143–149
4. Johnson JT, Myers EN, Hao SP, Wagner RL. Outcome of open surgical therapy for glottic carcinoma. Ann Otol Rhinol Laryngol 1993; 102:752–755
5. Levendag P, Sessions R, Vikram B, et al. The problem of neck relapse in early stage supraglottic larynx cancer. Cancer 1989; 63:345–348
6. Razack MS, Maipang T, Sako K, Bakamjian V, Shedd DP. Management of advanced glottic carcinomas. Am J Surg 1989; 158:318–320

FISTULA AFTER TOTAL LARYNGECTOMY

7. Hier M, Black MJ, Lafond G. Pharyngo-cutaneous fistulas after total laryngectomy: incidence, etiology and outcome analysis. J Otolaryngol 1993; 22:164–166
8. Johansen LV, Overgaard J, Elbrond O. Pharyngo-cutaneous fistulae after laryngectomy. Influence of previous radiotherapy and prophylactic metronidazole. Cancer 1988; 61:673–678
9. Krouse JH, Metson R. Barium swallow is a predictor of salivary fistula following laryngectomy. Otolaryngol Head Neck Surg 1992; 106:254–257
10. McCombe AW, Jones AS. Radiotherapy and complications of laryngectomy. J Laryngol Otol 1993; 107:130–132
11. Mendelsohn MS, Bridger GP. Pharyngocutaneous fistulae following laryngectomy. Aust N Z J Surg 1985; 55:177–179
12. Moses BL, Eisele DW, Jones B. Radiologic assessment of the early postoperative total-laryngectomy patient. Laryngoscope 1993; 103:1157–1160
13. Shemen LJ, Spiro RH. Complications following laryngectomy. Head Neck Surg 1986; 8:185–191

DYSPHAGIA AFTER TOTAL LARYNGECTOMY

14. Dey FL, Kirchner JA. The upper esophageal sphincter after laryngectomy. Laryngoscope 1961; 71:99–115
15. Jung TT, Adams GL. Dysphagia in laryngectomized patients. Otolaryngol Head Neck Surg 1980; 88:25–33

16. Kaplan JN. The incidence of hypopharyngeal stenosis after surgery for laryngeal cancer. Otolaryngol Head Neck Surg 1981; 89:956–959
17. Kirchner JA, Scatliff JH, Dey FL, Shedd DP. The pharynx after laryngectomy. Changes in its structure and function. Laryngoscope 1963; 73:18–33
18. McConnel FM, Cerenko D, Mendelsohn MS. Dysphagia after total laryngectomy. Otolaryngol Clin North Am 1988; 21:721–726
19. Schobinger R. Spasm of the cricopharyngeal muscle as cause of dysphagia after total laryngectomy. Arch Otolaryngol 1958; 67:271–275

SECOND PRIMARY CANCERS IN PATIENTS WITH HEAD AND NECK TUMORS

20. Lefor AT, Bredenberg CE, Kellman RM, Aust JC. Multiple malignancies of the lung and head and neck. Arch Surg 1986; 121:265–270
21. McGuirt WF. Panendoscopy as a screening examination for simultaneous primary tumors in head and neck cancer: a prospective sequential study and review of the literature. Laryngoscope 1982; 92:569–576
22. Shons AR, McQuarrie DG. Multiple primary epidermoid carcinomas of the upper aerodigestive tract. Arch Surg 1985; 120:1007–1009

CONTRAST PHARYNGOGRAPHY

23. Balfe DM, Koehler RE, Setzen M, Weyman PJ, Baron RL, Ogura JH. Barium examination of the esophagus after total laryngectomy. Radiology 1982; 143:501–508
24. Gibbons RG, Halvorsen RA, Foster WL Jr, et al. Esophageal lesions after total laryngectomy. AJR 1985; 144:1197–1200
25. Muller-Miny H, Eisele DW, Jones B. Dynamic radiographic imaging following total laryngectomy. Head Neck 1993; 15:342–347

Notes

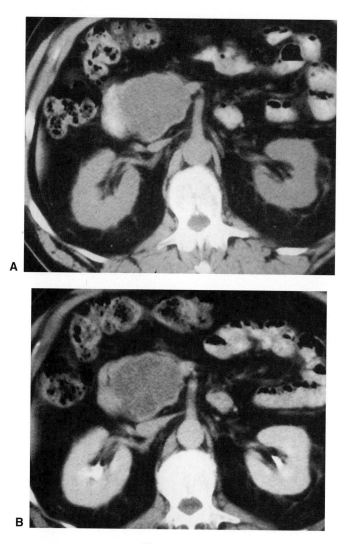

Figure 20-1

Figures 20-1 and 20-2. This 50-year-old man has vague upper abdominal discomfort. You are shown pre- and postcontrast CT images (Figure 20-1) and T1- and T2-weighted MR images (Figure 20-2).

Case 20: Serous Cystadenoma

Question 60

Which *one* of the following is the MOST likely diagnosis?

(A) Mucinous cystic neoplasm
(B) Adenocarcinoma
(C) Serous cystadenoma
(D) Solid and papillary epithelial neoplasm
(E) Mucin-hypersecreting tumor of the pancreatic duct

The CT images (Figure 20-1) and MR images (Figure 20-2) show a large, well-defined mass occupying the region of the pancreatic head (Figures 20-3 and 20-4). The interior of the mass appears homogeneous on noncontrast CT (Figure 20-3A), but the postcontrast image (Figure 20-3B) shows faintly enhancing curvilinear septa within the lesion. The perimeter of the mass is outlined on both CT images by a rim of tissue that has a slightly higher density than that of the interior. The contour of the mass is mildly lobular.

The well-defined margin, lobular contour, and heterogeneous composition of the mass are also apparent on the MR images (Figure 20-4). Both images show the outer wall and some internal septa as structures of low signal intensity. On the T1-weighted image (Figure 20-4A), the interior spaces are also of relatively low signal intensity, although not as low as the intensities of the surrounding capsule or visualized internal septa. On the T2-weighted image (Figure 20-4B), the material occupying the interior of the mass has very high signal intensity at the window setting displayed. The pattern of septation is obscured in all but the posterior portion of the mass. On both pulse sequences the signal intensity of the interior spaces of the mass is similar to that of the lumen of the gallbladder (Figure 20-4). The lesion therefore has features of an encapsulated pancreatic tumor, divided internally into thin-walled, fluid-filled spaces. The extent of septation and the number of cystic compartments are not completely shown on any of the test images, but the composite picture is that of a tumor composed of numerous small cysts. The compo-

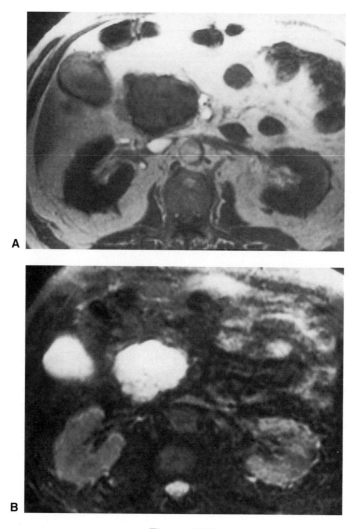

Figure 20-2

sition and structure of the tumor are most characteristic of one of the major types of cystic pancreatic tumor—serous cystadenoma, also known as microcystic adenoma **(Option (C) is correct).**

Mucinous cystic neoplasms (Option (A)), which constitute the other major class of cystic pancreatic tumors, have some features in common with the tumor in the test patient. They, too, are typically large masses—spherical, well defined, encapsulated, and cavitary. The mucinous material that occupies the cystic spaces in mucinous cystic neoplasms is similar in CT density and MR signal intensity to the clear intracystic fluid of serous cystadenomas.

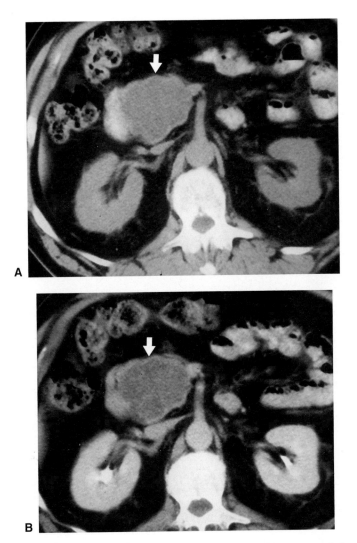

Figure 20-3 (Same as Figure 20-1). Serous cystadenoma of the pancreatic head. Noncontrast (A) and postcontrast (B) CT images show a large, well-defined, mildly lobular mass (arrows) in the region of the pancreatic head. Both images show a thin capsule of relatively high-density tissue at the perimeter of the mass. A pattern of internal septation is suggested on the postcontrast image.

There are, however, morphologic characteristics of mucinous cystic neoplasms that differ from those of the tumor illustrated in the test images. Mucinous cystic neoplasms are either unilocular or divided by septations into only a few (rarely more than six) cystic compartments (Figure 20-5). Moreover, the cystic spaces in mucinous cystic neoplasms

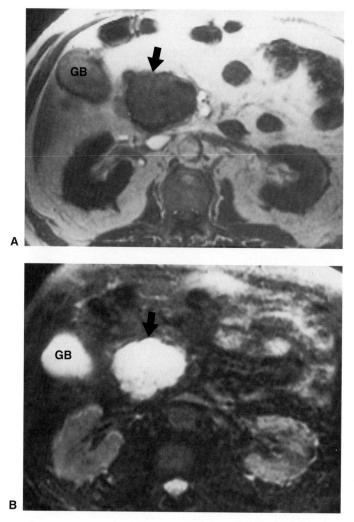

Figure 20-4 (Same as Figure 20-2). Serous cystadenoma of the pancreatic head. T1-weighted (A) and T2-weighted (B) MR images show the
pancreatic tumor (arrows) as a well-defined, encapsulated mass of mildly
lobular contour. On each of the pulse sequences, the interior of the tumor
has a signal intensity similar to that of the gallbladder (GB). A pattern of
internal septation is visible on the T1-weighted image and to a lesser
extent on the T2-weighted image.

are larger than those in the tumor depicted in Figures 20-1 and 20-2,
usually exceeding 2 cm in diameter. For that reason, the term "macrocystic" is sometimes applied to these tumors. Mural nodules or papillary
excrescences sometimes protrude into the cystic spaces from the outer
wall or internal septa (Figure 20-5). Calcification, which occurs only

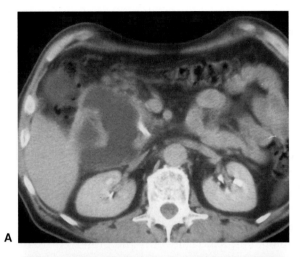

A

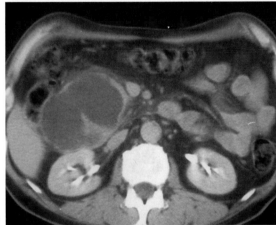

B

Figure 20-5. Multiloculated mucinous cystic neoplasm of the pancreatic head. Postcontrast CT images show the tumor to be composed of large cystic cavities. (A) A soft tissue papillary protrusion containing a tiny fleck of calcification projects into the dominant cyst from the lateral wall. Dense calcification is present in a thickened portion of the medial wall. (B) At a lower level, a thin septum separates adjacent cysts. Histologically, the tumor was a mucinous cystadenoma.

occasionally, is usually peripheral (Figure 20-5). Mucinous cystic neoplasms occur predominantly in middle-aged women, and most tumors are located in the tail of the pancreas. However, these tumors are found in men and women of all age groups and can occur in any part of the pancreas. Therefore, although the sex of the test patient and the location of his tumor are not typical for mucinous cystic neoplasm, they are not sufficiently unusual to disqualify mucinous cystic neoplasm from serious diagnostic consideration. Rather, the morphologic characteristics of the tumor in the test patient make mucinous cystic neoplasm an unlikely candidate for the diagnosis.

The practical reason to distinguish mucinous cystic neoplasms from serous cystadenomas relates to differences in biologic behavior between the two types of cystic pancreatic tumor. Unlike serous cystadenomas, mucinous cystic neoplasms have a high malignant potential. Mucinous cystic tumors that are already malignant at the time of discovery are designated as mucinous cystadenocarcinomas, whereas those that are not malignant can be classified as mucinous cystadenomas. However, even tumors without malignant histology, especially those that exhibit epithelial atypia, are considered to have the capacity for malignant transformation. Furthermore, a tumor that is otherwise histologically benign can harbor foci of malignancy. For these reasons, it has become customary to refer to all tumors of this class as mucinous cystic neoplasms. Unless there is evidence of extrapancreatic invasion or of metastatic disease associated with the pancreatic tumor, it is not possible to distinguish the malignant form of this tumor from its benign counterpart by radiologic imaging. Complete surgical removal is the preferred treatment for all resectable mucinous cystic neoplasms.

The most common tumor of the pancreas is an adenocarcinoma that arises from ductal epithelium of the organ. Statistically, adenocarcinoma (Option (B)) is by far the most likely pancreatic neoplasm to develop in an individual of the age and sex of the test patient. However, the tumor in the test images has several features that are inconsistent with pancreatic adenocarcinoma. Ordinary-type adenocarcinomas of the pancreas are unencapsulated, solid, scirrhous tumors with diminished vascularity relative to the remainder of the gland. As such, they usually undergo a uniformly low degree of enhancement relative to the enhancement of normal pancreas on dynamic postcontrast CT (Figure 20-6). The appearance of the tumor in the test patient does suggest solid composition on the precontrast CT image (Figure 20-1A), and for the most part it shows a low degree of enhancement on the postcontrast CT image (Figure 20-1B). However, the tumor has a capsular covering in both CT images and internal septation is visible in the postcontrast image. The cystic nature of the mass is shown most convincingly on the MR images, which demonstrate signal intensities typical of a fluid-filled structure on both pulse sequences. Solid adenocarcinomas of the pancreas are typically hypointense on T1-weighted images but isointense relative to normal pancreas on T2-weighted MR images. The intense signal on the T2-weighted image in the test patient (Figure 20-2B) is not characteristic of pancreatic adenocarcinoma, and neither are the external capsule and internal septations, which are demonstrated by MRI as well as by CT. Another feature of the tumor in the test patient that is uncharacteristic of adenocarcinoma is the size of the mass. Most adenocarcinomas, especially those of the pancreatic head, are considerably smaller than the tumor in Figures 20-1 and 20-2 at the time they come to clinical attention (Figure 20-6).

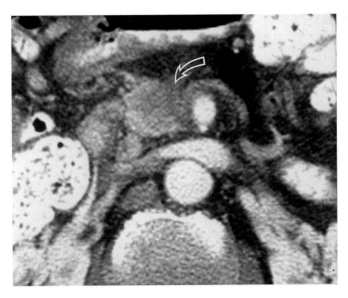

Figure 20-6. Adenocarcinoma of the pancreatic head. A postcontrast CT scan shows the tumor as a lesion of low enhancement in the region of the uncinate process (arrow). Unlike typical cystic neoplasms of the pancreas, this solid tumor is small and unencapsulated. It extends medially beyond the pancreas to involve the adjacent wall of the superior mesenteric artery.

Solid and papillary epithelial neoplasm (Option (D)) can practically be excluded from diagnostic consideration on the basis of the sex and age of the test patient. More than 95% of these rare pancreatic neoplasms are found in young females, specifically adolescent or postadolescent girls and young women. Few have been reported in individuals over 40 years of age, and fewer still occur in men. Solid and papillary epithelial neoplasms are discussed further in Question 62.

Mucin-hypersecreting tumors of the pancreatic duct (Option (E)) are recently described neoplasms that are closely related histologically and in biologic behavior to mucinous cystic neoplasms of the pancreas. One form of this tumor, which results in mucinous cystic dilatation of one or more branches of the main pancreatic duct (and which was first recognized to occur in the uncinate process of the pancreatic head), could in many respects resemble the tumor in the test patient. However, mucin-hypersecreting tumors of the pancreatic duct do not produce the internal architectural arrangement that is displayed by the tumor on the test images. Mucin-hypersecreting intraductal tumors are discussed further in Question 63.

Question 61

Concerning serous cystadenoma,

  (A) it usually arises in the pancreatic tail
  (B) calcification is typically central
  (C) its epithelium is rich in glycogen
  (D) the septa are well vascularized
  (E) its malignant potential is high

Serous cystadenomas of the pancreas have been recognized as being distinct from mucinous cystic neoplasms since the publication of landmark articles in 1978 by Compagno and Oertel and by Hodgkinson and associates. In recognition of the small sizes of the cystic compartments that typically occupy the interior of these cystadenomas, Compagno and Oertel coined the term microcystic adenoma, a name that remains synonymous with serous cystadenoma. The latter designation has recently gained favor because the cystic fluid within these lesions is consistently serous, whereas an occasional tumor of this type is made up of cysts too large to qualify as "microcystic." Another name applied to the tumor, glycogen-rich cystadenoma, refers to a constituent of the epithelial cells that line the cysts.

Serous cystadenomas can occur in any part of the pancreas, with perhaps a slight predilection for the pancreatic head **(Option (A) is false).** In a series of 40 patients with serous cystadenoma reported by Pyke et al., 25 had tumors located primarily in the pancreatic head or neck, 16 had tumors in the body, and 3 had tumors in the tail (7 patients had multiple tumor sites). This distribution is consistent with that reported in other series. These tumors grow slowly and usually reach a large size before producing symptoms or clinical signs. They are found, however, in an enormous range of sizes, from less than 1 cm in diameter to more than 25 cm.

Serous cystadenomas are sharply circumscribed, more or less spherical tumors, defined peripherally by a fibrous capsule that is often made lobular by underlying cysts. In their typical form, serous cystadenomas are composed of innumerable small cysts, a composition that gives the interior a honeycomb or spongelike appearance (Figure 20-7). Typical cysts range in size from microscopic to between 1 and 2 cm in diameter. The largest of these cysts tend to be located at the periphery of the tumor. Fibrous bands within the tumor often converge centrally to form a stellate scar (Figure 20-7), which is sometimes calcified. Peripheral elements in this tumor do not become calcified **(Option (B) is true).** Microscopically, the cysts that make up serous cystadenomas are lined with flattened or cuboidal epithelial cells (Figure 20-8) that, with appropriate

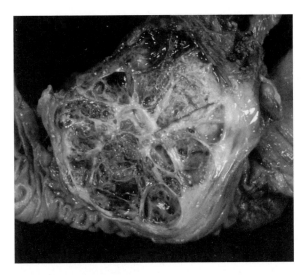

Figure 20-7. Serous cystadenoma. A cut surface of a pancreatic tumor removed by the Whipple procedure shows the tumor to be composed of innumerable small cysts. Within some of the larger cysts are several smaller cysts. A fibrous capsule surrounds the tumor, and internal fibrous bands converge to form a central stellate scar. Larger cysts at the periphery produce a slightly lobular contour.

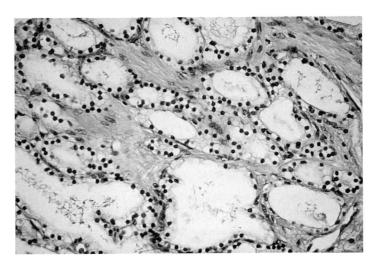

Figure 20-8. Serous cystadenoma. A photomicrograph shows microscopic cystic spaces lined by low cuboidal epithelium. Intervening septa are composed of collagenous tissue.

staining, are shown to contain large amounts of glycogen **(Option (C) is true).** A rich capillary network is usually present within the stromal septa **(Option (D) is true).**

Exceptions to the typical forms of serous cystadenoma include infrequently encountered unilocular cystic tumors or tumors composed exclusively or predominantly of cysts greater than 2 cm in diameter. More important deviations include recently reported tumors that may represent a malignant variety of serous cystic neoplasm. Throughout most of the years since serous cystadenomas were classified as distinct neoplasms, they were believed to have virtually no potential for malignant transformation. In 1989, however, George et al. reported histologic documentation of metastasis from a cystic pancreatic tumor that was microscopically identical to serous cystadenoma. In 1991, Kamei et al. described a patient with multifocal pancreatic serous cystadenomatous tumors that exhibited cellular atypia and perineural invasion on microscopic examination. Reports of tumors that appear to be serous cystadenocarcinomas cast strong doubt on the previously held concept that serous cystadenomas have practically no potential for malignant transformation. Nevertheless, it remains true that in all but very exceptional cases, serous cystadenomatous neoplasms are benign at discovery and, as far as is known, remain so. Evidence to date indicates that malignant transformation of serous cystadenomas must be exceedingly unusual **(Option (E) is false).**

Clinical presentations of pancreatic serous cystadenomas vary. The tumor is found most often in women over 60 years of age, but serous cystadenomas are encountered in both sexes and in all adult age groups. In most reported series, men account for more than one-third of cases. Serous cystadenomas are among the pancreatic lesions that occur in some patients with von Hippel-Lindau disease, but that association is uncommon.

Symptoms and signs of pancreatic serous cystadenomas are usually related to local pressure effects of the tumor and include abdominal pain or fullness, nausea, weight loss, and palpable mass. Tumors of the pancreatic head can obstruct the extrahepatic bile duct and produce jaundice, but biliary obstruction is present in only a few patients with serous cystadenoma of the pancreatic head. Tumors in the pancreatic head can also cause pancreatic insufficiency or pancreatitis by obstructing the main pancreatic duct, but consequences of pancreatic-duct obstruction are not common clinical presentations. Acute complications of serous cystadenoma are uncommon but potentially serious sources of presentation. Acute complications include hemorrhage from gastric or duodenal ulcers located adjacent to a tumor or from varices caused by portal or splenic vein occlusion. At least two cases of intraperitoneal hemorrhage from serous cystadenoma have been reported. The incidental discovery of a pancreatic serous cystadenoma at surgical exploration or autopsy has long been recognized. Increasing numbers of these tumors are now discovered as incidental findings on abdominal imaging procedures performed for indications unrelated to a pancreatic lesion.

Radiologic features of pancreatic serous cystadenomas vary according to the size, location, and architecture of the tumor. Some larger masses are apparent on radiographs or barium studies owing to their displacement of hollow viscera. Calcification of the central scar, when present, is often visible on conventional radiographs. Angiography is seldom used to evaluate cystic pancreatic tumors in contemporary practice, but classic angiographic reports describe displacement of major vessels, large feeding arteries, and a blush reflecting the rich stromal vascularity of the tumor. Hypovascular serous cystadenomas have also been observed.

Cross-sectional imaging demonstrates a well-defined, often lobulated mass. In general, depiction of internal architecture is related to the size of the cysts; groups of larger cysts are more accurately displayed than are collections of smaller cysts. Ultrasonography readily displays much of the solid structure and in most cases demonstrates the multicystic composition of the tumor as well (Figure 20-9A). Masses composed of myriads of extremely small cysts, however, can appear completely echogenic owing to the concentration of interfaces within such tumors. In some of these cases, the cystic nature of the tumor is indicated by enhanced through transmission of the sound beam.

The appearance of a serous cystadenoma on CT is influenced by the technique of scanning. As in the test image (Figure 20-1A), many of these tumors appear almost homogeneous on images made without contrast enhancement (Figure 20-9B). Depending on whether the cystic spaces or the solid elements make up the greater part of the tumor volume, the density of the mass on noncontrast images can be low (near that of water) or relatively high (near that of soft tissue). Careful inspection of the images will usually reveal at least a suggestion of multilocularity within the tumor (Figure 20-10A). The architecture of serous cystadenomas is best displayed by CT on postcontrast images, especially those acquired during a phase of relatively dense vascular opacification when perfused septa and other stromal components undergo greatest enhancement (Figures 20-1B, 20-9C, and 20-10B). Thin-section scanning, which improves spatial resolution, is also advantageous. Even with the best of techniques, however, CT often fails to reveal the full extent of fine internal septations.

The MR appearance of typical serous cystadenomas is that of sharply defined, encapsulated, lobulated masses of multilocular internal composition (Figure 20-2). Like CT, MRI often fails to demonstrate fully the fine internal architectural structure. The method can, however, indicate the largely liquid composition of the tumor. Typical of fluid-filled struc-

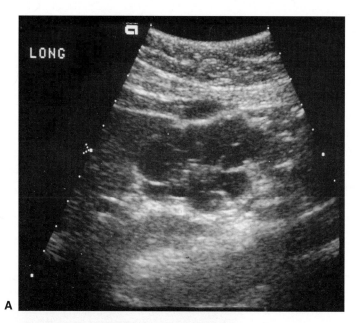

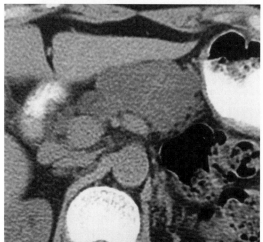

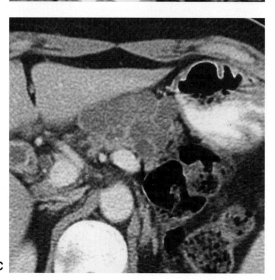

Figure 20-9. Serous
cystadenoma. (A) An
ultrasonogram also
shows the multicystic
composition of the tu-
mor, with anechoic
cysts outlined by
echogenic septa. (B) A
noncontrast CT scan
shows a well-defined
mass that arises from
the pancreatic body.
The tumor is of almost
homogeneous soft tis-
sue density but has a
mildly lobular contour.
(C) A 5-mm postcon-
trast CT section shows
the multicystic compo-
sition of the tumor,
with enhancing septa
and nonenhancing cys-
tic spaces.

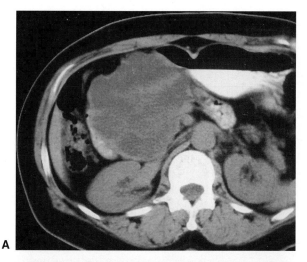

A

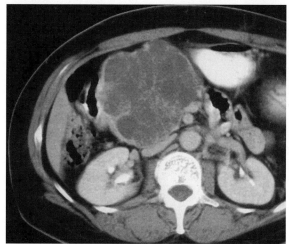

B

Figure 20-10. Serous cystadenoma of the pancreatic head. (A) A noncontrast CT scan shows a large lobular mass in the region of the pancreatic head. Faintly visible septa outline a few larger peripheral cysts within the mass. (B) A postcontrast CT scan clearly shows the multicystic architecture of the tumor, with smaller cysts and fine septal structures concentrated toward the center of the tumor and larger cysts at the periphery.

tures, the cystic spaces in these tumors are depicted as having relatively low signal intensity on T1-weighted images (Figure 20-2A) and high signal intensity on T2-weighted images (Figure 20-2B). Visible stromal components have low signal intensity on both sequences.

A component of some serous cystadenomas that is not displayed by MRI but can be shown by radiography, ultrasonography, and CT is internal calcification. CT and ultrasonography show the central location of the calcification. Because this calcification occurs within the central fibrous scar, which often has a stellate configuration, the calcification also has been noted on occasion to have a stellate or "sunburst" configuration. The shape of the central calcification in serous cystadenomas,

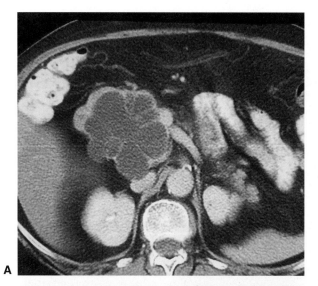

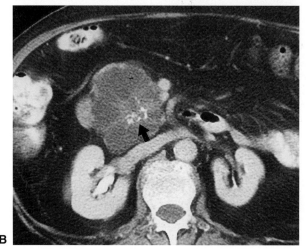

Figure 20-11. Serous cystadenoma with relatively large cysts and central calcification. Postcontrast CT images show a well-defined lobular tumor composed of numerous thin-walled cysts. Many of the cysts are more than 2 cm in diameter (larger than usual for a serous cystadenoma), but numerous cysts are present and their uniformly thin septal walls converge toward a central calcified scar (arrow in panel B); this arrangement is typical of serous cystadenoma.

however, is variable and nonspecific. It is often nodular. Calcification is easily recognized by its radiographic density on conventional radiographs and CT (Figure 20-11). On ultrasonography it produces a focal zone of bright echoes with or without shadowing.

Discussions of the radiologic differential diagnosis of pancreatic serous cystadenomas have tended to focus on distinguishing these tumors from mucinous cystic neoplasms, probably because the two types of cystic tumor were only relatively recently recognized to be pathologically distinct. However, typical serous cystadenomas, with their innumerable small internal cysts (Figures 20-7 through 20-10), do not closely resemble typical mucinous cystic neoplasms, in which the cysts are few and relatively large (Figure 20-5). Papillary excrescences and mural nodules are not present in serous cystadenomas but are common in mucinous cystic neoplasms (Figure 20-5). The central scar seen in many serous cystadenomas is not a feature of mucinous cystic neoplasms. Calcification in a serous cystadenoma is located within the central scar (Figure 20-11), whereas calcification that occasionally occurs in a mucinous cystic neoplasm is usually within a peripheral nodule (Figure 20-5).

Other cystic tumors generally can be dismissed from serious consideration in the differential diagnosis of a serous cystadenoma. Nonfunctioning islet cell carcinomas can undergo cystic degeneration, and about 20% of these tumors develop calcification. Necrotic islet cell carcinomas, however, do not have a microcystic morphology, and they usually retain significant components of solid soft tissue. Solid and papillary epithelial neoplasms of the pancreas, discussed in Question 62, usually do not resemble serous cystadenomas in internal architecture.

Thus, the radiologic diagnosis of typical forms of serous cystadenomas, which constitute the vast majority of these tumors, depends on accurate depiction of their structural morphology. When a typical microcystic composition is demonstrated, a confident radiologic diagnosis can be offered. Diagnosis is also possible in mildly atypical forms, such as masses containing peripheral cysts larger than 2 cm in diameter, as long as the dominant picture is a typical microcystic pattern (Figure 20-10) or an arrangement of cysts about a central scar (Figure 20-11).

A serous cystadenoma with microcystic morphology is probably more likely to be confused with a solid tumor than with another type of cystic mass at radiologic imaging. In that situation, it is particularly important to distinguish serous cystadenoma from pancreatic adenocarcinoma. As noted above, tumors of microcystic composition can resemble solid masses on ultrasonography or CT. The highly echogenic sonographic pattern of such a tumor, however, is not characteristic of solid pancreatic neoplasms such as adenocarcinomas, which are usually hypoechoic relative to normal pancreatic parenchyma. On CT, serous cystadenomas are most likely to resemble solid pancreatic tumors when images are made with inadequate contrast enhancement or spatial resolution to demonstrate the internal architecture of the tumor. Particularly when a pancreatic mass of indeterminate nature is discovered unexpectedly on a CT examination that was not designed to display fine anatomic detail, it is often worthwhile to repeat the examination with special attention devoted to display of the pancreatic lesion. This usually involves thin-section scanning combined with adequate delivery of intravenous contrast material. In some cases it is useful to obtain complementary information from other imaging procedures (Figures 20-1 and 20-2).

Clues that an incidentally discovered pancreatic tumor is something other than ordinary pancreatic adenocarcinoma and therefore deserving of further investigation include unusually large tumor size, presence of calcification within the mass, notable enhancement of the tumor after administration of intravenous contrast material, and presence of a peripheral capsule. The fact that a pancreatic tumor is asymptomatic is itself a clue that the lesion is probably something other than adenocarcinoma, because ordinary cancers of the pancreas are almost always symptomatic at the time of discovery.

The role of percutaneous needle biopsy under sonographic or CT guidance has not been established in regard to serous cystadenomas. Use of the procedure in a small number of cases is mentioned in several published series, but no comprehensive evaluation has been reported. A microscopic diagnosis can be made if the aspirate provides histologically or cytologically demonstrable glycogen-containing low cuboidal epithelial cells with clear cytoplasm and intranuclear inclusions. The frequency with which material of this kind can be obtained by needle biopsy is not known. Analysis of intracystic fluid can also be useful. Fluid from serous cystadenomas contains neither mucin nor a high concentration of amylase, characteristics that distinguish these tumors from mucinous cystic neoplasms and pseudocysts, respectively. A few authors have expressed concern about the potential risk of hemorrhage after puncture of a highly vascularized tumor, but experience accumulated to date is insufficient to determine whether this concern is warranted.

For most patients with serous cystadenoma of the pancreas, the main purpose of radiologic investigation is to establish an accurate diagnostic basis for appropriate management of the disease. Determination of the most appropriate form of management, however, is not always straightforward. For patients whose tumors are symptomatic, surgical intervention is usually recommended. When feasible, this usually involves complete resection of the tumor, but biliary or gastric bypass can be carried out in patients with obstructive tumors who are not considered candidates for major pancreatic resection. For patients whose tumors are not causing symptoms, determination of management involves a consideration of the risks and benefits of surgical intervention versus those of nonoperative observation. Several issues are relevant to this decision, including the age and condition of the patient, the type of operation required, and the natural history of the neoplasm. Complicating the last of these issues somewhat is the recently publicized evidence that these generally indolent tumors, although of very low malignant potential, are not invariably benign.

Question 62

Concerning solid and papillary epithelial neoplasm,

    (A) it occurs most often in elderly individuals
    (B) it is associated with von Hippel-Lindau disease
    (C) cystic degeneration is common
    (D) calcification is typically central
    (E) metastasis is usual at the time of discovery

Like other uncommon neoplasms of the pancreas, the tumor most often called solid and papillary epithelial neoplasm is known by a variety of descriptive names. Synonyms include papillary epithelial neoplasm, papillary cystic neoplasm, solid and cystic acinar-cell tumor, and solid and cystic tumor. The lesion was first described by Hamoudi et al. in a 1970 case report of a 12-year-old girl. Fewer than 200 additional cases of the tumor have been reported in the ensuing 25 years. Consistent with the initial case report, most solid and papillary epithelial neoplasms of the pancreas are discovered in adolescent or postadolescent girls or young women **(Option (A) is false).** More than 95% of the reported tumors have occurred in females, all but a few of them younger than 40 years. Early reports from the United States suggest a strong predilection toward African Americans, but subsequent reports, including series from Asia, indicate a wide racial and geographic distribution. There is no known association with other medical disorders. Specifically, this tumor is not associated with von Hippel-Lindau disease; pancreatic lesions observed most commonly in von Hippel-Lindau disease are simple cysts, islet cell tumors, and serous cystadenomas **(Option (B) is false).**

Solid and papillary epithelial neoplasms were initially thought to arise from the epithelium of small pancreatic ducts or acini, but recent evidence suggests that they originate from multipotential primordial cells. They can occur in any part of the pancreas, although a disproportionate number originate in the pancreatic tail. The tumors grow slowly and, like other indolent neoplasms of the pancreas, usually do not produce symptoms until they become large. The tumors become encapsulated by fibrous tissue and thus appear sharply demarcated on macroscopic inspection. The internal structure varies. Occasional tumors are homogeneously solid and others are almost completely cystic, but most are of mixed solid and cystic composition. (Considering the uncertain cellular origin of this neoplasm and its usual structural composition, "solid and cystic tumor" may be the most appropriate name among those commonly applied to the tumor. It is the term currently favored in Japanese publications.) The tumors apparently begin as solid lesions but undergo various degrees of cystic degeneration as a result of necrosis and hemorrhage **(Option (C) is true).** Degeneration of solid neoplastic tissue accounts for formation of both papillae and cysts, and it also results in internal hemorrhage, which, in turn, leads to further cystic degeneration. This process often produces a multicystic composition, but the internal organization of these tumors is not like that of intrinsically multicystic tumors such as serous cystadenomas; there are no well-defined septa, and there is no central scar. Calcification is relatively uncommon in solid and papillary neoplasms and, when it occurs, involves the fibrous capsule rather than interior components **(Option (D) is false).**

Microscopically, the neoplastic cells exhibit minimal mitotic activity, and therefore the neoplasm is classified as a tumor of low-grade malignancy. This designation is consistent with the clinical behavior of the tumor. Penetration of the fibrous capsule by neoplastic cells is a common microscopic feature; however, neither gross extracapsular invasion nor metastasis is common at the time the tumor is discovered **(Option (E) is false).** Metastasis from solid and papillary epithelial neoplasm is so uncommon that only a few cases of nodal, hepatic, or peritoneal dissemination have been reported. Most of these neoplasms can be excised, and surgical excision is usually curative.

Symptoms of solid and papillary epithelial neoplasm are usually related to local effects of the upper abdominal mass. Vague abdominal discomfort or the presence of a palpable mass may cause the patient to seek attention. Acute pain, probably related to intratumoral hemorrhage, is sometimes the presenting complaint. In some patients the tumor is discovered incidentally by surgical exploration or radiologic examination. Reviews of medical records of older patients found to have solid and papillary epithelial neoplasm provide evidence that some of these tumors were present many years before diagnosis. As an example, Ohtomo et al. described a 73-year-old woman with hepatic metastasis from a tumor that had been seen as a calcified mass on radiography 50 years before diagnosis. These authors point out that the reported incidence of metastatic or locally advanced disease from solid and papillary epithelial neoplasms tends to be highest in older patients, at least some of whom have had undiagnosed masses known to have been present for several years. The likelihood of clinically malignant behavior, therefore, appears related to the duration of the tumor, and it appears justified to remove these neoplasms when they are discovered, before they extend beyond the confines of the pancreas.

Radiologic manifestations of solid and papillary epithelial neoplasms of the pancreas are those of a large pancreatic mass with individual features related to the morphology of the tumor and the method of imaging. On conventional radiographs the tumor can cause recognizable compres-

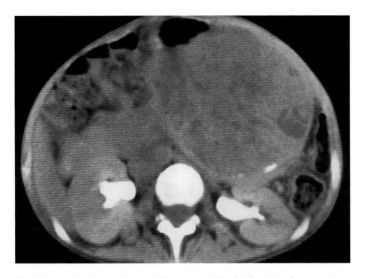

Figure 20-12. Solid and papillary epithelial neoplasm in a young woman. A postcontrast CT image shows a huge, spherical, encapsulated mass in the left side of the abdomen that contains both solid and cystic elements, with a predominance of solid tissue. Low-density cystic areas represent regions of liquefactive necrosis. A peripheral capsule contains foci of calcification posteriorly. The mass is so large that its pancreatic origin is difficult to ascertain, but the location of the tumor is consistent with a mass arising from the pancreatic tail.

sion or displacement of adjacent organs. If capsular calcification is present, a curvilinear or eggshell calcific density may be seen.

With ultrasonography, CT, or MRI, the pancreatic origin of the tumor is usually demonstrable, as are most of the salient architectural features. In some patients with larger masses, however, the organ of origin is impossible to determine with certainty (Figure 20-12), although the pancreas should be recognized as a likely source. The fibrous capsule is displayed as a structure of variable thickness. Calcification, best depicted by CT, is clearly shown to be within the capsule (Figure 20-12). The uncalcified capsule is of soft tissue density (Figure 20-13). The fibrous capsule appears as a rim of low signal intensity on T1- and T2-weighted MR images. CT and ultrasonography demonstrate different proportions and numbers of hypoechoic or low-density components within these tumors, depending on the degree of cystic degeneration (Figures 20-12 and 20-13). The solid components, on the other hand, are within the range of soft tissue density on CT (Figure 20-12). They undergo little enhancement with intravenous contrast material. Foci of hemorrhage within the tumor sometimes have a higher density. Regions of liquefactive necrosis generally have low density, near that of water,

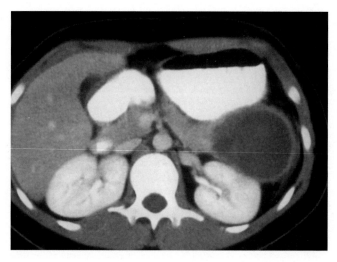

Figure 20-13. Solid and papillary epithelial neoplasm as a predominantly cystic tumor. A postcontrast CT scan in a 15-year-old girl shows a thick-walled unilocular cystic mass arising from the pancreatic tail.

but the admixture of solid debris or extravasated blood can elevate the density within a necrotic region. Hemorrhagic necrosis is best displayed by MRI, which shows the affected regions to have high signal intensity on T1-weighted images and variable intensities on T2-weighted images.

The differential diagnosis of solid and papillary epithelial neoplasms includes the other cystic tumors of the pancreas. Solid and papillary epithelial neoplasms, however, do not have the clearly septated, organized internal architecture that characterizes serous cystadenomas. Calcification, if present, is capsular in solid and papillary tumors and central in serous cystadenomas. A solid and papillary epithelial neoplasm of the highly cystic variety (Figure 20-13) could be indistinguishable from a mucinous cystic neoplasm (Figure 20-5), although mucinous cystic neoplasms rarely occur in patients younger than 30 years. Pancreatoblastoma is a tumor of childhood that can closely resemble solid and papillary neoplasm on cross-sectional images; however, pancreatoblastoma is very rare, and it occurs in children younger than those who typically develop solid and papillary epithelial neoplasm. Some forms of nonfunctioning islet cell carcinoma can also closely resemble solid and papillary epithelial neoplasms. Duct cell adenocarcinoma, which is rarely cystic and is usually relatively small at presentation, is not likely to resemble solid and papillary epithelial neoplasm. With the exception of a serous cystadenoma, which might be monitored without surgical resection, all the tumors likely to be considered in the differential diagnosis of solid and papillary epithelial neoplasm are best treated by complete surgical resection. In that respect, a precise preoperative diagnosis may not be critical. Nevertheless, a correct diagnosis is always desirable, and it is usually possible for this neoplasm. Solid and papillary epithelial neoplasm should be a primary consideration when a large, encapsulated tumor of solid and cystic composition is encountered in an adolescent girl or young woman.

Question 63

Concerning mucin-hypersecreting tumors of the pancreatic duct,

    (A) they rarely involve ductal side branches
    (B) histologically, they resemble mucinous cystic neoplasms
    (C) most are surgically resectable when discovered
    (D) pancreatitis is a common clinical presentation
    (E) intraductal filling defects are a characteristic finding on endoscopic retrograde pancreatography

Since they were first described by Japanese investigators in the 1980s, mucin-hypersecreting tumors of the pancreatic duct have been recognized with increasing frequency. Reports from Japan continue to dominate the literature on these tumors, but growing numbers of cases are reported from North America and Europe as well. To a large extent, recognition of these tumors and their clinical behavior can be attributed to expanded application and refined techniques of radiologic imaging.

Classification and nomenclature of mucin-hypersecreting tumors of the pancreatic duct have not been standardized, and lesions that fall within this category of neoplasm have been reported under a variety of names. These designations include mucin-producing tumor, mucin-hypersecreting tumor, ductectatic cystadenoma and cystadenocarcinoma, mucinous ductal ectasia, and intraductal mucin-hypersecreting neoplasm. Two forms were described in initial radiologic reports: the first, characterized by mucinous cystic dilatation of pancreatic ductal branches in the uncinate process, was called ductectatic mucinous cystadenoma or cystadenocarcinoma in a report published in 1986; and the second, characterized by mucinous distension of the main pancreatic duct, was called mucin-secreting carcinoma of the pancreatic duct in an article published in the following year. Subsequently, both types of tumor have come to be regarded as manifestations of the same pathologic process, which is now recognized to occur in an even greater variety of forms.

Mucin-hypersecreting neoplasia of pancreatic ductal epithelium can arise within the main pancreatic duct, in one or more ductal side branches, or in a combination of main and side-branch ducts. In comprehensively reported series, the main duct has been involved in most patients, but side branches have been involved in nearly one-half of patients **(Option (A) is false).** Involvement of the main pancreatic duct can be segmental or generalized, and the tumor can arise in or involve any part of the gland. Histologically, the condition occurs in a spectrum ranging from benign epithelial hyperplasia to overt carcinoma. Different degrees of cellular differentiation can coexist within the same tumor. Regardless of the site of origin or histologic grade, all forms of this condition are characterized by mucinous transformation of the affected ductal epithelium and consequent secretion of mucin into the lumen of the duct. Epithelial proliferation can produce nodular excrescences of tumor that also protrude into the ductal lumen.

The degree of mucinous luminal distension varies, but ducts can become spherically dilated, so that they resemble cysts. When mucinous distension of the main pancreatic duct extends to the ampulla of Vater, mucin can protrude through a dilated ductal orifice. When a side branch is involved, it usually communicates with the main pancreatic duct, although mucin plugs can cause them to be occluded.

The relationship between mucin-hypersecreting tumors of the pancreatic duct and classic mucinous cystic neoplasms (mucinous cystadenoma and cystadenocarcinoma) of the pancreas has been a matter of considerable discussion. Microscopically, the two conditions are indistinguishable **(Option (B) is true),** and although they differ in typical clinical presentation, they are similar in biologic behavior. Both are mucin-hypersecreting epithelial neoplasms that occur in benign and malignant forms. Some authorities therefore consider mucin-hypersecreting intraductal tumors to be variants of mucinous cystic neoplasms, with mucin-hypersecreting ductal tumors arising from the main pancreatic duct or intermediate-sized side branches and classic mucinous cystic neoplasms arising from parenchymal ductules. There are, however, demographic differences between these tumors. Most patients with mucin-producing tumor of the pancreatic duct are older men, whereas mucinous cystic neoplasms occur most commonly in middle-aged women. From a practical standpoint, determining the relationship of these two tumors is probably not very significant. Both are relatively slowly growing neoplasms, considered even in their histologically benign forms to have a potential for malignant transformation. For that reason, the current treatment of choice for both conditions is complete surgical resection of the neoplasms when feasible.

Most mucin-hypersecreting tumors of the pancreatic duct are confined to the pancreas at the time of discovery and therefore are amenable to surgical resection **(Option (C) is true).** Although data concerning long-term survival after resection of these neoplasms are limited, information available to date indicates that most patients whose tumors are resected are cured of the disease. Subsequent development of metastasis has been observed, but this almost always occurs in patients whose pancreatic tumors were histologically malignant. For patients who suffer from pancreatitis, resection of the tumor eliminates the cause of that complication.

Presenting clinical symptoms are variable in patients with mucin-hypersecreting tumor of the pancreatic duct. Abdominal pain, weight loss, and steatorrhea are common. Recurrent pancreatitis, attributed to mucinous blockage of the main pancreatic duct, is a common presentation **(Option (D) is true).** Chronic pancreatitis and pancreatic insufficiency can result from long-standing occlusion of the duct. The disease occurs predominantly in elderly men but is not limited to that age group or sex. In a series of 18 patients with the tumor studied at the Mayo Clinic (unpublished data), the median age was 69.5 years (range, 52 to 90 years) and 13 patients (72%) were men. These demographic characteristics are similar to those in series reported from Japan.

Whether nonspecific or indicative of pancreatitis, the clinical presentation of a mucin-hypersecreting tumor of the pancreatic duct is likely to lead to radiologic investigation of the pancreas. The radiologist who is familiar with the morphologic manifestations of this disease is therefore likely to have the first opportunity to provide the diagnosis. The radiologic features of mucin-hypersecreting intraductal pancreatic tumors vary according to the gross pathologic manifestations of the individual lesions. Endoscopic retrograde pancreatography (ERP), ultrasonography, CT, and MRI have all demonstrated features of this disease, but observations by ERP and CT have been most extensively reported.

These tumors are well suited for investigation by ERP because they arise from the pancreatic ductal system. Moreover, because patients often present with symptoms of chronic or recurrent pancreatitis, ERP is likely to be used early in their evaluation. In patients with tumors of the main pancreatic duct, endoscopic inspection of the duodenum prior to ductal cannulation can reveal evidence of the tumor in the form of gelatinous material protruding from a dilated ductal orifice. Injection of contrast material into the pancreatic duct usually demonstrates ductal dilatation (Figure 20-14A), which can be segmental or generalized. Uncalcified filling defects within the opacified duct, representing either globular collections of mucin or excrescences of tumor, are characteristic findings **(Option (E) is true).** Mucinous globules are sometimes demon-

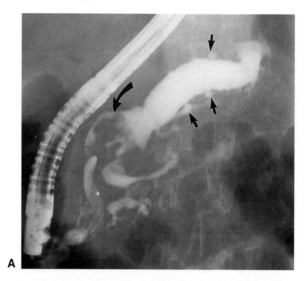

A

Figure 20-14. Mucin-hypersecreting tumor of the pancreatic duct. (A) ERP shows marked dilatation of the main pancreatic duct, which contains a large intraluminal filling defect (curved arrow) representing a collection of mucin. Side branches of the main pancreatic duct are also dilated (small arrows). (B and C) Contrast-enhanced CT images show the mucin-filled, markedly distended main pancreatic duct (arrows) in the head of the pancreas (B) and in the body and tail (C). Most of the surrounding pancreatic parenchyma is severely thinned.

strably mobile within the duct, changing location under fluoroscopic observation or on serial radiographs. Complete retrograde filling of the main pancreatic duct is often blocked by thick mucinous material occupying the ductal lumen. When the disease involves side branches, the affected ducts appear as cystic lesions that communicate with the main pancreatic duct. These can be seen as solitary cavities, a cluster of a few cysts, or multiple separate cystic structures. As in main-duct tumors, filling defects within dilated side-branch ducts represent collections of mucin or nodules of tumor. Internal septations are sometimes seen.

On CT, the dilated mucin-filled ducts are of low density. Parenchyma surrounding the affected duct tends to be thinned to a degree proportional to the degree of ductal dilatation (Figures 20-14 and 20-15A). Papillary excrescences of tumor are sometimes visible as protrusions of tissue within the distended lumen. The features are shown to best advantage on thin-section scans made with intravenous contrast enhancement. The other methods of cross-sectional imaging, ultrasonography and MRI, can also demonstrate morphologic alterations caused by these tumors. Ultrasonography has shown mainly ductal dilatation, and

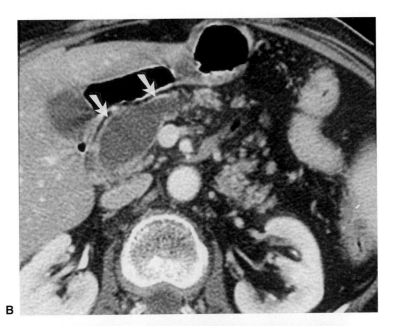

B

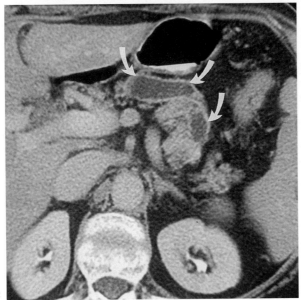

C

MRI, although used infrequently, has demonstrative capabilities similar to those of CT (Figure 20-15B and C). The mucin-filled ducts are hypointense on T1-weighted images (Figure 20-15B) and hyperintense on T2-weighted images (Figure 20-15C).

In the absence of evidence of extrapancreatic metastasis or invasive extrapancreatic extension of tumor, it is not possible by cross-sectional

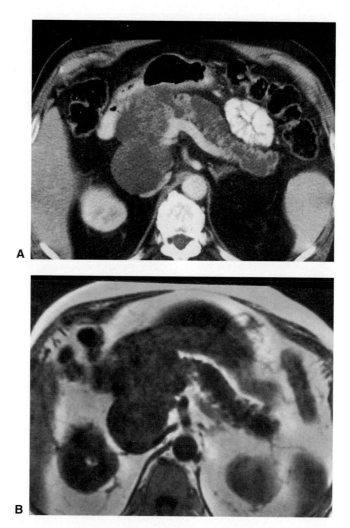

Figure 20-15. Mucin-hypersecreting tumor of the pancreatic duct involving the entire pancreatic duct as well as ductal branches within the pancreatic head. CT (A) and MR (B and C) images show large, rounded, cystic-appearing masses in the pancreatic head and a markedly dilated main pancreatic duct with irregular contours in the body and tail. The mucin-filled ductal structures are of low density on CT (A), low signal intensity on T1-weighted MRI (B), and high signal intensity on T2-weighted MRI (C). Thinning of the surrounding pancreatic parenchyma is pronounced. At resection, papillary portions of the tumor in the pancreatic head were found to be malignant (grade 2 mucin-secreting carcinoma).

imaging to distinguish histologically benign mucin-producing tumors from those with malignant histology. Complete surgical removal is the

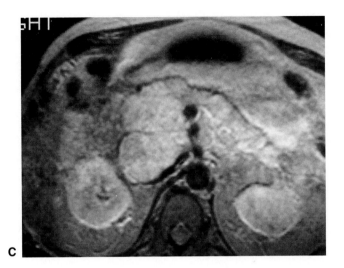

c

preferred treatment for all mucin-hypersecreting tumors of the pancreatic duct, so such a distinction is of little clinical relevance. In that regard, as in other respects, these tumors are similar to classic mucinous cystic neoplasms of the pancreas.

David H. Stephens, M.D.

SUGGESTED READINGS

SEROUS CYSTADENOMA (MICROCYSTIC ADENOMA)

1. Bennett GL, Chew FS. Serous cystadenoma of the pancreas. AJR 1993; 161:786
2. Buck JL, Hayes WS. From the archives of the AFIP. Microcystic adenoma of the pancreas. RadioGraphics 1990; 10:313–322
3. Compagno J, Oertel JE. Microcystic adenomas of the pancreas (glycogen-rich cystadenomas): a clinicopathologic study of 34 cases. Am J Clin Pathol 1978; 69:289–298
4. George DH, Murphy F, Michalski R, Ulmer BG. Serous cystadenocarcinoma of the pancreas: a new entity? Am J Surg Pathol 1989; 13:61–66
5. Hodgkinson DJ, ReMine WH, Weiland LH. Pancreatic cystadenoma. A clinicopathologic study of 45 cases. Arch Surg 1978; 113:512–519
6. Itai Y, Ohhashi K, Furui S, et al. Microcystic adenoma of the pancreas: spectrum of computed tomographic findings. J Comput Assist Tomogr 1988; 12:797–803

7. Kamei K, Funabiki T, Ochiai M, Amano H, Kasahara M, Sakamoto T. Multifocal pancreatic serous cystadenoma with atypical cells and focal perineural invasion. Int J Pancreatol 1991; 10:161–172

8. Lewandrowski K, Warshaw A, Compton C. Macrocystic serous cystadenoma of the pancreas: a morphologic variant differing from microcystic adenoma. Human Pathol 1992; 23:871–875

9. Nodell CG, Freeny PC, Dale DH, Ryan JA. Serous cystadenoma of the pancreas with a metachronous adenocarcinoma. AJR 1994; 162:1352–1354

10. Posniak HV, Olson MC, Demos TC. Coexistent adenocarcinoma and microcystic adenoma of the pancreas. Clin Imaging 1991; 15:220–222

11. Pyke CM, van Heerden JA, Colby TV, Sarr MG, Weaver AL. The spectrum of serous cystadenoma of the pancreas. Clinical, pathologic, and surgical aspects. Ann Surg 1992; 215:132–139

12. Rubin GD, Jeffrey RB Jr, Walter JF. Pancreatic microcystic adenoma presenting with acute hemoperitoneum: CT diagnosis. AJR 1991; 156:749–750

13. Zirinsky K, Abiri M, Baer JW. Computed tomography demonstration of pancreatic microcystic adenoma. Am J Gastroenterol 1984; 79:139–142

MUCINOUS CYSTIC NEOPLASMS

14. Compagno J, Oertel JE. Mucinous cystic neoplasms of the pancreas with overt and latent malignancy (cystadenocarcinoma and cystadenoma). A clinicopathologic study of 41 cases. Am J Clin Pathol 1978; 69:573–580

CYSTIC NEOPLASMS OF THE PANCREAS

15. Friedman AC, Lichtenstein JE, Dachman AH. Cystic neoplasms of the pancreas. Radiological-pathological correlation. Radiology 1983; 149:45–50

16. Fugazzola C, Procacci C, Bergamo Andreis IA, et al. Cystic tumors of the pancreas: evaluation by ultrasonography and computed tomography. Gastrointest Radiol 1991; 16:53–61

17. Johnson CD, Stephens DH, Charboneau JW, Carpenter HA, Welch TJ. Cystic pancreatic tumors: CT and sonographic assessment. AJR 1988; 151:1133–1138

18. Lewandrowski KB, Southern JF, Pins MR, Compton C, Warshaw A. Cyst fluid analysis in the differential diagnosis of pancreatic cysts. A comparison of pseudocysts, serous cystadenomas, mucinous cystic neoplasms, and mucinous cystadenocarcinoma. Ann Surg 1993; 217:41–47

19. Mathieu D, Guigui B, Valette PJ, et al. Pancreatic cystic neoplasms. Radiol Clin North Am 1989; 27:163–176

20. Minami M, Itai Y, Ohtomo K, Yoshida H, Yoshikawa K, Iio M. Cystic neoplasms of the pancreas: comparison of MR imaging with CT. Radiology 1989; 171:53–56

21. Ros PR, Hamrick-Turner JE, Chiechi MV, Ros LH, Gallego P, Burton SS. Cystic masses of the pancreas. RadioGraphics 1992; 12:673–686

22. Warshaw AL, Compton CC, Lewandrowski K, Cardenosa G, Mueller PR. Cystic tumors of the pancreas. New clinical, radiologic, and pathologic observations in 67 patients. Ann Surg 1990; 212:432–445

SOLID AND PAPILLARY EPITHELIAL NEOPLASM

23. Balthazar EJ, Subramanyam BR, Lefleur RS, Barone CM. Solid and papillary epithelial neoplasm of the pancreas. Radiographic, CT, sonographic, and angiographic features. Radiology 1984; 150:39–40
24. Choi BI, Kim KW, Han MC, Kim YI, Kim CW. Solid and papillary epithelial neoplasms of the pancreas: CT findings. Radiology 1988; 166:413–416
25. Farman J, Chen CK, Schulze G, Teitcher J. Solid and papillary epithelial pancreatic neoplasm: an unusual tumor. Gastrointest Radiol 1987; 12:31–34
26. Friedman AC, Lichtenstein JE, Fishman EK, Oertel JE, Dachman AH, Siegelman SS. Solid and papillary epithelial neoplasm of the pancreas. Radiology 1985; 154:333–337
27. Hamoudi AB, Misugi K, Grosfeld JL, Reiner CB. Papillary epithelial neoplasm of pancreas in a child. Report of a case with electron microscopy. Cancer 1970; 26:1126–1134
28. Kim SY, Lim JH, Lee JD. Papillary carcinoma of the pancreas: findings of US and CT. Radiology 1985; 154:338
29. Ohtomo K, Furui S, Onoue M, et al. Solid and papillary epithelial neoplasm of the pancreas: MR imaging and pathologic correlation. Radiology 1992; 184:567–570
30. Phillips GW, Chou ST, Mulhauser J. Papillary cystic tumour of the pancreas: findings at computed tomography and ultrasound. Br J Radiol 1991; 64:367–369

MUCIN-HYPERSECRETING TUMOR OF THE PANCREATIC DUCT

31. Agostini S, Choux R, Payan MJ, Sastre B, Sahel J, Clement JP. Mucinous pancreatic duct ectasia in the body of the pancreas. Radiology 1989; 170:815–816
32. Furukawa T, Takahashi T, Kobari M, Matsuno S. The mucus-hypersecreting tumor of the pancreas. Development and extension visualized by three-dimensional computerized mapping. Cancer 1992; 70:1505–1513
33. Itai Y, Kokubo T, Atomi Y, Kuroda A, Haraguchi Y, Terano A. Mucin-hypersecreting carcinoma of the pancreas. Radiology 1987; 165:51–55
34. Itai Y, Ohhashi K, Nagai H, et al. Ductectatic mucinous cystadenoma and cystadenocarcinoma of the pancreas. Radiology 1986; 161:697–700
35. Itoh S, Ishiguchi T, Ishigaki T, Sakuma S, Maruyama K, Senda K. Mucin-producing pancreatic tumor: CT findings and histopathologic correlation. Radiology 1992; 183:81–68
36. Kawarada Y, Yano T, Yamamoto T, et al. Intraductal mucin-producing tumors of the pancreas. Am J Gastroenterol 1992; 87:634–638
37. Lee MG, Auh YH, Cho KS, Chung YH, Han DJ, Yu ES. Mucinous ductal ectasia of the pancreas: MRI. J Comput Assist Tomogr 1992; 16:495–496

38. Obara T, Saitoh Y, Maguchi H, et al. Papillary adenoma of the pancreas with excessive mucin secretion. Pancreas 1992; 7:114–117

39. Ohta T, Nagakawa T, Akiyama T, et al. The duct-ectatic variant of mucinous cystic neoplasms of the pancreas: clinical and radiologic studies of seven cases. Am J Gastroenterol 1992; 87:300–304

40. Rattner DW, Pins MR. Case records of the Massachusetts General Hospital: Case 23–1994. N Engl J Med 1994; 330:1671–1676

41. Rickaert F, Cremer M, Deviere J, et al. Intraductal mucin-hypersecreting neoplasms of the pancreas. A clinicopathologic study of eight patients. Gastroenterology 1991; 101:512–519

42. Tian FZ, Myles J, Howard JM. Mucinous pancreatic ductal ectasia of latent malignancy: an emerging clinicopathologic entity. Surgery 1992; 111:109–113

43. Yamada M, Kozuka S, Yamao K, Nakazawa S, Naitoh Y, Tsukamoto Y. Mucin-producing tumors of the pancreas. Cancer 1991; 68:159–168

PANCREATIC LESIONS IN VON HIPPEL-LINDAU DISEASE

44. Binkovitz LA, Johnson CD, Stephens DH. Islet cell tumors in von Hippel-Lindau disease: increased prevalence and relationship to the multiple endocrine neoplasias. AJR 1990; 155:501–505

45. Hough DM, Stephens DH, Johnson CD, Binkovitz LA. Pancreatic lesions in von Hippel-Lindau disease: prevalence, clinical significance, and CT findings. AJR 1994; 162:1091–1094

Notes

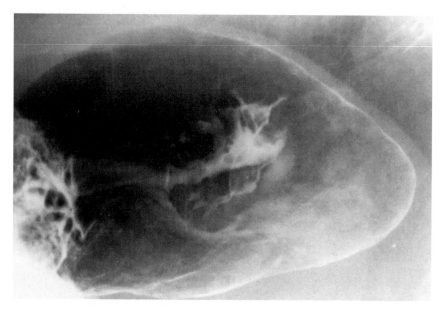

Figure 21-1. This 60-year-old man has dysphagia and heme-positive stools. You are shown a radiograph from an upper gastrointestinal examination.

Case 21: Carcinoma of the Cardia

Question 64

Which *one* of the following is the MOST likely diagnosis?

(A) Lymphoma
(B) Varices
(C) Carcinoma of the cardia
(D) Metastatic squamous cell carcinoma
(E) Benign gastric ulcer

A double-contrast radiograph of the gastric fundus with the patient in a right lateral recumbent position (Figure 21-1) shows an ulcerated mass in the fundus that has obliterated the normal anatomic landmarks at the cardia (Figure 21-2). These findings are characteristic of a malignant lesion at the cardia. The major diagnostic considerations include a carcinoma of the gastric cardia or an esophageal adenocarcinoma arising in Barrett's mucosa that has invaded the gastric cardia. However, Barrett's carcinoma is not listed as an option. Thus, carcinoma of the cardia is the most likely diagnosis **(Option (C) is correct).**

Tumors arising at the cardia are notoriously difficult to detect on single-contrast barium studies. The overlying rib cage precludes manual palpation or compression of the fundus, and so even large lesions can be obscured by relatively opaque barium that prevents adequate visualization of this region. With the double-contrast technique, however, it is possible to evaluate the normal anatomic landmarks at the cardia for signs of malignancy. As a result, double-contrast barium studies can detect lesions at the cardia that are missed on single-contrast examinations.

When viewed *en face*, the normal cardia is often recognized on double-contrast studies by the presence of four or five stellate folds that radiate to a central point at the gastroesophageal junction (the cardiac rosette) (Figure 21-3). Some malignant tumors at the cardia can be recognized only by relatively subtle nodularity, mass effect, or ulceration in this region with distortion or obliteration of these landmarks (Figures

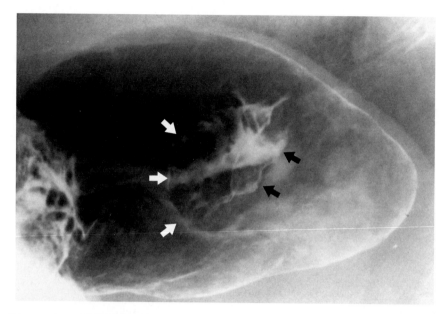

Figure 21-2 (Same as Figure 21-1).   Carcinoma of the cardia. The normal anatomic landmarks at the cardia have been obliterated and replaced by an irregular mass (white arrows) containing several areas of ulceration (black arrows). The normal cardia is shown in Figure 21-3 for comparison.

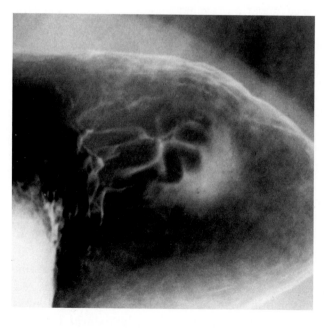

Figure 21-3 (left). Normal cardia. The gastric cardia is recognized by the presence of four or five stellate folds that radiate to a central point at the gastroesophageal junction; this structure is also known as the cardiac rosette. These normal anatomic landmarks can be distorted or obliterated by tumor at the cardia, as in Figures 21-1 and 21-4.

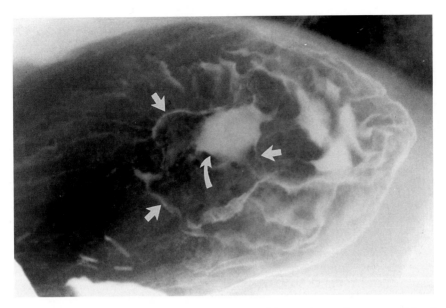

Figure 21-4. Carcinoma of the cardia. In this patient, the normal landmarks at the cardia have been replaced by a plaquelike lesion that is etched in white (straight arrows). Note that this lesion contains a large area of central ulceration (curved arrow). (Reprinted with permission from Gore RM, Levine MS, Laufer I [eds]. Textbook of gastrointestinal radiology. Philadelphia: WB Saunders; 1994.)

21-1 and 21-4). When a malignant lesion at the gastric cardia is suspected, endoscopy should be performed for a definitive diagnosis. However, radiographically demonstrated lesions at the cardia are occasionally missed at endoscopy. The barium study should therefore be repeated after a negative endoscopic examination if the initial study suggests a malignant lesion. Rarely, some patients with continuing radiologic evidence of malignancy require surgery without preoperative histologic confirmation.

Advanced carcinomas of the gastric cardia or fundus are usually exophytic or infiltrating lesions. Exophytic tumors appear as bulky, lobulated intraluminal masses in the gastric fundus and often contain irregular areas of ulceration. In contrast, infiltrating lesions are usually manifested by thickened folds and decreased distensibility of the fundus. Eventually, advanced tumors can encase the fundus, producing a linitis plastica appearance with a small, irregular residual lumen.

Gastric lymphoma (Option (A)) is manifested by infiltrative, ulcerative, nodular, or polypoid lesions. Infiltrative gastric lymphomas are characterized by focal or diffuse enlargement of rugal folds as a result of

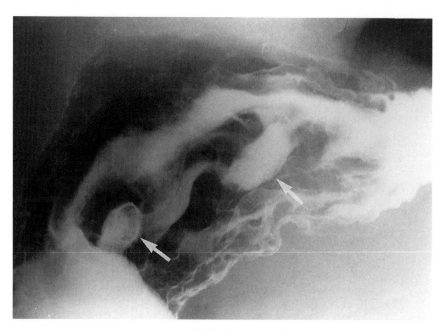

Figure 21-5. Gastric lymphoma. Several discrete ulcers (arrows) are seen in the fundus. There also are thickened, lobulated folds in the adjacent stomach. (Reprinted with permission from Gore RM, Levine MS, Laufer I [eds]. Textbook of gastrointestinal radiology.)

submucosal spread of tumor. Ulcerative lymphomas are characterized by one or more ulcerated lesions in the stomach (Figure 21-5). The nodular form of gastric lymphoma is characterized by multiple submucosal nodules or masses ranging from several millimeters to several centimeters in size. These submucosal masses often undergo central necrosis and ulceration, resulting in typical bull's-eye or target lesions. Occasionally, gastric lymphoma is manifested by polypoid lesions, appearing as lobulated intraluminal masses that are indistinguishable from polypoid carcinomas. The ulcerated mass lesion at the cardia in Figure 21-1 could conceivably represent gastric lymphoma; however, this patient is more likely to have gastric carcinoma, a much more common malignant neoplasm in the stomach.

Gastric varices (Option (B)) are usually manifested radiographically by a cluster of discrete submucosal defects in the gastric fundus that have been likened to the appearance of a bunch of grapes (Figure 21-6). Gastric varices that are associated with esophageal varices are usually caused by portal hypertension, whereas isolated gastric varices can be caused by either portal hypertension or splenic vein obstruction. Occa-

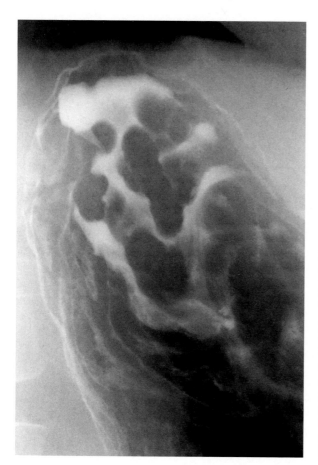

Figure 21-6. Gastric varices. Multiple large submucosal defects are present in the gastric fundus in a patient with portal hypertension. The radiographic findings are characteristic of gastric varices. This patient also had esophageal varices. (Reprinted with permission from Levine [8].)

sionally, a conglomerate of varices in the region of the gastric cardia is manifested by a polypoid mass that could be mistaken radiographically for a gastric carcinoma or even a gastric leiomyosarcoma. However, the lesion at the cardia in Figure 21-1 contains areas of irregular ulceration, so varices would not be likely.

Squamous cell carcinoma of the esophagus or pharynx occasionally metastasizes to the gastric cardia or fundus. These metastases (Option (D)) typically appear as smooth submucosal masses, often containing central areas of ulceration (Figure 21-7). The lesion illustrated in Figure 21-1 therefore does not have the typical appearance of a squamous cell carcinoma metastasis to the cardia.

More than 90% of benign gastric ulcers (Option (E)) are located in the gastric antrum or body. Benign ulcers are rarely found in the region of the gastric cardia. Furthermore, the ulcerated mass lesion seen at the cardia in Figure 21-1 does not have the radiographic features of a benign

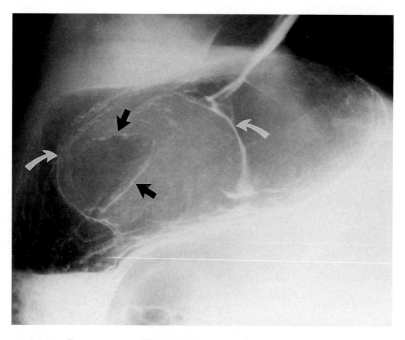

Figure 21-7. Squamous cell carcinoma metastasis to the cardia. There is a giant submucosal mass (white arrows) in the gastric fundus, containing a triangular area of central ulceration (black arrows). Although a leiomyoma or leiomyosarcoma could produce similar findings, this patient had a squamous cell carcinoma of the esophagus that had metastasized to the cardia. (Reprinted with permission from Glick et al. [22].)

gastric ulcer. Benign gastric ulcers classically appear as round or ovoid ulcer craters with a smooth surrounding mound of edema and/or regular, symmetric folds that radiate directly to the edge of the crater. None of these features is present in the test image.

Question 65

Concerning carcinoma arising at the cardia,

    (A) it makes up less than 10% of all gastric cancers
    (B) it is more common in men than in women
    (C) at surgery, the esophagus is involved by tumor in less than 10% of patients
    (D) referred dysphagia to the upper esophagus or pharynx is a symptom
    (E) affected individuals have a better prognosis than patients with carcinoma arising in a Barrett's esophagus that invades the gastroesophageal junction

During the past four or five decades there has been a gradual shift in the distribution of gastric cancer proximally from the antrum and body of the stomach to the cardia and fundus, so that carcinomas of the gastric cardia and fundus are now thought to make up between 30 and 40% of all gastric cancers **(Option (A) is false)**. These tumors are more common in men than in women by a ratio of about 7:1 **(Option (B) is true)**. For reasons that are unclear, a small but significant percentage of patients with carcinoma of the cardia are under the age of 40, so that radiologists should not be lulled into a false sense of security about the possibility of malignancy because of the patient's age.

Carcinoma of the cardia has a marked tendency to invade the distal esophagus by contiguous spread of tumor. Esophageal involvement is found at surgery in more than 50% of patients with this disease **(Option (C) is false)**. Whether or not the esophagus is invaded by tumor, carcinoma of the cardia has become an increasingly common cause of dysphagia in the adult population. Some patients complain of food sticking behind the lower sternum, but others have referred dysphagia to the upper esophagus or even the pharynx **(Option (D) is true)**, so that the gastric cardia and fundus should be carefully evaluated radiographically to detect these lesions in all patients with dysphagia.

Carcinoma of the cardia invading the distal esophagus can be indistinguishable radiographically from a primary adenocarcinoma in Barrett's esophagus invading the gastric cardia and fundus. However, cardiac carcinomas often have a disproportionate degree of gastric involvement in relation to that of the esophagus, whereas esophageal adenocarcinomas arising in Barrett's mucosa have a greater degree of esophageal involvement. A significant history of reflux symptoms should also suggest a carcinoma arising in Barrett's esophagus. In any case, these tumors have similar morphologic features in terms of pattern of growth, degree of differentiation, and depth of invasion, so that they have a similar long-term prognosis **(Option (E) is false)**.

Question 66

Concerning gastric metastases from squamous cell carcinoma of the esophagus,

(A) they are found at autopsy in about 50% of patients who die of esophageal carcinoma
(B) they are caused by tumor emboli that seed the gastric fundus via submucosal esophageal lymphatics
(C) they rarely occur in patients with carcinoma of the upper esophagus or midesophagus
(D) barium studies usually demonstrate multiple lesions
(E) they are often indistinguishable from gastric leiomyomas

Between 2 and 15% of patients who die of esophageal cancer have gastric metastases at autopsy **(Option (A) is false).** These metastases are probably caused by tumor emboli that seed the gastric fundus via submucosal esophageal lymphatics extending subdiaphragmatically to the stomach **(Option (B) is true).** This hypothesis is supported by the observation that the primary carcinoma is often located in the upper esophagus or midesophagus **(Option (C) is false)** at a considerable distance from the gastroesophageal junction, with a normal esophageal segment below the lesion.

Squamous cell carcinoma metastases to the stomach are usually manifested radiographically by solitary giant masses involving the gastric cardia and/or fundus **(Option (D) is false).** These lesions typically appear as large submucosal masses, often containing central areas of ulceration; therefore, they can be indistinguishable from ulcerated leiomyomas or leiomyosarcomas (Figure 21-6) **(Option (E) is true).** Less frequently, they are mistaken for primary gastric carcinomas. The appropriate treatment for esophageal cancer depends on the stage of the tumor, and so the gastric cardia and fundus should be carefully examined radiographically in all patients with esophageal cancer to rule out unsuspected metastases to the stomach.

Marc S. Levine, M.D.

SUGGESTED READINGS

CARCINOMA OF THE CARDIA

1. Antonioli DA, Goldman H. Changes in the location and type of gastric adenocarcinoma. Cancer 1982; 50:775–781
2. Balthazar EJ, Goldfine S, Davidian MM. Carcinoma of the esophagogastric junction. Am J Gastroenterol 1980; 74:237–243

3. Cady B, Rossi RL, Silverman ML, Piccione W, Heck TA. Gastric adenocarcinoma: a disease in transition. Arch Surg 1989; 124:303–308

4. Freeny PC. Double-contrast gastrography of the fundus and cardia: normal landmarks and their pathologic changes. AJR 1979; 133:481–487

5. Freeny PC, Marks WM. Adenocarcinoma of the gastroesophageal junction: barium and CT examination. AJR 1982; 138:1077–1084

6. Herlinger H, Grossman R, Laufer I, Kressel HY, Ochs RH. The gastric cardia in double-contrast study: its dynamic image. AJR 1980; 135:21–29

7. Kalish RJ, Clancy PE, Orringer MB, Appelman HD. Clinical, epidemiologic, and morphologic comparison between adenocarcinomas arising in Barrett's esophageal mucosa and in the gastric cardia. Gastroenterology 1984; 86:461–467

8. Levine MS. Gastroesophageal junction. In: Levine MS (ed), Radiology of the esophagus. Philadelphia: WB Saunders; 1989:247–265

9. Levine MS, Caroline D, Thompson JJ, Kressel HY, Laufer I, Herlinger H. Adenocarcinoma of the esophagus: relationship to Barrett mucosa. Radiology 1984; 150:305–309

10. Levine MS, Laufer I, Thompson JJ. Carcinoma of the gastric cardia in young people. AJR 1983; 140:69–72

11. Milnes JP, Hine KR, Holmes GK, Cohen ME. Limitations of endoscopy in the diagnosis of carcinoma of the cardia of the stomach. Br J Radiol 1982; 55:593–595

GASTRIC LYMPHOMA

12. Fork FT, Ekberg O, Haglund U. Radiology in primary gastric lymphoma. Acta Radiol [Diagn] (Stockh) 1984; 25:481–488

13. Hricak H, Thoeni RF, Margulis AR, Eyler WR, Francis IR. Extension of gastric lymphoma into the esophagus and duodenum. Radiology 1980; 135:309–312

14. Menuck LS. Gastric lymphoma, a radiologic diagnosis. Gastrointest Radiol 1976; 1:157–161

15. Zornoza J, Dodd GD. Lymphoma of the gastrointestinal tract. Semin Roentgenol 1980; 15:272–287

GASTRIC VARICES

16. Anderson MF, Dunnick NR. Pseudotumor caused by gastric varices. Am J Dig Dis 1977; 22:929–932

17. Kaye JJ, Stassa G. Mimicry and deception in the diagnosis of tumors of the gastric cardia. AJR 1970; 110:295–303

18. Levine MS, Kieu K, Rubesin SE, Herlinger H, Laufer I. Isolated gastric varices: splenic vein obstruction or portal hypertension? Gastrointest Radiol 1990; 15:188–192

19. Muhletaler C, Gerlock AJ Jr, Goncharenko V, Avant GR, Flexner JM. Gastric varices secondary to splenic vein occlusion: radiographic diagnosis and clinical significance. Radiology 1979; 132:593–598

20. Rice RP, Thompson WM, Kelvin FM, Kriner AF, Garbutt JT. Gastric varices without esophageal varices. An important preendoscopic diagnosis. JAMA 1977; 237:1976–1979

SQUAMOUS CELL CARCINOMA METASTASES TO THE CARDIA

21. Allen HA, Bush JE. Midesophageal carcinoma metastatic to the stomach: its unusual appearance on an upper gastrointestinal series. South Med J 1983; 76:1049–1051
22. Glick SN, Teplick SK, Levine MS. Squamous cell metastases to the gastric cardia. Gastrointest Radiol 1985; 10:339–344
23. Glick SN, Teplick SK, Levine MS, Caroline DF. Gastric cardia metastasis in esophageal carcinoma. Radiology 1986; 160:627–630

BENIGN GASTRIC ULCER

24. Gelfand DW, Dale WJ, Ott DJ. The location and size of gastric ulcers: radiologic and endoscopic evaluation. AJR 1984; 143:755–758
25. Levine MS, Creteur V, Kressel HY, Laufer I, Herlinger H. Benign gastric ulcers: diagnosis and follow-up with double-contrast radiography. Radiology 1987; 164:9–13
26. Thompson G, Stevenson GW, Somers S. Distribution of gastric ulcers by double-contrast barium meal with endoscopic correlation. J Can Assoc Radiol 1983; 34:296–297

Notes

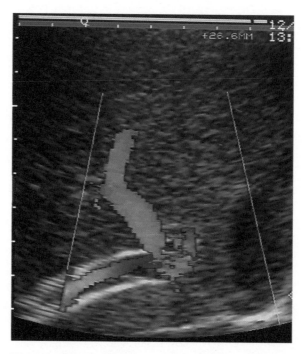

Figure 22-1. This 48-year-old man with idiopathic cirrhosis underwent a transjugular intrahepatic portosystemic shunt (TIPS) procedure for intractable variceal bleeding 6 months ago. You are shown a color Doppler sonogram performed as a routine follow-up study to evaluate the shunt.

Case 22: Transjugular Intrahepatic Portosystemic Shunt

Question 67

Concerning this patient,

(A) flow within the shunt is in the normal direction
(B) the direction of flow in the portal vein branches suggests shunt malfunction
(C) there is evidence of pseudointimal hyperplasia within the shunt
(D) the patient is at risk for recurrent variceal bleeding

Figure 22-1 was obtained during a color-flow Doppler ultrasound examination of a patient in whom a transjugular intrahepatic portosystemic shunt (TIPS) had been placed 6 months earlier. The highly echogenic metallic fibers making up the wall of the stent are easily visible (Figure 22-2). Flow within the shunt lumen is in the expected direction (color-coded blue, or away from the transducer), carrying portal venous blood posteriorly into the distal portion of the right hepatic vein, near the inferior vena cava **(Option (A) is true)**.

With a normally functioning stent, flow within major portal vein branches is usually directed toward the shunt. In the test patient, flow within the right portal vein is color-coded red, indicating that it is in the direction of the transducer (hepatopedal) and away from the shunt (Figure 22-3). This reversal of portal venous flow has been shown to be a sign of shunt malfunction **(Option (B) is true)**.

Additionally, there is a layer of intermediately echogenic material on the posterior wall of the shunt that continues throughout its observed length. Pathologically, this represents pseudointimal hyperplasia **(Option (C) is true)** and is the likely cause of the increased resistance to flow within the shunt (Figure 22-4). Multiple studies have shown that shunt obstruction (occlusion or stenosis) is directly related to recurrence of variceal bleeding **(Option (D) is true)**. A portal venogram can confirm the presence of shunt stenosis and provide a road map for repair (Figure 22-5).

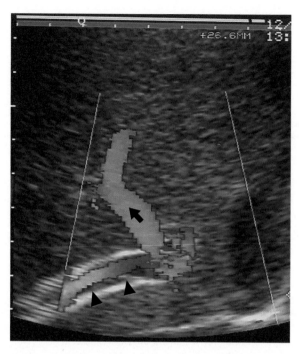

Figure 22-2 (Same as Figure 22-1). Pseudointimal hyperplasia within a transjugular intrahepatic portosystemic shunt (TIPS). A color Doppler sonogram shows moderate narrowing of the luminal diameter within the TIPS (arrowheads). Also note antegrade flow within the adjacent portal vein (arrow) in this patient who previously had retrograde portal venous flow direction.

Hemorrhage from esophageal varices that occur due to portal hypertension is a serious medical problem; the mortality during the first bleeding episode approaches 80%, and up to 80% of those surviving will bleed again. There have been two major therapeutic methods to halt the initial bleeding. Endoscopic sclerotherapy has recently been used and is almost always effective in arresting acute variceal hemorrhage. However, in up to 20% of cases, there are procedural complications, such as esophageal perforation, mediastinitis, and aspiration. The other major alternative is the creation of a portosystemic shunt (until the introduction of TIPS, this was a surgical shunt). This surgical procedure is effective in preventing rebleeding episodes but has a high perioperative mortality.

Accordingly, efforts to develop other therapeutic alternatives continued. In 1969, Rösch performed the first intrahepatic portocaval shunt via a percutaneous approach in a swine model. In 1982, Colapinto successfully performed intrahepatic portocaval shunting in 15 patients with

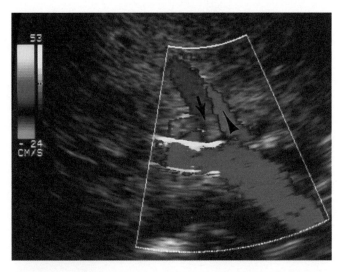

Figure 22-3. Normal functioning TIPS stent. A color Doppler sonogram of the junction between the stent and the main right portal vein reveals reversal of flow (arrow identifies flow direction) within the portal vein distal to the stent. The flow in the stent is from portal vein to hepatic vein. Note the antegrade flow within the adjacent right hepatic artery (arrowhead).

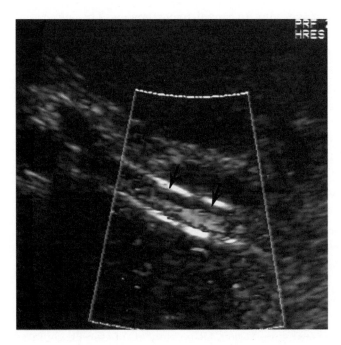

Figure 22-4 (left). Pseudointimal hyperplasia. A longitudinal color Doppler sonogram of a TIPS stent shows moderate narrowing (arrows) of the patent lumen throughout the length of the stent.

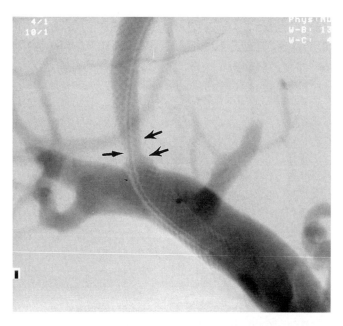

Figure 22-5. Pseudointimal hyperplasia. A digital subtraction venogram of a TIPS stent demonstrates the presence of luminal narrowing (arrows) due to pseudointimal hyperplasia.

severe variceal hemorrhage due to portal hypertension. The success of this procedure was limited by the absence of a permanent conduit and incomplete decompression of portal venous pressure, so that rebleeding was common.

Palmaz and colleagues were the first to effectively maintain patency of the intrahepatic parenchymal shunt in a series of dogs by implanting expandable shunts. The Palmaz stent was first placed in a human by Richter in 1988. Since that time, a number of centers have developed a large clinical experience. It has been established that the TIPS procedure is a relatively safe method of achieving portal decompression; its clinical value relative to alternative therapies for variceal hemorrhage is still under study.

The high technical success rate and low morbidity of the TIPS procedure have led to broadening of the indications for its use. Initially, the TIPS procedure was used only for therapy of recurrent variceal hemorrhage in the group with the highest surgical mortality (Child's class C) (Table 22-1). As more experience was gained, some patients with Child's class A or B portal hypertension underwent TIPS placement, some in anticipation of hepatic transplantation. Other indications for TIPS placement currently under study are treatment of refractory ascites, decom-

Table 22-1: Child's-Pugh classification of severity of liver disease[a]

Clinical and biochemical measurements	Points scored for increasing abnormality		
	1	2	3
Encephalopathy (grade)	None	1 and 2	3 and 4
Ascites	Absent	Slight	Moderate
Bilirubin (mg/100 mL)	1 to 2	2 to 3	>3
Albumin (g/100 mL)	3.5	2.8 to 3.5	<2.8
Prothrombin time (sec. prolonged)	1 to 4	4 to 6	>6

Class:
  A: 5 to 6 total points
  B: 7 to 9 total points
  C: ≥10 total points

[a] Adapted with permission from Pugh RN, Murray-Lyon IM, Dawson JL, Pietroni MC, Williams R. Transection of the oesophagus for bleeding oesophageal varices. Br J Surg 1973; 60:646–649.

pression of intestinal varices, and as a primary treatment for hepatorenal syndrome.

The typical candidate for a TIPS procedure has known portal hypertension and is actively bleeding from the upper gastrointestinal tract. Since other causes of bleeding are possible, patients should undergo endoscopy to verify that varices are, in fact, the source of bleeding. Doppler sonography is obtained to confirm that the portal vein is patent.

Puncture of the jugular vein is employed to avoid the complications inherent in transhepatic puncture of a cirrhotic patient with coagulopathy. Zemel et al. have artfully described and illustrated the technical aspects of TIPS placement. A sheath (typically 9 or 10 French diameter) is placed in the right internal jugular vein, and all subsequent catheter manipulations are performed through the sheath. A hepatic venogram is then performed to identify an appropriate systemic vein candidate and to ensure that no significant anomaly exists. The selected vein is then cannulated, and the catheter is replaced over a guidewire with a long 16-gauge Colapinto needle. After removal of the guidewire, an appropriate hepatic venous puncture site (usually about 2 cm proximal to the junction of the hepatic vein with the inferior vena cava) is chosen. The needle is then passed through the hepatic parenchyma in the direction of the right portal vein. Successful cannulation is documented by injection of intravenous contrast material. Once the portal vein is punctured, a guidewire is passed into the portal vein and a catheter is advanced over it through the parenchymal tract. Baseline mean pressure measurements are obtained in the portal vein and within the suprahepatic inferior vena cava to determine the pressure gradient. The tract is then dilated with a low-profile balloon catheter 8 to 10 mm in diameter. An implantable intravascular stent is placed across the parenchymal tract, and repeat pressure measurements are obtained to verify reduction in the portosystemic gradient. A splenoportogram is then performed to determine whether there is persistent variceal opacification. If varices fill despite reduction of the portosystemic gradient below 12 mm Hg, they can be electively embolized at this point.

Despite the apparent hazards in performing interventional procedures in patients with (often marked) coagulopathy, the TIPS procedure has a high technical success rate (average 97%) and a low procedural morbidity (average 7%). The relatively "blind" nature of the needle puncture is associated with penetration of the liver capsule or with laceration of the hepatic artery or biliary branches. Many of the reported short- or midterm complications also occur in surgically shunted patients; hepatic decompensation, encephalopathy, and acute congestive heart failure due to central venous fluid overload are examples.

Ultimate evaluation of the clinical merit of the TIPS procedure in patients not selected for hepatic transplantation will depend on the frequency of long-term complications and on its 5-year survival rate compared with that of standard surgical treatment. The major midterm complications encountered thus far have been related to stenosis or occlusion of the conduit. Haskal et al. defined the term "shunt stenosis" as "... a reduction in shunt diameter that results in either recurrent symptoms and/or venographic evidence of variceal filling and elevation of the portosystemic gradient beyond 15 mm Hg." Using this functional definition, they found the frequency of shunt stenosis to be 25% at 6 months, 50% at 1 year, and 68% at 2 years. Stenosis can occur within either the shunt or the hepatic vein and is the result of pseudointimal hyperplasia. Pseudointimal hyperplasia represents growth of collagenous tissue deep to the endothelial surface of the lumen of the vein or the shunt and occurs to a varying degree after every TIPS procedure. Close monitoring is therefore mandatory to detect hemodynamic alterations within the shunt before recurrent variceal hemorrhage or complete shunt occlusion occurs.

Color flow and duplex Doppler sonography have been effectively utilized as noninvasive means to detect blood-flow changes suggesting functional shunt stenosis. Despite the metallic nature of the shunt material, sonography is capable of depicting the lumen of the shunt without significant ringdown artifact. Some low-level echoes within the shunt lumen are frequently evident on gray-scale images, however, and are difficult to differentiate from pseudointimal hyperplasia.

In a normally functioning TIPS, there is high-velocity (100 to 200 cm/second) intraluminal flow in the direction of the hepatic vein. Resistance to flow in the hepatic sinusoids is greater than the resistance to flow in the shunt. Thus, reversal of flow is identified within the intrahepatic branches of the portal system and there is a marked increase in hepatopedal flow velocity (10 to 70 cm/second) within the main portal vein compared with the velocity before TIPS placement. Doppler sonography of the portal veins, hepatic veins, and hepatic arteries is normally obtained as a baseline the day after the shunt placement. Current practice recommends follow-up sonographic evaluation at 3- to 6-month intervals in the first year and 6- to 9-month intervals thereafter. Documentation of the absence of flow within the shunt is compelling evidence of shunt occlusion. Shunt or hepatic vein stenosis is suggested by (1) a decrease in flow velocity within the proximal (portal venous side) of the shunt, often associated with focally increased flow velocity in the region of shunt stenosis; (2) a restoration of hepatopedal flow within intrahepatic portal vein branches; and (3) reversal of flow in the hepatic vein draining the stent. Observation of any of these sonographic findings should prompt a venogram, with dilation of areas of stenosis or insertion of additional TIPS shunts performed as indicated.

Question 68

Concerning Doppler sonography of the portal vein,

- (A) the normal waveform is triphasic in nature
- (B) flow reversal is an early sign of portal hypertension
- (C) a hepatic mass is a cause of focal flow reversal
- (D) flow within intrahepatic branches adjacent to the shunt is reversed (hepatofugal) after TIPS placement
- (E) flow velocity in the main portal vein is expected to increase after a successful TIPS procedure

Many investigators have shown Doppler sonography to be an efficient method to evaluate a variety of vascular structures, including the major hepatic vessels. In normal subjects, the portal venous system supplies approximately 75% of total hepatic blood flow. The main portal vein and branches have a monophasic waveform **(Option (A) is false)** that is slightly pulsatile or undulating and courses toward the liver (hepatope-

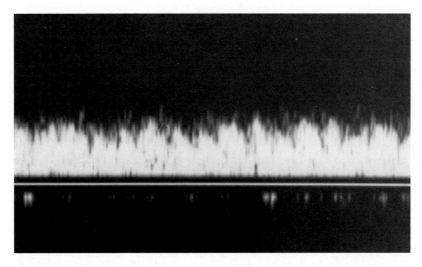

Figure 22-6. Normal portal vein. A duplex Doppler interrogation of the main portal vein reveals a mildly pulsatile portal venous waveform; the signal is registered above the baseline, indicating that flow is in a hepatopedal direction.

dal) at approximately 15 to 20 cm/second (Figure 22-6) rather than away from the liver (hepatofugal). Minimal variations in portal vein velocity on duplex Doppler sonography are noted during breathholding. These phase-related variations are due to transmitted right atrial pressure changes that occur throughout the cardiac cycle. These transmitted cardiac pulsations have largely been dampened by the intervening hepatic parenchyma.

The suprahepatic inferior vena cava and hepatic vein waveforms reflect right atrial pressure changes and therefore manifest a triphasic waveform. In patients with significantly elevated right atrial pressures secondary to congestive heart failure with or without subsequent tricuspid regurgitation, the portal vein can also display triphasic pulsatility similar to that of the hepatic veins. This is due to increased transmission of cardiac pulsations (Figure 22-7). The hepatic artery supplies the remainder of the blood volume to the liver. The resistance to arterial flow is minimal, as in other intra-abdominal organs such as the spleen or kidney. Duplex Doppler waveforms show high diastolic flow with broad systolic peaks. Mild portal hypertension caused by hepatic cirrhosis allows normal velocity portal venous flow and maintenance of its hepatopedal flow direction **(Option (B) is false).** However, in the late stages of disease, hepatic fibrosis significantly increases the resistance to

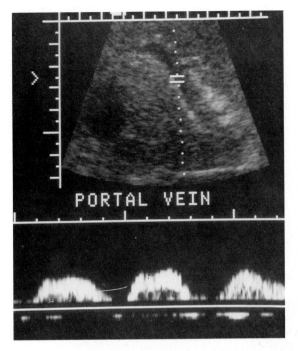

PORTAL VEIN

Figure 22-7. Pulsatile portal venous waveform secondary to congestive hepatopathy. A longitudinal view of the main portal vein reveals prominent portal vein pulsatility. A portion of the Doppler signal is registered below the baseline, indicating that flow is in the hepatofugal direction.

hepatic arterial and portal venous flow. The portal venous velocity therefore decreases and the flow direction can even reverse when the disease is severe.

Focal variations in portal venous waveform, velocity, and direction can occur and are often related to portal hypertension. Reversal of flow in certain vessels appears to be associated with specific collaterals. Reversal to a hepatofugal direction in the right portal vein is commonly identified in patients with enlarged paraumbilical veins. In fact, bidirectional hepatopedal and hepatofugal portal vein flow can be seen in patients with marked portal hypertension as a prelude to frank flow reversal. Isolated left portal vein reversal can be seen in patients with flow reversal in the coronary (left gastric) vein. Splenic vein reversal occurs in patients with splenorenal collaterals or surgically placed shunts.

Miller et al. have observed that the presence of an intrahepatic mass lesion can also produce flow reversal in the portal vein adjacent to the mass. The mass presumably alters pressure gradients within the liver relating to the extrinsic pressure of the mass on the portal vein (Figure 22-8) **(Option (C) is true).** A finding with the same etiology has been observed for some time on contrast-enhanced CT. Several investigators have described transient hepatic attenuation differences (see Case 26) in segments of the liver that contain mass lesions. The presence of

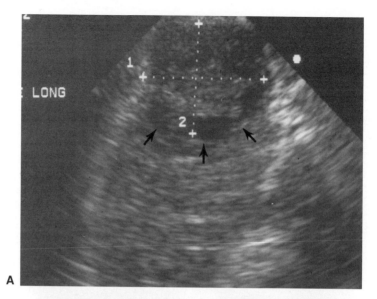

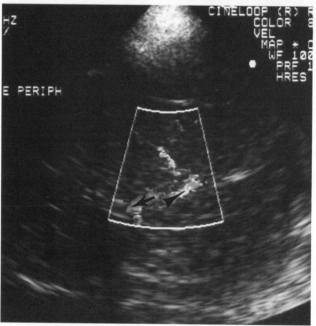

Figure 22-8. Focal portal vein flow reversal. (A) A gray-scale sonogram of the left hepatic lobe shows a complex, predominantly hypoechoic mass (arrows) in the subcapsular region consistent with a hematoma. (B) Duplex Doppler insonation displays flow reversal within the peripheral left portal vein (arrow shows flow direction) near the subcapsular hematoma. All other portal veins, including the proximal left portal vein, show normal hepatopedal flow direction. The adjacent left hepatic artery shows antegrade flow (arrowhead displays flow direction).

increased pressure within a lobe or segment produces shunting of the portal venous blood away from that region. The hepatic arterial flow supplying that segment of liver compensates by increasing.

As noted above, the resistance to venous flow in hepatic sinusoids is higher than flow within the TIPS in patients with portal hypertension. Therefore, TIPS placement generally alters flow (reversing it to hepatofugal) in the intrahepatic branches of the portal veins adjacent to the shunt **(Option (D) is true).** The main portal vein velocity, which is normally between 10 and 20 cm/second, usually decreases in patients with severe portal hypertension and can even reverse in the late stages of disease; this is due to increased resistance to flow within the fibrotic liver. However, the portal venous velocity uniformly increases after TIPS placement in patients with portal hypertension due to the markedly decreased resistance to flow within the patent TIPS stent **(Option (E) is true).**

Shawn P. Quillin, M.D.
Dennis M. Balfe, M.D.

SUGGESTED READINGS

TIPS: COLOR-FLOW DOPPLER EVALUATION

1. Chong WK, Malisch TA, Mazer MJ, Lind CD, Worrell JA, Richards WO. Transjugular intrahepatic portosystemic shunt: US assessment with maximum flow velocity. Radiology 1993; 189:789–793
2. Feldstein VA, LaBerge JM. Hepatic vein flow reversal at duplex sonography: a sign of transjugular intrahepatic portosystemic shunt dysfunction. AJR 1994; 162:839–841
3. Ferral H, Foshager MC, Bjarnason H, et al. Early sonographic evaluation of the transjugular intrahepatic portosystemic shunt (TIPS). Cardiovasc Intervent Radiol 1993; 16:275–279
4. Foshager MC, Ferral H, Finlay DE, Castañeda-Zuñiga WR, Letourneau JG. Color Doppler sonography of transjugular intrahepatic portosystemic shunts (TIPS). AJR 1994; 163:105–111
5. Longo JM, Bilbao JI, Rousseau HP, et al. Transjugular intrahepatic portosystemic shunt: evaluation with Doppler sonography. Radiology 1993; 186:529–534
6. Surratt RS, Middleton WD, Darcy MD, Melson GL, Brink JA. Morphologic and hemodynamic findings at sonography before and after creation of a transjugular intrahepatic portosystemic shunt. AJR 1993; 160:627–630

TIPS: TECHNIQUES, RESULTS, AND COMPLICATIONS

7. Echenagusia AJ, Camuñez F, Simo G, et al. Variceal hemorrhage: efficacy of transjugular intrahepatic portosystemic shunts created with Strecker stents. Radiology 1994; 192:235–240

8. Ferral H, Bjarnason H, Wegryn SA, et al. Refractory ascites: early experience in treatment with transjugular intrahepatic portosystemic shunt. Radiology 1993; 189:795–801
9. Freedman AM, Sanyal AJ, Tisnado J, et al. Complications of transjugular intrahepatic portosystemic shunt: a comprehensive review. RadioGraphics 1993; 13:1185–1210
10. Haskal ZJ, Pentecost MJ, Soulen MC, Shlansky-Goldberg RD, Baum RA, Cope C. Transjugular intrahepatic portosystemic shunt stenosis and revision: early and midterm results. AJR 1994; 163:439–444
11. Hausegger KA, Sternthal HM, Klein GE, Karaic R, Stauber R, Zenker G. Transjugular intrahepatic portosystemic shunt: angiographic follow-up and secondary interventions. Radiology 1994; 191:177–181
12. LaBerge JM, Ring EJ, Gordon RL, et al. Creation of transjugular intrahepatic portosystemic shunts with the wallstent endoprosthesis: results in 100 patients. Radiology 1993; 187:413–420
13. Nazarian GK, Ferral H, Castañeda-Zuñiga WR, et al. Development of stenoses in transjugular intrahepatic portosystemic shunts. Radiology 1994; 192:231–234
14. Uflacker R, Reichert P, D'Albuquerque LC, de Oliveira e Silva A. Liver anatomy applied to the placement of transjugular intrahepatic portosystemic shunts. Radiology 1994; 191:705–712
15. Zemel G, Becker GJ, Bancroft JW, Benenati JF, Katzen BT. Technical advances in transjugular intrahepatic portosystemic shunts. Radio-Graphics 1992; 12:615–622

HEPATIC SONOGRAPHY

16. Abu-Yousef MM. Duplex Doppler sonography of the hepatic vein in tricuspid regurgitation. AJR 1991; 156:79–83
17. Abu-Yousef MM, Milam SG, Farner RM. Pulsatile portal vein flow: a sign of tricuspid regurgitation on duplex Doppler sonography. AJR 1990; 155:785–788
18. Becker CD, Cooperberg PL. Sonography of the hepatic vascular system. AJR 1988; 150:999–1005
19. Dodd GD III, Zajko AB, Orons PD, Martin MS, Eichner LS, Santaguida LA. Detection of transjugular intrahepatic portosystemic shunt dysfunction: value of duplex Doppler sonography. AJR 1995; 164:1119–1124
20. Kerlan RK Jr, LaBerge JM, Gordon RL, Ring EJ. Transjugular intrahepatic portosystemic shunts: current status. AJR 1995; 164:1059–1066
21. Koslin DB, Berland LL. Duplex Doppler examination of the liver and portal venous system. JCU 1987; 15:675–686
22. Miller MM, Middleton WD, Balfe DM. Peripheral portal venous blood flow alterations induced by hepatic masses: a color Doppler sonographic analysis. Scientific Session, ARRS annual meeting, 1993
23. Ralls PW. Color Doppler sonography of the hepatic artery and portal venous system. AJR 1990; 155:517–525

Notes

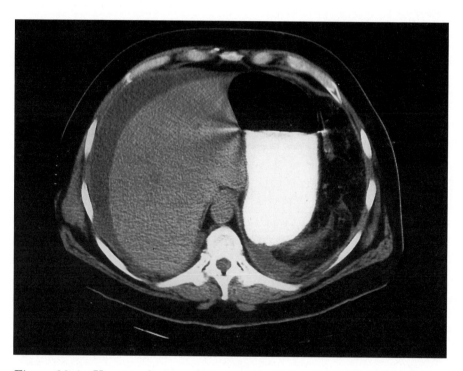

Figure 23-1. You are shown a CT scan of a 50-year-old man with abdominal pain and distension 1 week after laparoscopic cholecystectomy.

Case 23: Laparoscopic Cholecystectomy

Question 69

Which *one* of the following complications is the MOST likely cause of the CT findings in the test patient?

    (A) Duodenal perforation
    (B) Intraperitoneal hematoma
    (C) Intraperitoneal abscess
    (D) Bile leakage from the cystic duct remnant
    (E) Ligation of the common hepatic bile duct

Figure 23-1, a CT section through the mid-liver, shows a homogeneous low-density perihepatic fluid collection. There is no intrahepatic bile duct dilatation. Given the history of recent laparoscopic cholecystectomy, the peritoneal fluid is most probably bile and the most likely cause is leakage from the cystic duct remnant (Figure 23-2) **(Option (D) is correct).** Bile produces a chemical peritonitis, which is the cause of the patient's abdominal pain and distension.

According to Kang et al., small postoperative fluid collections in the gallbladder fossa are seen in about half of patients after laparoscopic cholecystectomy and are usually insignificant; it is likely that the collections spontaneously resolve within a few days. Larger fluid collections (greater than 20 mL of fluid) and those that extend perihepatically or elsewhere in the peritoneal cavity almost always indicate a postoperative complication.

Abnormal intraperitoneal fluid collections after laparoscopic cholecystectomy may be bilomas or bile ascites, hematomas, abscesses, or fluid from a bowel perforation. Imaging by CT or sonography is seldom specific but frequently suggests the nature of the fluid collection. Large peritoneal fluid collections that are homogeneous and of low density, like that in Figure 23-1, usually result from bile accumulation, particularly when there are no other reasons for ascites.

Leaked bile can be distributed diffusely throughout the peritoneal cavity, resulting in bile ascites, or localized and encapsulated, forming a

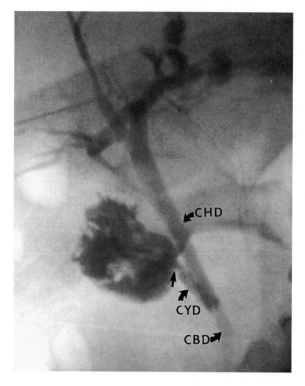

Figure 23-2. Same patient as in Figure 23-1. A transhepatic cholangiogram shows the bile leak from the cystic duct remnant (straight arrow) causing the bile ascites seen in the test figure. CHD = common hepatic duct; CBD = common bile duct; CYD = cystic duct.

biloma (Figure 23-3). Bilomas that occur after laparoscopic cholecystectomy form most commonly in the gallbladder fossa, the subhepatic space, or the left posterior perihepatic space behind the left lobe of the liver. Less often, they form in the peritoneal cavity remote from the liver. Bile ascites and bilomas are of low density on CT scans and have few internal echoes on sonograms. Thin septations, which are often better seen on sonograms than on CT scans, sometimes form within bile collections.

The presence of a bile collection after laparoscopic cholecystectomy indicates that leakage of bile has occurred; the underlying cause of the spillage must be found, since some causes are associated with important clinical consequences. About 25% of people have small ducts (called ducts of Luschka) extending from the right hepatic lobe to the gallbladder or cystic duct. At cholecystectomy these structures are severed and bile leakage results. Bile leaks from these small ducts tend to be small and to close spontaneously within several days of surgery. Occasionally, bile spills during the cholecystectomy, usually from laceration of a thin-walled gallbladder. In these cases, the surgeon attempts to aspirate bile from all visualized spaces before removing the laparoscope, and so the spilled bile collection is usually either small or in a remote location. Bile

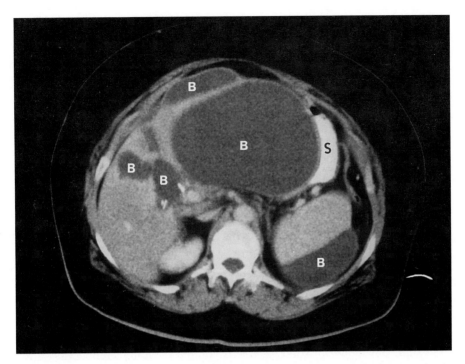

Figure 23-3. Biloma. A CT scan obtained 2 weeks after laparoscopic cholecystectomy shows multiple bilomas (B) in the gallbladder fossa and perihepatic spaces and posterior to the spleen. The large perihepatic biloma displaces the contrast-filled stomach (S) to the left. A transection of the common hepatic bile duct was repaired by choledochojejunostomy.

spillage occurring during the surgical procedure becomes important only if the bile is infected and an abscess subsequently develops. Another complication is bile leakage from the cystic duct stump. This occurs when surgically placed clamps or ligatures come off the cystic duct stump. Increased pressure in the cystic duct (in most cases because of a retained common duct stone) sometimes aggravates the cystic duct leak. Finally, the rarest but most significant cause of bile leakage is a tear or transection of central bile ducts.

Hepatobiliary scintigraphy is a highly sensitive method for identifying bile leaks after laparoscopic cholecystectomy. Trerotola et al. examined 9 patients and Peters et al. examined 11 patients with hepatobiliary scintigraphy. All patients had bile leaks, and all bile leaks were seen with scintigraphy. Cross-sectional imaging can demonstrate the size and location of the bile collection, and aspiration under CT or sonographic guidance can confirm that the fluid collection is bilious. If the bile leak is small and the patient is asymptomatic, no treatment is necessary. However, if the patient is symptomatic or a major leak is suspected, further investigation is warranted. Contrast cholangiography, either endoscopic retrograde cholangiography or transhepatic cholangiography, reliably demonstrates leakage from the cystic duct stump or major injuries to the central bile ducts. Endoscopic retrograde cholangiography is preferred because it allows therapeutic interventions including sphincterotomy and stone removal. If this procedure is unsuccessful at visualizing the entire biliary system, transhepatic cholangiography is needed to evaluate the bile leak. The diagnosis and treatment of these major bile leaks are discussed in Question 70.

Duodenal perforation (Option (A)) could cause the homogeneous fluid collection seen in the test image, but it is a much less likely cause than bile ascites secondary to cystic duct remnant leak. Bowel perforation occurs during laparoscopic cholecystectomy in 0.3% of patients, according to the study by the Southern Surgeons Club. The stomach, small bowel, and colon are all susceptible to injury; however, perforations occur most frequently in the duodenum, particularly in patients with dense inflammatory adhesions between the gallbladder and duodenum.

When bowel perforation occurs, abdominal radiographs almost always show a hydroperitoneum, pneumoperitoneum (Figure 23-4), or hydropneumoperitoneum. In patients with large leaks, an upper gastrointestinal contrast examination will show leakage of contrast material at the site of bowel perforation. CT shows a hydropneumoperitoneum or intraperitoneal fluid. The site of leakage can be identified on CT by detection of oral contrast material leaking from the bowel and associated high-density oral contrast material in the peritoneal cavity (Figure 23-5). Bowel perforations can become walled off and create a focal abscess rather than a hydropneumoperitoneum (Figure 23-6).

The appropriate examination to order when bowel perforation is suspected is controversial. It is often unclear clinically why the patient is doing poorly after cholecystectomy, and bowel perforation is often only one of several possible explanations. CT is usually performed first because it is the best postoperative survey examination and detects the vast majority of bowel perforations. If the CT findings are unclear, an upper gastrointestinal contrast examination may be done.

Intraperitoneal hematomas (Option (B)) are sometimes indistinguishable from bilomas, but the CT or sonographic findings can usually differentiate between the two. On CT scans, acute and subacute hematomas usually have central hyperdense components mixed with areas of lower density. Sonograms of hematomas contain more internal echoes, debris, and septations than are seen in sonograms of most bilomas. Serial sonograms obtained over several days show an echo pattern char-

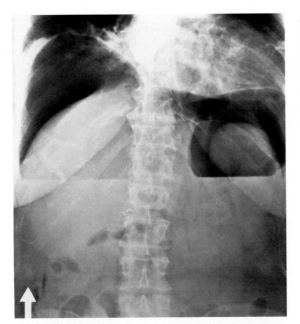

Figure 23-4 (left). An abdominal film obtained 2 days after laparoscopic cholecystectomy shows a large pneumoperitoneum. A perforated duodenum was surgically repaired.

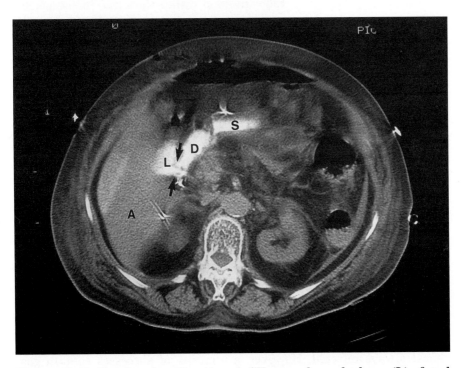

Figure 23-5. Duodenal perforation. A CT scan shows leakage (L) of oral contrast material from a duodenal perforation (arrows). The ascites (A) has a higher density, as a result of oral contrast material and gastrointestinal contents, than the bilomas in Figure 23-3. S = stomach; D = duodenum.

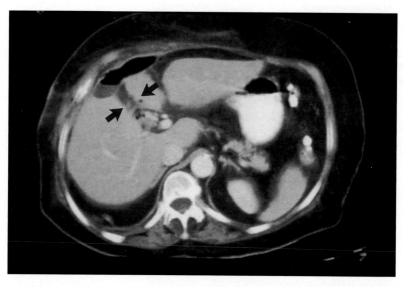

Figure 23-6. A CT scan obtained 2 weeks after laparoscopic cholecystectomy shows a fistula (arrows) from the duodenum to a gas-filled abscess. The duodenal perforation was contained rather than free in the peritoneum.

acteristic of an evolving hematoma. The hematoma is initially echogenic or of mixed echogenicity with solid and cystic components. Over several days to weeks, the echo pattern of a hematoma becomes less echogenic and more cystic, reflecting lysis of the blood clot. The test figure has no regions of hyperdensity, debris, or septation, and hematoma is therefore not the most likely diagnosis.

An abscess (Option (C)) can develop from spillage of infected bile, gallstones, or bowel contents or from secondary infection of undrained fluid collections such as bilomas or hematomas (Figure 23-7). Abscesses have a wide range of CT and sonographic appearances, but they most commonly appear as complex fluid collections that have some mass effect, compressing or displacing nearby structures. On CT, abscesses are uni- or multiloculated fluid collections, sometimes with septations or debris. Sonograms often show some internal echoes and septations. If imaging studies show that a fluid collection contains gas, the fluid is almost always infected. However, a minority of abscesses contain gas. Accordingly, abscesses are often indistinguishable from their uninfected counterparts. Aspiration of the fluid collection followed by Gram stain and culture of the aspirate will distinguish infected from uninfected fluid collections. The absence of fever in the history of the test patient and the

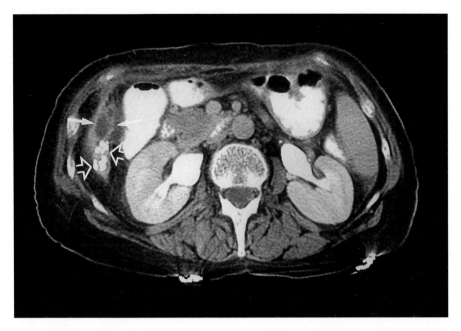

Figure 23-7. Abscess. A CT scan 2 weeks after laparoscopic cholecystectomy shows an abscess (solid arrows) containing spilled gallstones (open arrows).

absence of mass effect associated with the fluid collection make abscess less likely than biloma.

Ligation of the common hepatic bile duct (Option (E)) usually causes intrahepatic bile duct dilatation, a feature not seen in the test figure. When major injury to the bile duct occurs during cholecystectomy, bile leakage can accompany bile duct obstruction, in which case both a fluid collection (composed of leaked bile) and bile duct dilatation may be seen. Sometimes the bile duct leak is so large that it effectively decompresses the biliary system, preventing immediate duct dilatation. In these patients, bile duct dilatation develops days to weeks after the injury. Obstruction of the common hepatic duct after laparoscopic cholecystectomy is most often due to surgical injury or retained common duct calculi. If bile duct obstruction is suspected, cholangiography is indicated.

Question 70

Concerning laparoscopic cholecystectomy and its complications,

   (A) the site of a bile duct injury can usually be determined by CT
   (B) most bile duct injuries involve the proximal extrahepatic bile ducts (within 2 cm of the confluence of the right and left hepatic ducts)
   (C) most bile duct injuries occur in patients with anomalous bile duct anatomy
   (D) intraoperative cholangiography is technically possible in less than 50% of laparoscopic cholecystectomies
   (E) hepatobiliary scintigraphy is useful to distinguish cystic duct remnant leak from common hepatic duct injury
   (F) leaks from the cystic duct remnant usually require surgical repair
   (G) ligation of the hepatic artery rarely leads to hepatic infarction

Laparoscopic cholecystectomy was introduced by Mouret in France in 1987. Patients undergo a short hospitalization (mean, 1 day), resume normal activities rapidly (1 to 2 weeks), endure minimal pain, and have only a small abdominal scar; therefore, the procedure has rapidly replaced open cholecystectomy as the routine procedure for removal of the gallbladder.

The surgeon begins a laparoscopic cholecystectomy by creating a pneumoperitoneum. A trocar is placed through a 10-mm umbilical incision, and a laparoscope is then placed through the umbilical canal. Two 5-mm incisions in the right upper quadrant and a 1-cm subxyphoid incision are made for operating instruments (Figure 23-8). The peritoneal cavity is examined to exclude visceral injury from the trocars. The gallbladder is retracted anteriorly, and the fibroareolar tissues are stripped from the gallbladder wall. The cystic duct, gallbladder junction, and cystic artery are identified. Intraoperative cholangiography is performed in some patients. The cystic duct and cystic artery are clamped or ligated and divided. The gallbladder is dissected from the gallbladder bed and removed through the umbilical port. After final inspection of the abdomen, the laparoscope is removed and the pneumoperitoneum is decompressed.

The most important complication of open or laparoscopic cholecystectomy is injury to major bile ducts, resulting in bile leakage, ductal obstruction, or both. Intraperitoneal bile causes abdominal pain and distension, and undrained bile collections often become infected. Bile duct obstruction causes jaundice and cholangitis and, if untreated, eventually results in hepatic cirrhosis. The severe consequences of bile duct injury mean that the continued success of the technique depends on establishing that the frequency of bile duct injury during laparoscopic cholecystectomy approaches the low frequency of injury associated with open chole-

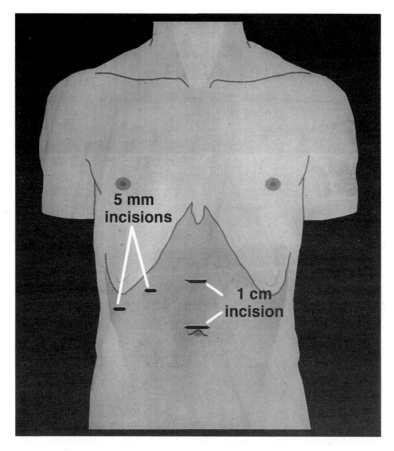

Figure 23-8. Diagram of the anatomic sites for the four cannulas used for laparoscopic cholecystectomy. The two right ports are used for instruments to retract the gallbladder. The umbilical port is used for the video laparoscope and for removal of the gallbladder. The incision in the epigastrum is used for the operating instruments.

cystectomy. Moreover, when bile duct injury occurs, prompt evaluation and therapy are imperative.

Reports to date suggest that laparoscopic cholecystectomy has a slightly higher frequency of major bile duct injuries than does traditional open cholecystectomy. Long-term data are limited; however, the relatively high frequency of major bile duct injuries associated with the laparoscopic technique reported in the early 1990s tended to occur early in the experience of each surgical group. In one report by the Southern Surgeons Club, 20 surgical groups performed 1,518 laparoscopic cholecystectomies. The frequency of bile duct injury was 2.2% in the initial cohort of

260 patients that represented the first 13 patients operated by each of the 20 groups. In contrast, the frequency of bile duct injury was only 0.1% in subsequent patients. The overall rate of bile duct injury was 0.5%. By comparison, the frequency of bile duct injury during open cholecystectomy is 0.1 to 0.2%. It is expected that, as surgeons are trained in and experience is gained with laparoscopic cholecystectomy, the frequency of bile duct injuries will decrease. Regardless of the frequency, the radiologist must be prepared to identify, characterize, and treat bile duct injuries that occur as complications of cholecystectomy.

Only a small number of injuries to the extrahepatic bile ducts are recognized at the time of cholecystectomy. Most patients become symptomatic within days to weeks after cholecystectomy, but bile duct strictures may not become clinically obvious until months to years after cholecystectomy. In patients undergoing open cholecystectomy, more than 25% of strictures occur more than 6 months after the surgery.

Bile duct injuries include strictures, ligations or staple occlusions, tears, transections, and combinations of injuries. Therefore, CT scans and sonograms will show dilated ducts if the obstructed component is dominant or normal-caliber ducts if bile leakage decompresses the obstructed ducts. In our experience, half of major bile duct injuries cause bile duct dilation. Eighty percent of patients with bile duct injuries have bilomas or bile ascites at CT or sonography. Cholangiography is the only accurate method to determine the exact site of bile duct injury **(Option (A) is false).** Endoscopic retrograde cholangiography is usually done first, primarily because it allows endoscopic therapy if the underlying cause is cystic duct leakage or choledocholithiasis. If major bile duct injury is present, the bile ducts proximal to the injury often cannot be visualized by endoscopic retrograde cholangiography because of complete duct occlusion by surgical staples. In these cases, transhepatic cholangiography is usually needed to evaluate the proximal biliary tree and accurately determine the level of bile duct injury prior to surgical anastomosis.

Bile duct injuries are categorized by their location in the biliary tree according to the Bismuth classification (Figure 23-9). The Bismuth classification was originally designed to classify strictures only, but by common usage it has been extended to classify bile duct tears, transections, strictures, and a combination of injuries. The level of bile duct injury is important because it determines the type of surgical repair required. Bismuth type IV injuries may require separate right and left hepatojejunostomy anastomoses (Figure 23-10).

Most bile duct injuries occurring during laparoscopic cholecystectomy are Bismuth II, III, or IV injuries, occurring within 2 cm of the biliary hilus **(Option (B) is true).** These high injuries generally cannot be

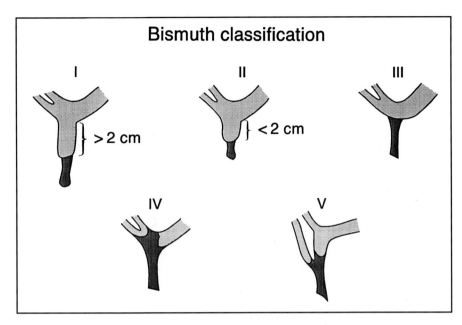

Figure 23-9. The Bismuth classification of bile duct injuries is used to identify the level of bile duct injury by describing the length of the intact proximal biliary stump (light-gray duct). This is the most important information determined from a cholangiogram because it determines the type of surgical repair that is necessary. Bismuth type I injury has more than 2 cm of intact common hepatic duct. Bismuth type II has 2 cm or less of intact common hepatic duct. Bismuth type III injury is at the hilus, and Bismuth type IV injury has isolated right and left ducts. Bismuth type V describes the rare situation of an anomolous right duct inserting low in the common hepatic duct. Eighty percent of bile duct injuries from laparoscopic cholecystectomy are Bismuth type II, III, or IV. (Adapted with permission from Bismuth [1].)

treated successfully by primary bile duct repair. Bile duct injuries from laparoscopic cholecystectomy often involve ligation and removal of some length of common hepatic duct (Figure 23-11). This makes primary duct repair impossible because of insufficient length of bile duct. Either chole-dochojejunostomy or hepaticojejunostomy is necessary for surgical repair of most bile duct injuries occurring at laparoscopic cholecystectomy.

Percutaneous transhepatic decompression is sometimes performed to treat sepsis or to identify bile duct anatomy before surgical repair. Endo-scopic or percutaneous decompression, stricture dilatation, or stent placement may be done instead of choledochojejunostomy if the bile duct stricture is short, symmetric, and negotiable by endoscopic or transhe-patic methods. Unfortunately, these features are present in only a few

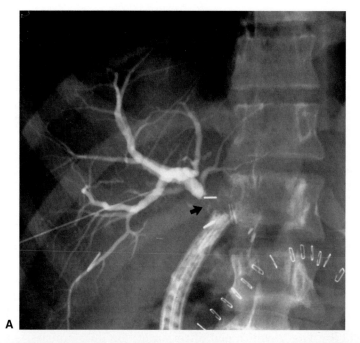

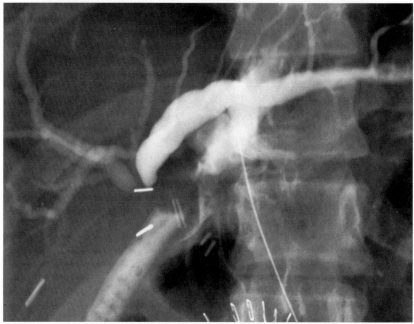

Figure 23-10. Bismuth type IV injury. Right (A) and left (B) transhepatic cholangiograms show a Bismuth type IV bile duct injury with contrast leaking into a surgical drain. Surgical repair was performed by separate right and left hepaticojejunostomies. (A) Only the right ducts fill from the right transhepatic injection. The right ducts are relatively undilated since contrast material leaks into a surgical drain (arrow). (B) Left ducts are markedly distended with no bile leak.

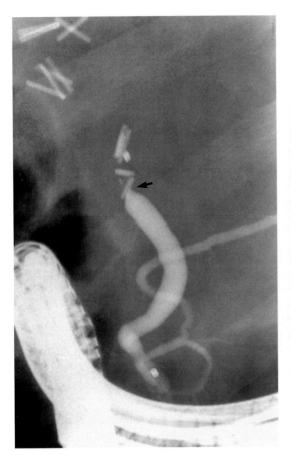

A

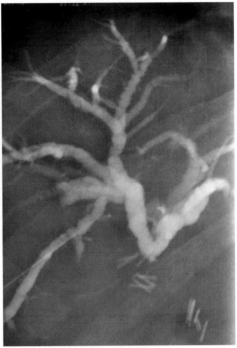

B

Figure 23-11. Bismuth type III injury. (A) An endoscopic retrograde cholangiogram shows surgical clips obstructing the common hepatic bile
duct (arrow). There is no opacification of the biliary tree proximal to the
obstructing surgical clips, so the level of the most proximal injury
remains unknown. (B) A transhepatic cholangiogram shows a Bismuth
type III injury. Note that 2 cm of bile duct is not opacified on either study.
Bile duct injury was repaired by hepaticojejunostomy.

strictures. Percutaneous methods have long-term patency rates of 76 to
88%, nearly identical to patency rates reported for surgical reconstruction of bile duct strictures. Percutaneous stricture dilatation and stenting are particularly helpful in treatment of strictures complicating bil-
iary-enteric anastomoses that occur months to years after the surgical
repair.

    As with traditional cholecystectomy, most bile duct injuries with lap-
aroscopic cholecystectomy occur when no bile duct anomalies are present

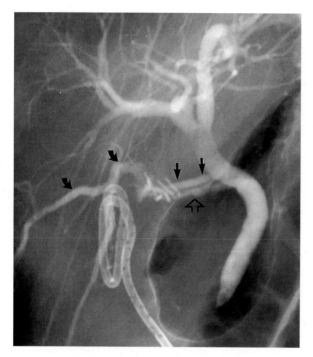

Figure 23-12. Bile duct injury in a patient with an anomalous bile duct. An endoscopic retrograde cholangiogram shows an anomalous right bile duct entering low in the common hepatic duct (straight solid arrows) parallel to the cystic duct (open arrow). It is obstructed by surgical clips. A percutaneously placed drainage catheter is in a biloma created by the bile leak from the anomalous right bile duct (curved solid arrows).

(Option (C) is false). Bile duct injuries occur when the common hepatic duct or right hepatic duct is misidentified as the cystic duct and then ligated or clipped. Chartrand-Lefebvre et al. reported a series of 33 patients with bile duct injuries from laparoscopic cholecystectomy. Only 2 of the 33 (6%) injuries resulted from bile duct anomalies. Injury associated with anomalous ducts occurs when a right duct inserts into the cystic duct or unusually low into the common hepatic duct or when there is a low junction of the right and left bile ducts (Figure 23-12).

Intraoperative cholangiography during laparoscopic cholecystectomy is technically possible in 80 to 90% of patients **(Option (D) is false).** A small catheter or probe is inserted into the cystic duct, 5 to 15 ml of contrast material with 15% iodine concentration is injected, and radiographs are taken at 63 kVp (Figure 23-13). Cholangiograms should be examined not only for choledocholithiasis but also to evaluate bile duct anatomy and search for unsuspected abnormalities such as primary sclerosing cholangitis or pancreatic carcinoma. A few surgeons perform intraoperative cholangiography routinely; however, most perform cholangiography only in selected patients in whom choledocholithiasis is suspected or in whom the bile duct anatomy is distorted or obscured by inflammation. Information gained from cholangiography is thought to

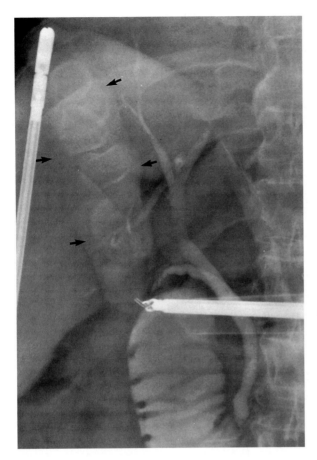

Figure 23-13. Normal intraoperative cholangiogram in a patient with normal bile duct anatomy and no choledocholithiasis. The gallstone-filled gallbladder is retracted upward (arrows).

reduce the frequency of bile duct injuries by outlining bile duct anatomy and by identifying aberrant duct anatomy, although bile duct injury can occur even after a normal intraoperative cholangiogram.

Hepatobiliary scintigraphy with either Tc-99m disofenin or mebrofenin is a very sensitive method for detecting bile leakage or obstruction after laparoscopic cholecystectomy, but the exact site of bile leakage cannot be reliably identified **(Option (E) is false).** Trerotola et al. evaluated 13 patients with biliary complications after laparoscopic cholecystectomy. Of the 13, 9 were studied with hepatobiliary scintigraphy. Hepatobiliary scintigraphy showed bile leak in all seven patients with bile leak but underestimated the severity of the leak in the one patient with bile duct transection. The same scintigraphic techniques and principles that are used to evaluate complications of open cholecystectomy can also be used to evaluate complications of laparoscopic cholecystectomy. The radiopharmaceutical is injected intravenously, and sequential imag-

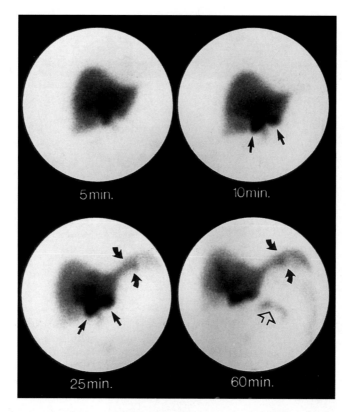

Figure 23-14. Leakage of bile into the peritoneal cavity. Hepatobiliary scintigraphy shows bile leakage. The leakage of radiopharmaceutical is first seen in the subhepatic space at 10 minutes (straight arrows). On the 25- and 60-minute images, radiopharmaceutical is seen in the subhepatic space (straight solid arrows) and in the paracolic gutter (curved arrows). There is a small amount of radiopharmaceutical in the small bowel (open arrow). Bile leakage was from the cystic duct remnant.

ing is performed for 60 to 90 minutes. Delayed images at 2 to 4 hours, or later, after injection are helpful in identification of smaller bile leaks. Views in oblique, lateral, or posterior projections may be helpful in distinguishing tracer in bile duct and bowel from leaked tracer. Serial hepatobiliary scintigraphy can be used to monitor closure of bile leaks, particularly after sphincterotomy.

Hepatobiliary scintigraphy after open cholecystectomy has shown a surprisingly large number of small bile leaks: 42% in a study by Gilsdorf et al. Nearly all these bile leaks are clinically insignificant and result from severance of small bile ducts (ducts of Luschka) in the gallbladder bed. With these small bile leaks, radiopharmaceutical accumulates in the gallbladder fossa, sometimes spilling into other peritoneal locations. These small leaks are often seen on delayed imaging done more than 1 hour after injection of the radiopharmaceutical. Clinically significant bile leaks are usually seen on early imaging (<1 hour) and result in a moderately large amount of radiopharmaceutical in the peritoneal cavity compared with the amount in the bowel (Figure 23-14).

The major limitation of hepatobiliary scintigraphy is that it cannot accurately identify the site of a bile leak. Therefore, a less significant problem such as cystic duct leak may be indistinguishable from a bile duct tear or transection. Massive leaks from the cystic duct remnant have been misinterpreted as duct transections when no radiopharmaceutical was seen in the small bowel because of preferential flow through the cystic duct remnant into the peritoneal cavity. Conversely, bile leakage from an injury to the common hepatic duct can be misinterpreted as bile leakage from the cystic duct remnant. Cholangiography is necessary for accurate identification of the site of bile leakage and for therapeutic treatment such as sphincterotomy or biliary stenting.

Hepatobiliary scintigraphy is a sensitive method for identifying bile duct obstruction after cholecystectomy, but it is not useful in determining the cause of obstruction. Cholangiography is necessary to identify a specific cause.

Most fluid collections after cholecystectomy are detected by CT or sonography. In many cases, aspiration of fluid to determine whether it is bile is faster and less expensive than performing hepatobiliary scintigraphy. Cholangiography is then done to find the site of bile leak and to aid therapeutic intervention.

Leakage from the cystic duct remnant occurs after laparoscopic cholecystectomy when ligatures or clips slip off the cystic duct remnant. These leaks are aggravated by distal obstructing lesions such as choledocholithiasis, papillary stenosis, or unsuspected pancreatic carcinoma.

There are several nonsurgical treatments for cystic duct remnant leak, and one of these is usually done in lieu of surgical repair (**Option (F) is false).** Bilomas or bile ascites can be drained under CT or sonographic guidance in anticipation of spontaneous closure of the cystic duct remnant. More commonly, after drainage of the bilomas, endoscopic sphincterotomy with or without biliary stenting is done, usually producing rapid resolution of the leak. Endoscopic sphincterotomy with or without stenting has been shown to cure the cystic duct remnant leak in more than 75% of patients. If endoscopic methods are not possible, transhepatic biliary drainage can be used to drain bile into the duodenum rather than through the cystic duct stump. In the unusual case in which these methods fail, the cystic duct is closed surgically.

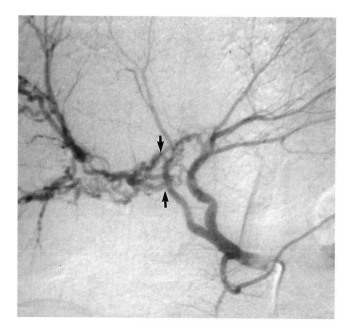

Figure 23-15. Arterial injury during laparoscopic cholecystectomy. An arteriogram shows ligation of the right hepatic artery with collateral filling of the peripheral right hepatic arteries (arrows). There was also a Bismuth type IV injury of the right hepatic bile duct.

Arterial vascular injuries during laparoscopic cholecystectomy result either from trocar injuries or from ligation of the hepatic artery (Figure 23-15). Inadvertent insertion of a trocar into the aorta, iliac arteries, and lumbar arteries has been reported and has required immediate surgical repair. The most common sequela of arterial injury seen on imaging studies is a hematoma, although pseudoaneurysm or arteriovenous fistula can result from trocar injury. Bismuth reported that 40% of bile duct injuries from open cholecystectomy had associated hepatic artery injury. The frequency of hepatic artery injury with bile duct injury during laparoscopic cholecystectomy remains unknown.

In a large autopsy series, Halasz reported that 7% of cadavers who had undergone open cholecystectomy at least 1 year previously had ligation of the right or proper hepatic artery. No liver infarctions were seen. The resistance of the liver to infarction has traditionally been attributed to the dual blood supply of the liver from the portal vein, which accounts for approximately 85% of the blood supply, and from the hepatic artery, which delivers the remaining 15%. In fact, the low frequency of hepatic infarction in the liver after hepatic artery ligation may be due to extensive arterial collateral flow to the liver from intercostal, phrenic, and gastric arteries, as well as from increased portal vein flow. Hepatic artery thrombosis after liver transplantation results in hepatic infarction when the portal vein is patent, supporting the importance of collateral arterial flow. Whatever the source of oxygenated blood flow to the liver, hepatic infarction rarely develops from hepatic artery ligation during cholecystectomy **(Option (G) is true).**

Ellen M. Ward, M.D.

SUGGESTED READINGS

1. Bismuth H. Postoperative strictures of the bile duct. In: Blumgart LH (ed), Biliary tract. Clinical Surgery International Series, vol. 5. New York: Churchill Livingstone; 1983:209–218
2. Brugge WR, Alavi A. Cholescintigraphy in the diagnosis of complications of laparoscopic cholecystectomy. Semin US CT MR 1993; 14:368–374
3. Cuschieri A, Dubois F, Mouiel J, et al. The European experience with laparoscopic cholecystectomy. Am J Surg 1991; 161:385–387
4. Gilsdorf JR, Phillips M, McLeod MK, et al. Radionuclide evaluation of bile leakage and the use of subhepatic drains after cholecystectomy. Am J Surg 1986; 151:259–262
5. Halasz NA. Cholecystectomy and hepatic artery injuries. Arch Surg 1991; 126:137–138
6. Kang EH, Middleton WD, Balfe DM, Soper NJ. Laparoscopic cholecystectomy: evaluation with sonography. Radiology 1991; 181:439–442
7. Chartrand-Lefebvre C, Dufresne MP, Lafortune M, Lapointe R, Dagenais M, Roy A. Iatrogenic injury to the bile duct: a working classification for radiologists. Radiology 1994; 193:523–526
8. Peters JH, Ollila D, Nichols KE, et al. Diagnosis and management of bile leaks following laparoscopic cholecystectomy. Surg Laparosc Endosc 1994; 4:163–170
9. Ponchon T, Gallez JF, Valette PJ, Chavaillon A, Bory R. Endoscopic treatment of biliary tract fistulas. Gastrointest Endosc 1989; 35:490–498
10. Southern Surgeons Club. A prospective analysis of 1518 laparoscopic cholecystectomies. N Engl J Med 1991; 324:1073–1078
11. Spaw AT, Reddick EJ, Olsen DO. Laparoscopic laser cholecystectomy: analysis of 500 procedures. Surg Laparoscopy Endoscopy 1991; 1:2–7
12. Trerotola SO, Savader SJ, Lund GB, et al. Biliary tract complications following laparoscopic cholecystectomy: imaging and intervention. Radiology 1992; 184:195–200
13. vanSonnenberg E, D'Agostino HB, Easter DW, et al. Complications of laparoscopic cholecystectomy: coordinated radiologic and surgical management in 21 patients. Radiology 1993; 199:399–404
14. Walker AT, Shapiro AW, Brooks DC, Braver JM, Tumeh SS. Bile duct disruption and biloma after laparoscopic cholecystectomy: imaging evaluation. AJR 1992; 158:785–789
15. Ward EM, LeRoy AJ, Bender CE, Donohue JH, Hughes RW. Imaging of complications of laparoscopic cholecystectomy. Abdom Imaging 1993; 18:150–155
16. Wright TB, Bertino RB, Bishop AF, et al. Complications of laparoscopic cholecystectomy and their interventional radiologic management. RadioGraphics 1993; 13:119–128

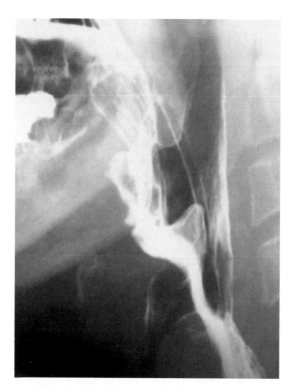

Figure 24-1. This 70-year-old man has a chronically sore throat. He received full-course radiation therapy for an epidermoid cancer of the right true vocal cord 7 years ago and continued to smoke and drink alcohol after therapy. You are shown a lateral radiograph from an air-contrast barium pharyngogram.

Case 24: Pharynx after Radiation

Question 71

Which *one* of the following is the MOST likely diagnosis?

    (A) Expected appearance of the pharynx after irradiation
    (B) Recurrent carcinoma
    (C) New primary epidermoid carcinoma
    (D) Radiation-induced ulceration
    (E) Pharyngeal diverticulum

The lateral view obtained during an air-contrast barium pharyngo-gram in the test patient (Figure 24-1) shows a barium collection within the base of the tongue immediately superior to the barium-filled vallec-ula (Figure 24-2). The radiographic appearance is that of a primary ulcerative process. Primary ulcerative processes in the pharynx are most commonly due to primary epidermoid carcinoma, but this is particularly true in the tongue base. Considering the patient's history of prior epider-moid cancer, his continued exposure to risk factors (tobacco and ethanol), and his symptomatic sore throat, new primary epidermoid carcinoma arising at the base of the tongue is the most likely diagnosis **(Option (C) is correct).**

The widening of the anteroposterior dimension of the epiglottis, the increase in the prevertebral soft tissue space (the space between the ver-tebral bodies and the posterior margin of the pharynx), and the small amount of barium in the anterior part of the vestibule all indicate vestib-ular penetration. These observations are to be expected in a patient who has previously received full-course radiation to the neck for definitive therapy of a laryngeal cancer. However, ulceration is not an expected fea-ture after pharyngeal irradiation (Option (A)).

Recurrent (or persistent) carcinoma (Option (B)) could produce the tongue base ulceration shown in the test image. However, the original primary tumor had been treated 7 years ago and was in a different ana-tomic location. In view of the patient's continued smoking, a new primary

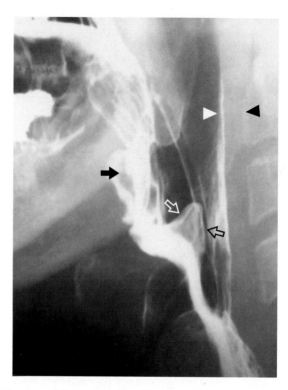

Figure 24-2 (Same as Figure 24-1). Primary carcinoma of the base of the tongue arising in an irradiated pharynx. A lateral radiograph obtained during an air-contrast pharyngogram shows mild thickening of the prevertebral stripe (arrowheads) and moderate thickening of the free margin of the epiglottis (open arrows). There is a triangular ulcer (solid arrow) in the tongue base. Biopsy of this ulcer showed epidermoid carcinoma. (Case courtesy of Seth N. Glick, M.D., Hahnemann University, Philadelphia, Pa.)

tumor is much more likely than a recurrence of the previous true vocal cord cancer.

Radiation therapy can induce mucosal ulceration (Option (D)), but the radiation-induced edema and ulceration generally arise within 6 months after completion of the therapy. Moreover, the necrosis that produces the radiographically visible ulceration usually occurs in the mucosa overlying the laryngeal cartilages and reflects chondronecrosis; this complication is now rarely seen when radiation therapy is appropriately chosen as the primary therapy for laryngeal cancer. Radiation-induced chondronecrosis is much more likely, however, when the primary tumor was extensive, when it invaded a laryngeal cartilage at the time of clinical presentation, or when radiation was administered to a site where previous surgery had been performed. The ulcer in the test image is far from the laryngeal cartilaginous skeleton and is therefore very unlikely to be due to chondronecrosis.

Pharyngeal diverticula (Option (E)) occur in two major locations. The more common is the lateral margin of the superior one-third of the hypopharyngeal wall (Figure 24-3). In this location, the lateral portion of the piriform sinus is supported only by the thyrohyoid membrane; the inferior two-thirds are supported by the thyroid cartilage. As individuals age, their thyrohyoid membrane weakens and allows mucosal protrusion, usually in a lateral and posterior direction. This process is accelerated in patients who develop unusually high pharyngeal pressures; trumpet players and glass blowers frequently develop diverticula for this reason. Pharyngeal pouches also develop from the vallecula and tend to protrude anteriorly, in the direction of the hyoid bone. In either case, the position of the barium collection would be different from that shown in the test image.

Radiation therapy has been effectively utilized for both primary and adjunctive therapy in the treatment of epidermoid cancers of the head and neck. Results in the study by Small et al. reported in 1992, dealing with a patient group restricted to T1 glottic carcinoma, showed that local control was achieved with radiation alone in 89%; when surgical salvage was performed for those patients with recurrence, the overall tumor control rate was 97%. Even when more-extensive (T2 to T4) tumors were included in the treatment group, radiation alone was quite successful in preventing local disease recurrence. In general, higher-stage, higher-grade tumors were more likely to recur, and tumors centered in the supraglottis recurred approximately twice as often as glottic tumors.

Lymph node recurrence depends on several factors, including the initial tumor T-stage and the overall medical condition of the patient. The detection of a recurrent node does not necessarily indicate that the patient will die of epidermoid cancer; 5-year disease-free survival in this group can be as high as 25%.

It is clear that early diagnosis of recurrence improves the chance for survival, since surgical salvage of low-stage recurrence has been quite successful. It is difficult, however, to make a confident diagnosis of tumor in a neck that has undergone full-course radiation therapy. Physical diagnosis is limited by the post-radiation edema that frequently results, and even biopsy is not 100% reliable in documenting the absence of cancer. In one series, the positive predictive value of biopsy was 91%, but its negative predictive value was only 25%. Moreover, biopsy of irradiated mucosa overlying laryngeal cartilage places the patient at risk for chondronecrosis. Radiologic studies are therefore an important part of the search for recurrent disease.

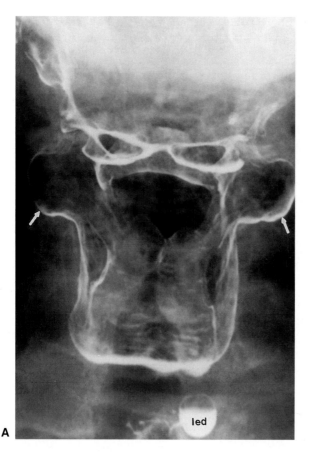

A

Figure 24-3. Pharyngeal diverticula. (A) An anteroposterior view from an air-contrast barium pharyngogram shows bilateral pharyngeal pouches (arrows) protruding through the thyrohyoid membrane in the upper third of the lateral hypopharyngeal wall. A lateral esophageal diverticulum (led) is also present. (B) A lateral view from the same examination shows the front surface of the pouches (arrowheads) projected over the superior portion of the vestibule (V) on the anterolateral surface of the hypopharynx.

Clinical studies suggest that all patients who undergo head and neck radiation therapy develop edema of the pharyngeal mucosa. Persistence or extension of the edema 6 months or more following the conclusion of radiation therapy is somewhat unusual, however, and should prompt careful evaluation for recurrent tumor. Accordingly, some of these patients are referred for pharyngographic examination. Interpretation of these studies requires a knowledge of the radiographic findings that should be expected in individuals with prior radiation therapy.

In a recent study, Quillin et al. found that all patients who had undergone full-course radiation therapy developed a degree of soft tissue thickening in the oro- and hypopharynx. This soft tissue thickening was most common in the posterior pharyngeal wall and the mucosa of the arytenoid cartilages (Figure 24-4). The latter are often asymmetrically swollen (the side of the treated tumor being larger), but the mucosal surface should be smooth (Figure 24-5). Irregularity or ulceration was a reliable sign of recurrent or persistent epidermoid carcinoma.

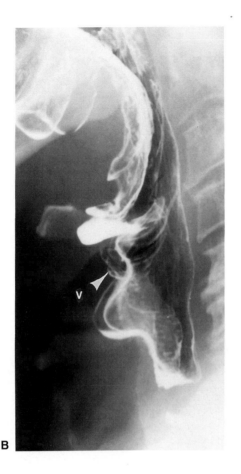

B

Almost all patients who undergo full-course radiation therapy also have some degree of functional swallowing difficulty. Reduced motion of the epiglottis was described in 12 of 13 patients in a series reported by Ekberg and Nylander; in 3 of their patients, the epiglottis was totally immobile. Accordingly, vestibular penetration of administered barium is common and is rarely associated with a cough reflex; this supports the contention that such penetration is chronic and can progress to produce pulmonary soilage. The same study also noted pharyngeal constrictor dysfunction in all of the examined patients. This leads to retention of the swallowed bolus in the hypopharynx, which places the patient at increased risk for subsequent aspiration.

When mucosal recurrence or persistence or new primary disease occurs in an irradiated pharynx, pharyngography shows mass effect with associated irregularity or ulceration of the affected mucosa; these findings are present in the vast majority of patients (17 of 19 patients in the study by Quillin et al.) (Figure 24-6).

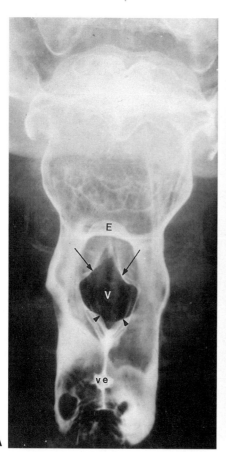
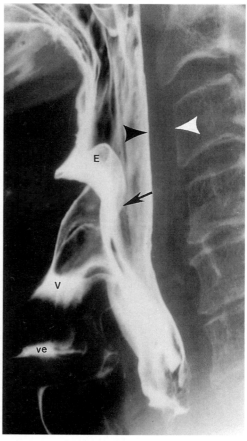

A

B

Figure 24-4. Expected appearance of the pharynx after full-course radiation therapy for carcinoma of the true vocal cord in an asymptomatic patient examined 6 months after completion of therapy. (A) An antero-posterior view obtained during an air-contrast pharyngogram shows marked thickening of the aryepiglottic folds (arrows), as well as thickening of the mucosa overlying the arytenoid cartilages (arrowheads). This has produced diminution in the size of the laryngeal vestibule (V). Though the patient reported no symptoms related to swallowing, there is barium within the supraglottic larynx, coating the medial surfaces of the true and false vocal cords and outlining the laryngeal ventricle (ve). This degree of laryngeal penetration was not accompanied by a cough reflex. E = epiglottis. (B) A lateral view obtained during the same examination shows thickening of the free margin of the epiglottis (E) and aryepiglottic folds (arrow). Moderate thickening of the prevertebral space (arrowheads) is also identified. Note barium outlining the laryngeal vestibule (V) and filling the ventricle (ve).

Although pharyngography is capable of detecting mucosal recurrence and persistence, nodal and local soft tissue recurrences are not reliably

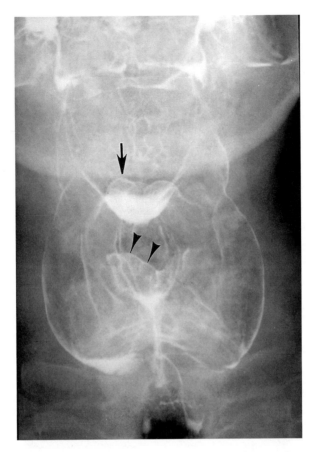

Figure 24-5. Asymmetric pharyngeal swelling after radiation therapy. An anteroposterior radiograph obtained during an air-contrast pharyngogram in a patient who received full-course radiation therapy for a right false vocal cord tumor shows swelling of the mucosa overlying the arytenoid cartilage (arrowheads) and epiglottis (arrow). Note that the right side is considerably more prominent than the left. The patient had no evidence of recurrent tumor.

depicted. Large nodes may be observed on pharyngography as smooth, extrinsic masses, most often detected on the lateral boundary of the oro- and hypopharynx (Figure 24-7). Cross-sectional imaging by CT or MRI has been helpful in the setting of a patient with suspected soft tissue disease (Figure 24-8). A study by Bronstein et al. reported the expected CT findings of pharyngeal irradiation of the neck; approximately half of the irradiated patients showed skin thickening, epiglottic enlargement, and stranding of the subcutaneous fat within the radiation port. However, the effects of radiation or surgery cannot be reliably distinguished from

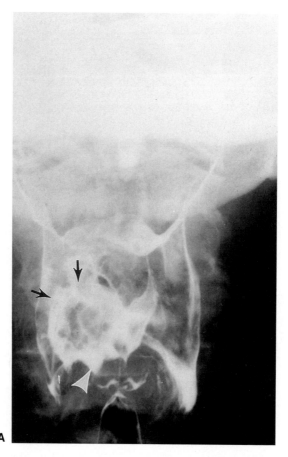

A

Figure 24-6. Pharyngographic appearance of epidermoid carcinoma in the irradiated pharynx. (A) This patient had undergone full-course radiation therapy for a primary epidermoid carcinoma of the left true vocal cord 18 months earlier. She has a persistently sore throat, with symptoms lateralized to the right side. An anteroposterior radiograph from an air-contrast pharyngogram shows a large spherical mass (arrows) arising from the false vocal cord, displacing the medial border of the piriform sinus. An ulcer crater (arrowhead) penetrates anteriorly into the paralaryngeal fat. Total laryngectomy showed epidermoid carcinoma. (B) This patient had undergone full-course radiation therapy for a glottic primary cancer. Note symmetrical swelling of the true vocal cords (C). There is an irregular mass (arrowheads), outlined by aspirated barium arising in the false vocal cords. A small superficial ulceration (arrow) is also present. Total laryngectomy documented primary epidermoid carcinoma.

tumor effects in every case. Obscuration of fat planes can occur as a result of either tumor recurrence or radiation-induced fibrosis. The presence of a discrete mass, however, reliably predicts tumor recurrence.

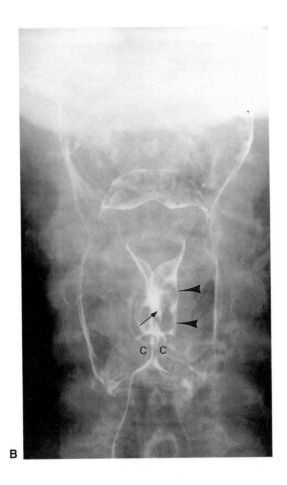

B

Mukherji et al., in a study of 61 patients, analyzed the expected CT findings after radiation therapy at sites away from the tumor. They found increased attenuation and infiltration of nearly all fat planes in the irradiated field. They also observed increased contrast enhancement of the mucosal surfaces of the oro- and hypopharynx, atrophy of lymphoid tissue and salivary glands, and thickening of the epiglottis, aryepiglottic folds, posterior pharyngeal wall, and subglottic region. With time, these findings tended to revert to normal in the paraglottic fat, but the change in the supraglottic region only occasionally reverted to normal.

MR studies on irradiated patients have shown posttreatment findings similar to those found on CT. In the study by Glazer et al., MR detection of areas of higher signal intensity allowed the radiologist to differentiate a recurrent tumor from surrounding low-intensity fibrosis. However, the same study noted that three patients with post-radiation

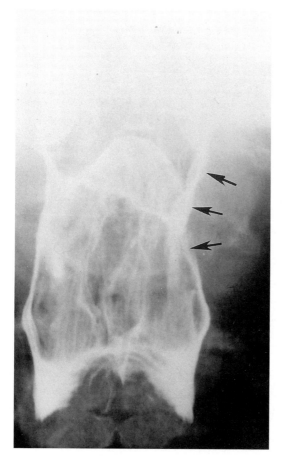

Figure 24-7. Large lymph node recurrence. An anteroposterior radiograph from an air-contrast pharyngogram in a patient treated with full-course radiation therapy for a left supraglottic epidermoid cancer shows extrinsic indentation (arrows) on the lateral wall of the pharynx, caused by a large lymph node recurrence.

edema (and associated high signal intensity on T2-weighted images) were misdiagnosed as having recurrent tumor.

There has been recent interest in using functional imaging geared to metabolic activity to distinguish radiation fibrosis from recurrent cancer. A recent study using PET with F-18 fluorodeoxyglucose (FDG) in 15 patients with suspected recurrence showed that malignant lesions accumulate significantly more FDG than do benign ones. The specificity of FDG-PET for diagnosing recurrent cancer was 86% in this relatively small series.

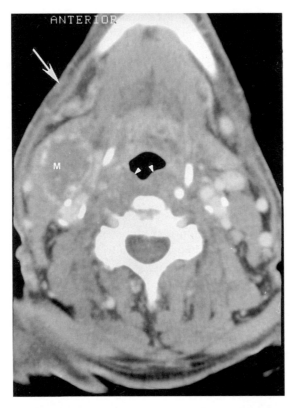

Figure 24-8. CT appearance of tumor recurrence after radiation therapy. This patient underwent CT for evaluation of a clinically palpable lymph node recurrence. A CT section through the oropharynx shows the low-attenuation lymph node mass (M) in the jugulodigastric chain, which proved to be recurrent epidermoid carcinoma. Generalized changes, expected after radiation therapy, are also present. There is thickening of the skin and platysma muscle, as well as infiltration of the subcutaneous fat (arrow). Slightly increased contrast enhancement of the mucosal surface of the posterior wall of the oropharynx (arrowheads) is also observed.

Question 72

Concerning the pharynx after radiation therapy,

    (A) chondronecrosis is a frequent complication of full-course therapy

    (B) asymmetry of the mucosa overlying the arytenoid cartilage is a sign of recurrent carcinoma

    (C) aspiration often occurs without associated coughing

    (D) the epiglottis often exhibits reduced motility

    (E) mucosal biopsy is not completely reliable in diagnosing recurrent cancer within an irradiated field

Radiation therapy is an attractive alternative to surgery for epidermoid cancer of the larynx and pharynx, primarily because it has a high rate of successful disease control and a very low rate of complications. In the series by Robson et al., 286 patients with glottic and supraglottic tumors were treated with no cases of chondronecrosis and no significant laryngeal edema. In a group of patients with no prior form of therapy, Viani et al. reported a radionecrosis rate of 1% for T1 tumors, 4% for T2 tumors, and 3% for T3 tumors. Extensive tumors with cartilaginous invasion and large radiation ports are more likely to develop this complication, but chondronecrosis remains a rare event **(Option (A) is false).**

Successful radiation therapy depends on selective destruction of tumor cells while normal epidermoid and other soft tissues remain relatively spared. The mucosal surfaces of the oro- and hypopharynx, however, have a relatively high radiation sensitivity, in part because of their normally high rate of replication. Death of the tumor therefore necessitates significant injury (and subsequent inflammation) to normal mucosal surfaces. The early-phase inflammatory response gives way to subacute and chronic edema, with proliferation of fibrous tissue in the submucosa of the irradiated tissues. The phase of progressive fibrosis lasts for months after therapy and does not regress. Swelling of all the mucosal surfaces is therefore expected. The inflammatory response is more pronounced on the side of the tumor, since cellular necrosis in the cancer induces a larger response. Accordingly, asymmetric swelling of the pharynx is quite common and does not, by itself, suggest the presence of recurrent carcinoma **(Option (B) is false).** As noted previously, and as illustrated by the test image, ulceration or irregularity of a pharyngeal mucosal surface is highly suggestive of recurrent cancer.

Histologic findings in the mucosa and submucosa in irradiated tissues include varying degrees of nuclear atypia, pleomorphism, and giant-cell formation, findings similar to those produced by cancer. This is one reason for the difficulty encountered by pathologists in establishing a histologic diagnosis of recurrent cancer by examining a biopsy specimen from a patient with an irradiated pharynx **(Option (E) is true).** Other factors include sampling error and the presence of tumor in the soft tissues deep to a superficial mucosal biopsy. In the study of Viani et al., the positive predictive value of biopsy was 91%. However, biopsy was a poor predictor of a negative result (50%) and had only a 25% specificity.

Another effect of the submucosal fibrosis induced by radiation therapy is reduction in the mobility of the affected tissues. Epiglottic thickening has been noted in both symptomatic patients and asymptomatic post-radiation volunteers; quite often there is attendant reduction in epiglottic motility **(Option (D) is true),** which in turn results in incomplete vestibular closure during swallowing. The study by Quillin et al. of patients who completed radiation therapy found that most demonstrated some degree of vestibular penetration and aspiration. Desensitization of the vestibular and proximal tracheal surface mucosa (a result of chronic stimulation by repeated aspiration) results in disappearance of the cough reflex **(Option (C) is true),** thus placing these patients at higher risk for aspiration pneumonia.

Dennis M. Balfe, M.D.
Shawn P. Quillin, M.D.

SUGGESTED READINGS

PHARYNGOGRAPHY AFTER IRRADIATION

1. Ekberg O, Nylander G. Pharyngeal dysfunction after treatment for pharyngeal cancer with surgery and radiotherapy. Gastrointest Radiol 1983; 8:97–104
2. Quillin SP, Balfe DM, Glick SN. Pharyngography after head and neck irradiation: differentiation of postirradiation edema from recurrent tumor. AJR 1993; 161:1205–1208

SUCCESS AND FAILURE OF RADIATION THERAPY

3. Fu KK, Woodhouse RJ, Quivey JM, Phillips TL, Dedo HH. The significance of laryngeal edema following radiotherapy of carcinoma of the vocal cord. Cancer 1982; 49:655–658
4. Kagan AR, Calcaterra T, Ward P, Chan P. Significance of edema of the endolarynx following curative irradiation for carcinoma. AJR 1974; 120:169–172
5. Meoz-Mendez RT, Fletcher GH, Guillamondegui OM, Peters LJ. Analysis of the results of irradiation in the treatment of squamous cell carcinomas of the pharyngeal walls. Int J Radiat Oncol Biol Phys 1978; 4:579–585
6. Nichols RD, Mickelson SA. Partial laryngectomy after irradiation failure. Ann Otol Rhinol Laryngol 1991; 100:176–180

7. Robson NL, Oswal VH, Flood LM. Radiation therapy of laryngeal cancer: a twenty year experience. J Laryngol Otol 1990; 104:699–703
8. Small W Jr, Mittal BB, Brand WN, et al. Results of radiation therapy in early glottic carcinoma: multivariate analysis of prognostic and radiation therapy variables. Radiology 1992; 183:789–794
9. Viani L, Stell PM, Dalby JE. Recurrence after radiotherapy for glottic carcinoma. Cancer 1991; 67:577–584

SECOND PRIMARY CANCERS

10. Teshima T, Inoue T, Chatani M, et al. Incidence of other primary cancers in 1,569 patients with pharyngolaryngeal cancer and treated with radiation therapy. Strahlenther Onkol 1992; 168:213–218

CROSS-SECTIONAL IMAGING AFTER RADIATION THERAPY

11. Bronstein AD, Nyberg DA, Schwartz AN, Shuman WP, Griffin BR. Soft-tissue changes after head and neck radiation: CT findings. AJNR 1989; 10:171–175
12. Glazer HS, Niemeyer JH, Balfe DM, et al. Neck neoplasms: MR imaging. Part II. Posttreatment evaluation. Radiology 1986; 160:349–354
13. Mukherji SK, Mancuso AA, Kotzur IM, et al. Radiologic appearance of the irradiated larynx. Part I. Expected changes. Radiology 1994; 193:141–148

HISTOPATHOLOGY OF THE IRRADIATED PHARYNX

14. Fajardo LFL-G (ed). Pathology of radiation injury. New York: Masson Publishing USA; 1982:47–50

Notes

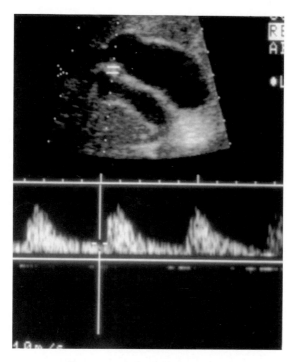

Figure 25-1

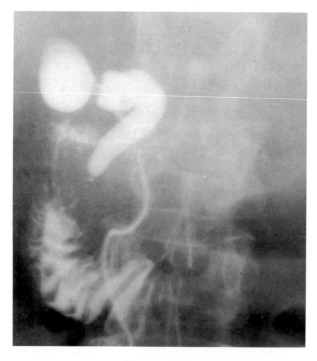

Figure 25-2

Figures 25-1 and 25-2. This 42-year-old woman received an orthotopic liver transplant 3 months ago. She now has abnormal liver function tests. You are shown a longitudinal oblique abdominal sonogram through the porta hepatis (Figure 25-1) and a T-tube cholangiogram (Figure 25-2).

Case 25: Anastomotic Biliary Stricture

Question 73

Which *one* of the following is the MOST likely cause of the finding?

(A) Hepatic artery stenosis
(B) Chronic rejection
(C) Cytomegalovirus infection
(D) Postsurgical fibrosis
(E) Sclerosing cholangitis

Sonographic examination of the region of the porta hepatis (Figure 25-1) demonstrates a markedly dilated bile duct but a normal flow pattern in the hepatic artery (Figure 25-3). Radiographs obtained during contrast infusion into the patient's T tube (Figure 25-2) show a very tight area of narrowing in the midportion of the common bile duct with limited filling of the dilated biliary system proximal to this lesion (Figure 25-4). This liver transplant recipient underwent end-to-end anastomosis of her native common bile duct to the donor duct (choledochocholedochostomy). This type of anastomosis is the most widely performed type of biliary reconstruction in adult liver transplantation. At the time of removal of the recipient liver, the native bile duct is ligated and divided above the insertion of the cystic duct, to provide an adequate length of duct for anastomosis with the donor duct. After placement of the allograft and establishment of portal and arterial reperfusion, a cholecystectomy is performed and the donor duct and recipient duct are then anastomosed in end-to-end fashion. A T tube is then inserted into the duct, with the upper limb of the T tube extending across the anastomosis and the lower limb of the T tube in the recipient bile duct. The lower limb of the T tube exits the recipient bile duct well below the level of the anastomosis (Figure 25-5).

A Roux-en-Y choledochojejunostomy is the second most commonly performed biliary anastomosis. It is used in children and in adults with primary biliary disease or with a discrepancy between the sizes of the donor and recipient ducts; it is also used in patients undergoing retrans-

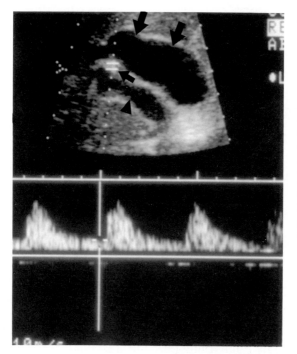

Figure 25-3 (left) (Same as Figure 25-1). Anastomotic stricture. A sonogram of the porta hepatis demonstrates a markedly dilated common bile duct (large arrows). The main portal vein (arrowhead) and the hepatic artery in which the Doppler gate has been placed (small arrow) are also seen. Normal arterial flow is seen in the hepatic artery.

Figure 25-4 (right) (Same as Figure 25-2). Anastomotic stricture. Contrast infusion into the patient's T tube shows a very tight area of narrowing in the mid-common bile duct (arrows) in the region of the surgical anastomosis. There is poor filling of a dilated biliary system proximal to the stricture.

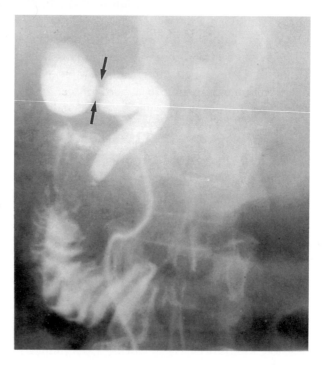

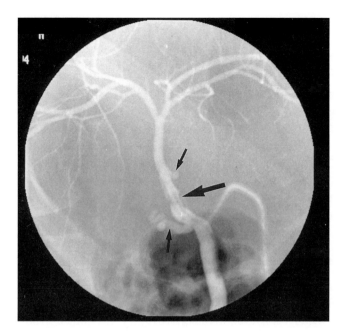

Figure 25-5. Normal T-tube cholangiogram 1 week after liver transplantation. A choledochocholedochostomy has been performed. The T tube enters the recipient duct, with one limb bridging the anastomosis between the recipient duct and donor duct (large arrow). Note two cystic duct remnants (small arrows).

plantation. At surgery, a Roux limb is fashioned and the donor common bile duct is anastomosed to it. External drainage may or may not be performed.

The narrowing evident in the midportion of the duct in the test patient represents a stricture at the surgical anastomosis. Stricture formation at the site of the surgical anastomosis is most probably due to the surgical procedure itself with resultant fibrosis and scar formation **(Option (D) is correct).** These strictures occur weeks to years after transplantation.

Complications involving the biliary ducts after transplantation are common, occurring in 11.6% of patients in a recent review of 1,792 transplants performed at the University of Pittsburgh. Most (69.5%) of these complications were either biliary strictures or bile leaks. Most biliary strictures after transplantation are anastomotic strictures (87% in the Pittsburgh series). Other biliary complications in that series included ampullary dysfunction, bile cast syndrome, bilomas, and choledocholithiasis.

The other options listed are potential causes of strictures but involve the intrahepatic donor bile ducts within the graft rather than the anastomotic site. Intrahepatic strictures are usually multiple (76% in the series reported by Campbell et al.). They occur less frequently than anastomotic strictures. Ischemia due to hepatic artery stenosis (Option (A)) or occlusion has been demonstrated to be a major cause of intrahepatic biliary strictures. The intrahepatic biliary tree in the allograft is dependent solely on the hepatic artery for its blood supply, because collateral blood supply, which is normally present from the gastroduodenal artery, has been severed during surgery. Zajko et al. reported finding bile duct abnormalities on cholangiography in 84% of patients with complete or partial occlusion of the hepatic artery. The most common abnormalities in this series were nonanastomotic bile leakage, due to ductal necrosis, and nonanastomotic strictures. Both are probably due to a vascular insult. Bile duct necrosis results from transmural ischemia, whereas a stricture forms after mucosal or submucosal ischemic injury. Although intrahepatic biliary strictures can result from hepatic artery occlusion or significant stenosis, a stricture isolated to the site of anastomosis is unlikely to be due to that cause.

Ischemic injuries produced by mechanisms other than compromise of the main hepatic artery also cause nonanastomotic biliary strictures. These mechanisms include prolonged donor liver ischemia times, chronic rejection (Option (B)) with associated arteriopathy, and ABO blood group incompatibility. A stricture at the surgical anastomosis, as seen in the test images, is unlikely to be due to any other cause than fibrosis around the surgical site itself.

Cytomegalovirus (CMV) infection (Option (C)) had previously been suggested to be a cause of a nonanastomotic biliary stricture. Dolmatch et al. reported stricture formation, similar to that seen associated with sclerosing cholangitis, in patients with AIDS and proposed that infection with CMV or *Cryptosporidium* species was the cause. Ward et al., however, have reported that the frequency of CMV infection was no greater in liver transplant recipients with hilar biliary strictures than in those without such strictures. This raises some doubt about the role of opportunistic infection in biliary stricture formation in liver transplant patients. CMV infection, a common opportunistic infection following transplantation, can be asymptomatic, detected only by positive blood or urine culture, or can result in fever and specific organ system disease. CMV hepatitis is common and can be difficult to differentiate clinically from rejection, requiring liver biopsy. Interstitial pneumonia due to CMV is also common following transplantation. CMV can also affect the bowel, leading to diarrhea and abdominal pain.

There is evidence suggesting that patients who undergo transplantation for primary sclerosing cholangitis (Option (E)) have a higher incidence of biliary strictures after transplantation than do patients who undergo transplants for other causes. In a review of 10 years of experience at the University of Pittsburgh, Sheng et al. found that intrahepatic and nonanastomotic strictures were more common in patients who underwent transplantation for sclerosing cholangitis than in other transplant recipients. In most centers, patients with sclerosing cholangitis undergo a biliary anastomosis, which consists of anastomosis of the donor common bile duct to the jejunum (choledochojejunostomy) rather than the choledochocholedochostomy seen in the test patient, making sclerosing cholangitis an unlikely cause of the findings in the test patient. The frequency of strictures at the anastomosis, as opposed to strictures at nonanastomotic sites, in patients undergoing a choledochojejunostomy during transplantation for sclerosing cholangitis was not significantly different from that in patients undergoing a choledochojejunostomy during transplantation for other indications.

Cholangiography via an indwelling T tube, by percutaneous transhepatic cholangiography, or by endoscopic retrograde cholangiography is the definitive examination for detection of biliary abnormalities in transplant recipients. The biliary dilatation in the test patient is evident sonographically; however, sonography is generally not as useful as cholangiography for detection of biliary complications. The close postoperative laboratory monitoring of most liver transplant recipients may result in detection of a biliary complication before biliary dilatation occurs, making cholangiography mandatory in patients with suspected biliary complications. This is particularly important since early graft dysfunction due to rejection is not easily differentiated from a biliary tract complication.

The interventional radiologist plays an integral role in the management, as well as the diagnosis, of patients with biliary complications by performing both percutaneous biliary drainage and dilatation of anastomotic stenoses. In patients with nonanastomotic biliary strictures, particularly strictures due to ischemia or chronic rejection, retransplantation may be necessary, but percutaneous biliary drainage can be an effective temporizing measure.

Liver transplantation has become an accepted treatment for end-stage liver disease and is being performed with increasing frequency at a number of institutions worldwide. Despite improvement in the post-transplantation survival rate, most notably as a result of advances in immunosuppressive therapy, the frequency of complications following this procedure is high. Graft dysfunction can result from a number of possible causes. In addition to biliary complications, vascular and infectious complications, graft rejection, drug-related hepatic injury, and various miscellaneous complications can occur.

Graft failure in the immediate preoperative period is usually due to one of four general causes: technical (surgical) complications, ischemic injury to the graft during donor death or organ harvesting, accelerated rejection, or, rarely, unrecognized disease in the donor liver. In the early postoperative period, causes of graft dysfunction include rejection, suboptimal revascularization, biliary leakage, infection (with a variety of organisms, including CMV, herpes simplex virus, Epstein-Barr virus, adenovirus, bacteria, and fungi), and drug hepatotoxicity. Late complications include biliary strictures due to defects in biliary reconstruction, recurrence of hepatic disease in the graft, infection by hepatitis B virus, and chronic rejection. Acute rejection and chronic rejection of the allograft are diagnosed by liver biopsy and histologic evaluation; imaging studies have not been shown to be reliable in diagnosing rejection. However, the radiologist is still called upon to exclude causes of graft dysfunction that can mimic rejection, particularly vascular and biliary causes. Diagnosis of complications following transplantation is often difficult because the clinical data and laboratory findings are nonspecific. The radiologist is often intensively involved with these patients and frequently provides valuable information for the assessment of transplant recipients with graft dysfunction.

Question 74

Concerning the portal vein in liver transplant recipients,

(A) a normal Doppler sonographic examination demonstrates continuous flow with variation due to respiration
(B) thrombosis of this vessel is the most common vascular complication after transplantation
(C) the site of anastomosis cannot be visualized by ultrasonography
(D) stenosis at the anastomosis is characterized on Doppler sonography by low-velocity blood flow in the main portal vein distal to the anastomosis

Doppler ultrasonography is widely used to evaluate the vessels supplying the liver allograft. Doppler examination allows noninvasive evaluation of vascular patency, so that angiography can be reserved for confirmation of Doppler findings in selected patients. Real-time and Doppler sonographic evaluation of the main portal vein and right and left branches are performed with special attention to the vascular anastomosis. The addition of color Doppler imaging expedites the identification of vessels and visualization of flow within them, but spectral Doppler is essential for quantifying stenoses, measuring volume flow rates, and assessing vascular impedance.

On Doppler sonography, the normal portal vein demonstrates continuous flow with variation due to respiration (Figure 25-6) **(Option (A) is true).** Portal vein complications of liver transplantation, including thrombosis or stenosis, are reported to occur in 1 to 2% of patients. Portal

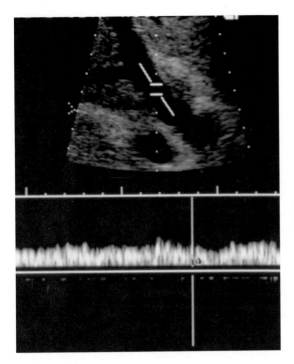

Figure 25-6. Normal Doppler examination of the portal vein in a liver transplant recipient, obtained while the patient is in suspended respiration. The time-velocity spectrum shows continuous blood flow in the portal vein directed toward the liver.

vein complications are less frequent than hepatic artery complications **(Option (B) is false)**, which are reported to occur in 11 to 13% of transplant recipients. The main portal vein and the surgical anastomosis are readily visualized on sonographic examination **(Option (C) is false)**. Complete thrombosis is demonstrated by the identification of echogenic material within the lumen of the portal vein and by the absence of Doppler flow signals. Nonoccluding thrombus is identified as an echogenic filling defect within the lumen, often occurring adjacent to the anastomosis (Figure 25-7). Stenosis at the end-to-end portal vein anastomosis can be diagnosed on Doppler examination by demonstration of a high-velocity jet through the anastomosis and by evidence of distal turbulence. Low-velocity blood flow is not a specific finding **(Option (D) is false)**. Indeed, portal venous flow rates are extremely variable, and flow rate has not been shown to be a reliable indicator of allograft function.

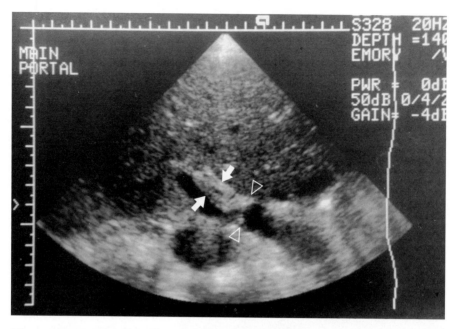

Figure 25-7. Nonoccluding portal vein thrombus. A rounded echogenic mass (arrows) is seen within the lumen of the portal vein adjacent to the surgical anastomosis (arrowheads). Doppler evaluation confirmed the presence of flow within the portal vein.

Question 75

Concerning hepatic artery thrombosis in liver transplant recipients,

    (A) it is more common in adults than in children
    (B) massive hepatic necrosis is the most common initial clinical presentation
    (C) retransplantation is often necessary
    (D) it occasionally presents clinically with bile leakage

Patency of the hepatic artery is critical to graft survival in the early post-transplantation period. Thrombosis of the hepatic artery is the most common and most significant vascular complication of hepatic transplantation. The frequency of hepatic artery thrombosis has been reported to range from 3 to 12% in adults and 12 to 42% in children **(Option (A) is false).** The higher frequency of thrombosis in children is probably related to the small size of the vessels and the necessity for more-complicated vascular anastomoses. Hepatic artery thrombosis can be clinically occult, presenting initially as elevation of liver function tests in 70 to 80% of graft recipients. More abrupt presentations, including massive hepatic necrosis, septic hepatic infarction with bacteremia, bile leaks, and bile duct rupture with bile peritonitis, are less common **(Option (B) is false).** In adults, emergent retransplantation is almost always necessary after a diagnosis of hepatic artery occlusion in the early postoperative period **(Option (C) is true).** In children, survival after hepatic artery occlusion because of development of adequate arterial collaterals has been reported. The biliary tree receives its blood supply from the hepatic artery, and so arterial occlusion can result in severe ischemic injury of the bile ducts with consequent necrosis and bile leakage **(Option (D) is true).** As noted above, ischemia can also lead to formation of biliary strictures.

Doppler sonography has become accepted as a screening method for the diagnosis of hepatic artery occlusion after transplantation, with high reported sensitivity and specificity. Occlusion is diagnosed by the inability to obtain an arterial Doppler tracing from the hepatic artery distal to the anastomosis. However, false-positive examinations (failure to obtain a hepatic artery Doppler tracing when the hepatic artery is patent) have been reported as a result of slow flow within a small patent vessel, a high-grade anastomotic stricture, or technical failure. Failure to obtain a technically adequate sonographic examination may be due to causes such as the patient's body habitus, motion, or an inability to obtain a sonographic window due to position of the surgical wound. False-negative examinations occur as a result of collateralized thrombosis. For this reason, angiographic confirmation of occlusion should be sought. Recently, Dodd et al. reported that the sensitivity of detection of hepatic artery stenosis or thrombosis could be improved by assessing the hepatic arterial resistive index (RI) and systolic acceleration time (SAT) and by combining these parameters with no-flow criteria or with elevated peak velocity (greater than 2 m/second). The use of threshold values of an RI of less than 0.5 and a SAT of 0.08 second or longer improved the sensitivity for stenosis by 30%, resulting in an overall sensitivity and specificity for marked hepatic artery disease of 97 and 64%, respectively (Figure 25-8).

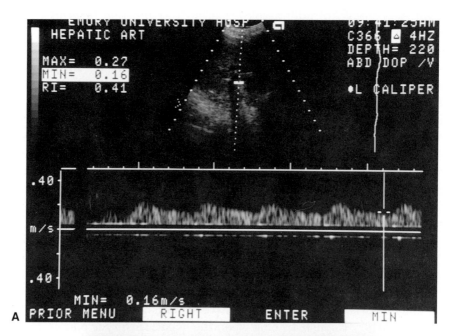

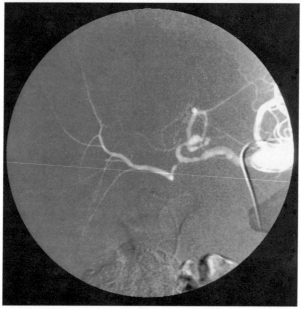

Figure 25-8. Hepatic artery stenosis. (A) A Doppler sonographic evaluation of the hepatic artery demonstrates an abnormal hepatic artery waveform, with a low RI (0.41) and a SAT of 0.2 second. The combination of these findings suggests that significant arterial disease is present. (B) An arteriogram obtained immediately following the sonographic examination demonstrates multifocal hepatic artery stenoses.

Question 76

Concerning post-transplantation lymphoproliferative disorder,

(A) it is related to Epstein-Barr virus infection
(B) it affects less than 1% of transplant recipients
(C) it is more likely to occur following liver transplantation than following heart-lung transplantation
(D) the mean interval between transplantation and development of the disease is 5 years
(E) treatment is the same as that for classic non-Hodgkin's lymphoma

The increased incidence of malignancy in organ transplant recipients, first reported by Penn et al. in 1969, is a well-documented complication of immunosuppression. Changes in immunosuppressive therapy, particularly the introduction of cyclosporine (in conjunction with steroids) as the standard immunosuppressive regimen following transplantation, have not changed the overall incidence of malignancy but have resulted in a change in the relative incidence of types of cancer, with a reported frequency of lymphoreticular tumors even higher than that in the non-cyclosporine-treated group. The disease process known as post-transplantation lymphoproliferative disorder (PTLD) is related to uncontrolled lymphoproliferation in the immunocompromised patient and has been reported to cover a spectrum of diseases from infectious mononucleosis to malignant non-Hodgkin's lymphoma, with B-cell non-Hodgkin's lymphoma the most common type. A strong association of PTLD with infection by Epstein-Barr virus has been documented by serologic evidence of primary Epstein-Barr virus infection **(Option (A) is true).**

The overall frequency of diagnosis of PTLD in the largest reported patient series is approximately 2%. This is probably a significant underestimation of the true incidence of PTLD, since some cases are not recognized until autopsy **(Option (B) is false).** Small differences in tumor frequency among recipients of different organs are reported, with kidney recipients having the lowest rate and heart-lung recipients having the highest (1% vs. 4.6% in the series reported by Nalesnik et al.) (higher than liver transplant recipients) **(Option (C) is false).** The time of onset of disease varies, ranging from within a month to years after transplantation, but most cases occur within a year; the mean and median times of diagnosis in the Pittsburgh series reported by Nalesnik et al. were 11.5 and 4.5 months, respectively, after transplantation **(Option (D) is false).**

PTLD can be confined to a single organ, but in many patients it is a diffuse disease involving multiple organ systems. Common sites of involvement include the brain, tonsils, lymph nodes, bowel, and lungs.

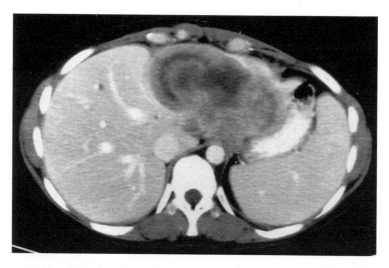

Figure 25-9. Post-transplantation lymphoproliferative disorder. This 30-year-old woman presented with cervical lymph node and tonsillar enlargement 2 years after transplantation. A CT scan demonstrates a large heterogeneous mass with central necrosis in the left lobe of the liver. Epstein-Barr virus titers were positive. After biopsy revealed PTLD, the patient was treated with surgical debulking of the tumor mass and a decrease in her immunosuppressive regimen.

The radiographic appearance of PTLD in the abdomen includes bulky enlarged nodal masses that may have central areas of necrosis; focal hepatic (Figure 25-9) and renal lesions; and focal bowel masses (Figure 25-10) or diffuse bowel wall thickening.

Therapy for PTLD, in contrast to non-transplant-associated tumors, is directed to restoring immunocompetence by reducing or discontinuing immunosuppression **(Option (E) is false),** which frequently results in regression of the disease. Clinical regression of tumor was seen in 10 of 43 patients treated with reduction in immunosuppression in the University of Pittsburgh series. Tumors resolved after treatment with surgical resection and reduced immunosuppression in 15 patients. Four patients had tumor response to chemotherapy or radiation therapy. There was no response to therapy in five patients. PTLD was diagnosed at autopsy in six patients. Large focal tumors, such as the one seen in Figure 25-9, may first be surgically resected to debulk the tumor mass. Untreated, PTLD has a high mortality.

Judith L. Chezmar, M.D.

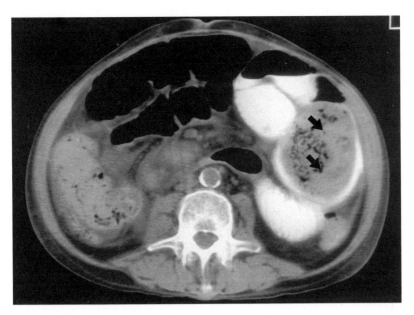

Figure 25-10. Post-transplantation lymphoproliferative disorder. This 50-year-old man underwent liver transplantation 7 months before this CT examination. This CT image, obtained with oral contrast only, demonstrates a large intraluminal mass, with a nodular soft tissue component involving the wall of the jejunum (arrows). At surgery, the small bowel lumen was filled with blood and contained ulcerated nodules involving the bowel wall. Pathologic evaluation demonstrated a malignant tumor with cellular features consistent with PTLD. Analysis for the presence of Epstein-Barr virus by colorimetric *in situ* hybridization was positive.

SUGGESTED READINGS

LIVER TRANSPLANTATION: BILIARY COMPLICATIONS

1. Campbell WL, Sheng R, Zajko AB, Abu-Elmagd K, Demetris AJ. Intrahepatic biliary strictures after liver transplantation. Radiology 1994; 191:735–740
2. Colonna JO II, Shaked A, Gomes AS, et al. Biliary strictures complicating liver transplantation. Incidence, pathogenesis, management, and outcome. Ann Surg 1992; 216:344–352
3. Dolmatch BL, Laing FC, Federle MP, Jeffrey RB, Cello J. AIDS-related cholangitis: radiographic findings in nine patients. Radiology 1987; 163:313–316
4. Greif F, Bronsther OL, Van Thiel DH, et al. The incidence, timing, and management of biliary tract complications after orthotopic liver transplantation. Ann Surg 1994; 219:40–45

5. Lerut J, Gordon RD, Iwatsuki S, et al. Biliary tract complications in human orthotopic liver transplantation. Transplantation 1987; 43:47–51

6. Sheng R, Zajko AB, Campbell WL, Abu-Elmagd K. Biliary strictures in hepatic transplants: prevalence and types in patients with primary sclerosing cholangitis vs those with other liver diseases. AJR 1993; 161:297–300

7. Ward EM, Kiely MJ, Maus TP, Wiesner RH, Krom RA. Hilar biliary strictures after liver transplantation: cholangiography and percutaneous treatment. Radiology 1990; 177:259–263

8. Zajko AB, Bron KM, Campbell WL, Behal R, Van Thiel DH, Starzl TE. Percutaneous transhepatic cholangiography and biliary drainage after liver transplantation: a five year experience. Gastrointest Radiol 1987; 12:137–143

9. Zajko AB, Campbell WL, Logsdon GA, et al. Cholangiographic findings in hepatic artery occlusion after liver transplantation. AJR 1987; 149:485–489

LIVER TRANSPLANTATION: VASCULAR COMPLICATIONS

10. Dalen K, Day DL, Ascher NL, et al. Imaging of vascular complications after hepatic transplantation. AJR 1988; 150:1285–1290

11. Dodd GD III, Memel DS, Zajko AB, Baron RL, Santaguida LA. Hepatic artery stenosis and thrombosis in transplant recipients: Doppler diagnosis with resistive index and systolic acceleration time. Radiology 1994; 192:657–661

12. Flint EW, Sumkin JH, Zajko AB, Bowen A. Duplex sonography of hepatic artery thrombosis after liver transplantation. AJR 1988; 151:481–483

13. Letourneau JG, Day DL, Ascher NL, et al. Abdominal sonography after hepatic transplantation: results in 36 patients. AJR 1987; 149:299–303

14. Segel MC, Zajko AB, Bowen A, et al. Hepatic artery thrombosis after liver transplantation: radiologic evaluation. AJR 1986; 146:137–141

15. Taylor KJ, Morse SS, Weltin GG, Riely CA, Flye MW. Liver transplant recipients: portable duplex US with correlative angiography. Radiology 1986; 159:357–363

16. Tzakis AG, Gordon RD, Shaw BW Jr, Iwatsuki S, Starzl TE. Clinical presentation of hepatic arterial thrombosis after liver transplantation in the cyclosporin era. Transplantation 1985; 40:667–671

17. Wozney P, Zajko AB, Bron KM, Point S, Starzl TE. Vascular complications after liver transplantation: a 5-year experience. AJR 1986; 147:657–663

LIVER TRANSPLANTATION: GENERAL

18. Starzl TE, Demetris AJ, Van Theil D. Liver transplantation. N Engl J Med 1989; 321:1014–1022, 1092–1099

POST-TRANSPLANTATION LYMPHOPROLIFERATIVE DISORDER

19. Day DL. The role of imaging in the evaluation of malignancy complicating transplantation. In: Letourneau JG, Day DL, Ascher NL (eds), Radiology of organ transplantation. St. Louis: Mosby-Year Book; 1991:60–67

20. Harris KM, Schwartz ML, Slasky BS, Nalesnik M, Makowka L. Posttransplantation cyclosporine-induced lymphoproliferative disorders: clinical and radiologic manifestations. Radiology 1987; 162:697–700

21. Honda H, Barloon TJ, Franken EA Jr, Garneau RA, Smith JL. Clinical and radiologic features of malignant neoplasms in organ transplant recipients: cyclosporine-treated vs untreated patients. AJR 1990; 154:271–274

22. Honda H, Franken EA Jr, Barloon TJ, Smith JL. Hepatic lymphoma in cyclosporine-treated transplant recipients: sonographic and CT findings. AJR 1989; 152:501–503

23. Nalesnik MA, Jaffe R, Starzl TE, et al. The pathology of posttransplant lymphoproliferative disorders occurring in the setting of cyclosporine A-prednisone immunosuppression. Am J Pathol 1988; 133:173–192

24. Penn I, Hammond W, Brettschneider L, Starzl TE. Malignant lymphomas in transplantation patients. Transplant Proc 1969; 1:106–112

25. Starzl TE, Nalesnik MA, Porter KA, et al. Reversibility of lymphomas and lymphoproliferative lesions developing under cyclosporin-steroid therapy. Lancet 1984; 1:584–587

26. Tubman DE, Frick MP, Hanto DW. Lymphoma after organ transplantation: radiologic manifestations in the central nervous system, thorax, and abdomen. Radiology 1983; 149:625–631

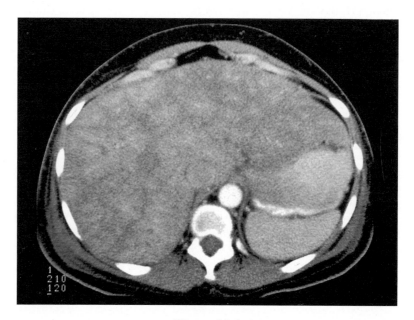

Figure 26-1

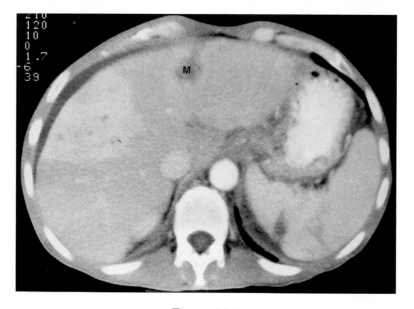

Figure 26-2

Case 26: Time-Related Contrast Enhancement Effects on Liver CT

Questions 77 through 80

Four patients underwent postcontrast CT for evaluation of abnormal liver function tests. For each numbered image listed below (Figures 26-1 through 26-4), select the *one* lettered explanation for the CT appearance (A, B, C, D, or E) that is MOST likely. Each lettered explanation may be used once, more than once, or not at all.

77. Figure 26-1
78. Figure 26-2 (Note: this patient has a known metastasis [M])
79. Figure 26-3
80. Figure 26-4

(A) Preferential segmental arterial flow
(B) Thrombosis of the main portal vein
(C) Hepatic venous outflow impairment
(D) Superior vena cava obstruction
(E) Focal fatty infiltration

The CT scan in Figure 26-1 was obtained during the arterial phase after rapid intravenous administration of contrast material. The enhancement pattern of the hepatic parenchyma is distinctly abnormal. There is a network of low-attenuation branching lines extending diffusely throughout the liver (Figure 26-5). These lucencies do not conform to segmental or subsegmental anatomic boundaries, and they are present in both peripheral and central hepatic regions. No identifiable branches of the hepatic veins are visible. This peculiar appearance is virtually pathognomonic of hepatic venous outflow impairment **(Option (C) is the correct answer to Question 77).**

Hepatic venous outflow impairment can be caused by several mechanisms. The patient whose CT scan is shown in Figure 26-1 had a long history of severe pulmonary hypertension and had recently exhibited

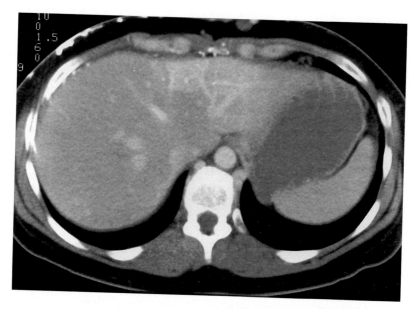

Figure 26-3

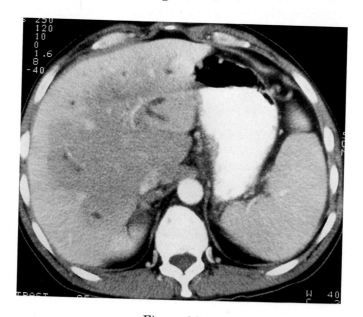

Figure 26-4

clinical evidence of right heart failure. Her hepatic veins were anatomically patent, but there was functional obstruction to hepatic venous outflow by the failing right ventricle. In a report of seven such patients, Moulton et al. noted the frequent occurrence of reflux of contrast mate-

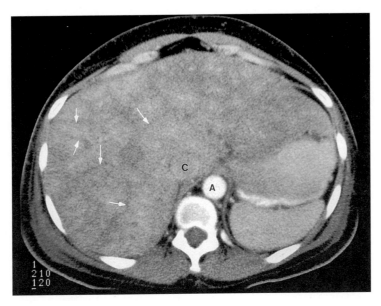

Figure 26-5 (Same as Figure 26-1). Passive congestion of the liver due to right heart failure. This 30-year-old woman has a congenital atrial septal defect, resulting in pulmonary hypertension and right ventricular failure. A CT section obtained during the hepatic artery-dominant phase (30 seconds after the beginning of rapid contrast infusion) shows a strikingly heterogeneous enhancement pattern characterized by multiple linear low-attenuation bands (arrows) throughout the hepatic parenchyma. The distribution of these bands does not conform to segmental boundaries. There is no enhancement of the inferior vena cava (C) or of any of the major hepatic veins, even though the aorta (A) is densely opacified.

rial into the inferior vena cava and hepatic veins, with enlargement of these structures (Figure 26-6). This finding is also explained by the presence of high right atrial filling pressure; reduced atrial compliance causes contrast-rich blood from the superior vena cava to be regurgitated into the inferior vena cava and main hepatic veins. A similar phenomenon occurs in patients with tricuspid valve regurgitation.

Anatomic obstruction of the inferior vena cava or hepatic veins (Budd-Chiari syndrome) causes this same enhancement pattern (Figure 26-7). This uncommon entity is most frequently related to hypercoagulable states; oral contraceptives and polycythemia are frequently associated with it. In children, congenital membranous webs may be the underlying cause. Up to 30% of cases are idiopathic. The parenchymal enhancement pattern is indistinguishable from that in Figure 26-1; however, the clinical features of Budd-Chiari syndrome are different from those of simple passive congestion. Patients with Budd-Chiari syndrome

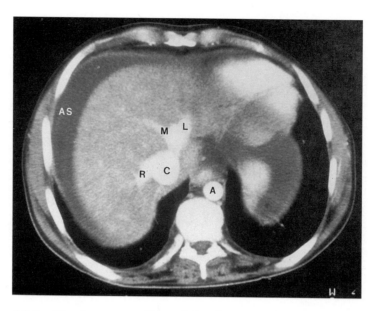

Figure 26-6. Passive congestion of the liver with elevated right atrial filling pressure. A CT section through the dome of the liver shows dense enhancement of the aorta (A), indicating that the scan was obtained in the arterial phase of contrast enhancement. Concentrated contrast material from the upper extremity has refluxed from the right atrium to opacify the inferior vena cava (C) and all three major hepatic veins, i.e., right (R), middle (M), and left (L). Note the presence of ascites (AS).

almost always present with abdominal pain and rapidly accumulating ascites. Biopsy specimens from patients with Budd-Chiari syndrome frequently show perivenular necrosis; this is an uncommon observation in patients with chronic passive congestion. The caudate lobe has a separate venous drainage (through multiple small veins directly into the inferior vena cava) and is therefore frequently spared when the major hepatic veins are occluded. Blood flow to the caudate typically increases in this situation, leading to marked enlargement of the lobe; the attenuation of the caudate can also differ from that of the remaining hepatic parenchyma. On scans obtained without contrast enhancement, it is usually hyperdense compared with the rest of the liver. In up to 20% of patients with Budd-Chiari syndrome, portal vein thrombosis is present as well and segmental liver infarction may be observed (Figure 26-8).

A pathologically closely related entity that can produce identical CT features is veno-occlusive disease. This entity was originally reported in Jamaican children with bush-tea poisoning. It can occur in any patient undergoing antimetabolite chemotherapy or immunosuppression; how-

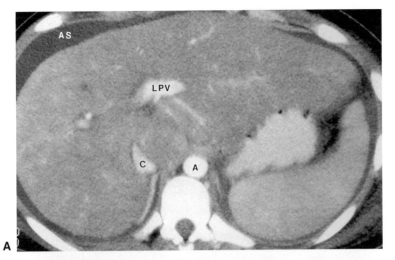

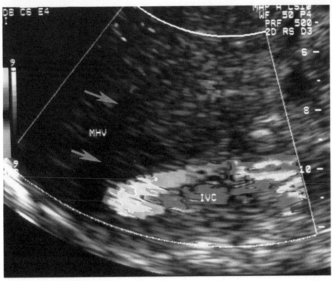

Figure 26-7. Budd-Chiari syndrome. This 38-year-old woman with a history of oral contraceptive use developed painful abdominal distension and deteriorating liver function. (A) A CT section through the liver immediately superior to the porta hepatis shows mottled hepatic parenchymal enhancement similar to but not as severe as the pattern shown in Figure 26-1. The inferior vena cava (C) is well opacified, but none of the major hepatic veins is identified. Note the peculiar distortion of the contour of the vena cava as a result of acute swelling of the liver from venous congestion. Ascites (AS) is present and is frequently associated with acute hepatic venous thrombosis. A = aorta; LPV = left portal vein. (B) A color flow Doppler sonogram obtained at the same time as the CT scan in panel A shows turbulent flow within the inferior vena cava (IVC) and complete absence of color signal within the middle hepatic vein (MHV; arrows). Subsequent evaluation also confirmed absence of flow in the left and right hepatic veins. The patient underwent liver transplantation, and the presence of hepatic vein thrombosis was confirmed at surgery.

447

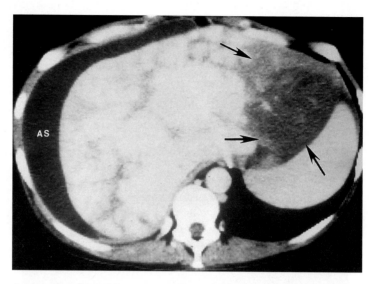

Figure 26-8. Combined hepatic and portal vein thrombosis in a 56-year-old woman with sudden onset of painful abdominal distension. A CT section through the dome of the liver demonstrates linear low-attenuation stripes similar to those seen in Figure 26-1. There is diffuse low attenuation involving the lateral segment of the left hepatic lobe (arrows). This proved to be segmental infarction; subsequent evaluation confirmed thrombosis of both the hepatic and portal veins. AS = ascites.

ever, it is most common in patients who have had bone marrow transplantation, in whom it is a major cause of morbidity. Major hepatic veins can be patent in veno-occlusive disease, but the terminal hepatic veins are filled with fibrous tissue, probably as a result of endothelial injury.

The pathologic correlate to the strikingly heterogeneous CT appearance shown in Figure 26-1 is not known. It has been established, however, that there is a marked increase in hepatic lymph flow when the hepatic veins are obstructed. Perilymphatic and perivenous edema could account for the widespread reticular pattern.

Preferential segmental arterial flow (Option (A)) is a response to decreased portal venous flow to a segment or lobe; as described below, this results in a homogeneously hyperdense segment or lobe, not the mottled appearance seen in Figure 26-1. Portal vein thrombosis (Option (B)) produces a pattern of central diminution of liver enhancement, not a diffuse pattern such as that seen in the test image. The liver enhancement abnormality seen in superior vena cava obstruction (Option (D)) affects only a part of the left lobe. Fatty infiltration (Option (E)) can be diffuse, segmental, or nodular but is unlikely to appear in a linear pattern, as seen in the test image.

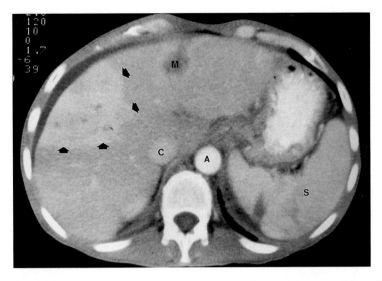

Figure 26-9 (Same as Figure 26-2). Transient hepatic attenuation difference due to preferential segmental arterial flow. This 57-year-old man with known metastases from a colorectal primary cancer was being evaluated for possible hepatic resection. A CT section obtained during the arterial dominant phase shows a low-attenuation metastasis (M) in the lateral segment of the left hepatic lobe. There is a wedge-shaped area of increased enhancement (arrows), whose margins conform to the boundaries of the anterior superior right hepatic segment (segment 8 in Couinaud's classification). There was a metastasis within this segment (shown on another section). A = aorta; C = inferior vena cava; S = spleen.

The CT scan in Figure 26-2 was obtained during the arterial phase after rapid intravenous infusion of iodinated contrast material. There is patchy enhancement of the spleen (a normal finding during the arterial phase). A rounded 2.5-cm low-attenuation lesion (M) present within the left hepatic lobe represents a metastatic deposit. Most of the anterior segment of the right hepatic lobe demonstrates hyperenhancement compared with the posterior segment (Figure 26-9). The straight boundaries of this regional enhancement and its anatomic segmental distribution are diagnostic of the so-called transient hepatic attenuation difference (THAD) due to preferential segmental arterial flow **(Option (A) is the correct answer to Question 78).** The transitory nature of this phenomenon is confirmed by rescanning the same anatomic section during the equilibrium phase (Figure 26-10)

Doppmann et al. have reported that, in primates, any intrahepatic process (benign or malignant) that increases the intraparenchymal pressure within a hepatic segment will result in portal flow away from that

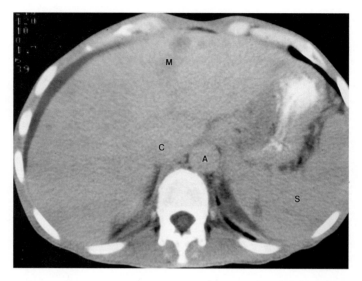

Figure 26-10. Same patient as in Figures 26-2 and 26-9. Transient hepatic attenuation difference due to preferential segmental arterial flow. A CT section at the same anatomic level obtained approximately 5 minutes after Figures 26-2 and 26-9. The attenuation of the anterior superior right segment is now the same as that of the surrounding liver. Note the diminished conspicuity of the metastasis (M) during this equilibrium phase. A = aorta; C = inferior vena cava; S = spleen.

segment. The decrease in portal blood flow produced by that segmental shunting will, in turn, produce an increase in hepatic artery flow to the same segment (Figure 26-11). The mechanism for that increase is multifactorial; in part, it is due simply to the removal of a slowly flowing stream (the portal vein), so that the resistance to hepatic artery flow to that segment is reduced and the volume of flow therefore increases. CT sections obtained during the arterial phase will therefore show hyperenhancement; scans obtained later, during the portal or equilibrium phase, will show no differential attenuation. This phenomenon was reported in 1982 by Itai et al., who suggested that it might be caused either by diversion of arterial flow ("steal") via arteriovenous communications or by an increase in reflex hepatic artery flow as a result of occlusion of the portal vein. Both arterioportal communications and hypervascular tumors can produce THAD (Figure 26-12); however, they are not necessary for its occurrence. Likewise, segmental portal vein occlusion will certainly produce an increase in hepatic artery blood flow (Figure 26-13), but occlusion is not necessary for this effect; THAD has been observed in patients with patent portal veins.

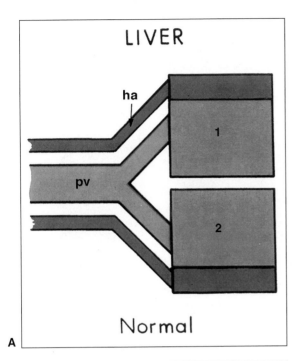

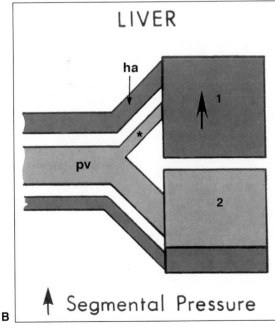

Figure 26-11. Line drawings depicting the mechanism responsible for transient hepatic attenuation difference. (A) Diagrammatic representation of blood flow to two segments (1 and 2) of normal liver. There is symmetric distribution of blood flow to the hepatic segments from the hepatic artery (ha) and portal vein (pv). The hepatic artery, however, supplies only about 25% of the oxygenated blood to the liver segments. (B) Diagrammatic representation of blood flow to the same segments as in panel A when there is increased pressure (↑) in segment 1. Flow within the portal vein (pv) of that segment (✷) is markedly reduced. Hepatic artery (ha) flow to the segment accordingly increases to compensate for loss of portal vein flow. Images obtained during the hepatic artery-dominant phase will therefore show increased enhancement of segment 1 compared with segment 2, since 75% of the blood flowing to segment 2 contains no contrast medium at that time.

The finding in Figure 26-2 is the imaging correlate to disordered hemodynamics. Other imaging methods capable of displaying physiologic information would be expected to show similar findings. CT arterial por-

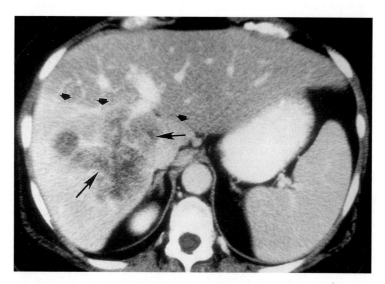

Figure 26-12. Transient hepatic attenuation difference due to arterio-portal shunting in a 55-year-old man with chronic active hepatitis, who developed a large hepatoma (long arrows) with angiographic evidence of arterioportal shunting. A CT image shows marked enhancement of the right lobe compared with the left, resulting from increased hepatic artery flow through the tumor into the portal system of the right lobe. The margins of the hyperenhanced region (short arrows) conform to the boundaries of the right lobe.

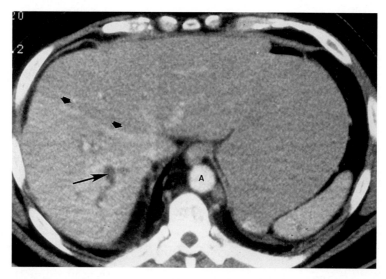

Figure 26-13. Transient hepatic attenuation difference due to portal vein thrombosis in a 35-year-old man recovering from acute pancreatitis. A CT section through the dome of the liver shows increased contrast enhancement of the right lobe compared with the left. The margins of the area of increased enhancement (short arrows) conform to the boundaries of the posterior superior segment of the right hepatic lobe (segment 7 in Couinaud's classification). A low-attenuation branching structure (long arrow) is identified in the center of the affected lobe. This proved to be segmental portal vein thrombosis. A = aorta.

tography (CTAP) is an example; in this technique, infusion of iodinated contrast material into a catheter placed in the superior mesenteric artery produces contrast-rich blood within the superior mesenteric vein, in turn leading to selective opacification of the normal hepatic parenchyma via the portal vein. Hepatic tumors and metastases are supplied by the hepatic artery, and therefore they become apparent as hypoattenuating lesions. The presence of a segmental portal flow defect on CTAP has been widely reported; like THAD, this defect can be related to segmental portal vein occlusion or simply to physiologic portal vein redistribution associated with increased segmental pressure. Accordingly, observation of a segmental or lobar flow defect is not compelling evidence for portal vein occlusion by tumor (Figure 26-14).

Alteration in portal blood flow may be the explanation for the frequent observation of pseudolesions on CTAP (see also Case 28) (Figure 26-15). The subcapsular portion of the medial segment of the left hepatic lobe, adjacent to the porta hepatis, is an area into which blood drains from the cystic veins and directly admixes with portal blood. Presumably because of this phenomenon, CTAP showed that normal portal opacification was absent in this segment in 14% of patients reported by del Pilar Fernandez and Bernardino.

Rapidly acquired contrast-enhanced MR images are now possible, and they display information similar to that obtained by dynamic CT. As expected, transient segmental hepatic intensity differences, analogous to the finding in Figure 26-2, have been found by this technique (Figure 26-16).

Color flow Doppler sonography has been of great value in assessing flow-related phenomena in a variety of anatomic regions. Analysis of portal vein flow patterns adjacent to large hepatic masses has shown that flow within the portal vein supplying the affected segment is reversed on some occasions. This almost certainly reflects the same hemodynamic alteration that produces THAD (Figure 26-17).

The physiologic effect of segmental absence of portal perfusion on the liver has not been completely studied, but Dwyer et al. have speculated that there may be alteration in regional metabolism, so that glycogen storage is suspended and fat deposition is increased. Over time, this could lead to alteration in segmental attenuation that could be observed without contrast administration (geographic focal fatty infiltration).

Moreover, it is not unlikely that focal sparing in a liver diffusely infiltrated with fat could occur in these regions of anomalous vascularity; metabolic activity in the liver is governed in part by hormonal stimulation from pancreatic glucagon and insulin, both of which reach the hepatic parenchyma via the portal vein. Areas in which portal flow is diminished or absent may then respond sluggishly to metabolic demands

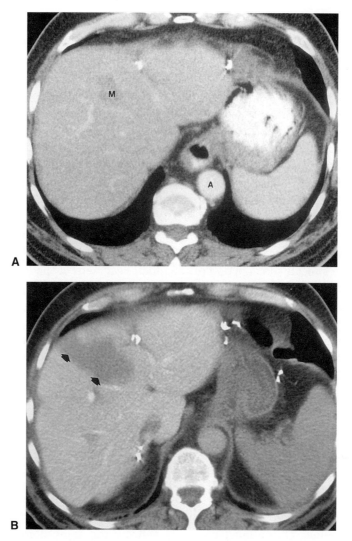

Figure 26-14. Effect of diminished portal flow during CT arterial portography. This 63-year-old man with known hepatic metastases from a colorectal carcinoma was being evaluated for potential resection of the metastases. (A) A CT section obtained during the portal vein-dominant phase of contrast enhancement shows an irregularly shaped low-attenuation metastasis (M) in the medial segment of the left hepatic lobe. A = aorta. (B) A CT image obtained during CTAP (contrast infusion into the superior mesenteric artery) at the same level as in panel A appears strikingly different from the standard CT image. A larger area of low attenuation is observed; its posterior border (arrows) delineates the interlobar fissure. This phenomenon, referred to as the "straight line sign," reflects reduced portal venous flow to the portion of the hepatic segment that contains tumor. The finding is not completely specific for portal vein invasion by tumor, since it can be produced by bland thrombus or by physiologic portal shunting due to segmentally increased pressure from the mass.

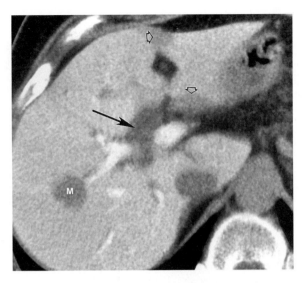

Figure 26-15. Flow-related "pseudotumor" during CT arterial portography. This 55-year-old man underwent CTAP for evaluation of possible liver resection to remove a colorectal cancer metastasis. A section through the porta hepatis shows the low-attenuation metastasis (M) in the posterior inferior right hepatic lobe. There is a wedge-shaped area of decreased attenuation (solid arrow) in the medial segment of the left hepatic lobe. Portal flow defects are commonly observed in this region and are probably related to systemic blood draining from the cystic veins. Two smaller but similar-appearing pseudotumors (open arrows) are present within the lateral segment of the left hepatic lobe, on its inferior surface, and adjacent to the falciform ligament. It is probable that regional flow variations affecting the portal vein account for these low-attenuation regions. In this patient, a single metastatic focus was successfully resected; no pathologic process was observed in any other location.

signaled by hormonal changes originating in the pancreas. Finally, it is also likely that hepatic atrophy is the end result of long-standing absence of portal flow to a given segment. That would explain the phenomenon illustrated in Figure 26-18, in which a lobe under increased pressure from a large solitary metastasis involutes over time.

Portal vein thrombosis (Option (B)) is a possible explanation for the findings in Figure 26-2; indeed, segmental portal vein thrombosis can produce the effect shown in the test image. However, thrombosis of the main portal vein does not produce attenuation differences in a single segment. As discussed above, hepatic vein obstruction (Option (C)) has a completely different CT appearance, with diffusely heterogeneous enhancement. Superior vena cava obstruction (Option (D)) can produce

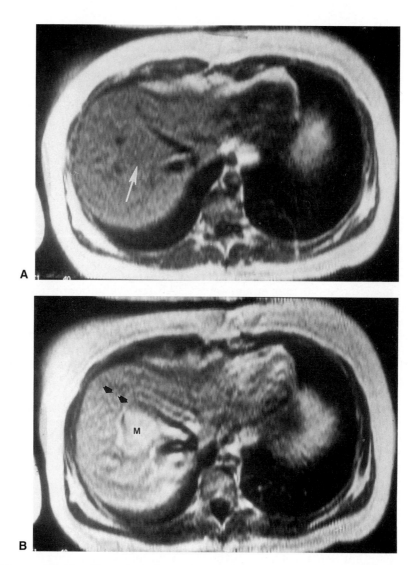

Figure 26-16. Transient hepatic intensity difference on MRI in a 29-year-old woman in whom a focal hypoechoic lesion was detected during an abdominal sonogram obtained for right upper quadrant pain. (A) A precontrast MR image through the dome of the liver shows a very slightly hypointense mass (arrow) in the anterior segment of the right hepatic lobe. (B) An MR image obtained 23 seconds after rapid administration of gadolinium DTPA shows intense contrast enhancement within the mass (M). The entire right lobe is observed to be hyperintense compared with the left lobe; the margin of the hyperintense zone outlines the major hepatic fissure (arrows). The mass was resected and proved to be focal nodular hyperplasia.

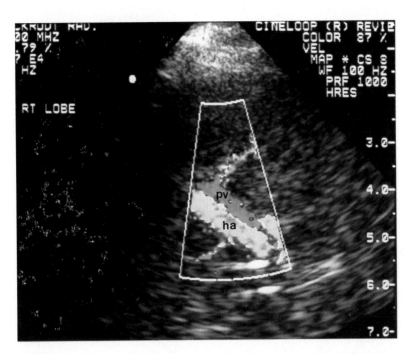

Figure 26-17. Flow reversal in a portal vein as a result of a mass in the same segment. A color flow Doppler sonogram of the anterior segment of the right hepatic lobe shows the right hepatic artery (ha); color-coding information indicates flow in the expected direction, toward the liver. The right anterior segment of the portal vein (pv), however, is coded blue, indicating reversal of flow. Other images demonstrated a mass within the same segment.

segmental hyperenhancement, but the abnormal segment is always the medial segment of the left hepatic lobe. Focal fatty infiltration (Option (E)) produces focal or diffuse diminution in liver attenuation, not focal segmental increase as in the test image.

The CT scan in Figure 26-3 was also obtained within the arterial phase of hepatic enhancement. It shows a geometric area of increased enhancement in the anterior portion of the medial segment of the left hepatic lobe (Figure 26-19). There are also numerous very dense, rounded structures just deep to the skin surface that clearly represent dilated venous collaterals. These findings are diagnostic of superior vena cava obstruction **(Option (D) is the correct answer to Question 79).**

The hyperdense enhancement of the left-lobe medial segment is also a transient phenomenon, observed during and immediately after contrast infusion; however, the mechanism of this enhancement is entirely different from that of preferential segmental arterial flow (described

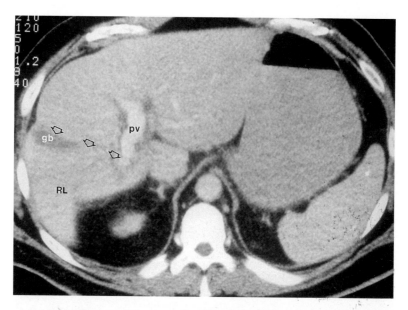

Figure 26-18. Same patient as in Figure 26-13. Atrophy due to portal vein thrombosis. The patient, who had segmental portal vein thrombosis, was reexamined 6 months after Figure 26-13 was obtained. A CT section somewhat inferior to the level shown in Figure 26-13 shows marked atrophy of the right lobe (RL), with posterior displacement of the gallbladder (gb) and interlobar fissure (arrows). pv = portal vein.

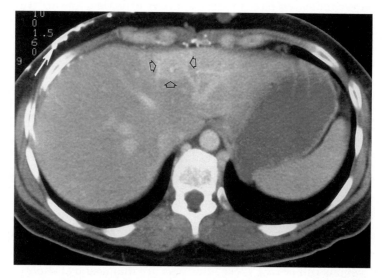

Figure 26-19 (Same as Figure 26-3). Superior vena cava obstruction. This 33-year-old woman with mediastinal involvement from histoplasmosis developed engorgement of venous collaterals in her chest and abdominal wall. A CT section through the dome of the liver shows an area of hyperenhancement (open arrows) within the anterior part of the medial segment of the left hepatic lobe. Also noted are numerous contrast-filled collateral channels (white arrow) on the surface of the abdomen.

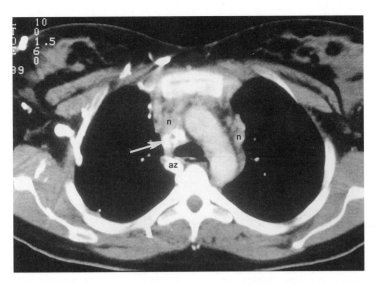

Figure 26-20. Same patient as in Figures 26-3 and 26-19. Superior vena cava obstruction. A CT section through the upper mediastinum shows multiple soft tissue attenuation nodes (n) and a large calcification (arrow) in the expected location of the superior vena cava. Concentrated contrast from the right upper extremity has entered the azygos vein (az) through collateral channels.

above). In patients with superior vena cava syndrome, contrast-rich upper extremity venous blood reaches the inferior vena cava by way of numerous collateral pathways. A posterior pathway, through the intercostal veins into the azygos and hemiazygos systems, directs blood into the iliac veins and thence to the inferior vena cava. An anterior channel (Figures 26-20 and 26-21) connects the anterior intercostal veins to the superficial epigastric veins, which in turn connect to paraumbilical collaterals to reach the left portal vein. This latter pathway occurs preferentially when the posterior communications are poorly developed or when the azygos/hemiazygos veins are themselves obstructed (as in the patient whose CT scan is shown in Figure 26-3, who has diffuse fibrosing mediastinitis) (Figure 26-20). During and just after contrast infusion, the undiluted contrast from the upper extremity enters the left portal vein and produces hyperenhancement of the medial segment parenchyma. This phenomenon has also been observed angiographically and by scintigraphy (Figure 26-22).

Superior vena cava obstruction is most commonly related to mediastinal invasion by malignant tumors but can also be a sequela of granulomatous disease, prolonged central venous catheterization, or trauma. The clinical presentation depends on the underlying disease, the rapidity

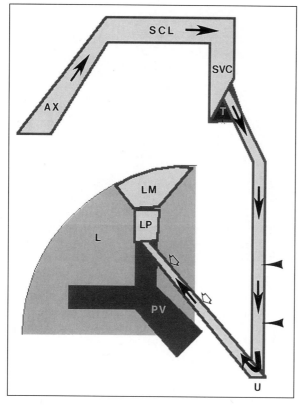

Figure 26-21. Diagrammatic representation of systemic-to-portal collaterals in patients with superior vena cava obstruction. Contrast material courses in the direction shown by the arrows, passing through the axillary (AX) and subclavian (SCL) veins to enter the superior vena cava (SVC). In this example, a thrombus (T) obstructs the superior vena cava. Contrast-rich blood is diverted into chest wall collaterals, specifically the lateral thoracic vein, which connects to the superficial epigastric veins (arrowheads) about the umbilicus (U). Collaterals recruited within the ligamentum teres (open arrows) direct blood into the liver (L) along the course of the umbilical vein. This collateral connects to the left portal vein (LP), and contrast entering at this site is preferentially directed toward the anterior portion of the medial segment (LM), producing the characteristic enhancement pattern shown in the test case. PV = portal vein.

with which obstruction develops, and the adequacy of collateral channels to direct upper extremity blood through alternative pathways. Sudden superior vena cava obstruction is typically heralded by venous engorgement of the neck and arm veins, with cyanosis and edema of the head and neck.

The CT scan in Figure 26-4 was obtained during the arterial phase after rapid injection of contrast material. There is a striking peripheral enhancement pattern with no clear segmental distribution (Figure 26-23). There are also tubular structures with low attenuation in all segments (best seen in the lateral segment). These structures represent intrahepatic branches of the portal vein and are filled with thrombus. The inferior vena cava is opacified, but there is no demonstrable opacifi-

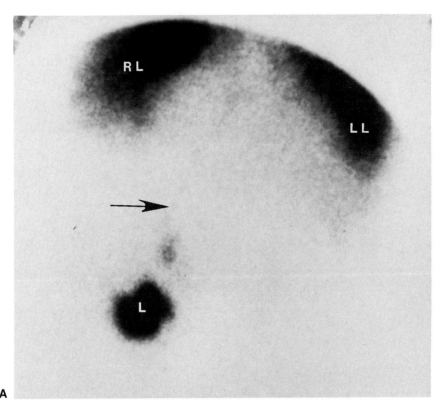

A

Figure 26-22. Superior vena cava obstruction incidentally discovered during pulmonary perfusion scintigraphy. (A) An anterior scintigram from a pulmonary perfusion study obtained after injection of Tc-99m macroaggregated albumin shows expected perfusion of the right lower (RL) and left lower (LL) lobes. There is an area of markedly increased activity corresponding to the left lobe of the liver (L). A linear area of increased activity (arrow) can be faintly seen extending down the anterior chest wall. (B) A right upper extremity radionuclide venogram (anterior projection) shows filling of collateral chest wall veins (arrow), consistent with central venous obstruction. (C) An anterior liver-spleen scintigram performed with Tc-99m sulfur colloid shows an intense focus of tracer uptake (arrow) in the inferior aspect of the left hepatic lobe. This patient had a thrombus occluding the innominate vein at its junction with the superior vena cava.

cation within a portal vein structure. These findings are diagnostic of main portal vein thrombosis **(Option (B) is the correct answer to Question 80).**

Portal vein thrombosis can be associated with hypercoagulable states, such as polycythemia vera, paraneoplastic syndromes, or oral contraceptive use. It is commonly observed as a complication of portal

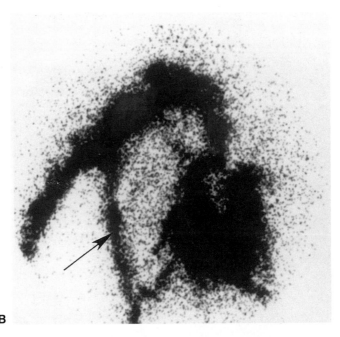

B

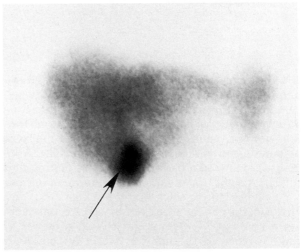

C

hypertension, and hepatocellular carcinoma frequently invades the portal system, causing either bland or tumor thrombosis. Roughly half of all cases are idiopathic.

Clinically, portal vein thrombosis can be completely asymptomatic or can produce symptoms of mild intestinal ischemia associated with nonspecific abdominal pain. In contrast to hepatic vein thrombosis, which frequently produces a tender liver, portal vein thrombosis rarely causes

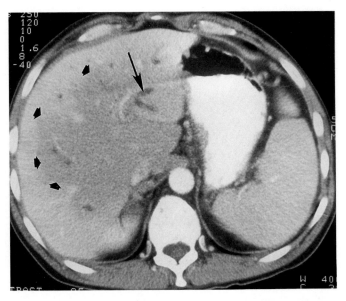

Figure 26-23 (Same as Figure 26-4). Main portal vein thrombosis. A CT section obtained just above the porta hepatis during the hepatic artery-dominant phase shows hyperenhancement of the periphery of the liver; the margins (short arrows) of the hyperenhancing region are nonsegmental in distribution. The central portal thrombus extended into all major hepatic segments and is best seen in the lateral segmental branch (long arrow).

symptoms in the right upper quadrant. If infection of the portal tributaries (pylephlebitis) is the underlying cause, focal pain can be due to a liver abscess and is usually associated with systemic signs of sepsis.

The CT findings of portal vein thrombosis include visualization of the thrombus. In patients with acute thrombosis, the thrombus has relatively high attenuation on unenhanced images (Figure 26-24) but fails to enhance after intravenous contrast material is administered. There may be peripheral enhancement around the thrombus, a finding attributed to contrast opacification of the vasa vasorum. Slight expansion of the lumen of the portal vein is sometimes observed. When patients are imaged in the hepatic artery-dominant phase, a pattern of peripheral enhancement is observed. It is speculated that the collateral vessels bypassing the thrombosed portal vein are effective only in supplying the central portion of the liver. The less well oxygenated periphery is supplied preferentially by the hepatic artery and therefore shows hyperenhancement during the arterial phase.

Collateral vessels develop rapidly within the porta hepatis after main portal vein thrombosis; veins draining the gallbladder can be

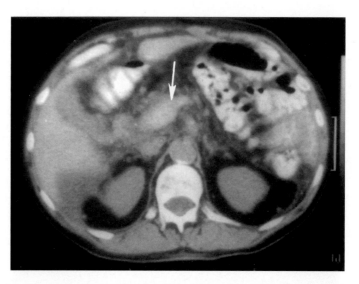

Figure 26-24. Acute portal vein thrombus. An unenhanced CT scan at the level of the confluence of the superior mesenteric vein with the splenic vein shows a high-attenuation thrombus (arrow) filling and slightly expanding the lumen of the main portal vein.

recruited as well. The serpentine contrast-filled channels surrounding a thrombosed portal vein have been (somewhat inaccurately) called "cavernous transformation of the portal vein." They have a striking and characteristic CT appearance (Figure 26-25).

Unusual CT appearances have been reported in patients with portal vein thrombosis; these include gas within a preexisting cavernoma (Figure 26-26) and calcification in the periphery of a chronic portal vein thrombus.

Diffuse fatty infiltration of the liver is a well-known feature of alcoholic liver disease, diabetes, obesity, and malnutrition disorders, including those in patients undergoing chemotherapy. Focal fatty infiltration (Option (E)) is, by contrast, a relatively poorly understood entity, which was not widely described until the routine use of abdominal CT. Pathologically, there is a reduction in glycogen stores and an associated increase in triglyceride content within hepatocytes in affected areas. The possible influence of regional changes in portal blood flow has been discussed above.

Tang-Barton et al. reported five different patterns of focal fatty infiltration: (1) a lobar or segmental distribution with uniform infiltration, (2) a lobar or segmental distribution with patchy or nodular infiltration, (3) fatty infiltration restricted to the perihilar region, (4) diffuse patchy

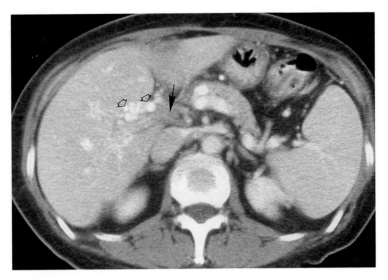

Figure 26-25. Collateral formation in a patient with long-standing portal vein thrombosis. A CT section at the level of the porta hepatis shows no enhancement of the thrombus-filled portal vein (long arrow). Multiple collateral vessels (short open arrows) are evident on the anterior surface of the portal vein. Their convoluted appearance has given rise to the description "cavernous transformation."

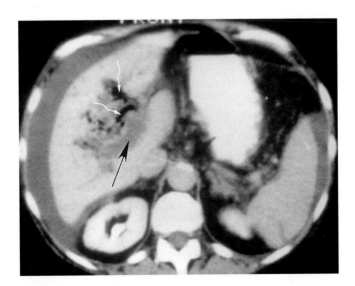

Figure 26-26. Portal vein thrombosis. A CT scan of a patient with long-standing polycythemia vera and known chronic portal vein thrombus (black arrow), who developed severe abdominal pain due to intestinal ischemia, shows that gas from the ischemic segment has entered the collateral vessels (white arrows) to produce this peculiar appearance.

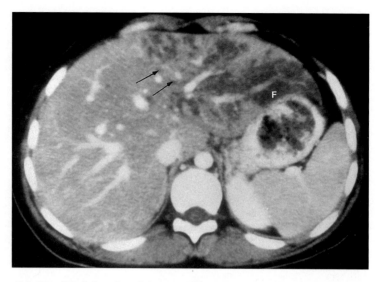

Figure 26-27. Nodular focal fatty infiltration. A CT section obtained in a patient evaluated for elevation of liver enzymes shows multiple low-attenuation zones within the left hepatic lobe. Regions of the lateral segment are confluent (F) and were confidently believed to represent focal fat. The medial segment is filled with nodular low-attenuation densities (arrows), whose nature was in doubt. Biopsy confirmed focal fatty infiltration.

infiltration, and (5) diffuse nodular infiltration (Figure 26-27). This last pattern is diagnostically the most troublesome, since it strikingly resembles other pathologic processes such as metastases, fungal abscesses, and sarcoidosis.

MRI has been particularly useful in evaluating problematic cases detected by CT. Proton spectroscopic imaging relies on the fact that the precession rate of protons in water molecules differs from that of protons within fat. Signals returning from protons in the different environments are thus out of phase with one another. Appropriate timing of radiofrequency pulses can lead to a situation in which the two signals are 180° out of phase when imaged. The resulting signal is thus related to the difference between the signal from water protons and that from fat protons. When this image is compared with the standard image, which represents the sum of the signal from water protons and that from fat protons, areas in which the signal intensity undergoes the greatest change can be reliably diagnosed as areas of increased fat content (Figure 26-28).

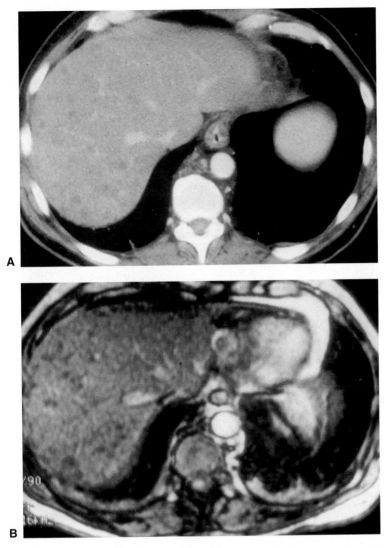

Figure 26-28. Focal fatty infiltration. Contribution of chemical-shift MRI. (A) A CT section obtained through the dome of the liver shows multiple rounded low-attenuation lesions throughout the parenchyma. The differential diagnosis in this patient included metastatic lesions and fungal infection. (B) MR section at the same level as in panel A. The pulse sequence has been adjusted so that the signal arising from fat is 180° out of phase with the signal arising from water. The nodular areas have very little signal, indicating that they are composed of approximately equal portions of fat and water. This condition occurs virtually only in patients with fatty infiltrated hepatocytes. Biopsy confirmed nodular focal fatty infiltration.

Discussion

The cases illustrated by Figures 26-1 through 26-4 are examples of the effect of the biologic distribution of intravenous contrast material during CT scanning. As our ability to acquire data rapidly has improved, most recently with the use of spiral and electron beam CT scanners, it has become even more important to understand the phases of contrast distribution and the effect of these contrast shifts on CT images of the liver.

For the moment, let us simplify the problem by assuming (unrealistically) that the entire intravenous contrast bolus is administered in a single instant into an antecubital vein; we will monitor the fate of that bolus over time. For the first few seconds, the bolus courses within the extremity veins before entering the superior vena cava and thereafter the right heart. It then exits through the pulmonary arteries, enters the capillary system of the lungs, and returns through the pulmonary veins to enter the left heart. No substantial loss of contrast occurs within normal pulmonary capillaries, since the extravascular fluid space within the pulmonary interstitium is small. This phase of the bolus transit takes only 10 to 15 seconds, depending on cardiac status.

As the bolus enters the left heart, it is rapidly distributed to every systemic capillary bed in the body. About 20% of the bolus enters the renal circulation, where a fraction (the filtration fraction) is effectively removed from the body. Another 20% enters the splanchnic circulation, where it perfuses the capillary beds of the gastrointestinal tract, pancreas, and spleen. Roughly 6% of the administered contrast courses through the hepatic artery, where it likewise perfuses the liver sinusoids. This phase of capillary perfusion is relatively brief, lasting 10 to 15 seconds after the bolus enters the arterial circulation. Images of the liver obtained during this period (the hepatic artery-dominant phase) will show a brisk rise in parenchymal attenuation but only moderate peak enhancement, since most of the blood perfusing the hepatic sinusoids at that moment is contrast-poor portal venous blood.

Once contrast material enters the capillary bed of the liver, spleen, pancreas, and gastrointestinal tract, it immediately begins to diffuse into the extravascular fluid space, so that its concentration within the veins draining these organs is considerably lower than the initial concentration of the bolus. The degree of dilution depends on the volume of the extravascular fluid space within the specific organ being perfused.

About 20 seconds after the bolus enters the arterial system, there is a second phase of contrast opacification of the liver parenchyma; this phase is produced by contrast material draining into the portal vein from the capillary beds of the pancreas, spleen, and gastrointestinal tract. The concentration of contrast material in this blood is lower than in arterial blood because of diffusion into the extravascular fluid space; however, the total volume of portal venous flow is three times that of the volume delivered via the hepatic artery. Imaging in this phase (the portal vein-dominant phase) demonstrates a relatively slower rise in parenchymal opacification but a much higher peak value than that reached during the hepatic arterial phase.

After this phase of parenchymal enhancement, a portion of the contrast material exits the liver through the hepatic veins and reenters the right heart. The remaining bolus recirculates, but its effect on parenchymal opacification is blunted because of contrast loss from renal excretion and contrast dilution within the extravascular fluid volume. Equilibrium between the extracellular fluid space and the blood occurs within a few minutes of intravenous administration of contrast material; imaging during this equilibrium phase provides information chiefly about the relative volume of extracellular fluid within a specific organ or pathologic process. The phenomenon of delayed enhancement (seen in patients with cholangiocarcinomas, for example) is explained by the fact that some tumors have a larger extracellular fluid space relative to their blood supply than does the surrounding liver (Figure 26-29).

The actual situation encountered in clinical practice is, unfortunately, even more complex than the model outlined above. The contrast agent is not administered intravenously as a huge bolus in a single instant but, instead, is infused over several seconds. Most clinically useful protocols for intravenous injection of contrast agent utilize flow rates of 3 to 5 mL/second, with total contrast doses of 125 to 150 mL. Clearly, administration of the bolus, even at the highest rates, requires 30 to 50 seconds. Accordingly, the time-density curve of hepatic enhancement after an intravenous contrast agent bolus shows a relatively slow rise during the arterial phase, a somewhat steeper rise at the beginning of the portal phase, a plateau at the end of the portal phase, and then a steady decline during the equilibrium phase (Figure 26-30).

From the above discussion, it is no surprise that certain pathologic processes can be seen best during one contrast enhancement phase but poorly (or not at all) during others (Figure 26-31). Clinical design of contrast-enhancement strategies aims toward optimizing detection of intrahepatic tumors, primary or secondary. A successful strategy will therefore produce the maximum contrast difference between the normal liver parenchyma and the tumor. Most tumors are supplied predominantly by the hepatic artery and receive little or no portal blood, and so the preferred strategy has been to obtain images during the portal vein-dominant phase. This leaves a relatively small "window of opportunity" for

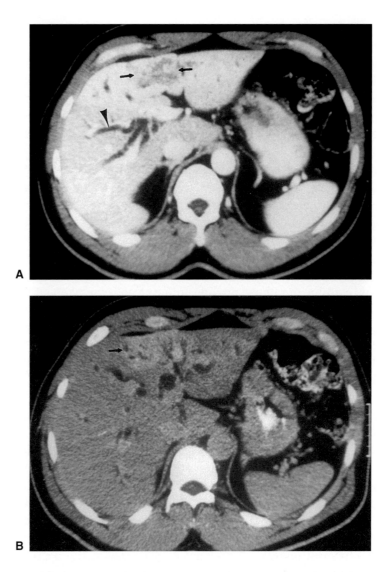

Figure 26-29. Delayed enhancement. This 67-year-old man has lymphoma of the bile duct, producing intrahepatic duct dilation. (A) A CT section through the porta hepatis shows a focal low-attenuation mass (arrows) in the medial segment of the left hepatic lobe. Note the intrahepatic ductal dilatation (arrowhead). (B) A delayed scan performed 4 minutes after the scan in panel A, through the same anatomic level, shows that the previously hypoattenuating lesion (arrow) is now hyperdense with respect to the surrounding hepatic parenchyma.

imaging, occurring after the hepatic artery-dominant phase and before equilibrium. Imaging solely during this time, however, risks failure to detect hypervascular tumors (whose arterial-phase opacification is more

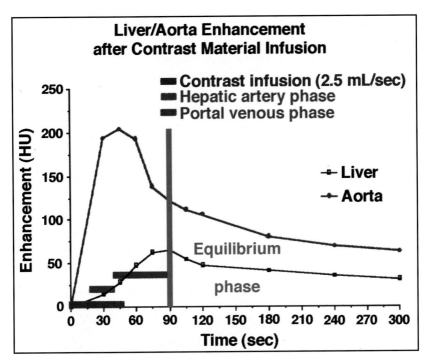

Figure 26-30. Graphic representation of contrast enhancement in the liver and aorta after rapid (2.5 mL/second) infusion of contrast agent. There is a rapid increase in attenuation of the abdominal aorta (green line) during the early phase of contrast infusion. Liver enhancement (black line), however, is much less brisk and attains a relatively lower peak value, because there is dilution of contrast agent by unopacified blood from the portal vein throughout this phase. Beginning about 40 seconds after the start of contrast medium injection, contrast-enhanced portal venous blood, returning from the spleen and intestine, produces marked hepatic enhancement, attaining a relatively high peak value. The portal venous phase (blue bar) lasts until the contrast enhancement curves for the aorta and liver become parallel. The onset of this so-called equilibrium phase varies with the volume and duration of contrast injection. In this example, it begins roughly 90 seconds after the beginning of contrast injection. Therefore, images obtained after 90 seconds reflect the distribution of contrast material into the extracellular fluid space and not differential vascularity.

intense than the surrounding normal liver but will fade to blend in with normal parenchyma during the portal vein-dominant phase) (Figure 26-32). A truly optimal strategy, designed to detect all liver tumors (and physiologic processes), has not yet been implemented; an understanding of the effects of intravenous contrast enhancement is therefore critical in evaluating individual cases.

Dennis M. Balfe, M.D.

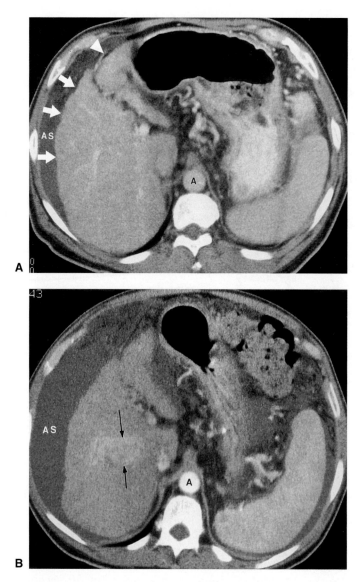

Figure 26-31. Hepatocellular carcinoma. Effect of image timing on lesion detection. This 63-year-old man with alcoholic cirrhosis has a rising α-fetoprotein level in serum. (A) A CT section through the liver, obtained during the portal vein-dominant phase, shows nodular surface irregularity (arrows), ascites (AS), and collateral vessels in the fissure for the ligamentum teres (arrowhead), suggesting cirrhosis with portal hypertension. No mass is identified. (B) The patient was reexamined 1 month later because of continuing hepatic decompensation. (Note the increase in ascites [AS].) A CT image at the same anatomic level as in panel A was obtained during the hepatic artery-dominant phase. A hyperenhancing mass (arrows) in the anterior segment of the right hepatic lobe is now evident. A = aorta.

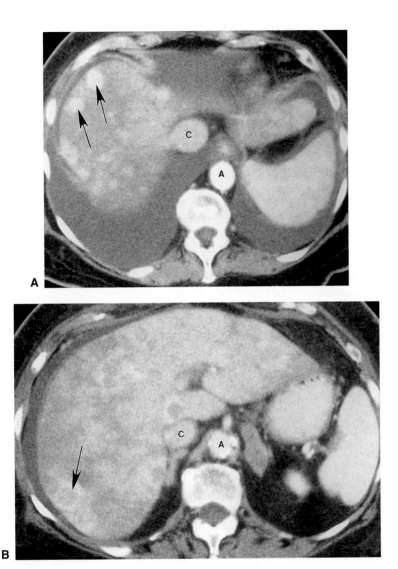

Figure 26-32. Metastatic islet cell carcinoma originating in the pancreas in a 60-year-old man. Effect of timing on the appearance of hypervascular hepatic metastases. (A) A CT section through the dome of the liver was obtained 40 seconds after the beginning of contrast infusion. At this time, near the end of the hepatic artery-dominant phase, there is clear demarcation of the hyperenhancing metastatic lesions (arrows) from the relatively hypoattenuating liver. (B) A CT section just above the porta hepatis was obtained 24 seconds after the section shown in panel A. At this time, during the portal vein-dominant phase, the metastatic lesions have an attenuation much closer to that of the surrounding liver parenchyma and are difficult to detect. Most lesions seen during this phase have slightly hyperattenuating rims (arrow), but their centers are nearly the same CT density as the liver. A = aorta; C = inferior vena cava.

SUGGESTED READINGS

HEPATIC VENOUS OUTFLOW IMPAIRMENT

1. Aspestrand F, Schrumpf E, Jacobsen M, Hanssen L, Endresen K. Increased lymphatic flow from the liver in different intra- and extrahepatic diseases demonstrated by CT. J Comput Assist Tomogr 1991; 15:550–554
2. Becker CD, Scheidegger J, Marincek B. Hepatic vein occlusion: morphologic features on computed tomography and ultrasonography. Gastrointest Radiol 1986; 11:305–311
3. Grant EG, Schiller VL, Millener P, et al. Color Doppler imaging of the hepatic vasculature. AJR 1992; 159:943–950
4. Holley HC, Koslin DB, Berland LL, Stanley RJ. Inhomogeneous enhancement of liver parenchyma secondary to passive congestion: contrast-enhanced CT. Radiology 1989; 170:795–800
5. Mathieu D, Vasile N, Menu Y, Van Beers B, Lorphelin JM, Pringot J. Budd-Chiari syndrome: dynamic CT. Radiology 1987; 165:409–413
6. Millener P, Grant EG, Rose S, et al. Color Doppler imaging findings in patients with Budd-Chiari syndrome: correlation with venographic findings. AJR 1993; 161:307–312
7. Mori H, Maeda H, Fukuda T, et al. Acute thrombosis of the inferior vena cava and hepatic veins in patients with Budd-Chiari syndrome: CT demonstration. AJR 1989; 153:987–991
8. Moulton JS, Miller BL, Dodd GD III, Vu DN. Passive hepatic congestion in heart failure: CT abnormalities. AJR 1988; 151:939–942
9. Vogelzang RL, Anschuetz SL, Gore RM. Budd-Chiari syndrome: CT observations. Radiology 1987; 163:329–333
10. Yang PJ, Glazer GM, Bowerman RA. Budd-Chiari syndrome: computed tomographic and ultrasonographic findings. J Comput Assist Tomogr 1983; 7:148–150

TRANSIENT PERFUSION-RELATED HEPATIC DENSITY ALTERATIONS: CTAP

11. Deflandre MF, Vilgrain V, Zins M, et al. Nontumorous attenuation changes on CT arterial portography. J Comput Assist Tomogr 1994; 18:761–767
12. del Pilar Fernandez M, Bernardino ME. Hepatic pseudolesion: appearance of focal low attenuation in the medial segment of the left lobe at CT arterial portography. Radiology 1991; 181:809–812
13. Peterson MS, Baron RL, Dodd GD III, et al. Hepatic parenchymal perfusion defects detected with CTAP: imaging-pathologic correlation. Radiology 1992; 185:149–155
14. Soyer P, Lacheheb D, Levesque M. False-positive CT portography: correlation with pathologic findings. AJR 1993; 160:285–289

TRANSIENT PERFUSION-RELATED HEPATIC DENSITY ALTERATIONS: DYNAMIC CT

15. Amin Z, Donald JJ, Masters A, et al. Hepatic metastases: interstitial laser photocoagulation with real-time US monitoring and dynamic CT evaluation of treatment. Radiology 1993; 187:339–347

16. Itai Y, Furui S, Ohtomo K, et al. Dynamic CT features of arterioportal shunts in hepatocellular carcinoma. AJR 1986; 146:723–727

17. Itai Y, Hachiya J, Makita K, Ohtomo K, Kokubo T, Yamauchi T. Transient hepatic attenuation differences on dynamic computed tomography. J Comput Assist Tomogr 1987; 11:461–465

18. Itai Y, Moss AA, Goldberg HI. Transient hepatic attenuation difference of lobar or segmental distribution detected by dynamic computed tomography. Radiology 1982; 144:835–839

19. Matsui O, Takashima T, Kadoya M, et al. Segmental staining on hepatic arteriography as a sign of intrahepatic portal vein obstruction. Radiology 1984; 152:601–606

20. Nakayama T, Hiyama Y, Ohnishi K, et al. Arterioportal shunts on dynamic computed tomography. AJR 1983; 140:953–957

21. Tyrrel RT, Kaufman SL, Bernardino ME. Straight line sign: appearance and significance during CT portography. Radiology 1989; 173:635–637

TRANSIENT PERFUSION-RELATED HEPATIC DENSITY ALTERATIONS: DYNAMIC MRI

22. Ito K, Choji T, Fujita T, Matsumoto T, Nakada T, Nakanishi T. Early-enhancing pseudolesion in medial segment of left hepatic lobe detected with multisection dynamic MR. Radiology 1993; 187:695–699

MORPHOLOGIC DENSITY ALTERATIONS

23. Doppman JL, Dwyer A, Vermess M, et al. Segmental hyperlucent defects in the liver. J Comput Assist Tomogr 1984; 8:50–57

24. Dwyer A, Doppman JL, Adams AJ, Girton ME, Chernick SS, Cornblath M. Influence of glycogen on liver density: computed tomography from a metabolic perspective. J Comput Assist Tomogr 1983; 7:70–73

25. Itai Y, Ohtomo K, Furui S, Minami M, Yoshikawa K, Yashiro N. Lobar intensity differences of the liver on MR imaging. J Comput Assist Tomogr 1986; 10:236–241

26. Lorigan JG, Charnsangavej C, Carrasco CH, Richli WR, Wallace S. Atrophy with compensatory hypertrophy of the liver in hepatic neoplasms: radiographic findings. AJR 1988; 150:1291–1295

27. Nishikawa J, Itai Y, Tasaka A. Lobar attenuation difference of the liver on computed tomography. Radiology 1981; 141:725–728

SUPERIOR VENA CAVA OBSTRUCTION

28. Engel IA, Auh YH, Rubenstein WA, Sniderman K, Whalen JP, Kazam E. CT diagnosis of mediastinal and thoracic inlet venous obstruction. AJR 1983; 141:521–526

29. Henke CE, Wolff JM, Shafer RB. Vascular dynamics in liver scan hot spot. Clin Nucl Med 1978; 3:267–270

30. Ishikawa T, Clark RA, Tokuda M, Ashida H. Focal contrast enhancement on hepatic CT in superior vena caval and brachiocephalic vein obstruction. AJR 1983; 140:337–338

31. Lee KR, Preston DF, Martin NL, Robinson RG. Angiographic documentation of systemic-portal venous shunting as a cause of a liver scan "hot spot" in superior vena caval obstruction. AJR 1976; 127:637–639

32. Muramatsu T, Miyamae T, Mashimo M, Suzuki K, Kinoshita S, Dohi Y. Hot spots on liver scans associated with superior or inferior vena caval obstruction. Clin Nucl Med 1994; 19:622–629

33. Okay NH, Bryk D. Collateral pathways in occlusion of the superior vena cava and its tributaries. Radiology 1969; 92:1493–1498

PORTAL VEIN THROMBOSIS

34. Lim GM, Jeffrey RB Jr, Ralls PW, Marn CS. Septic thrombosis of the portal vein: CT and clinical observations. J Comput Assist Tomogr 1989; 13:656–658

35. Marn CS, Francis IR. CT of portal venous occlusion. AJR 1992; 159:717–726

36. Mathieu D, Vasile N, Dibie C, Grenier P. Portal cavernoma: dynamic CT features and transient differences in hepatic attenuation. Radiology 1985; 154:743–748

37. Mathieu D, Vasile N, Grenier P. Portal thrombosis: dynamic CT features and course. Radiology 1985; 154:737–741

38. Miller VE, Berland LL. Pulsed Doppler duplex sonography and CT of portal vein thrombosis. AJR 1985; 145:73–76

39. Mori H, Hayashi K, Uetani M, Matsuoka Y, Iwao M, Maeda H. High-attenuation recent thrombus of the portal vein: CT demonstration and clinical significance. Radiology 1987; 163:353–356

40. Nakao N, Miura K, Takahashi H, et al. Hepatic perfusion in cavernous transformation of the portal vein: evaluation by using CT angiography. AJR 1989; 152:985–986

FOCAL FAT: CT

41. Arai K, Matsui O, Takashima T, Ida M, Nishida Y. Focal spared areas in fatty liver caused by regional decreased portal flow. AJR 1988; 151:300–302

42. Baker ME, Silverman PM. Nodular focal fatty infiltration of the liver: CT appearance. AJR 1985; 145:79–80

43. Flournoy JG, Potter JL, Sullivan BM, Gerza CB, Ramzy I. CT appearance of multifocal hepatic steatosis. J Comput Assist Tomogr 1984; 8:1192–1194

44. Gale ME, Gerzof SG, Robbins AH. Portal architecture: a differential guide to fatty infiltration of the liver on computed tomography. Gastrointest Radiol 1983; 8:231–236

45. Halvorsen RA, Korobkin M, Ram PC, Thompson WM. CT appearance of focal fatty infiltration of the liver. AJR 1982; 139:277–281

46. Lewis E, Bernardino ME, Barnes PA, Parvey HR, Soo CS, Chuang VP. The fatty liver: pitfalls in the CT and angiographic evaluation of metastatic disease. J Comput Assist Tomogr 1983; 7:235–241

47. Tang-Barton P, Vas W, Weissman J, Salimi Z, Patel R, Morris L. Focal fatty liver lesions in alcoholic liver disease: a broadened spectrum of CT appearances. Gastrointest Radiol 1985; 10:133–137

FOCAL FAT: MRI

48. Heiken JP, Lee JK, Dixon WT. Fatty infiltration of the liver: evaluation by proton spectroscopic imaging. Radiology 1985; 157:707–710

49. Lee JK, Dixon WT, Ling D, Levitt RG, Murphy WA Jr. Fatty infiltration of the liver: demonstration by proton spectroscopic imaging. Preliminary observations. Radiology 1984; 153:195–201

50. Levenson H, Greensite F, Hoefs J, et al. Fatty infiltration of the liver: quantification with phase-contrast MR imaging at 1.5 T vs biopsy. AJR 1991; 156:307–312

51. Mitchell DG. Focal manifestations of diffuse liver disease at MR imaging. Radiology 1992; 185:1–11

52. Thu HD, Mathieu D, Thu NT, Derhy S, Vasile N. Value of MR imaging in evaluating focal fatty infiltration of the liver: preliminary study. RadioGraphics 1991; 11:1003–1012

CONTRAST STRATEGIES: CTAP

53. Graf O, Dock WI, Lammer J, et al. Determination of optimal time window for liver scanning with CT during arterial portography. Radiology 1994; 190:43–47

CONTRAST STRATEGIES: DYNAMIC CT

54. Baron RL. Understanding and optimizing use of contrast material for CT of the liver. AJR 1994; 163:323–331

55. Claussen CD, Banzer D, Pfretzschner C, Kalender WA, Schorner W. Bolus geometry and dynamics after intravenous contrast medium injection. Radiology 1984; 153:365–368

56. Foley WD. Dynamic hepatic CT. Radiology 1989; 170:617–622

57. Foley WD, Berland LL, Lawson TL, Smith DF, Thorsen MK. Contrast enhancement technique for dynamic hepatic computed tomographic scanning. Radiology 1983; 147:797–803

58. Foley WD, Hoffmann RG, Quiroz FA, Kahn CE Jr, Perret RS. Hepatic helical CT: contrast material injection protocol. Radiology 1994; 192:367–371

59. Heiken JP, Brink JA, McClennan BL, Sagel SS, Forman HP, DiCroce J. Dynamic contrast-enhanced CT of the liver: comparison of contrast medium injection rates and uniphasic and biphasic injection protocols. Radiology 1993; 187:327–331

CONTRAST STRATEGIES: DELAYED ENHANCEMENT

60. Freeny PC, Marks WM. Patterns of contrast enhancement of benign and malignant hepatic neoplasms during bolus dynamic and delayed CT. Radiology 1986; 160:613–618

61. Itai Y, Ohtomo K, Kokubo T, et al. CT of hepatic masses: significance of prolonged and delayed enhancement. AJR 1986; 146:729–733

62. Yoshikawa J, Matsui O, Kadoya M, Gabata T, Arai K, Takashima T. Delayed enhancement of fibrotic areas in hepatic masses: CT-pathologic correlation. J Comput Assist Tomogr 1992; 16:206–211

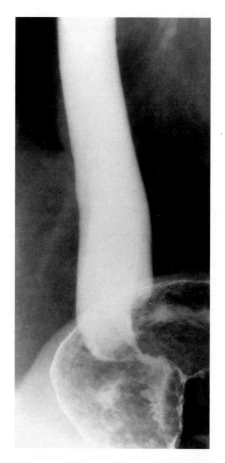

Figure 27-1. This 65-year-old man has recent onset of dysphagia and weight loss. You are shown a radiograph from an esophagram. There was no esophageal peristalsis at fluoroscopy.

Case 27: Secondary Achalasia

Question 81

Which *one* of the following is the MOST likely diagnosis?

(A) Primary achalasia
(B) Secondary achalasia (pseudoachalasia)
(C) Peptic stricture
(D) Esophageal carcinoma
(E) Scleroderma

Figure 27-1 is an esophagram that shows tapered narrowing of the distal esophagus adjacent to the gastroesophageal junction (Figure 27-2). There was no esophageal peristalsis at fluoroscopy. One might initially consider the possibility of primary or idiopathic achalasia (Option (A)), a motor disorder involving degeneration and loss of ganglion cells in Auerbach's plexus in the esophagus. Primary achalasia is manifested radiographically by smooth, tapered narrowing of the distal esophagus, producing a bird-beak appearance at the gastroesophageal junction (Figure 27-3). There is also no peristalsis in the body of the esophagus, with a variable degree of esophageal dilatation depending on the severity and duration of disease. However, the test image demonstrates areas of nodularity within the narrowed segment as well as irregular ulceration at the gastroesophageal junction. The test patient was also an elderly individual who had recent onset of dysphagia and weight loss, findings that historically suggest the presence of an occult neoplasm. Both the clinical and radiographic findings are highly suggestive of secondary achalasia or pseudoachalasia **(Option (B) is correct),** a condition that can closely resemble primary achalasia on clinical, radiographic, and manometric grounds. At surgery, this patient was found to have secondary achalasia due to a cardiac carcinoma invading the distal esophagus.

Most cases of secondary achalasia are caused by carcinoma of the gastric cardia or fundus directly invading the gastroesophageal junction or distal esophagus. Less frequently, blood-borne metastases from breast, lung, pancreatic, or other malignant tumors produce identical

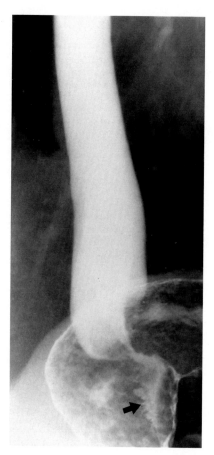

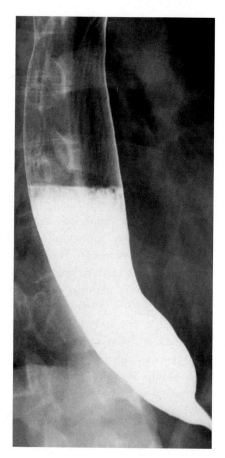

Figure 27-2 (left) (Same as Figure 27-1). Secondary achalasia. There is tapered narrowing of the distal esophagus adjacent to the gastroesophageal junction. However, irregular nodularity is seen within the narrowed segment, which has an asymmetric configuration. Ulceration (arrow) is also seen in the region of the cardia. These findings were caused by carcinoma of the cardia invading the distal esophagus.

Figure 27-3 (right). Primary achalasia. There is smooth, tapered narrowing of the distal esophagus adjacent to the gastroesophageal junction, producing a bird-beak appearance. Primary peristalsis was absent in the body of the esophagus. These findings are characteristic of primary achalasia.

findings. It is important to differentiate primary and secondary achalasia, because primary achalasia can be treated by pneumatic dilatation whereas secondary achalasia often necessitates exploratory laparotomy or other treatment for widespread metastatic disease.

The actual pathogenesis of secondary achalasia is uncertain. Some patients have tumor directly invading the distal esophagus with actual destruction of myenteric ganglia. However, others have tumor confined to the gastroesophageal junction without involvement of the neural plexus in the esophagus. It has therefore been suggested that this syndrome can also result from extraesophageal metastases to the vagus nerve or dorsal motor nucleus of the vagus nerve in the brain stem.

Dysphagia is present in both patients with primary achalasia and those with secondary achalasia, but other clinical features are often helpful in distinguishing these conditions. Most patients with primary achalasia are between 20 and 50 years of age, and they usually have dysphagia for 1 year or more before seeking medical attention. In contrast, most patients with secondary achalasia are older than 50 years, and the duration of symptoms at presentation is usually less than 6 months, as in the test patient. Also, secondary achalasia is more commonly associated with weight loss and upper gastrointestinal bleeding. An underlying malignancy should therefore be suspected whenever achalasia is diagnosed radiographically or endoscopically in elderly patients who have recent onset of dysphagia and weight loss.

Secondary achalasia is classically manifested on barium studies by absent peristalsis in the body of the esophagus associated with smooth, tapered narrowing of the distal esophagus, producing a bird-beak configuration. Although the radiographic appearance can closely resemble that of primary achalasia, certain morphologic features should suggest an underlying tumor. Irregular, eccentric, or asymmetric involvement of the narrowed segment, abrupt transitions, rigidity, and mucosal nodularity or ulceration can be found in patients with secondary achalasia as a result of infiltration of the distal esophagus by tumor (Figure 27-1). Another relatively subtle sign of malignancy is the length of the narrowed segment, which can extend several centimeters above the gastroesophageal junction in patients with secondary achalasia but rarely extends as far proximally in patients with primary achalasia (Figure 27-4).

Careful radiologic examination of the proximal stomach is essential in patients with secondary achalasia, because this condition is usually caused by carcinoma of the gastric cardia or fundus invading the distal esophagus. Not infrequently, an obvious polypoid, ulcerated, or infiltrating malignancy is demonstrated. Paradoxically, however, esophageal obstruction prevents adequate filling of the fundus with barium, so that it is not always possible to obtain a satisfactory examination of the gastric cardia and fundus in these patients. CT can also have a role in evaluating patients with suspected achalasia when the findings on barium studies are equivocal. The possibility of secondary achalasia should be

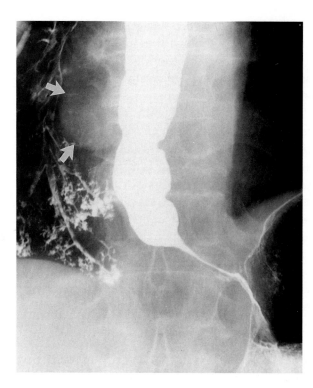

Figure 27-4. Secondary achalasia. Note how the narrowed segment extends several centimeters above the gastroesophageal junction. The area of narrowing rarely extends so far proximally in patients with primary achalasia. This patient has a right-sided bronchogenic carcinoma (arrows) that metastasized to the gastroesophageal junction, causing secondary achalasia. (Aspirated barium is also present in the right lung.) (Reprinted with permission from Levine [2].)

considered when there is asymmetric esophageal wall thickening or a soft tissue mass at the gastroesophageal junction. CT is also helpful in identifying the site of the primary tumor in patients with secondary achalasia.

Reflux-induced or peptic strictures (Option (C)) classically appear as smooth, tapered areas of concentric narrowing in the distal esophagus (Figure 27-5). Occasionally, asymmetric scarring from reflux esophagitis results in asymmetric strictures associated with one or more sacculations or outpouchings from the esophageal wall between areas of fibrosis. However, more than 95% of peptic strictures are associated with hiatal hernias. The test patient has irregular narrowing of the distal esophagus without evidence of a hiatal hernia, so the findings are not those of a peptic stricture.

Esophageal carcinoma (Option (D)) is usually characterized radiographically by an infiltrating lesion with irregular luminal narrowing, mucosal nodularity or ulceration, and relatively abrupt, shelf-like proximal and distal borders. The majority of esophageal cancers are squamous cell carcinomas, which tend to be located in the upper or midthoracic esophagus. However, 30 to 50% of esophageal cancers are adenocarcinomas arising in Barrett's mucosa. There is considerable evi-

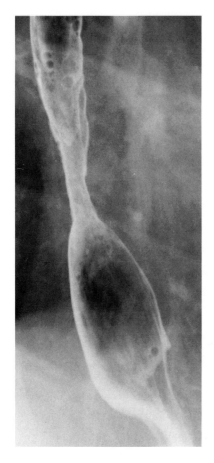

Figure 27-5. Peptic stricture. The stricture is seen as a smooth, tapered area of narrowing in the distal esophagus above a hiatal hernia.

dence that the incidence of adenocarcinoma in Barrett's esophagus has increased more rapidly than any other form of esophageal cancer in the United States during the past two decades. Esophageal adenocarcinomas tend to be located in the distal esophagus, and, unlike squamous cell carcinomas, these lesions have a marked tendency to spread distally into the gastric cardia and fundus. Esophageal adenocarcinoma invading the gastroesophageal junction could conceivably produce findings of secondary achalasia; however, most cases are caused by carcinoma of the gastric cardia or fundus invading the distal esophagus.

Esophageal involvement by scleroderma (Option (E)) is usually characterized by a patulous, incompetent lower esophageal sphincter and absent esophageal peristalsis with poor clearance of refluxed peptic acid from the esophagus once reflux has occurred. As a result, patients with scleroderma are at high risk for developing reflux esophagitis and peptic strictures. In these patients, however, there is almost always an associated hiatal hernia. The test patient did not have a hiatal hernia, making the diagnosis of scleroderma with an associated stricture unlikely. Because of the severity of esophagitis in patients with scleroderma, they are also at greater risk for developing Barrett's esophagus and even esophageal adenocarcinoma. Thus, scleroderma probably should be considered a premalignant condition of the esophagus.

Marc S. Levine, M.D.

SUGGESTED READINGS

SECONDARY ACHALASIA

1. Feczko PJ, Halpert RD. Achalasia secondary to nongastrointestinal malignancies. Gastrointest Radiol 1985; 10:273–276
2. Levine MS. Other malignant tumors. In: Levine MS (ed), Radiology of the esophagus. Philadelphia: WB Saunders; 1989:169–192
3. McCallum RW. Esophageal achalasia secondary to gastric carcinoma. Report of a case and a review of the literature. Am J Gastroenterol 1979; 71:24–29
4. Rabushka LS, Fishman EK, Kuhlman JE. CT evaluation of achalasia. J Comput Assist Tomogr 1991; 15:434–439
5. Seaman WB, Wells J, Flood CA. Diagnostic problems of esophageal cancer: relationship to achalasia and hiatus hernia. AJR 1963; 90:778–791
6. Simeone J, Burrell M, Toffler R. Esophageal aperistalsis secondary to metastatic invasion of the myenteric plexus. AJR 1976; 127:862–864
7. Tucker HJ, Snape WJ Jr, Cohen SC. Achalasia secondary to carcinoma: manometric and clinical features. Ann Intern Med 1978; 89:315–318

PRIMARY ACHALASIA

8. Katz PO, Castell DO. Esophageal motility disorders. Am J Med Sci 1985; 290:61–69
9. Laufer I. Motor disorders of the esophagus. In: Levine MS (ed), Radiology of the esophagus. Philadelphia: WB Saunders; 1989:229–246
10. Margulis AR, Koehler RE. Radiologic diagnosis of disordered esophageal motility: a unified physiologic approach. Radiol Clin North Am 1976; 14:429–439
11. Ott DJ. Radiologic evaluation of esophageal dysphagia. Curr Probl Diagn Radiol 1988; 17:1–33
12. Stewart ET. Radiographic evaluation of the esophagus and its motor disorders. Med Clin North Am 1981; 65:1173–1194

PEPTIC STRICTURE

13. Ho CS, Rodrigues PR. Lower esophageal strictures, benign or malignant? J Can Assoc Radiol 1980; 31:110–113

14. Levine MS. Reflux esophagitis. In: Levine MS (ed), Radiology of the esophagus. Philadelphia: WB Saunders; 1989:15–48
15. Ott DJ, Gelfand DW, Lane TG, Wu WC. Radiologic detection and spectrum of appearances of peptic esophageal strictures. J Clin Gastroenterol 1982; 4:11–15
16. Palmer ED. The hiatus hernia-esophagitis-esophageal stricture complex. Twenty-year prospective study. Am J Med 1968; 44:566–579

ESOPHAGEAL CARCINOMA

17. Agha FP. Barrett carcinoma of the esophagus: clinical and radiographic analysis of 34 cases. AJR 1985; 145:41–46
18. Blot WJ, Devesa SS, Kneller RW, Fraumeni JF Jr. Rising incidence of adenocarcinoma of the esophagus and gastric cardia. JAMA 1991; 265:1287–1289
19. Goldstein HM, Zornoza J, Hopens T. Intrinsic diseases of the adult esophagus: benign and malignant tumors. Semin Roentgenol 1981; 16:183–197
20. Keen SJ, Dodd GD, Smith JL Jr. Adenocarcinoma arising in Barrett esophagus: pathologic and radiologic features. Mt Sinai J Med 1984; 51:442–450
21. Levine MS. Esophageal carcinoma. In: Levine MS (ed), Radiology of the esophagus. Philadelphia: WB Saunders; 1989:131–168
22. Levine MS, Caroline D, Thompson JJ, Kressel HY, Laufer I, Herlinger H. Adenocarcinoma of the esophagus: relationship to Barrett mucosa. Radiology 1984; 150:305–309
23. Pera M, Cameron AJ, Trastek VF, Carpenter HA, Zinsmeister AR. Increasing incidence of adenocarcinoma of the esophagus and esophagogastric junction. Gastroenterology 1993; 104:510–513
24. Thompson JJ, Zinsser KR, Enterline HT. Barrett's metaplasia and adenocarcinoma of the esophagus and gastroesophageal junction. Hum Pathol 1983; 14:42–61

SCLERODERMA AND THE ESOPHAGUS

25. Halpert RD, Laufer I, Thompson JJ, Feczko PJ. Adenocarcinoma of the esophagus in patients with scleroderma. AJR 1983; 140:927–930
26. Recht MP, Levine MS, Katzka DA, Reynolds JC, Saul SH. Barrett's esophagus in scleroderma: increased prevalence and radiographic findings. Gastrointest Radiol 1988; 13:1–5
27. Zamost BJ, Hirschberg J, Ippoliti AF, Furst DE, Clements PJ, Weinstein WM. Esophagitis in scleroderma. Prevalence and risk factors. Gastroenterology 1987; 92:421–428

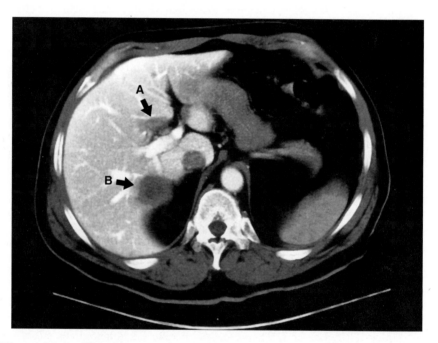

Figure 28-1. This 48-year-old woman with adenocarcinoma of the colon is being evaluated for possible resection of hepatic metastatic disease. You are shown one image from a CT arterial portogram.

Case 28: Nontumorous Perfusion Defect

Question 82

Which *one* of the following is the MOST likely explanation for the finding indicated by the arrow labeled A?

(A) Metastasis
(B) Hemangioma
(C) Benign perfusion defect
(D) Hepatic cyst
(E) Portal vein occlusion

The CT arterial portogram shown in Figure 28-1 demonstrates a hypoattenuating region (labeled A) in the medial segment of the left hepatic lobe just anterior to the porta hepatis (Figure 28-2). The location and appearance of this finding are most consistent with a benign perfusion defect rather than with a true mass lesion **(Option (C) is correct).**

CT during arterial portography (CTAP) is an invasive imaging technique for the detection of hepatic parenchymal lesions. It is usually reserved for patients who are candidates for surgical resection of hepatic tumors. The CT examination of the liver is performed during the portal phase of contrast agent injection through a catheter placed in the superior mesenteric artery or splenic artery. Most hepatic tumors receive their blood supply from the hepatic artery, so that selective enhancement of the portal venous system allows for improved contrast between the lesion and normal liver. CTAP has been shown to be the most sensitive technique currently available for preoperative evaluation of a candidate for hepatic resection of primary or metastatic hepatic tumors. The superiority of CTAP over standard contrast-enhanced CT and unenhanced MRI is a result of its improved detection of small (<2-cm) lesions.

Not infrequently, however, hypoattenuating defects that do not represent tumor are encountered during the CTAP examination. These include lesions due to abnormalities in hepatic perfusion that are unrelated to tumor. The specific benign perfusion abnormality seen in the test patient in the medial segment of the left hepatic lobe has been reported

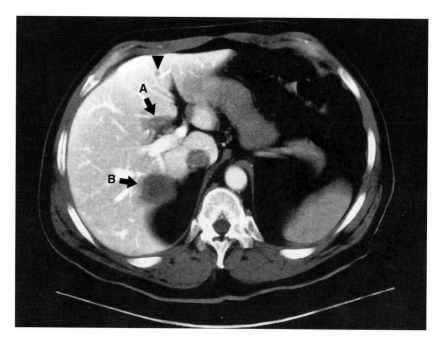

Figure 28-2 (Same as Figure 28-1). Benign perfusion defect and hepatic metastasis shown on a CT arterial portogram in a 48-year-old woman with adenocarcinoma of the colon. The lesion labeled A is located in the medial segment of the left hepatic lobe just anterior to the porta hepatis. This is a region in which a benign perfusion abnormality has been reported to occur in 14 to 25% of patients undergoing CTAP. It is postulated that this hypoperfused area is due to variant blood supply to this region. Lesion B is a metastasis from adenocarcinoma of the colon (see the text). An additional small lesion (arrowhead) is also seen in the medial segment of the left lobe (segment IVB). Unopacified blood is seen in the IVC.

to occur in 14 to 25% of patients undergoing CTAP. The defect can be elongated and somewhat rounded, as in the test patient, or even flatter and more plaquelike (Figure 28-3). It is postulated that this hypoperfused area is due to a variant blood supply to this region. Within this region of the medial segment of the left lobe of the liver, direct communications exist between portal vein radicals and capsular or cystic veins. These portal-systemic shunts may result in dilution or reversal of portal venous flow to this subsegment. Recognition of the existence of common perfusion abnormalities such as the one in the test patient is important to avoid incorrect interpretation of these studies and unnecessary exclusion of patients from potentially curative surgery.

Peterson et al. evaluated 245 perfusion defects detected by CTAP in 60 patients who subsequently underwent hepatic surgery. All 15 perfu-

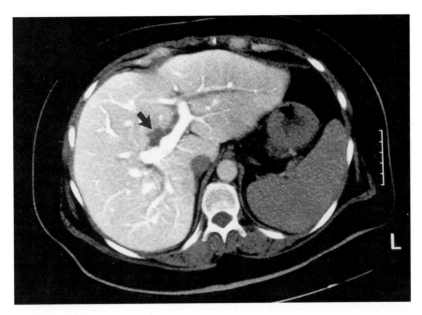

Figure 28-3. Benign perfusion defect. The CTAP examination in this 52-year-old woman with metastatic colon cancer demonstrates a flat hyper-perfused region (arrow) in the medial segment of the left lobe anterior to the portal vein. This is another characteristic appearance of the benign perfusion defect that occurs in this region.

sion defects in the posterior peripheral aspect of the medial segment, immediately anterior to the porta hepatis (as seen in the test image), were benign.

Other characteristic locations for benign perfusion defects have also been described (Figure 28-4). One of these locations is in the anterior aspect of the medial segment of the left lobe of the liver, adjacent to the intersegmental fissure. In the study of Peterson et al., seven perfusion defects identified adjacent to the intersegmental fissure were also found to be benign at pathology and were representative of focal fatty change or normal liver tissue. The region of the gallbladder fossa is another common location for benign perfusion abnormalities. Peripheral wedge-shaped defects are also common and are usually benign. Peterson et al. described six wedge-shaped perfusion defects with pathologic correlation; only one was found to be associated with tumor. These authors found that this perfusion defect could be differentiated from the benign wedge-shaped perfusion defects by the presence of a rounded central contour rather than a sharp apex.

While benign perfusion defects may have a variety of shapes, round perfusion defects were found to represent malignancies in the majority

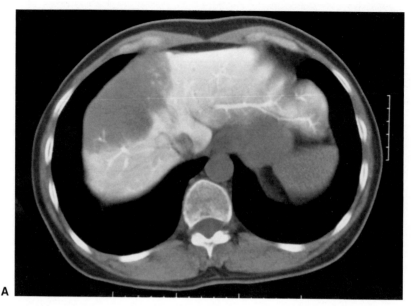

A

Figure 28-4. Benign perfusion defects. Three images from a CTAP examination in a 57-year-old woman with colon carcinoma metastatic to the liver demonstrate a single large metastasis and multiple benign perfusion defects. (A) The large metastasis occupies the medial segment of the left lobe of the liver. (B) A small perfusion defect is seen in the anterior aspect of the medial segment of the left lobe of the liver adjacent to the intersegmental fissure (long arrow). This is a common location for a benign perfusion defect and is also an area where focal fatty infiltration has been reported to occur. A wedgelike perfusion defect is also seen on the same section in the peripheral aspect of the right lobe of the liver (small arrows). This area was investigated at surgery by palpation and intraoperative ultrasonography, and no tumor was found. A portion of the metastatic lesion is also seen at this level. (C) Small perfusion defects are also seen adjacent to the gallbladder (arrows).

(58%) of patients in the Peterson et al. study. Pathologic diagnoses for benign round perfusion defects included cirrhotic nodules, normal liver, cysts, hemangiomas, focal nodular hyperplasia, focal fibrosis, focal fatty infiltration, and nonspecific regenerative change with an inflammatory exudate.

Metastasis (Option (A)) and hemangioma (Option (B)) would also appear as hypoattenuating defects on the CTAP study. Both of these of lesions would be expected to be rounder than the lesion in the test patient, and the characteristic location of the lesion makes a benign perfusion defect more likely.

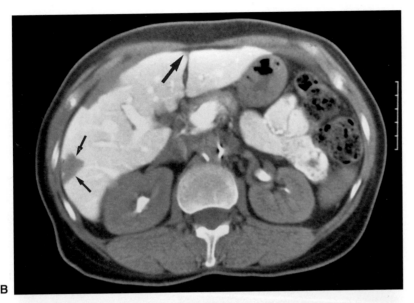

B

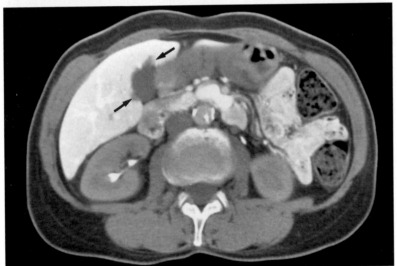

C

A hepatic cyst (Option (D)) would be expected to have an imaging appearance similar to that seen on routine CT, i.e., a sharply defined mass of water density, not the soft tissue attenuation mass seen in this case.

Occlusion of the portal vein or its branches (Option (E)) would be expected to result in a nonperfused region on CTAP. Most perfusion defects due to vascular occlusion have straight margins that parallel an

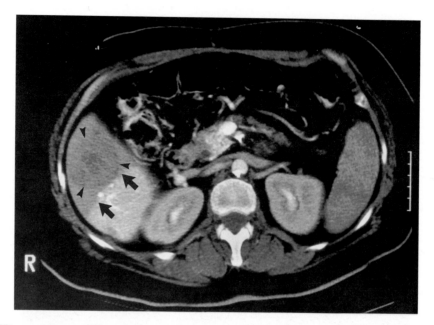

Figure 28-5. "Straight-line sign." The CTAP examination in this 52-year-old woman with colon cancer metastatic to liver demonstrates the straight-line sign (arrows), indicating involvement of the portal vein to the anterior segment of the right hepatic lobe (segment 5). The lesion itself (arrowheads) is seen within the nonperfused segment as a round lesion with central low attenuation consistent with necrosis.

expected vascular distribution (Figure 28-5), which is not the finding in the test image.

Question 83

Concerning the lesion marked with the arrow labeled B on the test image,

    (A) it is located in the anterior segment of the right hepatic lobe
    (B) it is located in Couinaud's segment VIII
    (C) it involves the inferior vena cava
    (D) its appearance excludes cavernous hemangioma

Patients who are candidates for hepatic resection undergo preoperative imaging studies to determine not only the size and number of hepatic lesions but also their segmental location and relationship to the hepatic vasculature. Hepatic segmental anatomy as described by Bismuth divides the liver transversely by a plane through the right and left

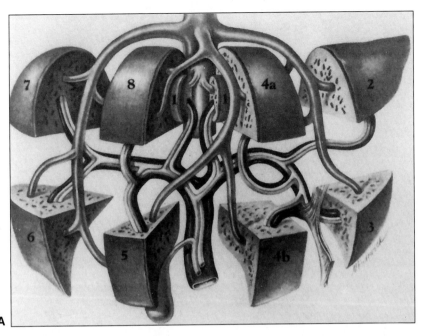

Figure 28-6. Hepatic segmental anatomy. (A) The liver is divided longitudinally by the hepatic veins and transversely by the right and left main portal pedicles (the transverse scissura). (Panel A is reprinted with permission from Nelson et al. [12].)

portal pedicles (the transverse scissura) and longitudinally by the three hepatic veins. All the hepatic segments except segment I, the caudate lobe, are defined by these planes. These segments are numbered I through VIII, using the numbering system established by Couinaud (Figure 28-6). This system is used by many hepatic surgeons to guide surgical resection of the liver, in order to decrease blood loss intraoperatively and decrease bile leaks and areas of devascularized parenchyma postoperatively. Therefore, knowledge of this system is required for the radiologist to describe the relevant anatomy precisely to the referring surgeon. Adoption of this surgically and radiologically relevant nomenclature by all radiologists has been advocated. Recent *in vivo* studies have demonstrated wide individual variation in portal and hepatic venous anatomy not described in the early radiologic literature on this subject; however, identification of major portal and hepatic venous branches and description of lesion location in relation to those vessels is clearly an essential part of preoperative decision-making in this population.

The test image (Figures 28-1 and 28-2) was obtained at the level of the right main portal vein, placing lesion B at the level of the transverse

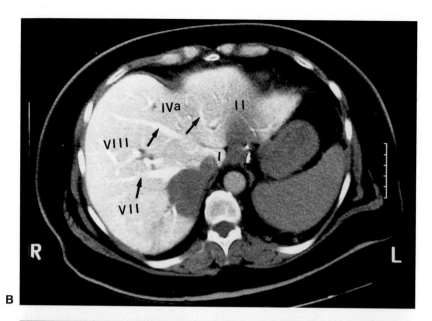

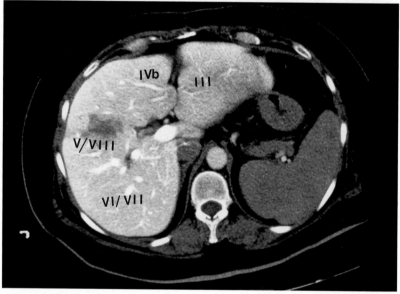

Figure 28-6 (Continued). Hepatic segmental anatomy. (B) Segmental anatomy above the transverse scissura. The hepatic segments are determined longitudinally by the hepatic veins (arrows). The lateral segment of the left lobe corresponds to segment II, the medial segment of the left lobe corresponds to segment IVa, the anterior segment of the right lobe corresponds to segment VIII, and the posterior segment of the right lobe corresponds to segment VII. A lesion is seen in segment VII, inseparable from the right hepatic vein and the IVC. (C) CTAP image at the level of the left portal pedicle. The right portal pedicle is located cephalad to this section. At this level, the lateral segment of the left lobe corresponds to segment III and the medial segment corresponds to IVb. (D) Hepatic segmental anatomy below the transverse scissura. The anterior segment of the right lobe corresponds to segment V, and the posterior segment corresponds to segment VI. A large lesion is seen occupying segment V.

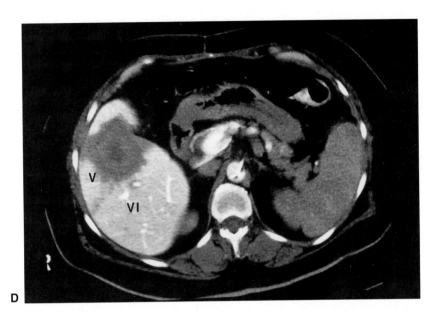

D

scissura. The lesion is located in the posterior segment of the right lobe of the liver, posterior to the right hepatic vein **(Option (A) is false).** The posterior segment of the right hepatic lobe corresponds to Couinaud's segments VI and VII, with the transverse scissura dividing the two (Table 28-1) **(Option (B) is false).** On this section, the lesion is remote from the inferior vena cava (IVC), which is not yet opacified with contrast material. Therefore, the low attenuation within the IVC represents unopacified blood and so the IVC is not involved by the tumor **(Option (C) is false).**

CTAP is a sensitive examination for lesion detection, but it is not specific. The characteristic globular peripheral enhancement associated with cavernous hemangioma on contrast-enhanced CT is not seen on CTAP examinations, since the hepatic arterial enhancement is not seen **(Option (D) is true).** Therefore, the identity of the lesion in the test image is indeterminate on the basis of the CTAP examination alone. Percutaneous biopsy of this lesion performed prior to this examination revealed adenocarcinoma consistent with a colonic primary tumor.

Table 28-1: Anatomic segments of the liver and corresponding nomenclature[a]

Anatomic segment	Nomenclature		
	Couinaud	Bismuth	Goldsmith & Woodburne
Caudate lobe	I	I	Caudate lobe
Left lateral superior	II	II	Left lateral segment
Left lateral inferior	III	III	Left lateral segment
Left medial	IV	IVa, IVb	Left medial segment
Right anterior inferior	V	V	Right anterior segment
Right anterior superior	VIII	VIII	Right anterior segment
Right posterior inferior	VI	VI	Right posterior segment
Right posterior superior	VII	VII	Right posterior segment

[a] Reprinted with permission from Soyer (13).

Question 84

Concerning surgical resection of hepatic metastases from a primary colorectal carcinoma,

- (A) approximately 30% of patients with newly diagnosed colorectal cancer meet the criteria for hepatic resection
- (B) only patients with solitary metastatic lesions are considered candidates
- (C) lymph node metastases are a contraindication to hepatic resection
- (D) the post-resection liver volume must be at least 50% of the preoperative volume
- (E) the 5-year survival rate is about 60%

Candidates for surgical resection of hepatic tumors must be carefully selected preoperatively to avoid the expense, morbidity, and mortality associated with surgery in a patient with little or no chance for cure. Isolated hepatic metastases from colorectal cancer are relatively uncommon, but the large number of patients diagnosed with this malignancy each year results in a large pool of potential resection candidates. It is estimated that 5% of the approximately 140,000 persons newly diagnosed with colorectal cancer each year will meet the criteria for hepatic resection **(Option (A) is false)**. Most patients are not candidates, for one of multiple reasons, with absence of metastatic disease at one end of the spectrum and disseminated metastatic disease at the other.

A retrospective analysis of a registry of patients who had successfully undergone removal of hepatic metastases from colorectal carcinoma determined the prognostic factors for survival of patients undergoing this surgery. A favorable outcome was associated with one to four hepatic metastases **(Option (B) is false)**, no extrahepatic metastases, a negative margin of resection of the primary tumor, and no spread of the intrahepatic metastases to lymph nodes draining the liver **(Option (C) is true)**. Factors found to be unimportant in survival included the number of metastases (one to three), bilobar versus unilobar disease, the type of surgery (removal of the metastasis only versus major hepatic resection), preoperative carcinoembryonic antigen level, the age or sex of the patient, and the size of the lesion. The functional liver volume after resection must be 30% or more of the preoperative volume to avoid postoperative hepatic failure **(Option (D) is false)**. Preoperative embolization of the involved hepatic segments prior to resection has been advocated as a means of inducing hypertrophy of the uninvolved liver to increase the post-resection hepatic volume in marginal cases. The radiologist must evaluate each surgical candidate with these factors in mind.

The rationale behind surgical resection of metastatic disease in selected cases is the concept of "metastatic insufficiency." According to this theory, tumor emboli from colon carcinoma that reach the liver via the portal vein become established as metastatic disease only when the number of cells overcomes the host's intrinsic resistance to tumor implantation. Once established, this metastatic deposit becomes a source of tumor emboli to the lung. By this reasoning, resection of hepatic metastases, if they are few in number, may completely interrupt cancer spread by removing isolated foci of disease, since the liver is the first capillary bed draining a primary colon cancer. Data from multiple individual series as well as multi-institutional studies have shown a 20 to 25% 5-year survival in patients undergoing resection of their metastases versus 0% in the nonresected group **(Option (E) is false)**. Unfortunately, postoperative tumor recurrence is common, usually due to disease already present at the time of surgery but not detected by current imaging techniques.

Judith L. Chezmar, M.D.

SUGGESTED READINGS

COMPUTED TOMOGRAPHY DURING ARTERIAL PORTOGRAPHY

1. del Pilar Fernandez M, Bernardino ME. Hepatic pseudolesion: appearance of focal low attenuation in the medial segment of the left lobe at CT arterial portography. Radiology 1991; 181:809–812
2. Heiken JP, Weyman PJ, Lee JK, et al. Detection of focal hepatic masses: prospective evaluation with CT, delayed CT, CT during arterial portography, and MR imaging. Radiology 1989; 171:47–51
3. Matsui O, Kadoya M, Suzuki M, et al. Work in progress: dynamic sequential computed tomography during arterial portography in the detection of hepatic neoplasms. Radiology 1983; 146:721–725
4. Matsui O, Takashima T, Kadoya M, et al. Dynamic computed tomography during arterial portography: the most sensitive examination for small hepatocellular carcinomas. J Comput Assist Tomogr 1985; 9:19–24
5. Nelson RC, Chezmar JL, Sugarbaker PH, Bernardino ME. Hepatic tumors: comparison of CT during arterial portography, delayed CT, and MR imaging for preoperative evaluation. Radiology 1989; 172:27–34
6. Nelson RC, Thompson GH, Chezmar JL, Harned RK Jr, Fernandez MP. CT during arterial portography: diagnostic pitfalls. RadioGraphics 1992; 12:705–718
7. Peterson MS, Baron RL, Dodd GD III, et al. Hepatic parenchymal perfusion defects detected with CTAP: imaging-pathologic correlation. Radiology 1992; 185:149–155

HEPATIC SEGMENTAL ANATOMY

8. Bismuth H. Surgical anatomy and anatomical surgery of the liver. World J Surg 1982; 6:3–9
9. Couinaud C. Controlled hepatectomies and exposure of the intrahepatic bile ducts: anatomical and technical study. Paris: Couinaud Press; 1981
10. Dodd GD III. An American's guide to Couinaud's numbering system. AJR 1993; 161:574–575
11. Mukai JK, Stack CM, Turner DA, et al. Imaging of surgically relevant hepatic vascular and segmental anatomy. Part 1. Normal anatomy. AJR 1987; 149:287–292
12. Nelson RC, Chezmar JL, Sugarbaker PH, Murray DR, Bernardino ME. Preoperative localization of focal liver lesions to specific liver segments: utility of CT during arterial portography. Radiology 1990; 176:89–94
13. Soyer P. Segmental anatomy of the liver: utility of a nomenclature accepted worldwide. AJR 1993; 161:572–573
14. van Leeuwen MS, Fernandez MA, van Es HW, Stokking R, Dillon EH, Feldberg MA. Variations in venous and segmental anatomy of the liver: two- and three-dimensional MR imaging in healthy volunteers. AJR 1994; 162:1337–1345

HEPATIC RESECTION

15. Freeny PC, Marks WM, Ryan JA, Bolen JW. Colorectal carcinoma evaluation with CT: preoperative staging and detection of postoperative recurrence. Radiology 1986; 158:347–353

16. Harned RK II, Chezmar JL, Nelson RC. Imaging of patients with potentially resectable hepatic neoplasms. AJR 1992; 159:1191–1194
17. Registry of Hepatic Metastases. Resection of the liver for colorectal carcinoma metastases: a multi-institutional study of indications for resection. Surgery 1988; 103:278–288
18. Seltzer SE, Holman BL. Imaging hepatic metastases from colorectal carcinoma: identification of candidates for partial hepatectomy. AJR 1989; 152:917–923
19. Sugarbaker PH. Surgical decision making for large bowel cancer metastatic to the liver. Radiology 1990; 174:621–626

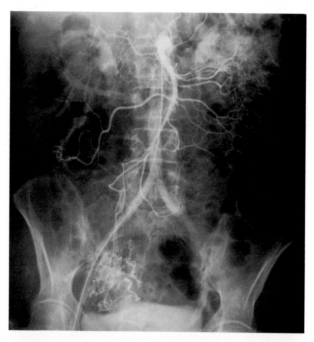

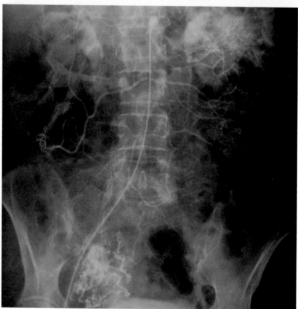

Figure 29-1. This 44-year-old woman has recurrent gastrointestinal hemorrhage. You are shown three radiographs from a superior mesenteric arteriogram.

Case 29: Bleeding Small Intestinal Leiomyosarcoma

Question 85

Which *one* of the following is the MOST likely diagnosis?

(A) Angiodysplasia
(B) Adenocarcinoma
(C) Leiomyosarcoma
(D) Small bowel diverticulum
(E) Carcinoid tumor

Radiographs from the early, middle, and late phases of a superior mesenteric arteriogram (Figure 29-1) show a moderately well-defined hypervascular mass in the distal small bowel (Figure 29-2). Intense neovascularity and capillary blush define a somewhat lobulated contour to the mass. The radiograph from the arterial phase shows no arterio-venous shunting and no vascular encasement. Extravasation of contrast material is not present, indicating by arteriographic criteria that the lesion is not actively bleeding. The location and arteriographic appearance are typical for a smooth muscle tumor of the small intestine (Figure 29-3). Arteriographic differentiation between a leiomyoma, the most common neoplasm of the small bowel, and leiomyosarcoma is often diffi-cult. Small tumors with a well-demarcated capillary blush are usually benign (Figure 29-4). Malignant lesions, that is, leiomyosarcomas, are larger and have less-distinct margins because of infiltration of adjacent structures. Sarcomas typically show intense neovascularity. Arterio-venous shunting may occur, and a large draining vein is often demon-strated. The intense neovascularity shown in Figure 29B favors a lei-omyosarcoma, and leiomyoma is not offered as an option **(Option (C) is correct).**

Angiodysplasia (Option (A)) is a common cause of chronic, recurrent lower gastrointestinal hemorrhage in older individuals. On occasion, angiodysplasias also bleed acutely. The lesion is composed of a small tan-

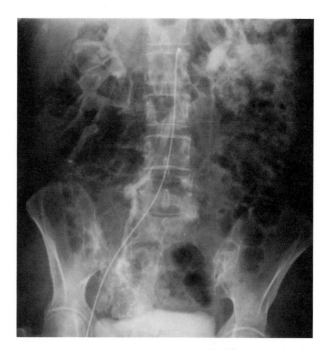

Figure 29-1 (Continued)

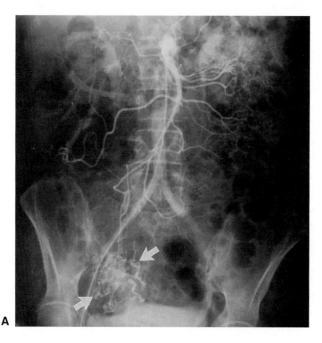

A

Figure 29-2 (Same as Figure 29-1). Ileal leiomyosarcoma. (A) A radiograph from the arterial phase of a superior mesenteric arteriogram shows a highly vascular mass (arrows) supplied by branches of the ileocolic artery.

gle of abnormally communicating arteries and veins in the mucosa and submucosa of the bowel. Typically, angiodysplasias are located on the

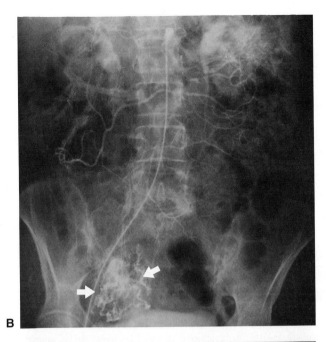

B

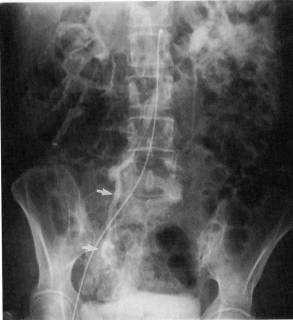

C

Figure 29-2 (Continued) (Same as Figure 29-1). Ileal leiomyosarcoma. (B) A radiograph from the capillary phase of the injection sequence shows intense staining of the lesion (arrows). Multiple large arteries within the mass are tortuous and irregular in contour, and they do not branch normally. These arteries have developed within the tumor, and this arteriographic pattern is referred to as neovascularity. No early-draining vein, indicating significant arteriovenous shunting, is seen. (C) A radiograph from the venous phase shows a large vein (arrows) draining blood from the tumor to the superior mesenteric vein.

antimesenteric border of the small intestine, cecum, or ascending colon. They can be multiple. The arteriographic appearance of angiodysplasia is characteristic, and arteriography is often diagnostic even if performed

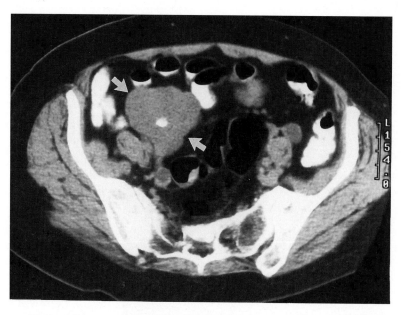

Figure 29-3. Same patient as in Figures 29-1 and 29-2. Ileal leiomyo-sarcoma. A CT scan shows a pelvic soft tissue mass (arrows) with a central area of high attenuation representing calcification. At operation, the surgeon resected a lobulated, 6-cm ileal mass that grossly resembled a leiomyoma. Foci of malignancy were found on histologic analysis.

when there is no bleeding. A small tangle of tortuous vessels is seen in the center of the lesion during the late arterial and capillary phases. These findings resemble those in the test patient, but there is no associated mass in patients with angiodysplasia. The *sine qua non* of angiodysplasia on arteriography is the appearance in the arterial phase of a densely opacified vein draining the lesion, a so-called "early draining vein" (Figure 29-5) (a finding not seen in the test patient's study). When angiodysplasia is suspected, the arteriographic injection should not last longer than 4 seconds. This minimizes the likelihood of arterial opacification lasting long enough to overlap the period during which veins normally become visible, an observation that could be misinterpreted as indicating an early-draining vein.

Primary malignant tumors of the small bowel account for only 1% of malignant tumors of the alimentary tract, with metastatic neoplasms being more frequent. Of the primary malignant tumors that occur in the small intestine, adenocarcinoma (Option (B)) is the most common. It is found most frequently in the distal duodenum and proximal jejunum and is rare in the ileum. Arteriographically, adenocarcinomas can appear hyper- or hypovascular; the latter appearance is more common. Encase-

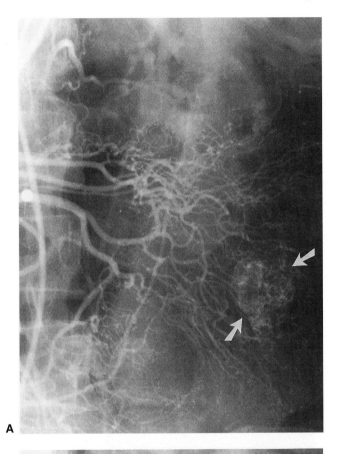

A

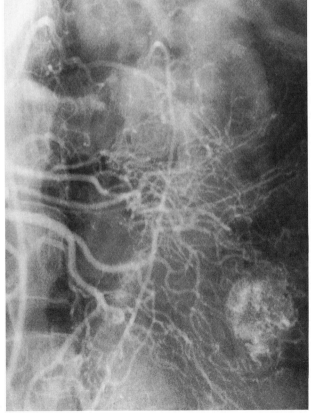

B

Figure 29-4. Arteriographic appearance of a jejunal leiomyoma in a 54-year-old woman with three episodes of gastrointestinal hemorrhage over a 2-year period. Barium studies and endoscopy were unrevealing. (A) In the arterial phase, there is early and focal opacification of small arteries and capillaries within a well-circumscribed, ovoid mass (arrows) in the left mid-abdomen. The mass is fed by jejunal branches of the superior mesenteric artery. (B) There is dense capillary staining in the late arterial phase. (C [following page]) In the venous phase, slow washout of contrast agent and a prominent vein (arrows) draining the tumor are seen. There is no extravasation to indicate active bleeding at the time of the arteriographic injection.

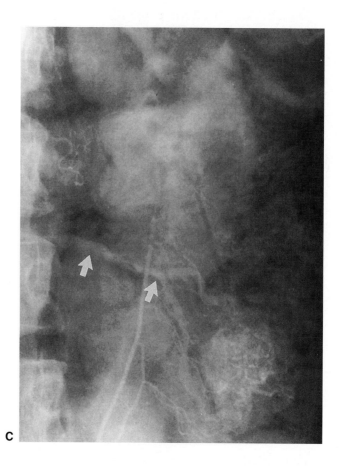

C

ment of small to medium-sized arteries is common but can be subtle. There can be arteriovenous shunting. Direct extension of the carcinoma to adjacent structures is common, and angiography shows an ill-defined border to the mass; in contrast, the lesion in the test figure appears as a well-defined mass. Small intestinal adenocarcinoma is more effectively demonstrated by CT or barium studies, particularly enteroclysis, than by arteriography, because of its subtle and variable arteriographic appearance.

A diverticulum (Option (D)) is another potential cause of bleeding from the small intestine, although hemorrhage is atypical (except from Meckel's diverticulum). Only rarely do small intestinal diverticula cause signs or symptoms. Acquired small bowel diverticula develop as a result of prolapse of mucosa through the muscularis propria on the mesenteric border of the bowel. In older persons, diverticula sometimes become large or numerous and can be sites of bacterial overgrowth, leading to

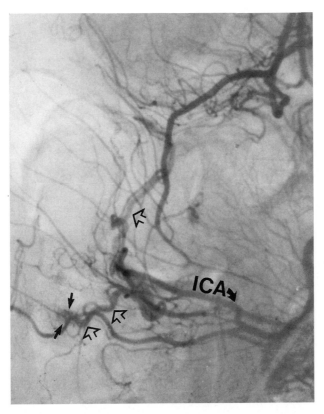

Figure 29-5. Angiodysplasia. An arteriogram in an elderly woman with recurrent, unexplained, gastrointestinal bleeding shows a small, ovoid tuft of tangled arteries (straight black arrows) supplied by a cecal branch of the ileocolic artery (ICA). Note the prominent vein (open arrows) draining the angiodysplasia. This vein is well opacified during the arterial phase of the filming sequence, well before other veins in the area, because of arteriovenous shunting in the angiodysplasia. The cecal location, vascular tuft, and early-draining vein establish the diagnosis.

malabsorption. The occasional hemorrhage from a small bowel diverticulum results from ulceration due to bacterial inflammation or to ischemia in a diverticulum with a stretched or twisted vascular supply. If bleeding occurs at a sufficient rate at the time of contrast injection, angiography shows a pool of extravasated contrast within the lumen of the diverticulum (Figure 29-6). This appearance can mimic that of a pool of contrast-enhanced blood in a patient with an aneurysm or pseudoaneurysm, and care must be taken to distinguish these entities. Contrast-induced opacification of an aneurysm remains constant in size and shape as it fades over a period of several seconds. Extravasated contrast agent within a

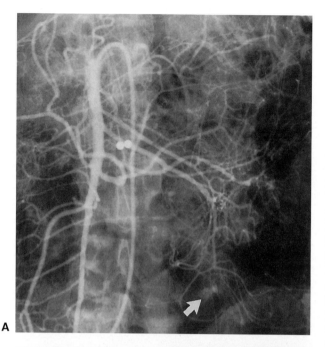

A

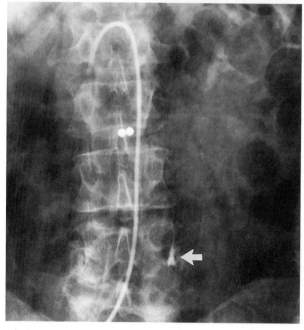

B

Figure 29-6. Hemorrhage from a jejunal diverticulum. The patient was a 61-year-old woman known to have numerous diverticula of the small and large bowel. (A) An arterial-phase arteriogram shows a pool of extravasated contrast material (arrow) beginning to form in the lumen of the bowel. The blood and contrast medium are leaking from the second branch that arises from the left side of the superior mesenteric artery, indicating a mid-jejunal location. (B) Late in the venous phase, there is persistence of the pool of contrast material in a confined space suggestive of a diverticulum. Bleeding was controlled with intraarterial infusion of vasopressin at a rate of 0.2 U/minute.

diverticulum persists much longer and changes in shape as it flows out of the diverticulum into the lumen of the adjacent bowel. In the absence of

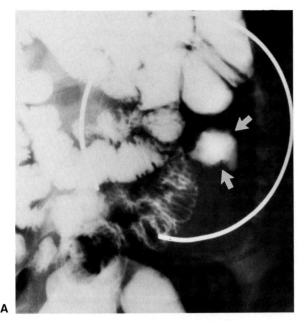
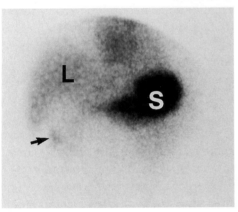

A

B

Figure 29-7. Meckel's diverticulum in a 25-year-old man with recurrent, unexplained gastrointestinal blood loss. (A) A compression radiograph from a small bowel series shows a 3-cm collection of barium (arrows) in the left lower abdomen. The diverticulum lacks mucosal folds, has a somewhat irregular contour, and did not change in size or shape from film to film. These features suggest ulceration, which was subsequently found at operation. (B) An anterior Tc-99m pertechnetate scintigram of the upper abdomen 15 minutes after injection of tracer. At the time of this study, the diverticulum was located in the right upper abdomen, where it appears as a focal area of increased uptake (arrow) due to secretion of the tracer by ectopic gastric mucosa within it. S = stomach; L = liver.

active bleeding at the time of the procedure, angiography in patients with diverticular hemorrhage is usually diagnostic.

Meckel's diverticulum occurs in 2% of the general population, making it the most common congenital anomaly of the gastrointestinal tract. These diverticula represent a vestige of the fetal vitello-intestinal duct and occur on or near the antimesenteric border of the ileum 45 to 90 cm proximal to the ileocecal valve (Figure 29-7A). Most are less than 5 cm long, but a few have been found to exceed 20 cm. They are often missed on routine barium studies of the small intestine. Enteroclysis is more sensitive than the conventional peroral examination.

Unlike acquired diverticula, Meckel's diverticula contain the mucosal, submucosal, and muscular layers of the bowel wall. Ectopic gastric mucosa occurs in 15 to 62% of Meckel's diverticula. This accounts for the most common clinical presentation, namely, gastrointestinal hemorrhage arising from peptic ulceration within a diverticulum containing gastric-type epithelium that secretes hydrochloric acid. Tc-99m pertechnetate scintigraphy is the most commonly used radiologic method of diagnosis and has a sensitivity of approximately 85% (Figure 29-7B). Mucus-secreting cells in the ectopic gastric mucosa within Meckel's diverticula secrete pertechnetate. For the scintigraphic study to be positive, there must be a sufficient number of these cells in the diverticulum. Rarely, a Meckel's diverticulum serves as the lead point for ileal intussusception. Eighty percent of patients with symptoms attributable to Meckel's diverticulum are under 10 years of age. It is rare for Meckel's diverticulum to cause symptoms in patients over 30 years of age.

Meckel's diverticula can sometimes be identified arteriographically even when they are not actively bleeding. The vitelline artery, which serves the diverticulum, is identified as an elongated branch of the ileal artery serving the affected segment of bowel. The vitelline artery terminates in tortuous vessels serving the ectopic gastric mucosa. Unlike the angiographic appearance of an arteriovenous malformation, no early draining vein is seen and the terminal vessels do not have communicating branches. There is no vascular encasement. A well-defined vascular mass, as seen in the test figure, is not present in a patient with Meckel's diverticulum.

Patients with carcinoid tumors of the small bowel (Option (E)) most often present with chronic, unexplained gastrointestinal hemorrhage. The great majority are ileal in location. Examination of the small intestine by conventional barium study, enteroclysis, or barium enema can, in some cases, detect carcinoid tumors; they are typically smooth, round, polypoid masses in the ileal lumen. The tumor has a propensity to spread to the adjacent mesentery, where it incites an intense desmoplastic response that causes kinking and fixation of the bowel. The fibrosis incited by the tumor also causes obstruction of mesenteric veins and lymphatics which, in turn, leads to thickening of the bowel wall and valvulae conniventes.

CT is also useful in demonstrating carcinoid tumors. If it is large enough to be visible on CT images, the primary tumor appears as a rounded, intraluminal ileal mass. Easier to detect on the CT scans, however, is the mesenteric component of the tumor, which usually appears as a 2- to 4-cm soft tissue mass with characteristic stellate or spiculated margins. Calcification can be seen in the primary tumor or in its mesenteric component.

Somatostatin-receptor scintigraphy with In-111 octreotide is effective in demonstrating a number of neuroendocrine tumors, including carcinoids. Approximately 80 to 90% of carcinoid tumors can be visualized in this way.

The arteriographic features of a small bowel carcinoid tumor are often quite characteristic. The vascular effects of mesenteric desmoplastic process incited by the tumor include kinking, straightening, and retraction of mesenteric arteries in and around the tumor, features not seen in the test arteriogram. Classically, the arteries in the affected mesentery radiate outward from a central nidus of tumor in a stellate or "sunburst" pattern (Figure 29-8). Venous occlusions also occur and can cause localized mesenteric varices.

Carcinoid syndrome occurs in less than 10% of patients. The classic symptoms of the syndrome include flushing of the head and neck, asthma-like attacks, and diarrhea. It is mediated by peptides, such as serotonin and precursors of bradykinin, that are produced by the tumor cells. Carcinoid tumors confined to the bowel release these peptides into the portal venous system. Passage through the liver then leads to their metabolism and deactivation. Only intestinal carcinoid tumors that have spread to the liver release their products into the systemic venous system, where they can cause carcinoid syndrome.

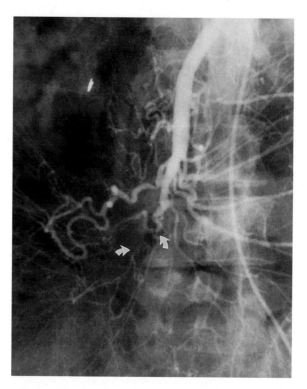

Figure 29-8. Carcinoid tumor of the ileum with spread to the mesentery. A radiograph from arterial phase of a superior mesenteric arteriogram shows that arterial branches in the area of the tumor are kinked and distorted. There are abrupt changes in arterial caliber and points of occlusion (arrows). Desmoplasia in the mesentery retracts the involved arteries toward the tumor, so that they appear to radiate out from its center.

Question 86

Concerning gastrointestinal angiodysplasia,

    (A) most occur in the descending colon
    (B) arteriography shows late opacification of the ileocolic vein
    (C) venous varices often lie adjacent to the lesion
    (D) it is a common cause of gastrointestinal bleeding in young adults
    (E) in individuals with Rendu-Osler-Weber syndrome, telangiectasias occur
        most often in the stomach and colon

Angiodysplasias, or vascular ectasias, are common lesions that are notoriously difficult to diagnose. Sheedy et al. and Foutch report acquired angiodysplastic lesions to be the most common explanation for obscure gastrointestinal bleeding. Most angiodysplasias are located in the small intestine, cecum, and proximal ascending colon **(Option (A) is false)**. They can be multiple. The lesion consists of a tuft or cluster of abnormal, thin-walled, vascular spaces in the submucosa. They vary in size from 1 or 2 mm to a few centimeters. They are visible endoscopically as one or more red spots seen through the bowel mucosa but cannot be seen on barium studies.

The arteriographic diagnosis is made by the demonstration of the vascular tuft along the antimesenteric border of the bowel in association with an early-draining vein **(Option (B) is false)**. The injection of contrast agent should last no longer than 4 seconds if an angiodysplastic lesion is suspected, to allow the early-draining vein to be identified accurately. There is no obstruction to flow in large or medium-sized veins, so varices are not a component of the angiographic appearance **(Option (C) is false)**. These lesions are thought to be degenerative in origin and are seldom encountered in young patients **(Option (D) is false)**. The reported prevalence of angiodysplasia in elderly patients is 27%. Often angiodysplasias are found incidentally in right colonic specimens resected for other reasons. If angiodysplasia is found arteriographically but does not show active bleeding (extravasation), the search should continue for another possible source of hemorrhage. Angiodysplastic lesions are so common in patients over the age of 50 years that they may coexist with another lesion responsible for bleeding.

Currently, the terminology related to angiodysplastic lesions of the gastrointestinal tract is somewhat confusing. Moore et al. in 1976 simplified the nomenclature of these lesions by dividing vascular abnormalities into three categories: acquired vascular ectasia, which occurs primarily in the elderly; arteriovenous malformations of developmental origin; and capillary angiomas associated with hereditary hemorrhagic telangiectasia (Rendu-Osler-Weber syndrome). Telangiectasias in patients with

Rendu-Osler-Weber syndrome are located most often in the small bowel **(Option (E) is false).** These patients can also have pulmonary arteriovenous malformations and vascular abnormalities of the hepatic arteries, including abnormal communications between hepatic and portal veins.

Question 87

Concerning patients with recurrent episodes of acute gastrointestinal bleeding with no etiology found by endoscopy or conventional barium studies,

    (A) arteriography is diagnostic only during periods of active bleeding
    (B) the small bowel is the most common location for an identifiable bleeding site
    (C) if the patient is actively bleeding, scintigraphy with Tc-99m erythrocytes is sensitive in localizing the site of bleeding
    (D) enteroclysis will identify the responsible lesion in about 20% of patients

Patients with intermittent, acute gastrointestinal hemorrhage can present a diagnostic dilemma. In the 1950s, the source of bleeding in 15 to 25% of these patients remained unexplained. With advances in endoscopy, double-contrast barium studies, and CT, the fraction of unexplained cases has fallen to about 10%. In half of these patients with unexplained sources of bleeding, the bleeding does not recur. For the 5% of patients who continue to bleed intermittently, sometimes with episodes of severe hemorrhage, arteriography has proven to be a valuable diagnostic and therapeutic tool. When active gastrointestinal bleeding is taking place, it is important that arteriography be performed as promptly as possible. This enables the radiologist to arteriographically demonstrate the extravasation of intravascular contrast material into the gut lumen.

Arteriography can demonstrate an etiology for the bleeding in 45 to 73% of patients with chronic, recurrent gastrointestinal blood loss of obscure origin, even when bleeding is not occurring at the time of the study **(Option (A) is false).** The small intestine is the most common part of the gastrointestinal tract in which to find such a lesion **(Option (B) is true),** probably because most bleeding lesions of the esophagus, stomach, duodenum, and colon are identified before they reach this stage. In patients presenting with iron deficiency anemia, heme-positive stools, negative findings on endoscopy and noninvasive imaging studies, and no history of episodic bleeding, the most common source of hemorrhage is a benign leiomyoma of the small intestine. Other sources of small intestinal bleeding include diverticula and primary and metastatic tumors. In the population over age 60, the most common lesion is

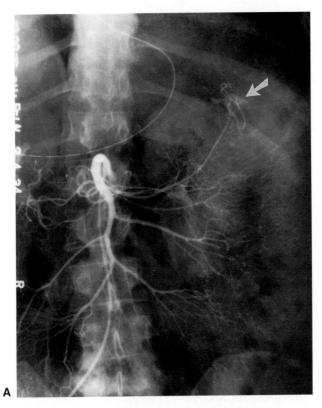

A

Figure 29-9. Arteriographic demonstration of brisk hemorrhage from a diverticulum of the splenic flexure in a patient with hematochezia. (A) An arterial-phase radiograph shows extravasation (arrow) from a branch of the middle colic artery.

acquired angiodysplasia, which occurs most commonly in the cecum and ascending colon, but also occurs in the jejunum and ileum.

It is known from animal studies that bleeding rates must be at least 0.5 to 1.0 mL/min for the radiologist to detect extravasation of contrast agent and therefore to detect a site of bleeding arteriographically. If an initial arteriogram is not revealing, a second arteriogram is warranted if bleeding recurs, since the bleeding site is sometimes visible only on the subsequent examination. Lou and co-workers found a repeat arteriogram to be positive in 5 (31%) of 16 patients whose bleeding recurred after a negative arteriogram was done on the previous day. Brisk hemorrhage can cause marked extravasation of contrast material into the bowel (Figure 29-9). A "pseudovein" appearance can be seen as contrast collects in the dependent portion of the bowel lumen between linear mucosal folds. This appearance can be distinguished from that of an opacified vein by

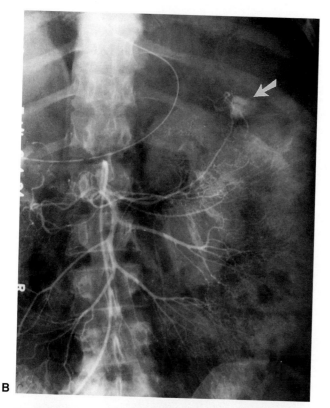

B

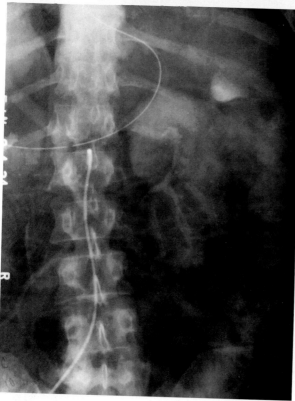

C

Figure 29-9 (Continued).
Arteriographic demon-
stration of brisk hemor-
rhage from a diverticu-
lum of the splenic flexure
in a patient with hema-
tochezia. (B) A few sec-
onds later, the pool of extravasated contrast
material (arows) has be-
gun to spread out in the
bowel lumen. (C) The last
radiograph in the injec-
tion sequence shows per-
sistence of the extrava-
sated contrast material at
a time when all but the
major veins have cleared.
This confirms that the
pool of contrast material
lies outside the vascular
system. Guided by the ar-
teriographic findings, the
surgeon performed a left
colectomy.

the lack of vascular washout and by gradual dispersion of the contrast pool into the adjacent bowel.

Radionuclide imaging plays a role in the evaluation of gastrointestinal hemorrhage. Imaging with Tc-99m erythrocytes is the most widely used scintigraphic method. Scintigraphy is more sensitive than arteriography and can detect active bleeding at rates as low as 0.05 to 0.1 mL/min. In the study of McKusick et al., scintigraphy correctly localized the bleeding site to the stomach/duodenum, small bowel, colon, or sigmoid/rectum in 31 of 39 instances (77%) **(Option (C) is true).** Occasional false-positive studies are a problem. These are minimized by use of the *in vitro* technique for erythrocyte labeling (since this method has the highest labeling efficiency and the lowest amounts of unbound Tc-99m). If surgery is contemplated, arteriography, endoscopy, or other studies are sometimes done to confirm the location of the bleeding site. For extravasation to be detectable, approximately 3 mL of radiolabeled blood must accumulate in a localized area of the bowel lumen. If the bleeding is very slow or intermittent, this can take 60 minutes or more. A distinct advantage of Tc-99m erythrocyte scintigraphy is its ability to label the blood (and therefore to monitor for bleeding) over a longer period than the few-second window afforded by arteriography. Patients can be reimaged repeatedly over 24 hours; reimaging is important if the study is initially negative. More than 70% of studies that are eventually positive fail to demonstrate extravasation in the first hour after injection. The site of bleeding can be difficult to define anatomically because of the poor spatial resolution of scintigraphic images, but the information gained in a positive study is helpful in directing future arteriographic or endoscopic examinations (Figure 29-10). Continuous data acquisition and cinematic display of images improve localization of the bleeding site.

Enteroclysis is an effective method for studying the small bowel with barium sulfate. The regulatory action of the pyloric sphincter is bypassed by instillation of barium through a tube passed into the distal duodenum or proximal jejunum, and so rapid infusion of barium suspension is possible. The small bowel is then distended and examined fluoroscopically with the aid of palpation. Enteroclysis has been reported to have about a 20% diagnostic yield in patients with gastrointestinal hemorrhage of obscure origin **(Option (D) is true).** The sensitivity of the conventional peroral barium examination of the small intestine probably approaches this level as well, if careful attention is paid to maintaining bowel distension and to performing fluoroscopy with palpation. The critical element in using barium studies to detect potential bleeding sites in the small intestine is the methodical fluoroscopic assessment of each segment of the bowel. Neither of these barium studies of the small bowel is appropriate during acute hemorrhage. It may take several days for barium to be

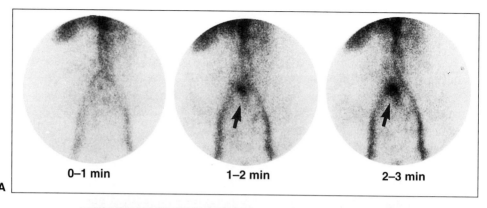

A

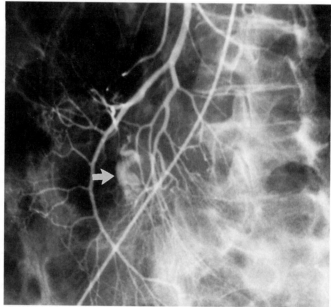

B

Figure 29-10. Ileal hemorrhage in a 53-year-old woman presenting with anemia and melena but no convincing evidence for active bleeding at the time. (A) During a scintigraphic study performed with Tc-99m erythrocytes, the patient became hypotensive. Three 1-minute images obtained over the first 3 minutes after injection show a rapidly expanding area of extravasation (arrows) in the lower mid-abdomen. This persisted and grew even larger on subsequent frames. The findings indicate brisk hemorrhage at a location most consistent with the small intestine. (B) Superior mesenteric arteriography was immediately performed and showed extravasation (arrow) from an ileal artery. At operation, the affected segment of ileum was resected. It was inflamed and necrotic, presumably on the basis of ischemia.

cleared completely from the gastrointestinal tract, and retained barium sulfate can conceal diagnostic findings on a subsequent arteriogram.

Question 88

Which *one* of the following is LEAST appropriate in a patient with acute hematochezia?

(A) Placement of a nasogastric tube
(B) Barium studies
(C) Colonoscopy
(D) Arteriography
(E) Tc-99m erythrocyte scintigraphy

The initial evaluation of a patient with acute hematochezia should be aimed at determining the most likely source of hemorrhage. Up to 90% of acute gastrointestinal hemorrhage originates proximal to the ligament of Treitz, so it is important to exclude hemorrhage from the stomach or proximal duodenum even when a patient presents with acute hematochezia. Since 10% of patients with hemorrhage from a gastrointestinal source proximal to the ligament of Treitz present with hematochezia, the placement of a nasogastric tube (Option (A)) is important in the initial evaluation of a patient with acute hematochezia. About 20% of patients with an acutely hemorrhaging gastroduodenal ulcer have a negative nasogastric aspirate, so the lack of blood in the aspirate does not exclude a source of bleeding proximal to the ligament of Treitz.

Accordingly, an upper gastrointestinal endoscopy is an appropriate examination in a patient with acute hematochezia. However, barium examinations should be avoided in this setting because the presence of barium in the bowel can interfere with endoscopy and obscure findings on arteriography, should either examination be required subsequently **(Option (B) is correct)**. Several factors support the use of endoscopy in patients with acute gastrointestinal bleeding. The most common etiology of acute gastrointestinal hemorrhage is gastritis, which can be difficult to diagnose by arteriography because of its diffuse nature. Many acutely hemorrhaging lesions can be treated transendoscopically by thermal coagulation, photocoagulation, or injection of epinephrine at the bleeding site. When a lesion is located endoscopically and local treatment is ineffective, the information gained can direct empirical transcatheter angiographic treatment even if the patient is no longer actively bleeding.

The role of colonoscopy (Option (C)) in the patient with acute hematochezia is less well defined. It is especially helpful if the source is located in the rectum or sigmoid colon. However, if bleeding is massive, colonoscopic identification of its source is difficult to impossible because of the amount of blood present throughout the colon. Colonoscopy is of greatest value in the patient with intermittent hematochezia who is clinically stable.

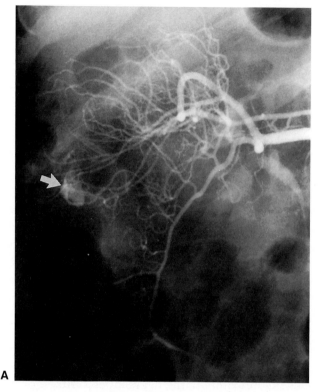

A

Figure 29-11. Hemorrhage from a diverticulum of the ascending colon in a 66-year-old man presenting with acute hematochezia. This selective middle colic artery injection was done after a superior mesenteric arteriogram suggested a right colonic bleeding site. (A) A radiograph from the arterial phase shows extravasation of contrast agent (arrow) from an arterial branch serving the proximal ascending colon. (B) The pool of extravasated contrast agent persists throughout the late venous phase, by which time it outlines the lumen of the diverticulum.

Arteriography (Option (D)) is quite valuable in the evaluation of acute lower gastrointestinal bleeding. Even though bleeding from lower gastrointestinal lesions is often intermittent, arteriography can be expected to identify the source in 40 to 50% of patients if care is taken to perform the arteriogram while there are clinical signs of active bleeding (falling hematocrit and passage of bright red blood per rectum) (Figure 29-11). By comparison, exploratory laparotomy can be expected to identify the source of hemorrhage in only 30% of patients and carries a higher morbidity and mortality. Colonic diverticula are the most common cause of acute lower gastrointestinal hemorrhage.

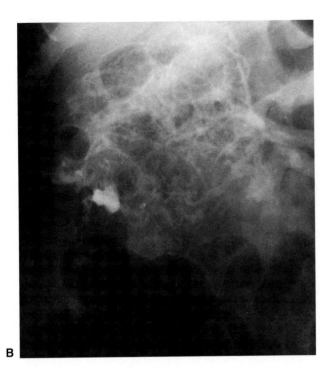

B

If bleeding is intermittent, scintigraphy with Tc-99m erythrocytes (Option (E)) is indicated even though 85% of patients will have to be imaged for more than 1 hour. In this clinical setting, scintigraphy is more sensitive than arteriography. Patients can be imaged repeatedly for up to 24 hours if the bleeding site is not detected on early images. A positive scintigraphic study can direct future arteriographic studies if brisk bleeding begins.

Question 89

Concerning transcatheter treatment of gastrointestinal hemorrhage,

(A) the treatment of choice in patients with acute colonic bleeding is usually pharmacologic therapy

(B) embolization is indicated for the treatment of hemorrhage due to duodenal ulcer

(C) metallic coils are not indicated for embolization of the upper gastrointestinal tract

(D) the standard intra-arterial dose of vasopressin is 20 to 40 U/minute

(E) unstable angina is a contraindication to vasopressin infusion

In most patients with acute gastrointestinal hemorrhage, the bleeding stops spontaneously. Only patients who are clinically unstable typically require arteriography on an emergent basis. Emergency abdominal surgery carries a high mortality in patients who are actively bleeding and hemodynamically unstable, and so transcatheter treatment is preferred. It is indicated both for definitive therapy and for stabilization prior to surgery.

Traditionally, pharmacologic methods are usually used to control bleeding from the stomach, small intestine, and colon **(Option (A) is true)**. Intra-arterial infusion of vasopressin for treatment of gastric bleeding results in control in approximately 70% of patients. Diffuse hemorrhagic gastritis responds particularly well to vasopressin infusion. When infused directly into the left gastric artery, vasopressin is effective in 82% of patients with this condition. More focal lesions of the upper gastrointestinal tract, such as chronic gastric ulcers, stress-induced gastric ulcers, and Mallory-Weiss tears, are better treated by arterial embolization. In some patients it is difficult to secure a catheter in the left gastric artery sufficiently well to allow for prolonged infusion over a period of hours or days. In addition, ventricular arrhythmias can develop as a result of vasopressin-induced constriction of pericardial branches of the inferior phrenic artery, which occasionally arises from the left gastric artery. The accepted treatment for acute hemorrhage in the mesenteric small bowel and colon is vasopressin infusion via the superior or inferior mesenteric artery depending on the site of bleeding (Figure 29-12).

Embolization is best for treatment of hemorrhage from the pyloroduodenal region. The rich collateral blood supply to the duodenum reduces the risk of infarction due to embolic arterial occlusion **(Option (B) is true)**. Embolotherapy also avoids the pharmacologic complications of vasopressin infusion. Because of the dual blood supply to the first and second portions of the duodenum from branches of the gastroduodenal and superior mesenteric arteries, control of bleeding may require embo-

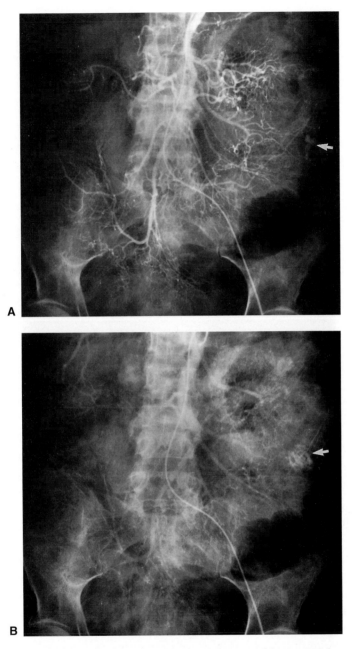

Figure 29-12. Jejunal hemorrhage in a 58-year-old man with sepsis and diffuse intravascular coagulation. Endoscopy revealed diffuse gastric bleeding. Celiac arteriography was performed and showed no extravasation into the stomach. The superior mesenteric artery was then studied, because of continued bleeding. (A) A radiograph from the arterial phase shows extravasation (arrow) from a jejunal branch in the left mid-abdomen. (B) A radiograph from the venous phase shows a pool of contrast material (arrow) outlining valvulae conniventes of the small bowel. (C) Repeated infusion of contrast agent after infusion of vasopressin into the superior mesenteric artery for 20 minutes shows no more bleeding.

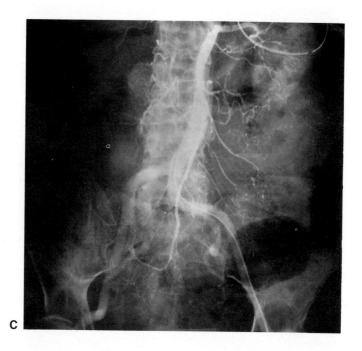

c

lization of the artery supplying the area of bleeding both distal and proximal to the site of hemorrhage (Figure 29-13).

Gelfoam is the embolic material of choice for arterial embolization in most patients with gastrointestinal hemorrhage. It provides a nidus for the formation of thrombus that occludes the embolized artery for a matter of weeks. The particle size can be tailored to the size of the artery to be occluded. Gelfoam embolization is associated with a low risk of infarction. Metallic 0.038-, 0.025-, and 0.018-inch embolic coils are available in a variety of configurations. Most have attached fibers of wool or dacron to stimulate thrombus formation. Occlusion is likely to be permanent. Embolization with a coil(s) and Gelfoam is effective in patients with hemorrhage refractory to occlusion with Gelfoam alone. Metallic coils are particularly well suited to the treatment of bleeding duodenal ulcers, since the propensity for collateral arterial supply to develop in the duodenum minimizes the risk of infarction due to the permanent occlusion by the embolic material **(Option (C) is false).**

Vasopressin, formerly known as antidiuretic hormone, is a vasoactive peptide produced by the posterior pituitary gland. It induces vasoconstriction by direct action on vascular smooth muscle, particularly at the arteriolar and capillary levels. Arterial infusion of vasopressin to control gastrointestinal bleeding is begun at a rate of 0.2 U/minute for 20 minutes. Another arterial contrast injection is then performed to look for

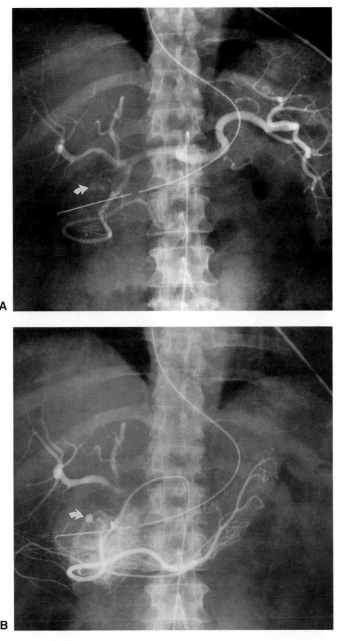

Figure 29-13. Embolization of a bleeding ulcer in the proximal duodenum. Previous endoscopy showed blood in the stomach and duodenum but did not demonstrate the site of bleeding. (A) A radiograph from a celiac arteriogram shows a faint area of extravasated contrast material (arrow) lateral to the gastroduodenal artery. (B) Selective injection of the gastroduodenal artery shows more obvious bleeding (arrow) from a small duodenal branch. (C) Arterial injection after embolization with Gelfoam and four metallic coils (arrow) shows occlusion of the gastroduodenal artery and cessation of bleeding.

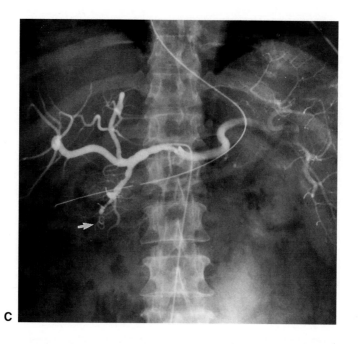

C

continued bleeding. If bleeding persists, the infusion rate is increased to 0.4 U/minute **(Option (D) is false)** for another 20 minutes. If this fails to stop the bleeding, vasopressin administration is discontinued. If hemorrhage stops after administration of vasopressin at 0.2 or 0.4 U/minute, intra-arterial infusion is continued at the effective rate for 24 hours and then tapered slowly to avoid rebound hyperemia. A 0.4-U/minute infusion is first decreased to 0.2 U/minute for 12 hours and then to 0.1 U/minute for another 12 hours before being stopped altogether.

Intra-arterial treatment with vasopressin causes serious complications in 9 to 43% of patients. These include ischemia of the heart, gastrointestinal tract, and distal extremities. The vasoconstrictor effect of vasopressin on the coronary circulation means that vasopressin is contraindicated in patients with symptomatic ischemic heart disease **(Option (E) is true).** Its antidiuretic effect also limits its use in patients with congestive heart failure. In patients receiving an infusion of vasopressin over several hours, a urethral catheter should be placed to allow careful monitoring of urinary output. Hyponatremia and cerebral edema have also been reported. Prior gastrointestinal embolization is a contraindication to the use of vasopressin because of a heightened risk of bowel infarction due to the previous occlusion of some of the arteries normally serving the area of hemorrhage. Vasopressin must also be used with caution in patients with prior surgical treatment for the same reason.

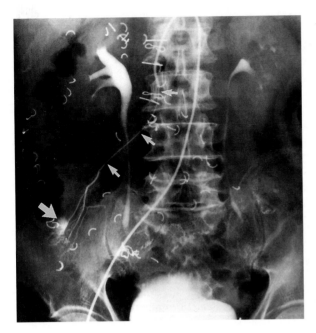

Figure 29-14. Subselective catheterization of an arterial branch supplying a bleeding arteriovenous malformation in the small intestine. There is extravasation (large arrow) into the bowel lumen. Note the 3 French coaxial catheter (small arrows) used to reach this small arterial branch. At operation, this catheter was used to inject methylene blue to assist in identification of the appropriate segment of bowel to resect.

The number and severity of complications of vasopressin infusion and the significant rate of recurrent hemorrhage (20 to 25%) after its use have renewed interest in the embolic treatment of bleeding lesions of the small intestine and colon. Several authors have recently reported success in embolizing both organs by superselective techniques with 3 French catheters, using polyvinyl alcohol particles, Gelfoam, or microcoils. Our current embolic agent of choice is polyvinyl alcohol particles with a diameter of 500 to 700 μm. To minimize the risk of bowel infarction, we exercise care in order to avoid using more embolic agent than is needed to stop the bleeding. Preoperative placement of superselective arterial catheters is also being used to label bleeding lesions in the bowel by injection of methylene blue intraoperatively (Figure 29-14). This allows quicker identification and more conservative resection of the abnormal segment of bowel.

Kay M. Hamrick, M.D.
Robert E. Koehler, M.D.

SUGGESTED READINGS

DIAGNOSTIC ANGIOGRAPHY IN PATIENTS WITH GASTROINTESTINAL HEMORRHAGE

1. Athanasoulis CA, Galdabini JJ, Waltman RA, Novelline RA, Greenfield AJ, Ezpeleta ML. Angiodysplasia of the colon: a cause of rectal bleeding. Cardiovasc Radiol 1978; 1:3–13
2. Baum S, Athanasoulis CA, Waltman AC, et al. Angiodysplasia of the right colon: a cause of gastrointestinal bleeding. AJR 1977; 129:789–794
3. Foutch PG. Angiodysplasia of the gastrointestinal tract. Am J Gastroenterol 1993; 88:807–818
4. Kadir S. Visceral angiography. In: Kadir S (ed), Diagnostic angiography. Philadelphia: WB Saunders; 1986:338–376
5. Lau WY, Yuen WK, Chu KW, Poon GP, Li AK. Obscure bleeding in the gastrointestinal tract originating in the small intestine. Surg Gynecol Obstet 1992; 174:119–124
6. Moore JD, Thompson NW, Appleman HD, Foley D. Arteriovenous malformations of the gastrointestinal tract. Arch Surg 1976; 111:381–389
7. Okazaki M, Higashihara H, Saida Y, et al. Angiographic findings of Meckel's diverticulum: the characteristic appearance of the vitelline artery. Abdom Imaging 1993; 18:15–19
8. Reuter S, Redman H, Kyung J. Gastrointestinal angiography, 3rd ed. Philadelphia: WB Saunders; 1986:128–156
9. Rollins ES, Picus D, Hicks ME, Darcy MD, Bower BL, Kleinhoffer MA. Angiography is useful in detecting the source of chronic gastrointestinal bleeding of obscure origin. AJR 1991; 156:385–388
10. Sheedy PF II, Fulton RE, Atwell DT. Angiographic evaluation of patients with chronic gastrointestinal bleeding. AJR 1975; 123:338–347
11. Spiller RC, Parkins RA. Recurrent gastrointestinal bleeding of obscure origin: report of 17 cases and a guide to logical management. Br J Surg 1983;70:489–493
12. Whitaker SC, Gregson RH. The role of angiography in the investigation of acute or chronic gastrointestinal haemorrhage. Clin Radiol 1993; 47:382–388

ENTEROCLYSIS

13. Herlinger H, Maglinte DD. Clinical radiology of the small intestine. Philadelphia: WB Saunders; 1989:119–145

SCINTIGRAPHY IN PATIENTS WITH GASTROINTESTINAL HEMORRHAGE

14. Bunker RS, Lull RJ, Tanasescu DE, et al. Scintigraphy of gastrointestinal hemorrhage: superiority of ^{99m}Tc red blood cells over ^{99m}Tc sulfur colloid. AJR 1984; 143:543–548
15. Jacobson AF, Cerqueira MD. Prognostic significance of late imaging results in technetium-99m-labeled red blood cell gastrointestinal bleeding studies with early negative images. J Nucl Med 1992; 33:202–207
16. Maurer AH, Rodman MS, Vitti RA, Revez G, Krevsky B. Gastrointestinal bleeding: improved localization with cine scintigraphy. Radiology 1992; 185:187–192

17. McKusick KA, Froelich J, Callahan RJ, Winzelberg GG, Strauss HW. ^{99m}Tc red blood cells for detection of gastrointestinal bleeding: experience with 80 patients. AJR 1981; 137:1113–1118

18. St George JK, Pollak JS. Acute gastrointestinal hemorrhage detected by selective scintigraphic angiography. J Nucl Med 1991; 32:1601–1604

19. Voeller GR, Bunch G, Britt LG. Use of technetium-labeled red blood cell scintigraphy in the detection and management of gastrointestinal hemorrhage. Surgery 1991; 110:799–804

SCINTIGRAPHY IN PATIENTS WITH SUSPECTED CARCINOID TUMOR

20. Krenning EP, Kwekkeboom DJ, Oei HY, et al. Somatostatin receptor scintigraphy in carcinoids, gastrinomas and Cushing's syndrome. Digestion 1994; 55(Suppl 3):54–59

21. Lamberts SW, Reubi JC, Krenning EP. Validation of somatostatin receptor scintigraphy in the localization of neuroendocrine tumors. Acta Oncologia 1993; 32:167–170

TRANSCATHETER TREATMENT IN PATIENTS WITH ACUTE GASTROINTESTINAL HEMORRHAGE

22. Bennett J, Kadir S. Treatment of colorectal bleeding. In: Kadir S (ed), Current practice of interventional radiology. Philadelphia: BC Decker; 1991:428–436

23. Cho K, Doenz F. Treatment of small intestinal bleeding. In: Kadir S (ed), Current practice of interventional radiology. Philadelphia: BC Decker; 1991:424–428

24. Encarnacion CE, Saadoon K, Beam CA, Payne CS. Gastrointestinal bleeding: treatment with gastrointestinal arterial embolization. Radiology 1992; 183:505–508

25. Guy GE, Shetty PC, Sharma RP, Burke MW, Burke TH. Acute lower gastrointestinal hemorrhage: treatment by superselective embolization with polyvinyl alcohol particles. AJR 1992; 159:521–526

26. Hilleren D. Treatment of gastric bleeding. In: Kadir S (ed), Current practice of interventional radiology. Philadelphia: BC Decker; 1991:414–418

27. Kadir S. Principles of management of gastrointestinal bleeding. In: Kadir S (ed), Current practice of interventional radiology. Philadelphia: BC Decker; 1991:408–411

28. Kadir S. Treatment of pyloroduodenal bleeding. In: Kadir S (ed), Current practice of interventional radiology. Philadelphia: BC Decker; 1991:418–424

29. Keller FS, Routh WD. Angiographic diagnosis and management. Hepato-Gastroenterology 1991; 38:207–215

30. Keller FS, Routh WD. Treatment of Mallory-Weiss tears. In: Kadir S (ed), Current practice of interventional radiology. Philadelphia: BC Decker; 1991:411–414

31. Moncure AC, Tompkins RG, Athanasoulis CA, Welch CE. Occult gastrointestinal bleeding: newer techniques of diagnosis and therapy. Adv Surg 1989; 22:141–178

32. Richter JM, Christensen MR, Kaplan LM, Nishioka NS. Effectiveness of current technology in the diagnosis and management of lower gastrointestinal hemorrhage. Gastrointest Endosc 1995; 41:93–98

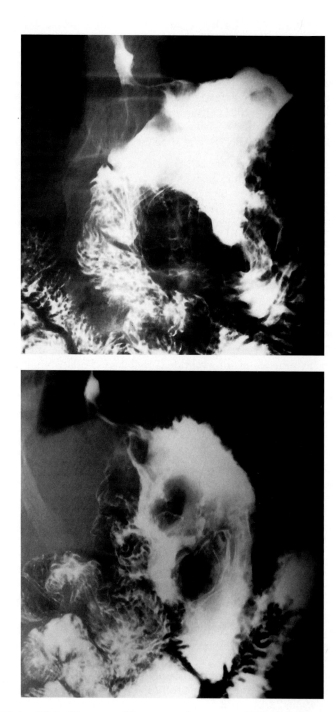

Figure 30-1. This 72-year-old man underwent a Billroth II procedure 31 years ago for peptic ulcer disease. He now has nausea and vomiting. You are shown two radiographs from an upper gastrointestinal study.

Case 30: Gastric Remnant Carcinoma

Question 90

Which *one* of the following is the MOST likely diagnosis?

    (A) Lymphoma
    (B) Carcinoma
    (C) Bile reflux gastritis
    (D) Bezoar
    (E) Jejunogastric intussusception

The two radiographs from the upper gastrointestinal series (Figure 30-1) show a markedly deformed gastric remnant (Figure 30-2, arrows). The proximal jejunum is also opacified but appears normal. There is no impairment of gastric emptying. A large, lobulated polypoid mass arises from the gastric wall and protrudes into the lumen as a filling defect. No normal gastric rugae are seen, and the entire gastric wall has an irregular, shaggy contour. These findings are most consistent with a malignant tumor of the gastric remnant. Of the two tumors listed, gastric carcinoma is more likely to show this degree of diffuse infiltration, and it is much more likely than lymphoma to develop in the postoperative stomach, especially after antrectomy **(Option (B) is correct).**

Partial gastrectomy for the treatment of gastric and duodenal ulcer disease is rapidly becoming a thing of the past. Medical treatment has all but replaced antrectomy and vagotomy for benign disease. However, carcinoma of the gastric remnant and many other complications that follow partial gastrectomy occur years after the surgical procedure. For gastric remnant cancer, this delay is typically 20 years or more. Despite the rarity of gastrectomy for ulcer disease today, radiologists will be called upon to recognize gastric remnant cancers for many years to come. The diagnosis should be considered whenever an irregular or lobulated mass or stricture involves the distal stomach in a patient who had gastric surgery for benign disease many years earlier. When detected, the tumor is typically widespread and diffuse and involves the anastomosis. The prognosis is poor. Even prospective endoscopic surveillance programs have

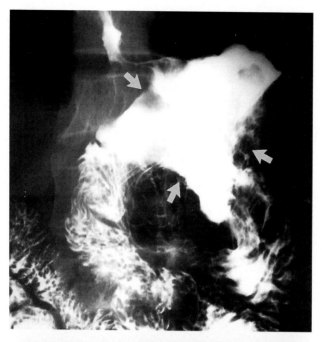

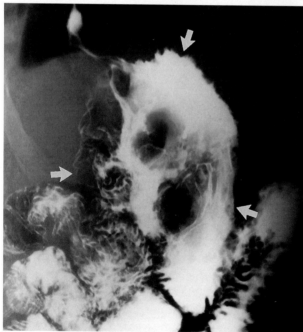

Figure 30-2 (Same as Figure 30-1). Primary adenocarcinoma of the gastric remnant. The entire gastric remnant (arrows) is markedly irregular and deformed. Large polypoid nodules of tumor protrude into its lumen.

failed to effect early detection. The rapid growth rate of gastric carcinomas and their tendency toward early metastatic spread are likely to defeat the value of any surveillance method used less often than every four months.

For years, there has been debate over the magnitude of heightened cancer risk after antrectomy. This controversy has been fueled by conflicting results of epidemiologic studies performed in different parts of the world. Analyses of European and North American data have shown an average of a 1.5- to 1.7-fold increase in gastric cancer incidence after gastrectomy, while published studies from Japan actually show a lower incidence, i.e., a protective effect. It has also been established that the increase in incidence of postoperative carcinoma in Americans and Europeans applies to the distal gastric remnant but not the gastric cardia. Also of interest is the fact that the relative risk of gastric cancer is lower in the first few postoperative years (presumably because a portion of the target organ has been removed) but rises continuously in later years. To summarize these results in relation to patients in the United States, there is a moderate increase in the risk of development of adenocarcinoma in the distal portion of the gastric remnant beginning 15 to 20 years after the operation. The risk is greater among patients who underwent gastrectomy for treatment of gastric ulcer than for treatment of duodenal ulcer.

Many theories have been proposed for the pathogenesis of cancer developing in the gastric remnant. Three that stand out are (1) intestinal metaplasia due to chronic gastric mucosal exposure to refluxed bile and pancreatic juice, (2) diminished ability to deactivate carcinogens from tobacco and other sources, and (3) chronic gastric infection with *Helicobacter pylori*. With regard to the first hypothesis, it is interesting that some studies have shown gastric remnant cancer to be more common after the Billroth II procedure, in which reflux of alkaline secretions is a greater problem; however, there is some increase in risk after the Billroth I procedure and even after gastrojejunostomy without antral resection. Arguing for the second hypothesis is a reported postgastrectomy increase in the incidence of several other malignant tumors including carcinomas of the lung, colon, pancreas, biliary tract, and gallbladder. Thirdly, there is increasing evidence that infection with *H. pylori* causes most gastric ulcers that are not due to chronic use of aspirin or other nonsteroidal anti-inflammatory drugs. Persistent infection with this organism after gastrectomy is thought to cause epithelial hyperplasia in which carcinoma sometimes develops.

Primary non-Hodgkin's lymphoma of the stomach (Option (A)) is rare, making up only 3% of gastric tumors. As with lymphoma elsewhere in the gastrointestinal tract, gastric lymphoma can have a variety of radiologic appearances. In both the operated and nonoperated stomach, it can present as diffuse or focal thickening of rugal folds, a lobulated or ulcerated mass, or multiple discrete nodules. As noted above, lymphoma is less likely than carcinoma in the test patient because of the greater relative frequency of the latter and because of the greater likelihood of diffuse infiltration of the gastric wall by the carcinoma.

There is little evidence that the risk of gastric lymphoma is increased after partial gastrectomy; however, this tumor does share with gastric carcinoma another pathogenetic link—both have a strong epidemiologic association with *H. pylori* infection. Gastric lymphoid tissue that developed in response to *H. pylori* infection (the normal stomach does not contain lymphoid tissue) appears to be the tissue in which non-Hodgkin's gastric lymphoma usually arises.

Bile reflux gastritis (Option (C)) is a common benign condition that occurs in patients who have previously undergone antrectomy with Billroth I or Billroth II anastomosis. It is due to reflux of bile back into the gastric remnant. The irritating effect of alkaline bile and pancreatic juice causes painful swelling of the gastric mucosa and rugal folds. Affected rugae typically appear smoothly thickened with straight, parallel margins. They do not have the bizarre, distorted appearance seen in the test images.

Chronically impaired gastric emptying of solid food is a common occurrence after vagotomy and antrectomy. In some series it occurs more often after anastomosis of the Billroth I type. Most often, the retained material appears on barium studies as multiple, irregularly shaped, freely movable filling defects in the lumen of the gastric remnant. The anastomosis can be narrowed but is more often widely patent, and there is no associated problem with gastric emptying of liquids. This type of gastric retention is usually asymptomatic.

Less common but more significant clinically is retention in the form of a single collection of compacted food, sometimes referred to as a foodball. Foodballs are typically 5 to 10 cm in size. Unlike most tumors, they tend to conform to the round or ovoid shape of the gastric stump. They move about in the lumen, and liquid flows around them into the small bowel. Patients with a foodball filling most of the gastric lumen often complain of epigastric fullness and early satiety. Foodballs are usually easy to break up endoscopically and may even resolve spontaneously with a clear liquid diet for a few days.

At the most severe and least common end of the spectrum of retained food is the bezoar (Option (D)). This is a gastric collection of ingested material consisting primarily of plant fibers (phytobezoar) that are tightly bound together and more difficult to break up. Citrus fruit fibers are an important component of the matrix of many postoperative bezoars. Gastric outlet obstruction is uncommon, and symptoms are similar to those caused by foodballs. On rare occasions, a bezoar will pass

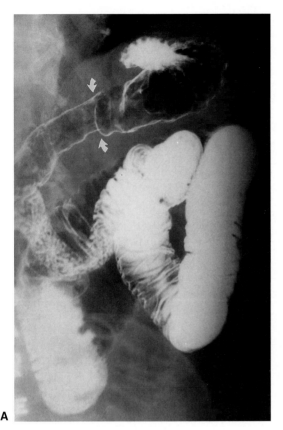

Figure 30-3. Small bowel obstruction due to a bezoar 10 years after vagotomy and antrectomy of the Billroth I type. (A) Normal postoperative appearance of the gastric remnant and gastroduodenal anastomosis (arrows). Note the dilatation of the jejunum, greater than that usually seen as a result of vagotomy alone.

A

through the gastric anastomosis to obstruct the small bowel, usually at the level of the distal ileum (Figure 30-3). Rare cases of postgastrectomy bezoars composed of a mass of monilial fibers have been reported. The irregularity of the gastric wall in the test patient is not a feature of a bezoar.

Jejunogastric intussusception (Option (E)) is another condition that presents as an intraluminal filling defect in the gastric remnant after vagotomy and antrectomy. Again, the gastric wall irregularity seen in the test patient would not be expected in a patient with this condition. Patients complain of intermittent abdominal pain. Barium upper gastrointestinal study shows filling and obstruction of the gastric remnant by a bulky, smoothly lobulated, intraluminal mass representing the coiled, intussuscepted segment of jejunum. Like all intussuscepted bowel, the intragastric segment of jejunum is inverted, with its mucosa and valvulae conniventes forming its outer surface. The radiologic find-

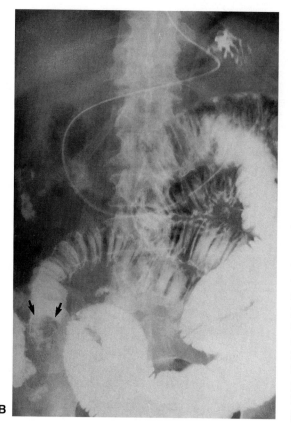

Figure 30-3 (Continued). Small bowel obstruction due to a bezoar 10 years after vagotomy and antrectomy of the Billroth I type. (B) By 2 hours later, barium had reached a point of obstruction in the mid-small bowel. Note the rounded, intraluminal filling defect (arrows) at the point of obstruction, about the same caliber as the gastroduodenostomy.

ing of an obstructing, intraluminal mass with a coiled-spring appearance to its surface is characteristic.

Question 91

Concerning combined vagotomy and antrectomy,

(A) over 90% of the acid-producing (parietal) cells of the stomach are typically removed
(B) the gastrin level in serum rises markedly in the postoperative period
(C) frequent vomiting in the first 10 days after operation usually indicates the presence of alkaline gastritis
(D) it virtually eliminates reflux esophagitis in patients prone to gastroesophageal reflux

Vagotomy has long been advocated as a treatment for duodenal and gastric ulcer disease, because it markedly reduces the neural stimulation of release of hydrochloric acid from the gastric mucosa. Truncal vagotomy also causes loss of peristaltic activity in the gastric antrum and failure of coordinated relaxation of the pyloric sphincter. To prevent consequent problems with gastric emptying, therefore, vagotomy is performed in combination with some form of gastric drainage procedure. This can be a pyloroplasty, an antrectomy with gastroduodenostomy (Billroth I), or an antrectomy with gastrojejunostomy (Billroth II). Antrectomy serves the added function of removing the gastrin-secreting cells (G-cells), almost all of which occur in the mucosa of the gastric antrum. Thus, combined vagotomy and antrectomy reduces both the neural and hormonal stimuli to gastric acid production. Parietal cells, which produce hydrochloric acid, lie in the fundus and body of the stomach. Few of these are removed at antrectomy **(Option (A) is false).**

Vagotomy without antrectomy leads to a moderate (two- to threefold) increase in fasting and postprandial levels of gastrin in serum. This is thought to be due to reduced gastric acid output and to decreased end-organ sensitivity to gastrin that follows vagal denervation. When vagotomy is combined with antrectomy, however, postoperative gastrin levels in serum rise little or not at all, depending on how much of the G-cell mass is removed **(Option (B) is false).** Marked hypergastrinemia after antrectomy should suggest the presence of ectopic gastrin production in a neoplasm or a retained antral remnant in an afferent limb (see below).

Recurrent vomiting in the first 1 to 2 weeks after antrectomy and vagotomy indicates early postoperative impairment of gastric emptying **(Option (C) is false).** This is usually due to a combination of gastric atony and narrowing of the gastric anastomotic outlet. Early postoperative narrowing of the gastroduodenal or gastrojejunal anastomosis can be due to surgical creation of too small an anastomosis; it is much more likely, however, that the anastomotic narrowing is due to transient edema that will resolve if treated for a few weeks with nasogastric suc-

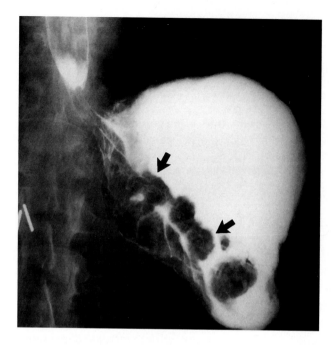

Figure 30-4. Gastric outlet obstruction 5 days after a Billroth II procedure. No barium left the stomach during a 1-hour period of observation. The gastrojejunostomy is occluded by edema. Note also the swelling of the gastric wall adjacent to the staple line (arrows). Gastric emptying improved markedly with 5 days of nasogastric suction.

tion and other conservative measures (Figure 30-4). Postoperative edema severe enough to impair gastric emptying often also affects the line of closure along the distal lesser curvature of the gastric remnant (Figure 30-5). In a patient with vomiting due to anastomic obstruction in the first or second postoperative week, the presence of a mass of swollen tissue in this area on early postoperative barium studies suggests that the anastomotic obstruction is due to edema. Swelling of the surgical line of closure and of the anastomosis usually subsides within the first two postoperative weeks. A severe complication of excessive gastric distension in the postoperative period is perforation and leak from the anastomosis or gastric staple (or suture) line (Figure 30-6).

Gastroesophageal reflux is common after both the Billroth I and Billroth II procedures. The postoperative reduction in gastric acid output almost eliminates the likelihood of acid-induced esophageal inflammation. However, refluxed bile and pancreatic secretions irritate the mucosa of the esophagus, so reflux esophagitis continues to be a problem in many patients **(Option (D) is false).** As many as one-third of patients have esophageal symptoms related to alkaline reflux. Alkaline reflux-induced esophagitis is not as easy to detect radiographically as is the more common acid-induced esophagitis. Patients can be quite symptomatic, despite normal findings on biphasic esophagography. Endoscopy

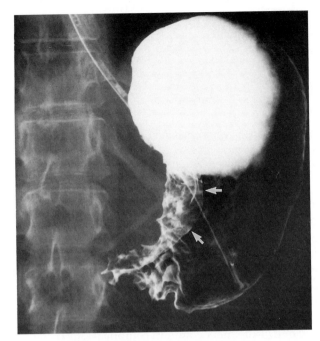

Figure 30-5 (left).
Gastric outlet obstruction after a Billroth I procedure. A radiograph obtained 15 minutes after instillation of barium via nasogastric tube in a patient with persistent vomiting 10 days after a Billroth I procedure shows that no barium has entered the duodenum. The rugal folds in the distal stomach are swollen, and swelling around the closure line on the lesser curvature mimics a mass (arrows).

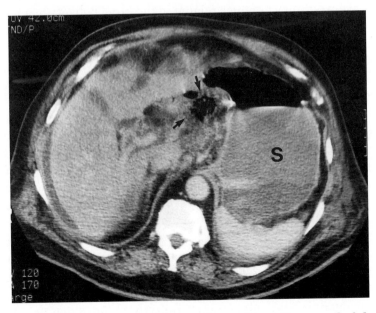

Figure 30-6. CT scan in a patient with vomiting, fever, and abdominal pain a few days after antrectomy. The gastric remnant (S) is distended with fluid, and there is a collection of extraluminal air (arrows) medial to the stomach. An upper gastrointestinal study performed with water-soluble contrast material the preceding day had shown partial gastric outlet obstruction but no leak.

and 24-hour monitoring of esophageal bile concentrations are more sensitive ways of establishing this diagnosis.

Question 92

Concerning postoperative complications of vagotomy and antrectomy,

    (A) dumping syndrome can be diagnosed by radiographic evaluation of gastric emptying

    (B) barium evaluation can distinguish alkaline gastritis from recurrent acid-peptic inflammation

    (C) afferent loop syndrome can be caused by narrowing of either the afferent or efferent jejunal loop

    (D) the most likely site of marginal ulcer after a Billroth II procedure is on the jejunal side of the anastomosis

    (E) the retained antrum syndrome is due to hyperplasia of gastrin-producing cells (G-cells) in the gastric remnant

Dumping syndrome is one of the most common complications of vagotomy and antrectomy. It is characterized by a constellation of vasomotor and gastrointestinal symptoms related to the rapid delivery of a high solute load (food and hypertonic liquid) from the stomach to the jejunum. Patients experience postprandial flushing, palpitations, diaphoresis, and postural hypotension. Crampy abdominal pain, nausea, vomiting, and diarrhea can also occur. Symptoms begin within 30 minutes after meals, especially meals with high liquid and/or carbohydrate content. It is evident on upper gastrointestinal barium studies that almost all patients with a previous antrectomy empty their stomachs of liquids rapidly, and patients with dumping syndrome cannot be distinguished radiographically from those without **(Option (A) is false).** Another form of dumping syndrome causes symptoms of rebound hypoglycemia 1 to 3 hours after a high carbohydrate meal. Symptoms are primarily vasomotor in nature, and, again, the condition is not detectable radiographically.

Alkaline gastritis is very common after vagotomy and antrectomy. Bile and pancreatic juice have an irritating effect when they contact the mucosa of the stomach. Reflux of these alkaline secretions into the gastric remnant occurs to some extent in all patients after antrectomy and is more common in patients with a Billroth II anastomosis. Affected patients may be asymptomatic or may complain of recurrent, burning epigastric pain for months to years following the operation. The occurrence of pain of alkaline gastritis often bears little relation to mealtime. Some patients vomit bilious material, and the vomiting may not relieve the symptoms.

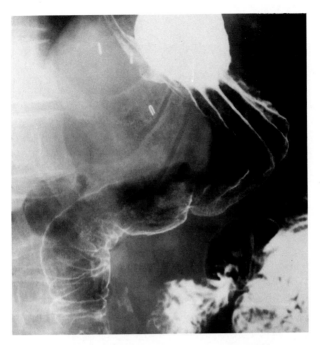

Figure 30-7. Reflux alkaline gastritis in a patient after a Billroth I procedure. There are thick, straight, swollen rugal folds in the gastric remnant. Endoscopically, the gastric folds were confirmed to be swollen and erythematous. The patient also had alkaline esophagitis proven by endoscopically detected esophageal erythema and by 24-hour photometric monitoring for the presence of bile in the esophagus. A barium esophagram showed gastroesophageal reflux but no morphologic abnormalities.

The radiographic appearance of alkaline gastritis is characteristic. Inflammatory abnormalities are confined to the gastric side of the anastomosis, since contact with bile and pancreatic juice has no adverse effect on the mucosa of the duodenum and jejunum. On barium upper gastrointestinal series, the rugal folds in the gastric stump are diffusely thickened and straightened (Figures 30-7 and 30-8), by comparison with the normal postgastrectomy appearance (Figure 30-9). The fold thickening creates an appearance somewhat like the impression left by closely apposed fingers pressed into modeling clay. Ulcers are not usually seen radiographically, although endoscopy can reveal small, superficial erosions. This appearance differs from the radiographic appearance of recurrent postoperative acid-peptic inflammation, in which edematous valvulae conniventes are seen on the intestinal side of the anastomosis **(Option (B) is true)**. Either condition can induce swelling of the anas-

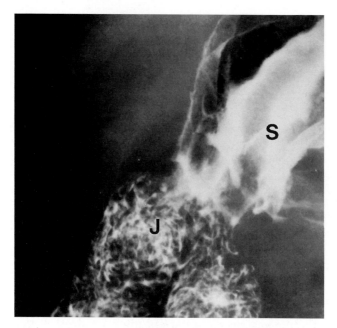

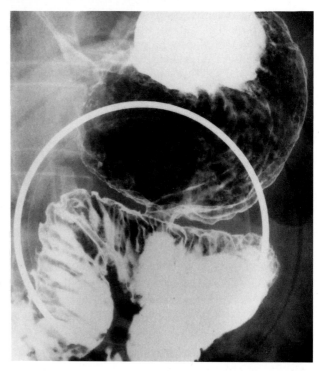

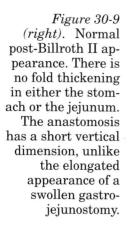

Figure 30-8 (left). Reflux alkaline gastritis after a Billroth II procedure. Note the thickened rugae in the gastric remnant (S) and the lack of swelling or other inflammatory change on the jejunal side (J) of the anastomosis.

Figure 30-9 (right). Normal post-Billroth II appearance. There is no fold thickening in either the stomach or the jejunum. The anastomosis has a short vertical dimension, unlike the elongated appearance of a swollen gastrojejunostomy.

tomosis itself, giving it a narrowed, elongated appearance. Alkaline gastritis is seldom severe enough to cause intractable symptoms. When it is, surgical conversion to Roux-en-Y gastric drainage is sometimes undertaken to reduce the frequency and volume of refluxed alkaline secretions.

"Afferent loop syndrome" is the term applied to postprandial upper abdominal pain due to distension of the afferent (duodenojejunal) limb after a Billroth II procedure. Vomiting is common and characteristically relieves the symptoms. The syndrome is rare and can be due to partial obstruction of either the afferent or efferent limb near the gastrojejunostomy **(Option (C) is true).** When the afferent limb is obstructed, it fills with bile and pancreatic juice. When the obstruction is at the level of the proximal efferent limb, the distended afferent limb is filled not only with bile and pancreatic juice but also with food, which moves back and forth from the gastric pouch to the afferent limb for hours after each meal.

Afferent loop syndrome is more often chronic than acute. The most common site of obstruction is in the efferent jejunal limb, immediately adjacent to the anastomosis (Figure 30-10). The blockage can be due to scarring and stricture following recurrent peptic ulcer (marginal ulcer), kinking as a result of postoperative adhesions, internal hernia, or gastric stump cancer. The same conditions can also cause obstruction on the afferent side of the gastrojejunostomy, usually in patients with a long afferent limb. In patients in whom the Billroth II procedure was originally done for resection of primary gastric carcinoma, recurrence of the original tumor tends to occur at the site where the afferent limb was brought through the transverse mesocolon to meet the stomach. When such tumor recurrence occurs, the picture is often that of afferent loop syndrome (Figure 30-11).

"Marginal ulcer" is a term applied to recurrent peptic ulcer disease in the perianastomotic area after vagotomy and antrectomy. Recurrent ulcer disease is very uncommon after the Billroth II procedure, occurring in no more than 1 to 2% of patients. Its causes fall into two major categories: those due to rare inadequacies in surgical technique and those developing on a hormonal, metabolic, or pharmacologic basis.

Incomplete vagotomy, especially failure to section the posterior vagal trunk, is the most common surgical inadequacy. Alternatively, too much of the antrum can be left in the gastric stump, leaving a large population of G-cells. These inadequacies in the performance of vagotomy and antrectomy can lead to inadequate suppression of gastric acid output and to recurrent inflammation on an acid-peptic basis. The intestinal mucosa on the jejunal side of the anastomosis is more sensitive to acid-peptic degradation than is the mucosa of the gastric remnant, so the jejunum, especially the proximal efferent limb, is the site of most marginal ulcer

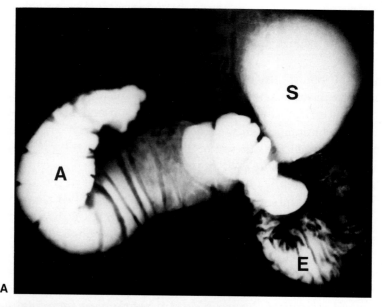

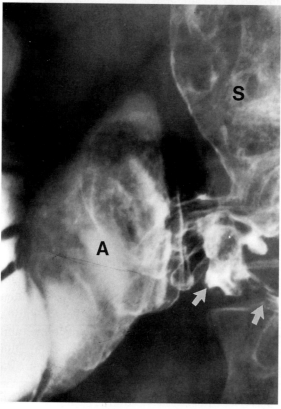

Figure 30-10. Afferent loop syndrome several years after a Billroth II procedure for benign peptic ulcer disease. (A) The afferent limb (A) is dilated from its proximal end to its junction with the stomach (S). Note how little barium has passed into the efferent limb (E) of the jejunum. (B) A spot radiograph of the anastomotic region shows the dilated stomach (S) and afferent loop (A) and narrowing and irregularity of the efferent loop (arrows). The abnormalities were due to scarring that followed a marginal ulcer.

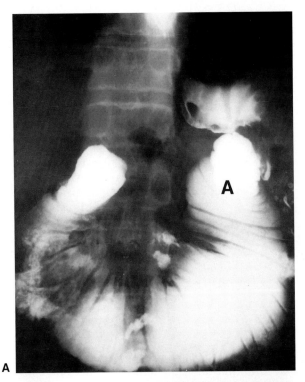

A

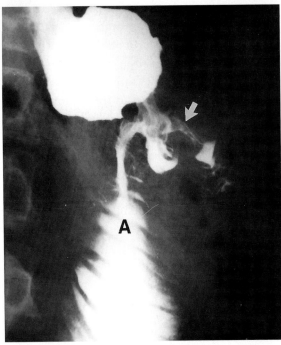

B

Figure 30-11. Recur-
rence of tumor after a
Billroth II resection
for gastric carcinoma.
(A) Marked afferent
loop (A) distension
with almost no filling
of the efferent loop.
(B) The tumor has en-
cased and mildly nar-
rowed the anastomosis
and afferent limb (A) of
the jejunum. The effer-
ent limb (arrow) is ob-
structed.

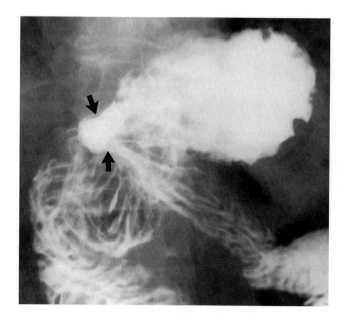

Figure 30-12. Marginal ulcer (arrows) occurring after a Billroth II procedure. The ulcer is in the efferent limb, immediately adjacent to the anastomosis.

disease (Figure 30-12) **(Option (D) is true).** Even more common than jejunal ulcer is the finding of inflammatory thickening of valvulae conniventes immediately adjacent to the anastomosis (Figure 30-13). This can extend for a variable distance down the efferent limb.

A rare but potentially severe problem related to operative technique is the retained antrum syndrome, which is due to retention of a remnant of antral mucosa at the proximal end of the afferent jejunal limb **(Option (E) is false).** The G-cells in this isolated antral remnant, isolated from any acid produced in the stomach, are chronically stimulated to secrete gastrin by their continued exposure to the alkaline milieu of the duodenum. With inability of the acid-gastrin feedback control loop to close, hypersecretion of both gastrin and hydrochloric acid continues, resulting in a situation that mimics the Zollinger-Ellison syndrome both clinically and chemically. The rarity of the retained antrum syndrome is partially because a complete truncal vagotomy significantly reduces the responsiveness of gastric parietal cells to gastrin stimulation. It is thought that some patients left with a small antral remnant at the end of the afferent limb have no significant return of gastric acid production even if moderate postoperative hypergastrinemia does develop. The antral remnant in patients with the retained antrum syndrome is usually quite small but is sometimes large enough to be recognized as such on a barium study. Radionuclide imaging with Tc-99m pertechnetate is

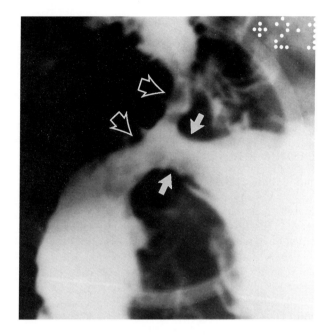

Figure 30-13. Compression spot radiograph of a Billroth II gastrojejunal anastomosis. Recurrent peptic inflammation produces narrowing and elongation of the anastomosis (solid arrows). Note also the thickening of the mucosal folds (open arrows) in the adjacent jejunum.

another way to demonstrate the presence of gastric mucosa in the afferent limb.

One additional form of recurrent ulcer disease related to problems with postoperative anatomy occurs in patients with gastric stasis. This can be due to a tight gastrojejunostomy or to high placement of the anastomosis in a position that does not promote drainage by gravity when the patient is upright. The resulting distension of the gastric remnant can promote gastric acid secretion. Postoperative ulcers in these patients tend to be superficial and on the gastric side of the anastomosis.

Ulcers due to any of these surgical technique-related problems are rare, and so metabolic and drug-related causes must be given serious consideration in patients who experience recurrence of ulcer disease after vagotomy and antrectomy. Gastrinoma (Zollinger-Ellison syndrome) is the underlying cause in about 2% of these patients. Hypercalcemia, usually related to hyperparathyroidism, is another potential cause. Probably most common in this category, however, is ulcer recurrence related to the use of nonsteroidal anti-inflammatory drugs, especially aspirin. Ulcers in these patients tend to be large and multiple. They are usually gastric in location but can occur anywhere from the lower esophagus to the jejunum. When excessive aspirin usage was a factor in the pathogenesis of the initial preoperative ulcer disease, it is especially important to exclude it in patients with postoperative recurrence.

Robert E. Koehler, M.D.

SUGGESTED READINGS

CARCINOMA OF THE GASTRIC REMNANT

1. Domellof L, Eriksson S, Janunger KG. Carcinoma and possible precancerous changes of the gastric stump after billroth II resection. Gastroenterology 1977; 73:462–468
2. Dougherty SH, Foster CA, Eisenberg MM. Stomach cancer following gastric surgery for benign disease. Arch Surg 1982; 117:294–297
3. Eide TJ, Viste A, Andersen A, Sooreide O. The risk of cancer at all sites following gastric operation for benign disease. A cohort study of 4,224 patients. Int J Cancer 1991; 48:333–339
4. Lechago J, Correa P. Prolonged achlorhydria and gastric neoplasia: is there a causal relationship? Gastroenterology 1993; 104:1554–1557
5. Lundegardh G, Adami HO, Helmick C, Zack M, Meirik O. Stomach cancer after partial gastrectomy for benign ulcer disease. N Engl J Med 1988; 319:195–200
6. Offerhaus GJ. Gastric stump cancer: lessons from old specimens. Lancet 1994; 343:66–67
7. Picton TD, Owen DA, MacDonald WC. Comparison of esophagocardiac and more distal gastric cancer in patients with prior ulcer surgery. Cancer 1993; 71:5–8
8. Stalsberg H, Taksdal S. Stomach cancer following gastric surgery for benign conditions. Lancet 1971; 2:1175–1177
9. Stemmermann GN, Nomura AM, Chyou PH. Cancer incidence following subtotal gastrectomy. Gastroenterology 1991; 101:711–715

GASTRIC LYMPHOMA

10. Ghahremani GG, Fisher MR. Lymphoma of the stomach following gastric surgery for benign peptic ulcers. Gastrointest Radiol 1983; 8:213–217
11. Isaacson PG. Gastric lymphoma and *Helicobacter pylori*. N Engl J Med 1994; 330:1310–1311
12. Parsonnet J, Hansen S, Rodriguez L, et al. *Helicobacter pylori* infection and gastric lymphoma. N Engl J Med 1994; 330:1267–1271

BENIGN POSTGASTRECTOMY CONDITIONS

13. Arends TW, Nahrwold DL. Gastric resection and reconstruction. In: Zuidema GD (ed), Schackelford's surgery of the alimentary tract, 3rd ed., vol II. Philadelphia: WB Saunders; 1991:149–172
14. Bondurant FJ, Maull KI, Nelson HS Jr, Silver SH. Bile reflux gastritis. South Med J 1987; 80:161–165

15. Cross R, Clements JL Jr, Weens HS. Jejunal monilial bezoar following total gastrectomy. Gastrointest Radiol 1979; 4:29–31

16. Fromm D. Postgastrectomy syndromes. In: Zuidema GD (ed), Schackelford's surgery of the alimentary tract, 3rd ed., vol II. Philadelphia: WB Saunders; 1991:173–187

17. Goldstein HM, Cohen LE, Hagen RO, Wells RF. Gastric bezoars: a frequent complication in the postoperative ulcer patient. Radiology 1973; 107:341–344

18. Jay BS, Burrell M. Iatrogenic problems following gastric surgery. Gastrointest Radiol 1977; 2:239–257

19. Meyer JH. Chronic morbidity after ulcer surgery. In: Sleisinger MH, Fordtran JS (eds), Gastrointestinal disease, 4th ed. Philadelphia: WB Saunders; 1989:962–987

20. Smith C, Deziel DJ, Kubicka RA. Evaluation of the postoperative stomach and duodenum. RadioGraphics 1994; 14:67–86

21. Waits JO, Beart RW Jr, Charboneau JW. Jejunogastric intussusception. Arch Surg 1980; 115:1449–1452

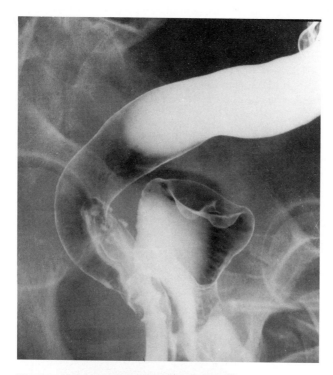

Figure 31-1

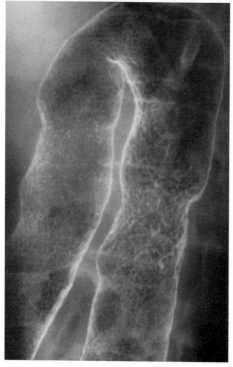

Figure 31-2

Case 31: Colitis

Questions 93 through 96

For each of the numbered barium enema radiographs from four different patients (Figures 31-1 through 31-4), select the *one* lettered diagnosis (A, B, C, D, or E) that is MOST closely associated with it. Each lettered diagnosis may be used once, more than once, or not at all.

    93. Figure 31-1
    94. Figure 31-2
    95. Figure 31-3
    96. Figure 31-4

        (A) Ischemic colitis
        (B) Radiation colitis
        (C) Ulcerative colitis
        (D) Granulomatous colitis
        (E) Pseudomembranous colitis

Figure 31-1, an oblique rectal spot radiograph from an air-contrast barium enema, demonstrates a smooth, featureless rectum with limited distensibility. The valves of Houston are absent. Communication with the vagina via a fistula on the anterior rectal wall is confirmed by the presence of barium and air outlining the vagina and cervix (Figure 31-5). The smooth, symmetric rectal narrowing and the presence of a rectovaginal fistula are characteristic findings in patients with radiation colitis **(Option (B) is the correct answer to Question 93).** Symmetric tapering of the rectum and obliteration of the rectal valves can also be seen in patients with chronic ulcerative colitis. However, the rectal mucosa shown in Figure 31-1 is smooth, not showing the granular texture commonly seen in patients with ulcerative colitis. Fistulae do not develop in patients with ulcerative colitis, in whom the inflammatory process tends to be confined to the mucosa. Granulomatous colitis (Crohn's disease) commonly involves the rectum and is associated with fistula formation, but the asymmetric, coarse mucosal irregularity characteristic of granulomatous colitis is not seen in Figure 31-1. Also lacking are other typical

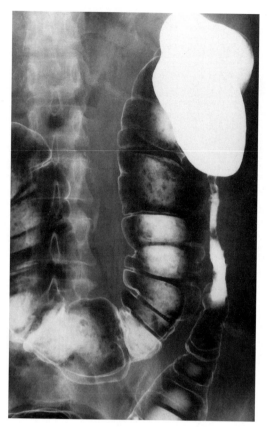
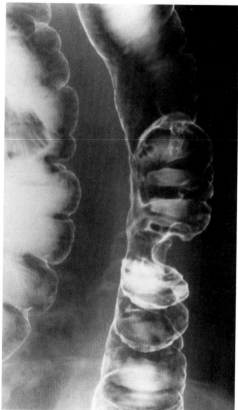

Figure 31-3   *Figure 31-4*

features of granulomatous colitis such as aphthous and linear ulcers. The rectum is rarely affected by ischemic disease, because of its dual arterial blood supply by both splanchnic and systemic arteries. The superior rectal artery is a branch of the inferior mesenteric artery. The middle and inferior rectal arteries arise from the internal iliac arteries bilaterally. The raised, plaque-like mucosal nodules typical of pseudo-membranous colitis are notably absent in this case. Pseudomembranous colitis is not associated with fistula formation.

Most patients with radiation colitis are women who have undergone radiation therapy for carcinoma of the uterine cervix. Approximately 5% of such patients develop radiation colitis involving the rectum. The likeli-hood of developing radiation colitis is greatest in patients treated with higher radiation doses. Doses of 70 Gy to the rectum, usually achieved by a combination of external beam and intracavitary radiation for carci-

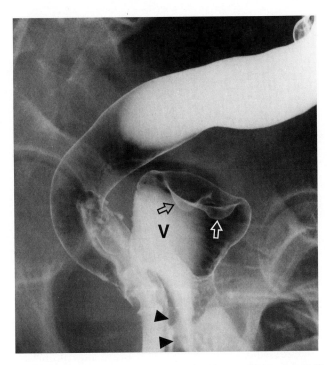

Figure 31-5 (Same as Figure 31-1).   Radiation colitis. An oblique radiograph of the rectum in a woman with chronic radiation colitis 15 years after radiation therapy for carcinoma of the cervix shows that the rectum is diffusely narrowed and the rectal valves are obliterated. There is a fistula (arrowheads) between the anorectal junction and vaginal introitus, with air-contrast demonstration of the vagina (V) and uterine cervix (arrows).

noma of the cervix, are associated with a 10% frequency of radiation colitis. Doses as low as 45 Gy can induce radiation colitis if a larger segment of the colon is exposed.

Barium enema is not usually performed during the acute inflammatory phase of radiation proctitis, during or immediately after the course of radiation treatments. When it is, radiographic findings include rectal spasm and edema manifested by thickening of rectal mucosal folds and a granular mucosal pattern.

More typically, patients experience rectal bleeding and changing bowel habits 2 to 24 months (or longer) after radiation therapy. It is at this stage that a barium enema shows smoothly tapered narrowing confined to the portion of the bowel that received the greatest radiation exposure (Figures 31-6 and 31-7). These abnormalities are due to an underlying small-vessel endarteritis resulting in progressive tissue

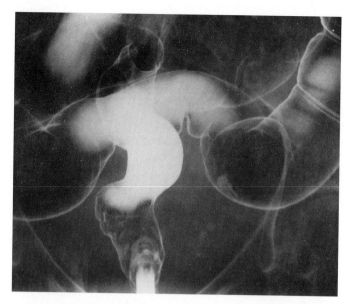

Figure 31-6. Radiation colitis involving the rectum. A radiograph from a barium enema study in a woman with hematochezia 14 months after radiation therapy for carcinoma of the cervix shows diffuse rectal narrowing with absence of the rectal valves, typical of chronic radiation colitis. The appearance is also consistent with long-standing ulcerative colitis, and correlation with the clinical status is important in distinguishing the two entities.

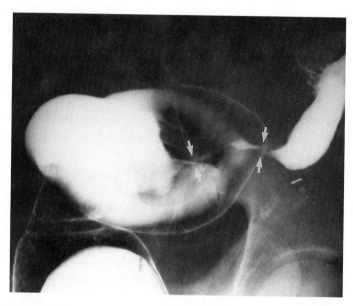

Figure 31-7. Radiation colitis. A radiograph of the sigmoid colon in a patient who received radiation therapy for Hodgkin's lymphoma 2 years earlier shows a smooth, 5-cm colonic stricture (arrows), typical of the late fibrotic effects of radiation colitis. A stricture resulting from ischemic colitis could also have this appearance.

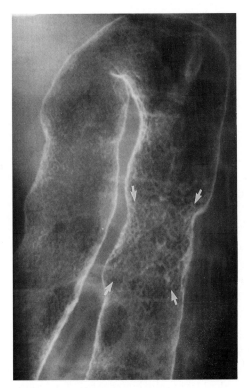

Figure 31-8 (Same as Figure 31-2). Ulcerative colitis. A spot radiograph of the splenic flexure from an air-contrast barium enema in a patient with ulcerative colitis for many years shows a diffuse, finely granular mucosal irregularity that is characteristic of this disease. The focal area in the proximal descending colon (solid arrows), showing a more coarse mucosal texture with a plaque-like or "mosaic tile" appearance, was found to represent mucosal dysplasia on colonoscopic biopsy.

ischemia, fibrosis, and telangiectasis. This process can progress relentlessly over a period of years with worsening stricture, bleeding, tenesmus, and pain. Rectal dilatation, diverting colostomy, and ultimately surgical resection of the abnormal segment may be required.

Figure 31-2, an oblique spot radiograph of the splenic flexure from an air-contrast barium enema, reveals continuous mucosal granularity with loss of haustration and narrowing of the colonic lumen (Figure 31-8). This appearance is typical of ulcerative colitis **(Option (C) is the correct answer to Question 94).** In addition, the coarser, nodular mucosal irregularity in the proximal descending colon suggests a focal area of mucosal dysplasia, an important complication of chronic ulcerative colitis. The term "mosaic tile" has been used to describe the mucosal surface texture in areas of colonic mucosal dysplasia.

The splenic flexure is the portion of the colon most often affected in patients with ischemic colitis; however, the thumbprinting, ulceration, and spasm typical of acute ischemic colitis are not present in Figure 31-2. Healing ischemic colitis can give rise to mucosal irregularity and stricture but not to the diffuse, fine granularity demonstrated in this image. The lack of discrete ulcers with normal or less-affected intervening mucosa makes granulomatous colitis unlikely. The left upper abdomen is rarely treated with sufficient therapeutic radiation to induce radiation colitis. The lack of stricture and the diffuse granular mucosal surface also make radiation colitis unlikely. Pseudomembranous colitis is a continuous inflammatory process usually involving the entire colon. It is characterized by marked colonic fold thickening and mucosal irregularity due to multiple plaque-like pseudomembranes, rather than the granularity and loss of haustration seen in this case.

Ulcerative colitis is a chronic inflammatory bowel disease with an annual incidence of 6 per 100,000, making it a slightly more frequent occurrence than granulomatous colitis. It has a white-to-nonwhite ratio of 4:1 and a slight female predominance. The age distribution of ulcerative colitis is bimodal, with a large peak at age 15 to 25 years and a smaller peak at 55 to 65 years. Etiologic factors remain unclear, but a definite genetic predisposition is known; 15% of patients have an affected first-degree relative. In most patients, ulcerative colitis is characterized clinically by recurrent episodes of diarrhea, rectal bleeding, abdominal pain, and weight loss. Chronic ulcerative colitis confers an increased risk of colonic carcinoma, especially atypical, scirrhous tumors. The risk of malignancy increases with the extent of colonic involvement and the duration of disease. Levin advises that patients with pancolitis for longer than 8 years undergo regular cancer surveillance or prophylactic colectomy.

Ulcerative colitis can be accompanied by extraintestinal manifestations that may or may not parallel the course of the colonic disease. Those that do not parallel the clinical severity or course of the colitis include sclerosing cholangitis (seen in 1 to 4% of patients), cholangiocarcinoma, pyoderma gangrenosum, ankylosing spondylitis, and sacroiliitis. Peripheral arthritis, uveitis, episcleritis, renal stone formation, amyloidosis, erythema nodosum, and fatty infiltration of the liver are more likely to parallel the course of the colonic involvement.

The barium enema findings of ulcerative colitis involve the rectum and extend proximally to a variable extent (Figure 31-9), often involving the entire colon. Mucosal abnormalities in acute or long-standing but active disease include granularity, mucosal stippling, collar button ulceration, and inflammatory pseudopolyp formation (Figure 31-10). The transition to normal colonic mucosa can be gradual. The granular appearance of the mucosal surface is a manifestation of mucosal edema and does not imply the presence of ulcers. Edema of the deeper layers of the colonic wall causes thickening of interhaustral folds and, if severe enough, flattening or loss of the normal haustral pattern. Mucosal stippling is caused when barium fills multiple tiny ulcers overlying and pro-

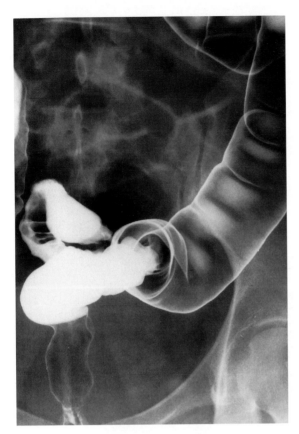

Figure 31-9. Ulcerative colitis involving the rectum and sigmoid region. A barium enema radiograph shows that a single, continuous segment is involved and has moderate narrowing. The rectal mucosa has a finely granular texture, and the rectal valves are obliterated.

duced by crypt abscesses. When the ulcers spread to the submucosa and undermine the inflamed mucosa, they take on the shape of a collar button. Inflammatory pseudopolyps represent islands of relatively spared mucosa that are raised with respect to the denuded areas surrounding them.

In patients with chronic ulcerative colitis, there can be permanent narrowing of the lumen (Figure 31-11). Loss of haustration and shortening of the colon (Figure 31-10) are due in part to alterations in muscle tone of the teniae coli and to hypertrophy of the muscularis mucosa. Thickening or obliteration of the rectal valves, widening of the presacral space, and postinflammatory polyps (Figures 31-11 and 31-12) can also be seen. Widening of the presacral space, defined as greater than a 1.5-cm separation between the anterior surface of the fifth sacral segment and posterior rectal mucosa on a lateral film of the rectum, is due to mural thickening and perirectal fat proliferation (Figure 31-13). Post-

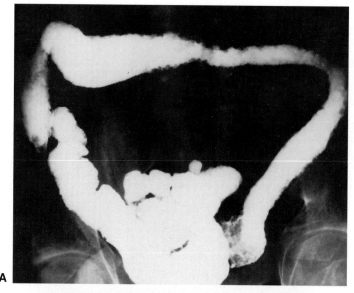

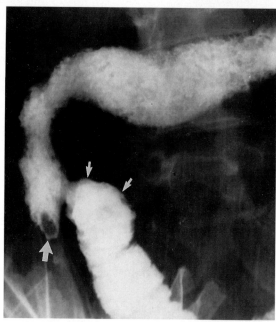

Figure 31-10. Chronic ulcerative colitis with backwash ileitis. (A) A single-contrast barium enema radiograph of a patient with recurrent bloody diarrhea for 10 years shows marked colonic shortening and narrowing and loss of the normal haustral contour. Coarse mucosal irregularity is due to a combination of ulceration and inflammatory pseudopolyps. (B) A spot radiograph of the right colon demonstrates diffuse dilatation of the terminal ileum with irregularity of the mucosa (small arrows) in its distal 2 cm. The ileocecal valve is widely patulous. Note also the polyp (large arrow) in the cecum. At operation, this was found to be an adenoma, but many random samples of the inflamed colonic mucosa were found to contain foci of adenocarcinoma on histologic analysis.

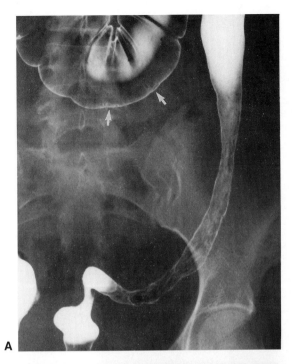

A

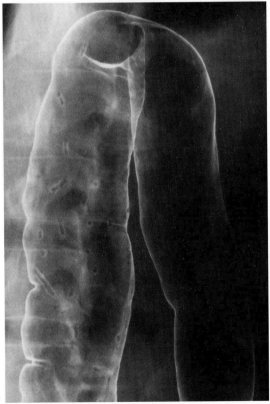

B

Figure 31-11. Ulcerative colitis. (A) A double-contrast enema radiograph in a patient with a 20-year history of ulcerative colitis who is presently asymptomatic shows a long, continuous segment of narrowing extending from the rectum to the mid-descending colon. The mucosal surface is minimally and uniformly irregular. The transverse colon contains several postinflammatory polyps (arrows), but the appearance of this area is otherwise normal. (B) A spot radiograph of the splenic flexure shows the postinflammatory polyps in greater detail. Many have the filiform shape typical of postinflammatory colonic polyps remaining after a severe bout of colonic inflammation.

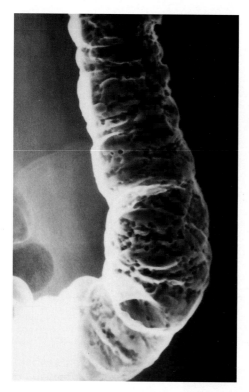

Figure 31-12. Ulcerative colitis. A barium enema radiograph performed 10 days after resolution of an acute, severe episode of ulcerative colitis in an asymptomatic 17-year-old girl shows numerous postinflammatory polyps. The radiograph shows only the distal descending region, but the remainder of the colon was similarly involved. The polyps vary from round to bifid to filiform and are seen on a background of normal mucosa. They represent overgrown regenerating mucosa in the healed phase of the disease. They can be seen not only after ulcerative colitis but also after healing of granulomatous or amoebic colitis.

inflammatory polyps represent overgrowth of regenerating mucosa in the healing phase of ulcerative colitis. They persist even after ulcerative colitis has healed, as does the loss of haustral markings in some patients.

The terminal ileum is most often normal in patients with ulcerative colitis. In up to 40% of patients with pancolitis, however, the terminal ileum is dilated and the ileocecal valve is patulous (Figure 31-10). The ileal mucosa may appear granular, but ileal ulcers are characteristically absent. This constellation of findings is referred to as backwash ileitis.

Mucosal dysplasia is a premalignant change in the colon that can occur in patients with long-standing ulcerative colitis. It is detected most often during colonoscopy for routine surveillance by biopsy of random areas not identifiable on the barium enema. Sometimes, however, the finding of an area of focally irregular, coarsened, raised nodular mucosa on barium enema can enable the radiologist to suggest the need for colonoscopy and biopsy of the suspicious area (Figure 31-8). Biopsy specimens of multiple, random areas of the colon in such a patient may show a mixture of dysplasia and unsuspected carcinoma.

Other radiographic features of ulcerative colitis are seen in patients with toxic megacolon, one of the most important complications of ulcer-

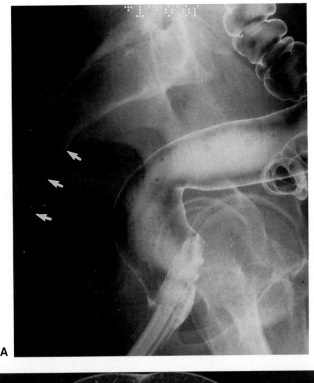

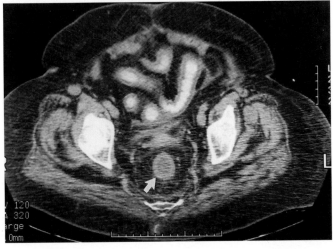

Figure 31-13. Ulcerative colitis. (A) A lateral rectal spot radiograph in a patient with chronic, clinically inactive ulcerative colitis demonstrates marked widening of the presacral space. The distance from the anterior edge of the sacrum (arrows) to the posterior rectal mucosa measured 4 cm (the normal distance is ≤1.5 cm). The widening of this space is due to mural thickening related to hypertrophy of the muscularis mucosa and to proliferation of perirectal fat. (B) CT scan with oral and intravenous contrast enhancement demonstrates the perirectal fat proliferation resulting in a widened presacral space in this patient with chronic ulcerative colitis. Note the thickened rectal wall (arrow); it has maintained a target appearance, which is typical of inflammatory thickening.

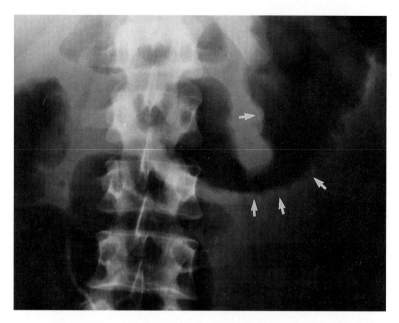

Figure 31-14. Toxic megacolon due to ulcerative colitis. The distal transverse colon shows dilatation and thumbprinting (arrows). These findings on a scout radiograph should alert the radiologist to the presence of fulminant colitis and the danger of performing a barium enema examination at this time.

ative colitis. This condition is characterized in abdominal radiographs by colonic dilatation. Air-fluid levels are seen on upright or lateral decubitus views. Most helpful in establishing the diagnosis on plain radiographs is an irregular contour to the colon (Figure 31-14). The normal haustral folds are thickened or absent. Irregular islands of soft tissue density represent inflammatory pseudopolyps projecting into the gas-filled lumen. Barium enema is contraindicated in patients with toxic megacolon, as it is in patients with fulminant colitis of any type, because of a significant risk of colonic perforation. Any patient with abdominal pain, bloody diarrhea, fever, and leukocytosis is better off being treated with corticosteroids and other medical therapy until clinically stable rather than undergoing an immediate barium enema. If the diagnosis is in question, a gentle endoscopic examination of the rectum is better tolerated and is usually sufficient to guide initial therapeutic decisions.

Figure 31-3, a supine view of the transverse and descending colon from an air-contrast barium enema, reveals a segmental stricture of the mid-descending colon. Mucosal irregularity in the affected segment indicates the presence of ulceration. The tapered, funnel-like margins of the stricture are best seen at its distal margin. The findings are characteristic of ischemic colitis **(Option (A) is the correct answer to Question 95).** Ischemic colitis typically occurs in patients over 50 years of age, often with signs of generalized atherosclerotic disease, and this clinical setting can be a clue to the diagnosis. The typical clinical features of ischemic colitis (which were present in the test patient) also serve to confirm the radiologic impression. These include sudden onset of severe localized abdominal pain, diarrhea, hematochezia, vomiting, and leukocytosis.

Granulomatous colitis can also cause focal colonic strictures such as the one shown in Figure 31-3. However, in the absence of the more specific mucosal abnormalities of granulomatous colitis, such as aphthous or linear ulcers, ischemia is the more likely etiology. The absence of colonic involvement distal to the stricture makes ulcerative colitis unlikely. The location is unusual for radiation-induced colitis. Pseudomembranous colitis does not cause focal left colonic strictures as seen in the test case. It usually involves the entire colon and, when focal, the right colon is more often affected.

Colonic ischemia occurs when insufficient oxygen is delivered to a region of colon. Underlying mechanisms include arterial occlusion, venous thrombosis, and nonocclusive ischemia. Atherosclerotic disease, embolus, and arteritis are the leading causes of colonic ischemia on an arterial occlusive basis. Cardiogenic shock and other severe low-flow states give rise to the nonocclusive form of colon ischemia. The area supplied by the inferior mesenteric artery, from splenic flexure to rectosigmoid junction, is the region of the colon most susceptible to ischemic injury on either an arterial occlusive or nonocclusive basis. Inferior mesenteric arterial supply to the rectum is supplemented by blood from the superior hemorrhoidal arteries, which renders the rectum relatively immune to ischemic injury.

Colonic ischemia due to venous occlusion is associated with various causes of mesenteric venous thrombosis, including inflammatory conditions such as diverticulitis and pancreatitis, and neoplastic mesenteric disease such as carcinoid tumor. Unlike arterial ischemic colitis, it is quite variable in distribution. Most patients are older than 50 years. Venous engorgement in the affected segment leads to intramural hemorrhage and edema that is usually more marked than in patients with ischemic colitis due to arterial occlusion.

Following an ischemic event, the colon can respond in several ways depending on the degree of ischemic insult. Complete healing occurs in 50% of patients, perforation occurs in 18%, stricture occurs in 12%, and persistent colitis occurs in 20%. Complete healing is most common in

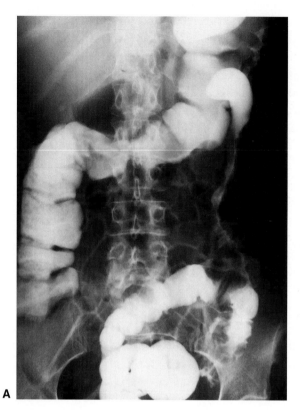

Figure 31-15. Ischemic colitis. (A) A single-contrast barium enema radiograph demonstrates thumbprinting and spasm of the entire descending colon. The thumbprinting is due to edema and hemorrhage within the colonic wall and is a common radiographic finding in acute ischemic colitis. (B) An abdominal CT scan shows marked thickening of the wall of the affected descending colon (small arrows). Areas of thumbprinting on the barium enema show mixed attenuation of the thickened bowel wall. Note the normal thickness of the wall of the unaffected transverse colon (large arrows).

A

patients who suffer only mucosal ischemia, whereas perforation, persistent colitis, and stricture arise after transmural ischemic injury.

In the acute phase, a single-contrast barium enema is useful in establishing the diagnosis (Figure 31-15A). Findings on barium enema frequently are characteristic and include thumbprinting, spasm, transverse ridging, ulceration, and intramural barium (Figure 31-16). "Thumbprinting" is a term applied to indentations of the barium-filled lumen that are caused by collections of blood and edema in the colonic wall. Thumbprinting can be made less evident or even obliterated by full colonic distension on a double-contrast barium enema. One of the radiographic hallmarks of bowel ischemia is serial changes in the appearance of the colon. Strictures begin forming in the subacute phase and may regress by 6 to 9 months. They usually show a short transition zone with the adjacent unaffected colon. Most strictures due to ischemic colitis are concentric, but asymmetric fibrosis sometimes leads to bizarre configurations with eccentric narrowing and marked sacculation within the involved segment (Figure 31-17).

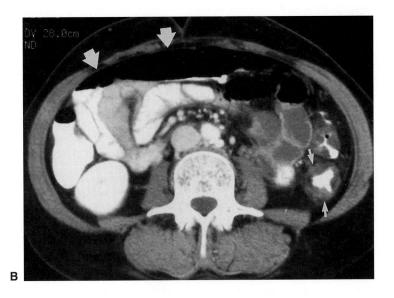

B

There is another form of colitis that is probably categorized most accurately as ischemic in nature, namely, the colitis that occurs proximal to an obstructing lesion of the colon. The pathogenesis is thought to be related to diminished mucosal perfusion resulting from increased intraluminal pressure. This form of colitis is seen in patients with an obstructing colonic adenocarcinoma and occasionally in patients with sigmoid volvulus. Typically, the underlying obstruction is long-standing. Barium enema studies reveal diffuse colonic edema that can be quite severe (Figure 31-18). Only the portion of the colon affected by preobstructive dilatation is involved. The findings are demonstrable on barium enema only when barium can be introduced above the site of obstruction. For this reason, the condition is most likely to be seen on barium studies done shortly after an obstructive process is relieved. Diffuse, edematous thickening of the colonic wall above a short, focal obstructing tumor can also be seen on CT and should not be confused with a long segment of colonic tumor or inflammatory stricture. The findings of preobstructive colitis slowly disappear over the several days following relief of the underlying obstructive process.

Figure 31-4 demonstrates an abnormal segment of descending colon containing two large linear ulcers and several aphthous ulcers scattered on a background of normal intervening mucosa (Figure 31-19). Ulcers with this appearance and the asymmetric, discontinuous nature of the findings are characteristic of granulomatous colitis (Crohn's disease) **(Option (D) is the correct answer to Question 96).**

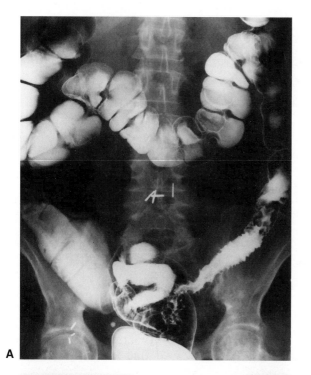

A

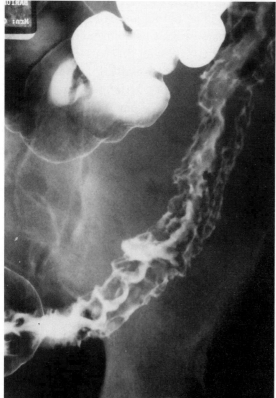

B

Figure 31-16. Ischemic colitis developing in a patient a few days after aortofemoral bypass surgery for severe atherosclerosis. (A) There is spasm and mucosal thickening of the distal descending and proximal sigmoid colon. (B) A spot radiograph of the distal descending region shows typical thumbprinting in more detail.

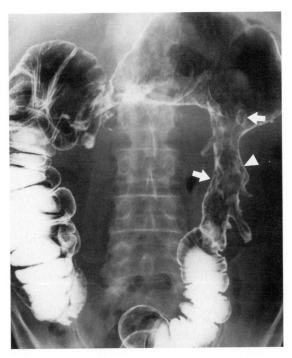

Figure 31-17. Ischemic colitis. The bizarre appearance of this double-contrast enema radiograph might initially be confusing; however, it reveals one abnormal segment of colon (left-sided) with abrupt funnel-like transitions to the normal mucosa, typical of stricture formation in colonic ischemia. The saccular and eccentric configuration of this strictured segment can be seen (but usually to a lesser degree). Note also the persistent ulceration (arrowhead) and sessile polyps (arrows) in this patient, whose colon was normal at laparotomy 6 weeks prior to this study.

Ulcerative colitis is not a serious diagnostic consideration in this patient. It is characterized by more uniform, concentric, and continuous mucosal involvement. Ulcers of the type seen in Figure 31-4 do not occur in patients with ulcerative colitis. The relative normality of the segment distal to the area of greatest abnormality also militates against this diagnosis. Ischemic colitis does tend to occur in the descending colon and does give rise to asymmetric strictures; however, the pattern of long linear and aphthous ulcers would be unusual and make this diagnosis less likely. In some patients, however, granulomatous colitis and ischemic colitis can be very difficult to distinguish, even when biopsy material is available for histologic analysis. The location and mucosal features in Figure 31-4 are not typical of radiation colitis. The aymmetric mucosal

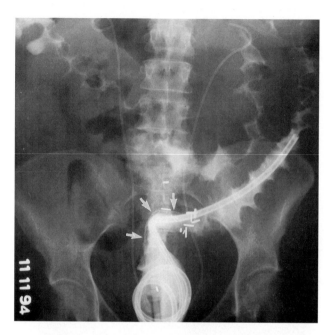

Figure 31-18. Colitis proximal to obstructing adenocarcinoma of the rectum. The tumor caused mechanical obstruction that progressively worsened over several weeks. This radiograph is part of a diagnostic enema study performed with iodinated, water-soluble contrast material 1 day after endoscopic placement of an expandable stent prosthesis (arrows) to relieve the obstruction. Throughout the colon, there is marked, diffuse thumbprinting and edema.

involvement, large linear ulceration, and segmental appearance seen in the test images are not compatible with pseudomembranous colitis.

Crohn's disease has an annual incidence of 4 cases per 100,000, with a bimodal age distribution peaking at 20 to 30 years and at 70 years. Most patients are affected during the earlier peak. Possible etiologic factors include genetic predisposition, immune mechanisms, infections (mycobacterial), and environmental causes. Patients with Crohn's disease are often more chronically ill and malnourished than their counterparts with ulcerative colitis. Surgical options for patients with Crohn's disease differ from those for patients with ulcerative colitis because of the transmural nature of Crohn's colitis, the tendency to form fistulae and strictures, the frequency of concomitant small bowel involvement, and the likelihood of recurrence after resection. Exclusive involvement of the colon is seen in only 15% of patients with Crohn's disease. Most have ileocolic disease (55%) or involvement limited to the small bowel (30%).

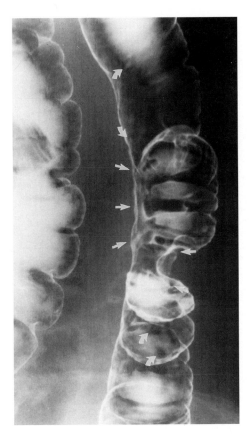

Figure 31-19 (Same as Figure 31-4). Granulomatous colitis. A spot radiograph of the descending colon reveals an abnormal segment of asymmetrically affected mucosa containing aphthous ulcers (curved arrows) and two long linear ulcers (straight arrows) on a background of normal colonic mucosa. The findings are typical of granulomatous colitis (Crohn's disease).

Anorectal disease occurs in approximately 50% of all patients with Crohn's disease (Figures 31-20 and 31-21).

The earliest radiographic changes seen on barium studies in patients with granulomatous colitis consist of aphthous ulcers on a background of normal intervening mucosa (Figure 31-20). Aphthous ulcers are tiny, superficial ulcers that form over enlarged colonic lymphoid follicles. On barium enema examination, they appear as punctate collections of barium surrounded by thin radiolucent halos. Aphthous ulcers are not specific for Crohn's disease, however, and can be seen in patients with other forms of colitis, including colitis due to infection with *Salmonella* spp., *Shigella* spp., herpesvirus, cytomegalovirus, *Yersinia* spp., and amoebae. Aphthous ulcers also occur in patients with Behçet's disease. They are not seen in patients with ulcerative colitis or radiation colitis.

Later in the course of granulomatous colitis, there is development of deeper ulcers that penetrate into the submucosa. These take the form of

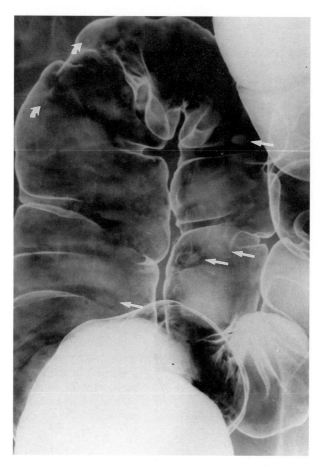

Figure 31-20. Granulomatous colitis with ulcerations. A close-up view of the sigmoid colon reveals aphthous ulcerations (curved arrows) as well as larger flat superficial ulcerations (straight arrows) in this young male patient who had already undergone ascending colectomy.

small, pointed ("rose thorn") ulcers, irregularly shaped (geographic) ulcers, and long, longitudinally oriented linear ulcers. The cobblestone mucosal pattern of Crohn's disease is formed by areas of edematous mucosa separated by numerous longitudinal ulcers and transverse fissures. Transmural extension of Crohn's disease through the muscularis propria and serosa leads to sinus tracts and fistulae (Figures 31-22 and 31-23). It also leads to a pattern of spread that is characteristic of Crohn's disease and easy to detect radiographically. The inflammatory process extends through the serosa to involve segments of bowel (or occasionally urinary tract) that lie nearby in immediate anatomic contact with the inflamed segment (Figure 31-24). This is quite unlike the pat-

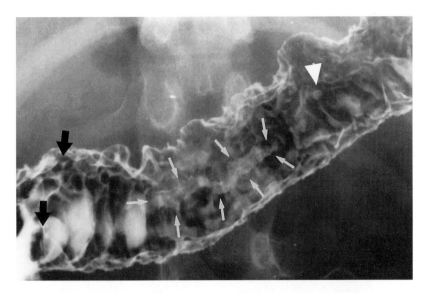

Figure 31-21. Granulomatous colitis with ulcerations. A close-up view of the transverse colon in this young male patient who is taking high-dose steroids reveals a long flat linear ulcer (white arrows), a shallow round ulcer (arrowhead), and pseudopolyps (black arrows), which at colonoscopy appeared identical to the radiographic findings.

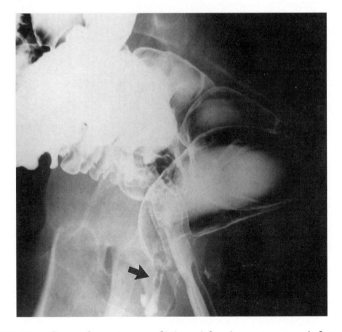

Figure 31-22. Granulomatous colitis with sinus tracts. A lateral spot radiograph in this 17-year-old woman, taking four medications for Crohn's disease, shows characteristic sinus tract formation at the anorectal junction (arrow). The rectal mucosa is normal, the presacral space is normal, and the rectal valves are preserved, excluding radiation proctitis or ulcerative proctitis in this patient.

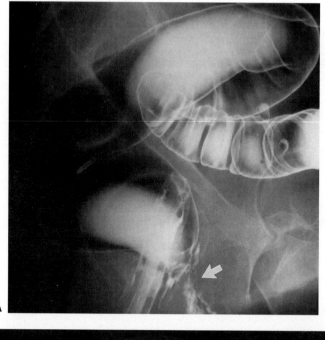

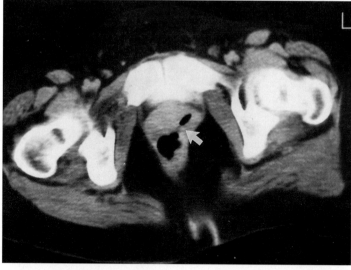

Figure 31-23. Granulomatous colitis with fistula. (A) A lateral spot radiograph reveals normal rectal mucosa with fistula formation from the anorectal junction to the vagina (arrow). (B) A CT scan at the level of the symphysis pubis also demonstrates the fistula, which contains air (arrow). Inserting the enema tip too proximally in the rectum may inhibit the visualization of anorectal sinus tracts and fistulae; CT is often helpful in evaluating this aspect of Crohn's disease.

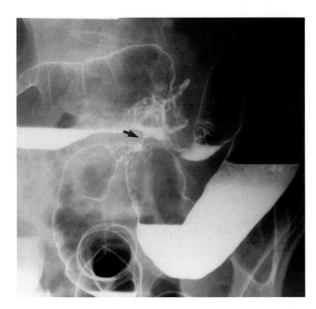

Figure 31-24. Granulomatous colitis with fistula. A spot radiograph from a double-contrast enema in this 81-year-old woman with long-standing Crohn's disease demonstrates distal transverse-to-sigmoid colocolic fistula formation (arrow). Adjacent, non-axially contiguous bowel loops are often affected by the transmural inflammation of granulomatous colitis.

tern of spread in patients with ulcerative colitis, which extends to involve previously unaffected areas by spreading along the length of the bowel.

Pseudomembranous colitis is most often associated with antibiotic usage, which alters the normal colonic flora and results in overgrowth of *Clostridium difficile*. Enterotoxin released by this pathogen causes the colitis. The clinical manifestations of pseudomembranous colitis include abdominal pain, watery diarrhea, leukocytosis, and fever. If left untreated, pseudomembranous colitis can result in toxic megacolon and perforation. The history of antibiotic usage may be remote or overlooked; occasionally, the appearance of radiographic abnormalities on conventional radiographs, barium enema images, or CT scans will be the first indicators for this disease. The definitive diagnosis is made by stool toxin assay or by endoscopy with visualization of the typical pseudomembranes.

Abdominal radiographs in patients with pseudomembranous colitis are most often normal or else show nonspecific gaseous distension of the colon. However, when the pseudomembranous colitis is severe, thumb-printing and thickening of the haustral folds can be seen. The thickened haustral folds sometimes result in a characteristic pattern of transverse banding (Figure 31-25). Differentiation from other causes of severe colonic edema such as ischemia, acute severe inflammatory bowel disease, or cytomegalovirus colitis is difficult on radiographic grounds alone.

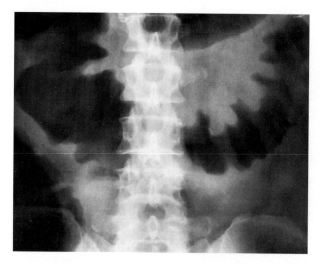

Figure 31-25 (left).
Abdominal radiograph in a patient with pseudomembranous colitis. The transverse colon shows extreme haustral thickening, producing a characteristic but infrequently seen pattern of transverse banding.

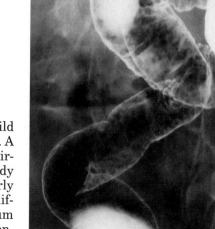

Figure 31-26 (right). Mild pseudomembranous colitis. A spot radiograph from an air-contrast barium enema study shows subtle, irregularly shaped, mucosal plaques diffusely blanketing the rectum and sigmoid colon.

The findings of pseudomembranous colitis on barium enema examination vary with the severity of the disease. In mild cases, irregular, small, nodular, or plaque-like mucosal filling defects are seen (Figure 31-26). As the disease progresses, thickened haustral folds, more numer-

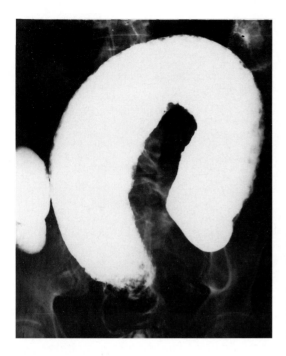

Figure 31-27 (left). Severe pseudomembranous colitis. A radiograph from a single-column barium enema study demonstrates marked, shaggy, plaque-like mucosal irregularities in the sigmoid colon.

ous and larger mucosal nodules and plaques, and marked colonic wall thickening develop (Figure 31-27). The distribution of mucosal irregularities in the colon is also variable. Pseudomembranous colitis is most often a pancolitis, but rectal sparing is not uncommon. When pseudomembranous colitis is focal, the right colon is most often affected (Figure 31-28).

CT is often the first imaging test used for patients with pseudomembranous colitis; it is frequently used to evaluate abdominal pain and fever prior to making a diagnosis. The sensitivity and specificity of CT in the detection of colon abnormalities in patients with pseudomembranous colitis have recently been reported to be 85 and 48%, respectively. Although somewhat nonspecific, the CT findings of diffuse or focal colonic wall thickening and irregular or shaggy mucosal contour should alert the radiologist and the referring physician to reevaluate the patient's history, assay the stool for enterotoxin, and begin appropriate therapy. The average colon wall thickness seen on CT in patients with pseudomembranous colitis is typically at least 1.5 cm and in many cases exceeds 2.0 cm. This is greater than the colonic wall thickening usually seen in patients with granulomatous or ulcerative colitis. With extensive thickening of the haustral folds, the lumen is nearly obliterated and luminal contrast is trapped between the folds; this has been described as

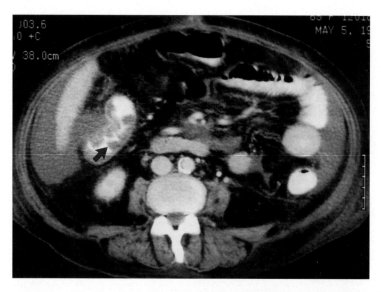

Figure 31-28. Pseudomembranous colitis developing after 3 weeks of intravenous antibiotic therapy. CT performed with administration of intravenous, oral, and rectal contrast media shows marked haustral fold thickening (arrow) of the hepatic flexure. The radiologic findings and clinical history suggest pseudomembranous colitis. When focal, pseudomembranous colitis more often involves the right colon than the left one.

the accordion pattern of pseudomembranous colitis (Figure 31-29). When severe diffuse wall thickening is present throughout the colon, differentiating pseudomembranous colitis from cytomegalovirus colitis may be difficult (Figure 31-30). Likewise, when focal right colonic wall thickening and fold enlargement are present, differentiating pseudomembranous colitis from typhlitis in immunosuppressed individuals is also difficult. The presence of pericolonic fluid in association with focal right colon wall thickening should suggest typhlitis, although pericolonic stranding and ascites may be seen in patients with pseudomembranous colitis. In a recent study, 39% of patients with pseudomembranous colitis had no detectable colonic abnormality on CT. Despite the nonspecific nature of the CT findings, the diagnosis of pseudomembranous colitis can and should be suggested in the appropriate clinical setting when colon wall thickening is seen.

CT is being shown to be increasingly useful in the evaluation of patients with colitis. Of the conditions discussed in this case, CT is most useful in evaluation of Crohn's disease. It is effective in detecting complications such as sinus tracts and abscesses (Figure 31-31). Perineal

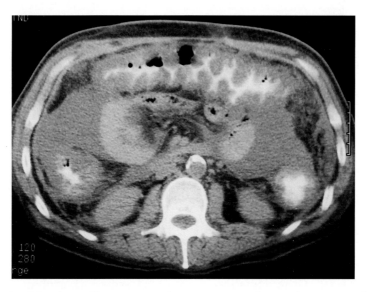

Figure 31-29. Accordion pattern in severe pseudomembranous colitis. A CT scan obtained with administration of oral, rectal, and intravenous contrast media demonstrates marked haustral fold thickening (accordion pattern) in the transverse colon. Extensive wall thickening of the ascending and descending colon is also present.

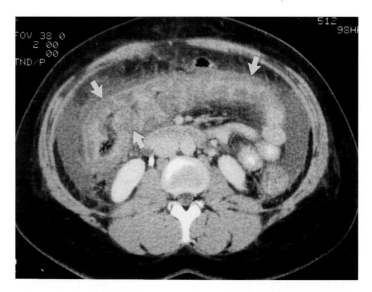

Figure 31-30. CT scan obtained with administration of intravenous and oral contrast media in a patient with severe pseudomembranous colitis. There is marked thickening of the colonic wall (arrows) with near complete obliteration of the lumen. Ascites is also present.

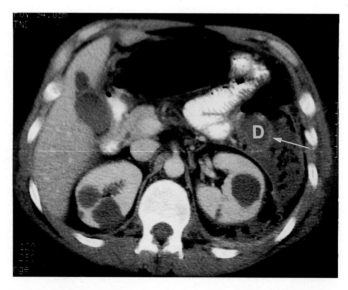

Figure 31-31. Granulomatous colitis. A CT scan with oral and intravenous contrast enhancement in a 32-year-old man with prior right colectomy for granulomatous colitis reveals a circumferentially thickened
descending colonic wall (D) with perforation and abscess formation in the
left anterior pararenal space. Note the target appearance of the thickened colonic wall (arrow), which is composed of enhancing mucosa and
serosa with a low-attenuation edematous submucosa.

pathology is well shown on CT (Figure 31-23B), as are thickening of the
bowel wall and luminal narrowing (Figure 31-32). In patients with
Crohn's disease and a palpable mass, CT can often aid in determination
of whether the palpable abnormality is due to fibrofatty proliferation
around an affected bowel loop, marked bowel wall thickening, or phlegmon and abscess (Figure 31-33). With CT, as with barium studies, however, there are often discrepancies between the severity of the radiologic
findings and the clinical indicators of disease activity in patients with
Crohn's disease. Normal bowel wall thickness can be seen in patients
with early but active granulomatous colitis, and marked mural thickening can be seen in patients with chronic but clinically inactive disease.

In the evaluation of ischemic colitis, CT can play a role not only in
detecting mural thickening and thumbprinting (Figure 31-15B) but also
in detecting intramural pneumatosis, portal venous gas, and intraperitoneal free air. Patients with radiation colitis often undergo CT evaluation
to assess clinically suspected recurrence of their primary neoplastic disease, during which the radiation-induced changes (Figure 31-34) can also
be demonstrated. The role of CT in the evaluation of ulcerative colitis is

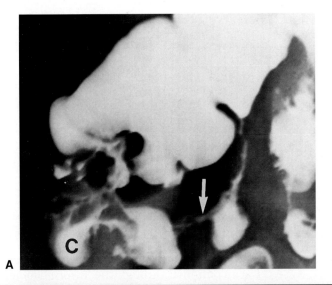

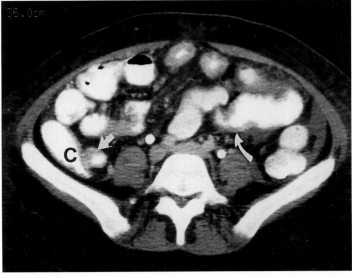

Figure 31-32. Crohn's disease, with large and small bowel involvement. (A) A digital spot radiograph from a small bowel follow-through demonstrates marked irregular narrowing of the terminal ileum (arrow) with persistent conical narrowing of the cecum (C). (B) A CT scan through the midabdomen with intravenous, oral, and rectal contrast enhancement reveals conical narrowing of the cecum (C) and wall thickening with narrowing of the terminal ileum (straight arrow). A dilated preobstructive small bowel loop with irregularly thickened walls (curved arrow) is seen in the left abdomen.

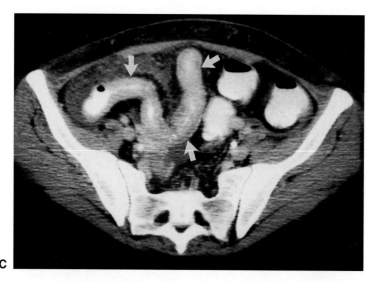

C

Figure 31-32 (Continued).   Crohn's disease, with large and small bowel involvement. (C) A CT scan obtained through the lower abdomen shows a long segment of irregularly thickened and narrowed ileum (arrows), an appearance characteristic of Crohn's disease.

minor. The utility of CT in pseudomembranous colitis lies in its ability to display the colonic wall thickening and thereby to alert the clinical team that colitis is present. As mentioned in the discussion of pseudomembranous colitis, patients with this condition sometimes have relatively nonspecific abdominal symptoms; CT is the first imaging method to visualize the colonic involvement. CT has no role in managing patients, however, once the diagnosis has been made.

Desiree E. Morgan, M.D.
Robert E. Koehler, M.D.

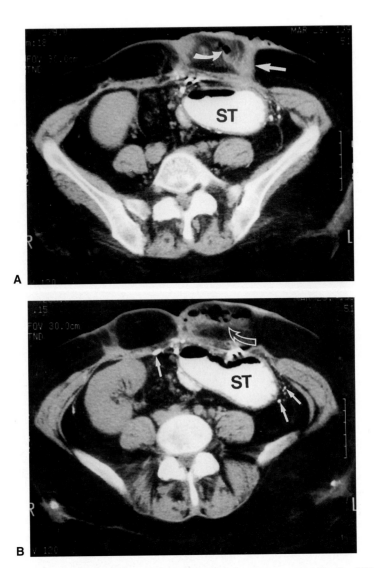

Figure 31-33. Crohn's disease, with local recurrence. Both CT scans were obtained with oral contrast agent administration in a patient with previous colectomy and ileostomy for Crohn's disease. (A) A CT scan through the lower abdomen shows the ileostomy (straight arrow) in the left lower quadrant. A fistula (curved arrow) extends from the ileostomy into the medial soft tissues of the anterior abdominal wall, indicating local recurrence of Crohn's disease. The most common site for postoperative recurrence is immediately proximal to the resection margin. ST = stomach. (B) A CT scan through a slightly higher level shows an abscess cavity (open arrow) extending from the fistulous tract. A scar from a previous ileostomy can be seen in the right lower quadrant. Barium droplets from a previous perforation are scattered throughout the peritoneal cavity (small arrows). ST = stomach.

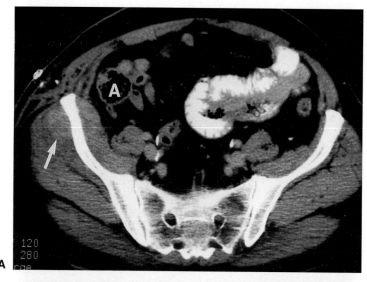

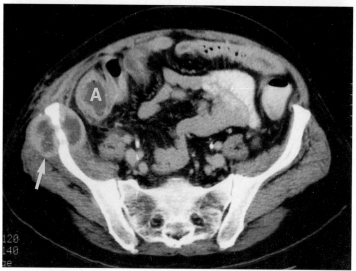

Figure 31-34. Radiation colitis. (A) A CT scan with oral and intravenous contrast enhancement in a 51-year-old male patient with metastatic adenocarcinoma involving the right iliac wing. Soft tissue enhancement (arrow) is present in the mass adjacent to the affected ilium. Note the normal thickness of the ascending colon (A). Postbiopsy changes are present in the right lateral abdominal wall. (B) A CT scan through the same level 1 month later, following radiation therapy to the right iliac region. Expansion of the right iliac metastasis (arrow) with central necrosis is noted. In addition, thickening of the abdominal wall muscles and ascending colon (A) can be seen due to their proximity to the radiation port.

SUGGESTED READINGS

INFLAMMATORY BOWEL DISEASE: GENERAL

1. Danzi JT. Extraintestinal manifestations of idiopathic inflammatory bowel disease. Arch Intern Med 1988; 148:297–302
2. Dubrow RA, Frank PH. Barium evaluation of the anal canal in patients with inflammatory bowel disease. AJR 1983; 140:1151–1157
3. Grimm IS, Friedman LS. Inflammatory bowel disease in the elderly. Gastrointest Clin North Am 1990; 19:361–389
4. Guillaumin E, Jeffrey RB Jr, Shea WJ, Asling CW, Goldberg HI. Perirectal inflammatory disease: CT findings. Radiology 1986; 161:153–157
5. Halpert RD. Toxic dilatation of the colon. Radiol Clin North Am 1987; 25:147–155
6. Kelly JK, Gabos S. The pathogenesis of inflammatory polyps. Dis Colon Rectum 1987; 30:251–254
7. Kirsner JB. Inflammatory bowel disease. I. Nature and pathogenesis. Disease-a-Month 1991; 37:605–666
8. Kirsner JB. Inflammatory bowel disease. II. Clinical and therapeutic aspects. Disease-a-Month 1991; 37:669–746
9. Lichtenstein JE. Radiologic-pathologic correlation of inflammatory bowel disease. Radiol Clin North Am 1987; 25:3–24
10. Philpotts LE, Heiken JP, Westcott MA, Gore RM. Colitis: use of CT findings in differential diagnosis. Radiology 1994; 190:445–449
11. Williams HJ Jr, Stephens DH, Carlson HC. Double-contrast radiography: colonic inflammatory disease. AJR 1981; 137:315–322

ISCHEMIC COLITIS

12. Alpern MB, Glazer GM, Francis IR. Ischemic or infarcted bowel: CT findings. Radiology 1988; 166:149–152
13. Bartram CI. Obliteration of thumbprinting with double-contrast enemas in acute ischemic colitis. Gastrointest Radiol 1979; 4:85–88
14. Bower TC. Ischemic colitis. Surg Clin North Am 1993; 73:1037–1053
15. Iida M, Matsui T, Fuchigami T, Iwashita A, Yao T, Fujishima M. Ischemic colitis: serial changes in double-contrast barium enema examination. Radiology 1986; 159:337–341
16. Wolf EL, Sprayregen S, Bakal CW. Radiology in intestinal ischemia. Plain film, contrast, and other imaging studies. Surg Clin North Am 1992; 72:107–124

RADIATION COLITIS

17. Meyer JE. Radiography of the distal colon and rectum after irradiation of carcinoma of the cervix. AJR 1981; 136:691–699

ULCERATIVE COLITIS

18. Bartram CI. Radiology in the current assessment of ulcerative colitis. Gastrointest Radiol 1977; 1:383–392

19. Frank PH, Riddell RH, Feczko PJ, Levin B. Radiological detection of colonic dysplasia (precarcinoma) in ulcerative colitis. Gastrointest Radiol 1978; 3:209–219
20. Levin B. Ulcerative colitis and colon cancer: biology and surveillance. J Cell Biochem Suppl 1992; 166:47–50

GRANULOMATOUS COLITIS (CROHN'S DISEASE)

21. Ni XY, Goldberg HI. Aphthoid ulcers in Crohn's disease: radiographic course and relationship to bowel appearance. Radiology 1986; 158:589–596

PSEUDOMEMBRANOUS COLITIS

22. Boland GW, Lee MS, Cats AM, et al. Antibiotic-induced diarrhea: the specificity of abdominal CT for the diagnosis of *Clostridium difficile* disease. Radiology 1994; 191:103
23. Fishman EK, Madhav K, Jones B, et al. Pseudomembranous colitis: CT evaluation of 26 cases. Radiology 1991; 180:57–60
24. Rubesin SE, Revine MS, Glich SN. Pseudomembranous colitis with rectosigmoid sparing on barium studies. Radiology 1989; 170:811–814
25. Stanley RJ, Melson GL, Tedesco FJ. Plain film findings in severe pseudomembranous colitis. Radiology 1976; 118:7–11

Notes

Index

Where there are multiple page references, **boldface** indicates the main discussion of a topic.

A

Abdominal radiography
closed-loop small bowel obstruction, 80
duodenal perforation after laparoscopic cholecystectomy, 394
small bowel obstruction, 75
Abscesses. *See also* Amebic liver abscesses; Fungal liver abscesses; Greater peritoneal sac abscesses; Lesser peritoneal sac abscesses; Periappendiceal abscesses
differential diagnosis
benign postoperative stricture of the neopharynx, 319
laparoscopic cholecystectomy and, 396–97
postoperative complication of laryngectomy, 322
Abscess sinography, **273–76**
Accidents. *See also* Trauma
duodenal hematomas and, 35
Achalasia. *See* Primary or idiopathic achalasia; Secondary achalasia
Acquired immunodeficiency syndrome. *See also* AIDS cholangiopathy; AIDS-related cholangitis; AIDS-related lymphoma; AIDS-related nephropathy; Human immunodeficiency virus
acalculous inflammation of the gallbladder and the biliary tract and, 232, 234
biliary stricture due to CMV after liver transplant, 430
Candida esophagitis and, 24, 157
cytomegalovirus colitis and, 167–70
erosive gastritis and, 145–46
gallbladder appearance, 234
gastrointestinal infections, **173–75**
gastrointestinal tumors, **175–79**
Pneumocystis carinii infection, **294–95**

Adenocarcinomas. *See also specific types by name*
Barrett's esophagus and, 7
differential diagnosis
leiomyosarcomas, 504, 506
serous cystadenomas, 338, 347
of the duodenum
differential diagnosis
duodenal hematomas, 33
of the small intestine
location and spread, 41–43
Adenomatous hyperplasia
differential diagnosis
hepatocellular carcinoma, 126, 128
Adhesions
differential diagnosis
strangulated hernia, 64
Afferent loop syndrome, 543
Age factors
achalasia, 481
angiodysplasia, 501
Budd-Chiari syndrome, 445
carcinoma of the cardia, 371
Crohn's disease, 568
diverticula, 506–7
diverticulosis, 57
fibrolamellar hepatocellular carcinoma, 137
focal nodular hyperplasia, 89
gastrointestinal angiodysplasias, 513, 514–15
gastrointestinal bleeding with no etiology found by endoscopy or conventional barium studies, 514–15
glycogenic acanthosis, 24
hepatic artery thrombosis, 434–35
hepatocellular adenoma, 87
herpes esophagitis, 160
inguinal hernias, 73
ischemic colitis, 563
Kaposi's sarcoma, 176, 177

Age factors *(cont'd)*
  laryngopharyngeal carcinoma, 319
  Meckel's diverticulum, 510
  mesenchymal hamartoma, 90–91
  mucin-hypersecreting tumors of the pancreatic duct, 354, 355
  mucinous cystic neoplasms, 337
  obturator hernias, 71
  serous cystadenomas, 342
  solid and papillary epithelial neoplasms, 339, 349
  type AL amyloidosis, 46
  ulcerative colitis, 556
AIDS. *See* Acquired immunodeficiency syndrome
AIDS cholangiopathy, **232**
  differential diagnosis
    cholangiocarcinoma, 232, 235
    gallbladder carcinoma, 230, 232
    Mirizzi's syndrome, 232
    nodal metastases, 232, 243
AIDS-related cholangitis, 294
AIDS-related lymphoma, **290–93**. *See also* Non-Hodgkin's lymphoma
  chemotherapy, 291
  differential diagnosis
    cytomegalovirus colitis, 170
    Kaposi's sarcoma, 283, 285
    lymphadenopathy in patients with HIV infection, 288
    mycobacterial infection of the liver, 285
    Pneumocystis carinii infection, 285–86
    pyogenic liver abscesses, 281
  fine-needle aspiration, 292
  gastrointestinal involvement, 175
  morphologic patterns of hepatic involvement, 291
AIDS-related nephropathy, 294
Alcoholic cirrhosis, and hepatocellular carcinoma, 132
Alcohol use, and
  epidermoid carcinoma of the pharynx, 411
  esophageal intramural pseudodiverticula, 12
  laryngopharyngeal carcinoma, 319, 327
Alkaline gastritis, 540–41, 543
Amebic dysentery, 256
Amebic liver abscesses
  differential diagnosis
    greater peritoneal sac abscesses, 256, 258–59
  pyogenic liver abscesses comparison, 282
Amoebae, and colitis, 569
Amyloidosis, **46–51**
  differential diagnosis
    duodenal hematomas, 33, 35

Anal cancer. *See also* Colorectal carcinoma
  AIDS patients and, 179
Anastomotic biliary stricture, and
  chronic rejection, 430
  cytomegalovirus infection, 430
  hepatic artery stenosis, 429–30
  interventional radiologist, 431
  postsurgical fibrosis, 429
  sclerosing cholangitis, 430–31
Anemia. *See also* Iron deficiency anemia
  attenuation value of blood and, 218
Aneurysms. *See also* Hepatic artery aneurysms; Pseudoaneurysms of the gastroduodenal artery
  contrast-induced opacification, 507
Angiodysplasias. *See* Gastrointestinal angiodysplasias
Angiography
  extravasation, 219–22
  serous cystadenomas, 343
Ankylosing spondylitis, and
  type AA amyloidosis, 47
  ulcerative colitis, 556
Antibiotics
  percutaneous abscess drainage, 271
  periappendiceal abscess treatment, 191–92
  phlegmon treatment, 191
  pseudomembranous colitis and, 171, 573
Antidiuretic hormone. *See* Vasopressin
Antrectomy
  combined with vagotomy, 537–38, 540
  postoperative complications, 540–48
Aphthous ulcers
  Behçet's disease and, 569
  Crohn's disease, 4–6, 117, 146, 552, 569
Appendiceal carcinoma, and mucoceles, 193
Appendiceal cystadenocarcinomas, 193
Appendiceal cystadenomas, 193
Appendiceal polyps, and mucoceles, 193
Appendicitis. *See also* Periappendiceal abscesses
  imaging workup, 186–90
Arteriography
  adenocarcinomas, 504, 506
  angiodysplasias, 504
  carcinoid tumors, 511
  gastrointestinal angiodysplasias, 513
  gastrointestinal bleeding with no etiology found by endoscopy or conventional barium studies, 514
  hematochezia and, 520
  leiomyosarcomas, 501
  Meckel's diverticulum, 510
  pseudoaneurysms of the gastroduodenal artery, 310

Arteriovenous malformations
  causes, 301
  differential diagnosis
    pseudoaneurysms of the gastroduodenal artery, 299–301
Aspirin. *See* Nonsteroidal anti-inflammatory drugs

B

Bacillary angiomatosis, and
  Kaposi's sarcoma, 290
  lymphadenopathy in patients with HIV infection, 288, 290
  pyogenic granuloma, 290
Bacteroides fragilis, pylephlebitis cause, 207
Barium enema studies
  colitis that occurs proximal to an obstructing lesion of the colon, 565
  cytomegalovirus colitis, 169
  diverticulitis, 57, 59
  granulomatous colitis (Crohn's disease), 551–52, 565, 568–73
  ischemic colitis, 555–56, 562–64, 567
  pancolitis, 560
  pseudomembranous colitis, 552, 556, 567–68, 573–75
  radiation colitis, 551, 552–55, 567
  toxic megacolon and, 562
  ulcerative colitis, 551, 555, 556–62, 567, 572–73
Barium studies. *See also specific studies by name*
  carcinoma of the cardia, 365
  hematochezia and, 519
Barrett's esophagus, **7–12**
  adenocarcinoma and, 483
  carcinoma of the cardia and, 371
  classification, 10–12
  differential diagnosis
    esophageal intramural pseudodiverticulosis, 6
    midesophageal strictures and, 8
  reticular mucosal pattern, 9–10
  scleroderma and, 483–84
Behçet's disease
  aphthous ulcers and, 569
  midesophageal ulceration cause, 21
Benign mucous membrane pemphigoid
  midesophageal stricture cause, 8
  midesophageal ulceration cause, 21–22
Benign perfusion defects
  CTAP appearance, 487–90
  hemangioma and, 490–91
  hepatic cysts and, 491
  locations for, 489
  metastasis and, 490–91

Benign perfusion defects *(cont'd)*
  portal vein occlusion and, 491–92
  shapes of, 489–90
Bezoars
  differential diagnosis
    gastric carcinoma, 534–35
Bile ascites, 391, 392, 407
Bile duct carcinoma
  differential diagnosis
    gallbladder carcinoma, 226–27, 230
Bile duct injury following laparoscopic cholecystectomy, 398–407
Bile leaks
  cholecystectomy and, 406–7
  laparoscopic cholecystectomy and, 391–93, 398, 405–8
  treatment, 394
Bile reflux gastritis
  differential diagnosis
    gastric carcinoma, 534
Biliary cystadenoma. *See* Hepatobiliary cystadenoma
Biliary obstruction. *See also* AIDS cholangiopathy; Anastomotic biliary stricture; Bile duct carcinoma; Gallbladder carcinoma; Mirizzi's syndrome; Nodal metastases
  patient management, 245–47
Billroth procedures, and
  afferent loop syndrome, 543
  alkaline gastritis, 540
  bile reflux gastritis, 534
  gastric remnant cancer, 533
  gastroesophageal reflux, 538, 540
  marginal ulcers, 543
Bilomas, 391, 392, 407
Bismuth classification of bile duct injury, 400–401
Bismuth nomenclature for anatomic segments of the liver, 492–93, 496
Blunt abdominal trauma, 215–17. *See also* Trauma
  intra-abdominal hemorrhage, 218–22
  "sentinel clot" sign, 218
Bone marrow transplantation, and veno-occlusive disease, 448
Bowel perforation. *See* Duodenal perforation
Breast carcinoma, metastasis to small bowel, 59, 62–64
Bronchogenic carcinoma
  metastasis to duodenum, 44
  metastasis to small bowel, 59
Brunner's gland hamartomas, 119
Brunner's gland hyperplasia, **118–19**
  differential diagnosis
    heterotopic gastric mucosa, 117
Budd-Chiari syndrome, 445–46

"Bull's eye" pattern of fungal liver abscesses, 266

Bush-tea poisoning, 446

C

Campylobacter jejuni infection
  differential diagnosis
    CMV colitis, 170
  drug resistance, 175
Campylobacter pylori. See Helicobacter pylori
Candida, esophageal intramural pseudodiverticula cause, 12
Candida albicans, and liver abscesses, 266
Candida esophagitis, **157–59**
  differential diagnosis
    HIV esophagitis, 154
  "shaggy" appearance of esophagus, 24, 158
  ulcer appearance, 19, 162
  ulcer location, 22
Carcinoid tumors
  differential diagnosis
    leiomyosarcomas, 510–11
  ischemic colitis and, 563
  sunburst pattern on arteriography, 511
Carcinoma of the cardia, **371**
  differential diagnosis
    gastric lymphoma, 367–68
    gastric ulcers, 369–70
    gastric varices, 368–69
    squamous cell metastasis, 369
Cardia. *See also* Carcinoma of the cardia
  normal appearance, 365
Caustic ingestion
  esophageal ulceration cause, 21, 161
  midesophageal stricture cause, 8
Cavernous hemangiomas
  differential diagnosis
    hepatocellular adenoma, 89–90
  of the liver, **96–103**
    complications following needle biopsy, 99–100
Cavernous transformation of the portal vein
  differential diagnosis
    hepatic artery aneurysm, 200
    periportal adenopathy, 201
    portal vein thrombosis, 199, 201–2, 204
    pylephlebitis, 200–201
Cecal carcinoma. *See also* Ruptured cecal carcinoma
  mucoceles and, 193
Cecal diverticulum. *See* Ruptured cecal diverticulum
Cervical carcinoma, and radiation colitis, 552–53

Chemotherapy
  AIDS-related lymphoma, 291
  Kaposi's sarcoma, 290
  mycobacterial infection, 290
  non-Hodgkin's lymphoma, 290
  veno-occlusive disease and, 446
Children. *See* Age factors
Child's-Pugh classification of severity of liver disease, 381
Cholangiocarcinoma, **235**, **237–42**
  differential diagnosis
    AIDS cholangiopathy, 232, 235
    gallbladder carcinoma, 235
    Mirizzi's syndrome, 235
    nodal metastases, 235, 243
  ulcerative colitis and, 556
Cholangiography
  AIDS cholangiopathy, 232, 234
  bile duct injury, 400
  bile leaks, 394
  biliary abnormalities, 431
  cholangiocarcinoma, 238–39
  gallbladder carcinoma, 225
  during laparoscopic cholecystectomy, 404–5
  nodal metastases, 243
Cholangitis. *See also* AIDS-related cholangitis
  pyogenic liver abscesses and, 266
Cholecystectomy
  bile leaks, 406–7
  laparoscopic cholecystectomy comparison, 399–400
Cholecystitis
  gallbladder carcinoma and, 230
  greater peritoneal sac abscesses and, 255
  pyogenic liver abscesses and, 266
Choledochal cysts, and cholangiocarcinoma, 235, 242
Choledochocholedochostomy, 427
Choledochojejunostomy, and bile duct injury, 401
Chondronecrosis following radiation therapy, 412–13, 422
Cirrhosis of the liver
  hepatocellular carcinoma and, 125–26, 132, 138
  regenerative nodules, 131
Clonorchis sinensis infestation, and cholangiocarcinoma, 242
Closed-loop small bowel obstruction, 78–83
Clostridium difficile infection
  differential diagnosis
    CMV colitis, 170
  pseudomembranous colitis and, 573
CMV. *See* Cytomegalovirus

Colitis. *See also* Cytomegalovirus colitis; *specific types of colitis by name*
AIDS and, 170
barium enema studies, 551–82
Colitis proximal to an obstructive lesion of the colon
barium enema studies, 565
Colon carcinoma. *See also* Colorectal carcinoma
metastasis to small bowel, 59, 62–64
Colonic hematomas
differential diagnosis
jejunal perforation, 214–15
Colonoscopy
hematochezia and, 519
ulcerative colitis, 560
Color Doppler sonography
cavernous transformation of the portal vein, 199
focal nodular hyperplasia, 92
hepatocellular carcinoma, 138
portal vein thrombosis, 207
Colorectal carcinoma
surgical resection of metastases to the liver, 496–97
ulcerative colitis and, 556
Common hepatic bile duct ligation, and laparoscopic cholecystectomy, 397
Computed tomography. *See also* CT arterial portography
abscesses following laparoscopic cholecystectomy, 396
achalasia, 481–82
adenocarcinomas, 338
adenomatous hyperplasia, 128
AIDS cholangiopathy, 232
amebic liver abscesses, 256, 258–59
appendicitis, 188–90
bile leakage after laparoscopic cholecystectomy, 391
biliary obstruction, 246
blunt abdominal trauma, 215–16, **216–17**
carcinoid tumors, 510–11
cavernous hemangiomas of the liver, 96, 98, 101
cholangiocarcinoma, 235, 239–40
closed-loop small bowel obstruction, 78–83
Crohn's disease, 576, 578
cytomegalovirus colitis, 167
distribution of intravenous contrast material, 468–71
diverticulitis, 59
duodenal hematomas, 29
duodenal perforation after laparoscopic cholecystectomy, 394
E. multilocularis, 259

Computed tomography.
extravasation, 219
focal nodular hyperplasia, 92–94
fungal liver abscesses, 266
gallbladder carcinoma, 230–32
gastrinomas, 40
greater peritoneal sac abscesses, 253
hepatic lymphoma, 291
hepatocellular carcinoma, 138
intra-abdominal hemorrhage, **218–22**
intraperitoneal hematomas, 394
ischemic colitis, 578
jejunal perforation, 213
mucin-hypersecreting tumors of the pancreatic duct, 356
mucoceles, 186, 193
neuroendocrine tumors of the pancreas, 308
nodal metastases, 242–43, 244
percutaneous drainage of periappendiceal inflammatory masses, 190–93
periappendiceal abscesses, 183
pharyngeal irradiation of the neck, 417–19
Pneumocystis carinii infection, 294
portal vein thrombosis, 204, 207–8, 463, 464
pseudomembranous colitis, 575–76, 580
radiation colitis, 578
serous cystadenomas, 333, 343, 345–46, 347
small bowel obstruction, **75–78**
solid and papillary epithelial neoplasms, 351–52
strangulated hernia, 55, 57
time-related contrast enhancement effects on liver CT
anatomic obstruction of the inferior vena cava or hepatic veins, 445–46
CT arterial portography, 453
fatty infiltration, 448, 453, 464, 466
hepatic vein obstruction, 455
hepatic venous outflow impairment, 443–45
portal vein thrombosis, 455, 461–64
preferential segmental arterial flow, 448, 457
superior vena cava obstruction, 448, 455, 457, 459–60
transient hepatic attenuation difference, 449–50, 453
veno-occlusive disease, 446, 448
ulcerative colitis, 578, 580

Contrast enema. *See also* Barium enema studies
  appendicitis, 190
  periappendiceal abscesses, 185
Contrast enhancement, time-related contrast enhancement effects on liver CT, 443–71
Cough reflex, disappearance following radiation therapy, 415, 423
Couinaud nomenclature for anatomic segments of the liver, 493, 496
Cricopharyngeal muscle, and neopharynx, 318–19, 325–26
Crohn's disease
  amyloidosis and, 48
  barium enema studies, 551–52, 565, 568–73
  cholangiocarcinoma and, 235
  cobblestone mucosal pattern, 570
  CT evaluation, 576, 578
  differential diagnosis
    duodenitis secondary to renal failure, 111–12
    esophageal intramural pseudodiverticulosis, 4–6
    heterotopic gastric mucosa, 117
    strangulated hernia, 65
  erosive gastritis cause, 146
  esophageal ulcer cause, 21, 161
  pattern of spread, 570
  "rose thorn" ulcers, 570
  surgical options, 568–69
  ulcer characteristics, 569–70
Cryptosporidium infection
  acalculous inflammation of the gallbladder and the biliary tract and, 234
  differential diagnosis
    CMV colitis, 170
CTAP. *See* CT arterial portography
CT arterial portography, 451, 453
  benign perfusion defect, 487–90
Cyclosporine, and malignancy in organ transplant recipients, 437
Cystadenomas. *See specific types by name*
Cystic pancreatic tumors. *See* Mucinous cystic neoplasms; Serous cystadenomas
Cytomegalovirus
  acalculous inflammation of the gallbladder and the biliary tract and, 234
  colitis and, 569
  drug resistance, 175
  erosive gastritis cause, 145–46
  interstitial pneumonia and, 430
  liver transplants and, 430
  microcalcifications and, 294
  treatment, 153
  ulcer appearance, 162, 163

Cytomegalovirus colitis, **167–70**
  differential diagnosis
    AIDS-related lymphoma, 170
    Campylobacter jejuni infection, 170
    Clostridium difficile infection, 170
    Cryptosporidium infection, 170
    gonococcal colitis, 171
    herpes simplex virus, 170–71
    Mycobacterium avium-intracellulare infection, 170
    pseudomembranous colitis, 171
    Shigella flexneri infection, 170
  "owl eye" appearance, 170

D

Decubitus ulcers, and type AA amyloidosis, 47–48
Dementia, and laryngectomy, 321
Diabetes mellitus, and
  Candida esophagitis, 157
  esophageal intramural pseudodiverticula, 12
  laryngectomy, 321
Dialysis. *See also* Hemodialysis
  duodenitis secondary to renal failure, 109
Diarrhea
  cytomegalovirus colitis and, 167
  gastrointestinal infection symptom, 173
Direct inguinal hernias, 73–75
Diverticula, and gastrointestinal bleeding with no etiology found by endoscopy or conventional barium studies, 514
Diverticula of the small bowel. *See also* Meckel's diverticulum; Pharyngeal diverticula
  differential diagnosis
    leiomyosarcomas, 506–10
Diverticulitis
  bowel obstruction and, 57
  differential diagnosis
    strangulated hernia, 57, 59
  ischemic colitis and, 563
Doppler sonography. *See also* Color Doppler sonography
  flow-related phenomena assessment, 453
  hepatic artery occlusion after transplantation, 435
  normal portal vein, 432
  portal vein, **383–87**
  portal vein in liver transplant recipients, 432–33
  transjugular intrahepatic portosystemic shunt, 377, 382–83
Doxycycline, esophagitis cause, 20, 161

Drug-induced esophagitis, 19, 20–21, 22
  differential diagnosis
    esophageal carcinoma, 21
  ulcer location, 22
Duct cell carcinoma
  differential diagnosis
    solid and papillary epithelial neo-
      plasms, 352
Ductectatic cystadenomas and cystadeno-
    carcinomas. *See* Mucin-hypersecret-
    ing tumors of the pancreatic duct
Ducts of Luschka, bile leaks from, 392, 406–
    7
Dumping syndrome, 540
Duodenal hematomas, **29, 35–37**
  differential diagnosis
    adenocarcinoma of the duodenum, 33
    amyloidosis, 33, 35
    duodenal leiomyosarcoma, 33
    pancreatic inflammatory mass, 29, 32–
      33
Duodenal leiomyomas, 44
Duodenal leiomyosarcomas
  description, 44
  differential diagnosis
    duodenal hematomas, 33
Duodenal lymphoma
  differential diagnosis
    duodenitis secondary to renal failure,
      110–11
Duodenal perforation
  greater peritoneal sac abscesses and, 255
  laparoscopic cholecystectomy, 394
Duodenal tumors, **38–45**. *See also* Adenocar-
    cinomas
  differential diagnosis
    adenomas, 38
    Brunner's gland hamartomas, 38
    neuroendocrine tumors, 38
  neurofibromatosis type 1 and, 40
  resectability rate, 43
Duodenal ulcers
  combined vagotomy and antrectomy
    treatment, 537–38, 540
  partial gastrectomy treatment, 531–33
Duodenal villous adenomas, 41
Duodenitis
  Brunner's gland hyperplasia and, 118
  differential diagnosis
    heterotopic gastric mucosa, 115
Duodenitis secondary to renal failure, **109**
  differential diagnosis
    Crohn's disease, 111–12
    duodenal lymphoma, 110–11
    ischemia of the small bowel, 110
    pancreatitis, 109–10

Duodenum
  blunt trauma injury site, 216
  mortality from delayed diagnosis of perfo-
    ration, 215

E

Echinococcosis
  differential diagnosis
    greater peritoneal sac abscesses, 259
  imaging features, 268
Echinococcus, 259
Elderly persons. *See* Age factors
Embolization
  gastrointestinal hemorrhage treatment,
    522, 524, 527
  pseudoaneurysms of the gastroduodenal
    artery treatment, 310
Emphysema, and laryngectomy, 321
Empyema, and amyloidosis, 47
Endoscopic catheterization and drainage,
  248
Endoscopic retrograde cholangiography, bile
  leaks, 394
Endoscopic retrograde pancreatography,
  mucin-hypersecreting tumors of the
  pancreatic duct, 355–56
Endoscopic sphincterotomy, bile leaks, 407
Endoscopy
  Barrett's esophagus, 7
  carcinoma of the cardia, 367
Enteroclysis
  closed-loop small bowel obstruction, 80
  contraindications, 77
  gastrointestinal bleeding with no etiology
    found by endoscopy or conven-
    tional barium studies, 517
  metastases to small bowel, 59
  small bowel obstruction, 76, 77
Enterocytozoon bieneusi infection, and acal-
    culous inflammation of the gallblad-
    der and the biliary tract, 234
Epidermoid anal cancer, and AIDS patients,
  179
Epidermoid carcinoma of the head and neck.
    See also New primary epidermoid
    carcinoma of the pharynx
  radiation therapy, 413–20, 422
Epidermolysis bullosa dystrophica
  midesophageal stricture cause, 8
  midesophageal ulceration cause, 21
Epstein-Barr virus, and PTLD, 437
Erosive gastritis
  Crohn's disease as cause, 146
  cytomegalovirus as cause, 145–46
  H. pylori as cause, 144–45
  nonsteroidal anti-inflammatory drugs as
    cause, 143–44

Erosive gastritis *(cont'd)*
  Zollinger-Ellison syndrome as cause, 146–48
ERP. *See* Endoscopic retrograde pancreatography
Escherichia coli
  pylephlebitis cause, 207
  pyogenic liver abscesses and, 256, 266
Esophageal adenocarcinoma, and Barrett's esophagus, 7
Esophageal carcinoma, 158. *See also* Squamous cell metastases
  differential diagnosis
    drug-induced esophagitis, 21
    secondary achalasia, 482–83
Esophageal intramural pseudodiverticula, **12–14**
  differential diagnosis
    esophagitis, 13–14
  treatment, 12–13
Esophageal intramural pseudodiverticulosis, **3**
  differential diagnosis
    Barrett's esophagus, 6
    esophageal Crohn's disease, 4–6
    herpes esophagitis, 3
    radiation esophagitis, 3–4
Esophagitis. *See also specific types of esophagitis by name*
  differential diagnosis
    esophageal intramural pseudodiverticula, 13–14
    "shaggy" esophagus, 24, 158
Esophagography
  esophagitis, 19–24
  herpes esophagitis, 160
  HIV esophagitis, 153, 154, 163
  intramural pseudodiverticulosis, 3
  secondary achalasia, 479
Esophagus. *See also* Barrett's esophagus
  amyloidosis and, 49
  bird-beak configuration due to achalasia, 481
Ethnic factors
  hepatocellular carcinoma, 134
  solid and papillary epithelial neoplasms, 349
  ulcerative colitis, 556
External hernias, 67–75

F

Familial adenomatous polyposis syndromes, 38
Familial amyloidosis. *See* Type AF amyloidosis

Familial polyposis coli, 38–39, 41
Fatty infiltration of the liver, 448, 453, 455, 457, 464–66
FDG-PET, recurrent cancer, 420
Fibrolamellar hepatocellular carcinoma, 95, **137–38**
  differential diagnosis
    hepatocellular carcinoma, 128, 131
Fistulas
  colitis and, 551–52
  formation following laryngeal radiation, 321–22
  percutaneous abscess drainage and, 271
FNH. *See* Focal nodular hyperplasia
Focal nodular hyperplasia, **92–95**
  differential diagnosis
    hepatocellular adenoma, 89
Foodballs, 534
Frequency. *See also* Incidence; Prevalence
  hepatic artery thrombosis, 434
Fungal liver abscesses, 266–67

G

Galactosemia, and hepatocellular adenoma, 103
Gallbladder carcinoma, **225–26, 230–32**. *See also* Cholecystitis; Laparoscopic cholecystectomy
  cholecystitis and, 230
  differential diagnosis
    AIDS cholangiopathy, 230, 232
    carcinoma of the bile duct, 226–27, 230
    cholangiocarcinoma, 235
    Mirizzi's syndrome, 230
    nodal metastases, 243
Ganciclovir, cytomegalovirus treatment, 153
Gardner syndrome, 38, 39
Gastrectomy. *See* Antrectomy; Billroth procedures; Partial gastrectomy; Vagotomy
Gastric carcinoma
  differential diagnosis
    bezoars, 534–35
    bile reflux gastritis, 534
    jejunogastric intussusception, 535–36
    non-Hodgkin's lymphoma of the stomach, 533–34
  metastasis to small bowel, 59, 62–64
  secondary achalasia and, 479–80, 481
Gastric lymphoma
  differential diagnosis
    carcinoma of the cardia, 367–68
Gastric perforation, and greater peritoneal sac abscesses, 255

Gastric ulcers. *See also* Duodenal ulcers
  combined vagotomy and antrectomy
    treatment, 537–38, 540
  differential diagnosis
    carcinoma of the cardia, 369–70
  partial gastrectomy treatment, 531–33
Gastric varices
  differential diagnosis
    carcinoma of the cardia, 368–69
Gastrin levels, and combined vagotomy and
    antrectomy, 537
Gastrinomas, 39–41, 146–47, 303, 547
Gastritis. *See specific types by name*
Gastroesophageal reflux following Billroth
    procedures, 538, 540
Gastrointestinal angiodysplasias, **513–14**
  differential diagnosis
    leiomyosarcomas, 501–4
Gastrointestinal bleeding with no etiology
    found by endoscopy or conventional
    barium studies, **514–18**
Gastrointestinal hemorrhage, transcatheter
    treatment, **522–27**
Gastrointestinal tumors in patients with
    AIDS, **175–79**
Gelfoam
  gastrointestinal hemorrhage emboliza-
    tion, 522, 524, 527
  pseudoaneurysms of the gastroduodenal
    artery, 310
Gender factors
  carcinoma of the cardia, 371
  cavernous hemangioma, 89
  focal nodular hyperplasia, 89, 92
  hepatobiliary cystadenoma, 90
  hepatocellular adenoma, 87
  herpes esophagitis, 160
  human papillomavirus, 179
  Kaposi's sarcoma, 176, 177
  mesenchymal hamartoma, 90–91
  mucin-hypersecreting tumors of the pan-
    creatic duct, 354, 355
  mucinous cystic neoplasms, 337
  obturator hernias, 71
  radiation colitis, 552
  serous cystadenomas, 342
  solid and papillary epithelial neoplasms,
    339, 349
  ulcerative colitis, 556
Genetic factors
  Crohn's disease, 568
  duodenal tumors, 38–39
  ulcerative colitis, 556
Geographic factors
  gastrointestinal infections in AIDS pa-
    tients, 173
  solid and papillary epithelial neoplasms,
    349

Glycogenic acanthosis
  description, 24
  ulcer appearance, 19–20
  ulcer location, 22
Glycogen-rich cystadenomas. *See* Serous
    cystadenomas
Glycogen storage disease type I, and hepato-
    cellular adenoma, 103
Goldsmith & Woodburne nomenclature for
    anatomic segments of the liver, 496
Gonococcal colitis
  differential diagnosis
    cytomegalovirus colitis, 171
Graded-compression sonography, appendici-
    tis, 186–88
Granulomatous colitis. *See* Crohn's disease
Granulomatous disease, and superior vena
    cava obstruction, 459
Granulomatous ileocolitis. *See* Crohn's dis-
    ease
Gray-scale sonography, portal vein thrombo-
    sis, 199
Greater peritoneal sac abscesses
  causes, 256
  description, 253, 255
  differential diagnosis
    amebic liver abscess, 256, 258–59
    echinococcosis, 259
    lesser peritoneal sac abscesses, 259
    pyogenic liver abscess, 256

H

H. pylori. See Helicobacter pylori
HCC. *See* Hepatocellular carcinoma
Helicobacter pylori
  erosive gastritis cause, 144–45
  gastric carcinoma and, 533
  non-Hodgkin's lymphoma of the stomach
    and, 534
Hemangiomas, and benign perfusion de-
    fects, 490–91
Hematochezia
  arteriography and, 520
  barium studies and, 519
  colonoscopy and, 519
  nasogastric tube placement and, 519
Hematomas. *See specific types of hematomas
  by name*
Hemobilia, percutaneous transhepatic bil-
    iary drainage complication, 248
Hemochromatosis, and hepatocellular carci-
    noma, 132
Hemodialysis. *See also* Dialysis
  amyloidosis and, 46, 48
Hepatic arterial resistive index, and hepatic
    artery stenosis, 435

Hepatic artery aneurysms
  differential diagnosis
    cavernous transformation of the portal vein, 200
Hepatic artery complications, occurrence in liver transplants, 433
Hepatic artery stenosis, and liver transplants, 429–30
Hepatic artery thrombosis. *See also* Portal vein thrombosis
  in liver transplant recipients, **434–35**
Hepatic cysts, and benign perfusion defects, 491
Hepatic hemangiomas. *See* Cavernous hemangiomas, of the liver
Hepatic segmental anatomy, 492–95
Hepatic vein obstruction, 455
Hepatic venous outflow impairment, 443–45
Hepatitis, and hepatocellular carcinoma, 132
Hepatobiliary cystadenoma
  differential diagnosis
    hepatocellular adenoma, 90
Hepatobiliary scintigraphy
  bile leaks, 393–94, 405–7
Hepatocellular adenoma, **87–88, 103–5**
  differential diagnosis
    cavernous hemangioma, 89–90
    focal nodular hyperplasia, 89
    hepatobiliary cystadenoma, 90
    mesenchymal hamartoma, 90–91
Hepatocellular carcinoma, **125–26**
  arterioportal shunting, 137
  differential diagnosis
    adenomatous hyperplasia, 126, 128
    fibrolamellar HCC, 128, 131
    nodular regenerative hyperplasia, 128
  encapsulation, 134–35
  expanding pattern, 132
  hepatocellular adenoma and, 88
  imaging features, 131–37
  intratumoral arterial flow signal, 136–37
  intratumoral septation, 135
  multifocal or diffuse growth pattern, 132
  portal vein thrombosis and, 462
  spreading growth pattern, 132
  vascular invasion, 132, 134
Hernias, **67–75**. *See also specific types of hernias by name*
Herpes esophagitis, **160–62**
  differential diagnosis
    esophageal intramural pseudodiverticulosis, 3
    HIV esophagitis, 155–56
  immunocompromised patients and, 19
  "shaggy" esophagus and, 24
  ulcer appearance, 162–63

Herpes simplex virus
  differential diagnosis
    cytomegalovirus colitis, 170–71
  drug resistance, 175
  herpes esophagitis cause, 155, 160
Herpesvirus, and colitis, 569
Heterotopic gastric mucosa, **115, 120**
  differential diagnosis
    Brunner's gland hyperplasia, 117
    Crohn's disease, 117
    duodenitis, 115
    lymphoid hyperplasia, 115, 117
HIV. *See* Human immunodeficiency virus
HIV esophagitis, **155–56, 162–63**
  differential diagnosis
    Candida esophagitis, 154
    herpes esophagitis, 155–56
    Kaposi's sarcoma, 156
    lymphoma, 156
Howship-Romberg sign, 72
Human immunodeficiency virus. *See also* HIV esophagitis
  lymphadenopathy, 288–90
  pyogenic liver abscesses and, 281
Human papillomavirus, 179
Hydatid disease. *See* Echinococcosis
Hypercalcemia, 547
Hypomotility, and amyloidosis, 48–49

I

Ibuprofen, erosive gastritis cause, 143
Idiopathic achalasia. *See* Primary or idiopathic achalasia
Immunocompromised patients
  Candida esophagitis and, 157
  esophageal intramural pseudodiverticula and, 12
  herpes esophagitis, 19, 160
  liver abscesses, 266
Immunosuppression, and
  malignancy in organ transplant recipients, 437, 438
  veno-occlusive disease, 446
Incidence
  adenocarcinoma in Barrett's esophagus, 483
  Crohn's disease, 568
  gastric carcinoma following gastrectomy, 533
  hepatocellular adenoma, 87
  hepatocellular carcinoma, 138
  Kaposi's sarcoma, 177–78
  malignancy in organ transplant recipients, 437
  ulcerative colitis, 556

Infectious bowel disease, and bowel wall thickening, 81

Inflammatory bowel disease. *See also specific types of bowel disease by name*
  amyloidosis and, 48
  bowel wall thickening, 81
  cholangiocarcinoma and, 235

Inguinal hernias, 72–75

[111]In-pentetreotide, neuroendocrine tumors, 40–41

Internal hernias, 67

Intraductal mucin-hypersecreting neoplasms. *See* Mucin-hypersecreting tumors of the pancreatic duct

Intraperitoneal hematomas, and laparoscopic cholecystectomy, 394, 396

Intraperitoneal hemorrhage
  differential diagnosis
    jejunal perforation, 213

Iron deficiency anemia, and gastrointestinal bleeding with no etiology found by endoscopy or conventional barium studies, 514

Irreducible hernias, 67

Ischemic colitis
  barium enema studies, 555–56, 562–64, 567
  causes, 563
  CT evaluation, 578
  response of colon to, 563–64
  thumbprinting characteristic, 564
  ulcer characteristics, 567

Islet cell tumors. *See* Neuroendocrine tumors of the pancreas

J

Jaundice. *See* AIDS cholangiopathy; Bile duct carcinoma; Biliary obstruction; Echinococcosis; Gallbladder carcinoma; Mirizzi's syndrome; Nodal metastases

Jejunal perforation, **213**
  differential diagnosis
    intramural hematomas of the small bowel or colon, 214–15
    intraperitoneal hemorrhage, 213
    mesenteric hematomas, 213–14
    small bowel obstruction, 214

Jejunogastric intussusception
  differential diagnosis
    gastric carcinoma, 535–36

Jejunum, blunt trauma injury site, 216

Juvenile polyposis, 38

K

Kaposi's sarcoma
  bacillary angiomatosis and, 290
  chemotherapy, 290
  cytologic features, 290
  differential diagnosis
    AIDS-related lymphoma, 283, 285
    HIV esophagitis, 156
    lymphadenopathy in patients with HIV infection, 288–89
  gastrointestinal involvement, 176–79
  lesion description, 178

Klatskin tumors, 239

L

Laparoscopic cholecystectomy
  abscesses, 396–97
  arterial vascular injuries, 408–9
  bile leaks following, 391–94
  complications, 398–409
  intraperitoneal hematomas, 394, 396
  technique, 398

Laryngectomy
  benign stricture of the neopharynx
    differential diagnosis
      abscess, 319
      expected postoperative appearance, 319
      recurrent mucosal carcinoma, 317–19
      ulceration of the mucosal surface of the neopharynx, 315–17
  complications, **321–28**
  features, 319
  tongue muscle strain on suture line, 316, 321, 324–25
  voice-conserving procedures, 319, 321

Laryngopharyngeal carcinomas. *See also* Epidermoid carcinoma of the head and neck
  laryngectomy, 321
  recurrence rates, 326–27

Leiomyomas. *See also* Duodenal leiomyomas
  gastrointestinal bleeding with no etiology found by endoscopy or conventional barium studies and, 514
  leiomyosarcomas and, 501
  squamous cell metastases and, 372

Leiomyosarcomas. *See also* Duodenal leiomyosarcomas
  differential diagnosis
    adenocarcinomas, 504, 506
    angiodysplasia, 501–4
    carcinoid tumors, 510–11
    diverticula of the small bowel, 506–10

Leiomyosarcomas *(cont'd)*
squamous cell metastases and, 372
Lesser peritoneal sac, **261–65**
Lesser peritoneal sac abscesses
catheter drainage, 264
differential diagnosis
greater peritoneal sac abscesses, 259
Liver. *See also* Benign perfusion defects; Portal vein occlusion; Portal vein thrombosis; Pyogenic liver abscesses; Transjugular intrahepatic portosystemic shunt
blood supply, 266
Child's-Pugh classification of severity of liver disease, 381
embryonic development, 262–64
hepatic segmental anatomy, 492–95
infarction resistance, 408–9
intrahepatic infectious lesions, **266–68**
metastatic insufficiency concept, 497
metastatic tumors, 490–91, 496–97
surgical resection of metastases from a primary colorectal carcinoma, **496–97**
time-related contrast enhancement effects on liver CT, 443–71
Liver transplants
anastomosis types, 427, 429
complications involving biliary ducts, 429
difficulty of complication diagnosis, 432
end-stage liver disease treatment, 431
frequency of complications, 431
graft failure, 431–32
portal vein complications, 432–33
post-transplantation lymphoproliferative disorder, **437–38**
role of opportunistic infection in biliary stricture formation, 430
Liver tumors. *See also* Hepatocellular adenoma
differentiation of for surgical resection, 88–89
Lung carcinoma, metastasis to small bowel, 59
Lymphadenopathy in patients with HIV infection
differential diagnosis
AIDS-related lymphoma, 288
Kaposi's sarcoma, 288–89
mycobacterial infections, 289
non-Hodgkin's lymphoma, 289
Lymphoid hyperplasia
differential diagnosis
heterotopic gastric mucosa, 115, 117

Lymphoma. *See also* AIDS-related lymphoma; Gastric lymphoma; *specific types of lymphoma by name*
differential diagnosis
HIV esophagitis, 156
Lymphoproliferation following liver transplantation, 437

M

Magnetic resonance imaging
adenocarcinomas, 338
adenomatous hyperplasia, 128
biliary obstruction, 246
blood breakdown product appearance, 210
cavernous hemangiomas of the liver, 98–99, 101, 103
fibrolamellar hepatocellular carcinoma, 95
focal nodular hyperplasia, 94–95
hepatocellular adenoma, 103–5
hepatocellular carcinoma, 125, 126, 138
mucin-hypersecreting tumors of the pancreatic duct, 357
pharyngeal irradiation of the neck, 419–20
portal vein thrombosis, 207, 208–10, 466
rapidly acquired contrast-enhanced images, 453
serous cystadenomas, 333, 343, 345
MAI. *See Mycobacterium avium-intracellulare* infection
Malignant melanoma, metastasis to duodenum, 44
Marginal ulcers, 543, 546–48
Meckel's diverticulum, 509–10
Mediastinal irradiation
midesophageal stricture cause, 8
midesophageal ulceration cause, 21
Melanoma. *See also* Malignant melanoma
metastasis to small bowel, 59
nodal metastases, 242–43
Mesenchymal hamartomas
differential diagnosis
hepatocellular adenoma, 90–91
Mesenteric hematomas
differential diagnosis
jejunal perforation, 213–14
Metastatic tumors. *See also* Liver, metastatic tumors
benign perfusion defects and, 490–91
differential diagnosis
strangulated hernia, 59, 62–64
Microcystic adenomas. *See* Serous cystadenomas

Mirizzi's syndrome, **244–45**
  differential diagnosis
    AIDS cholangiopathy, 232
    cholangiocarcinoma, 235
    gallbladder carcinoma, 230
    nodal metastases, 243
Mortality rates. *See also* Survival rates
  delayed diagnosis of perforation of the
    duodenum, 215
  endoscopic catheterization drainage of
    biliary obstruction, 248
  external hernias, 68
  gastrointestinal infections in AIDS pa-
    tients, 173
  hemorrhage from esophageal varices, 378
  percutaneous transhepatic biliary drain-
    age of obstruction, 248
  post-transplantation lymphoproliferative
    disorder, 438
Motor vehicle accidents, and duodenal hematomas, 35
Mucin-hypersecreting tumors of the pancreatic duct, **353–59**
  differential diagnosis
    serous cystadenomas, 339
Mucinous cystic neoplasms
  differential diagnosis
    serous cystadenomas, 334–38, 346–47
    solid and papillary epithelial neo-
      plasms, 352
Mucinous ductal ectasia. *See* Mucin-hypersecreting tumors of the pancreatic
  duct
Mucin-producing tumors. *See* Mucin-hypersecreting tumors of the pancreatic
  duct
Mucoceles of the appendix, **193–94**
Mucosal carcinoma
  differential diagnosis
    benign postoperative stricture of the
      neopharynx, 317–19
Multiple myeloma, and amyloidosis, 46
Mycobacterial infections. *See also specific
    infections by name*
  chemotherapy, 290
  cytologic features, 290
  differential diagnosis
    AIDS-related lymphoma, 285
    lymphadenopathy in patients with HIV
      infection, 289
Mycobacterium avium-intracellulare infection, 174–75
  differential diagnosis
    AIDS-related lymphoma, 285
    CMV colitis, 170
  microcalcifications and, 294

Mycobacterium tuberculosis infection
  differential diagnosis
    AIDS-related lymphoma, 285

N

Nasogastric tubes, and hematochezia, 519
Neopharynx. *See also* Laryngectomy
  expected postoperative appearance
    differential diagnosis
      benign postoperative stricture, 319
  stenosis and, 323–24
  tongue muscle strain on the surgical su-
    ture line, 316, 321, 324–25
  ulceration of the mucosal surface
    differential diagnosis
      benign postoperative stricture, 315–
        17
Neuroendocrine tumors of the duodenum,
  39–41
Neuroendocrine tumors of the pancreas
  differential diagnosis
    pseudoaneurysms of the gastroduode-
      nal artery, 303–9
    serous cystadenomas, 347
    solid and papillary epithelial neo-
      plasms, 352
Neurofibromatosis type 1, and duodenal tumors, 40
New primary epidermoid carcinoma of the
    pharynx
  differential diagnosis
    expected appearance of the pharynx af-
      ter irradiation, 411
    pharyngeal diverticula, 413
    radiation-induced ulceration, 412–13
    recurrent or persistent carcinoma,
      411–12
Nodal metastases
  differential diagnosis
    AIDS cholangiopathy, 232, 243
    cholangiocarcinoma, 235, 243
    gallbladder carcinoma, 243
    Mirizzi's syndrome, 243
Nodular regenerative hyperplasia
  differential diagnosis
    hepatocellular carcinoma, 128
Nodular transformation. *See* Nodular regenerative hyperplasia
Non-Hodgkin's lymphoma
  chemotherapy, 290
  cytologic features, 290
  differential diagnosis
    gastric carcinoma, 533–34
    lymphadenopathy in patients with HIV
      infection, 289
  gastrointestinal involvement, 41, 175–76

Non-Hodgkin's lymphoma *(cont'd)*
  H. pylori infection and, 534
Nonsteroidal anti-inflammatory drugs
  erosive gastritis cause, 143–44
  ulcer cause, 547–48
NRH. *See* Nodular regenerative hyperplasia
NSAIDS. *See* Nonsteroidal anti-inflammatory drugs

O

Obese patients
  graded compression sonography difficulties, 188
  hernia diagnosis, 68
Obturator hernias, 55, 57, 70–72
Occult gastrointestinal blood
  duodenal leiomyomas and duodenal leiomyosarcomas, 44
  duodenal villous adenomas, 41
Opportunistic infections. *See specific infections by name*
Oral contraceptives, and
  hepatocellular adenoma, 87, 103
  portal vein thrombosis, 461
Osler-Weber-Rendu disease, and arteriovenous malformations, 301
Osteomyelitis, and amyloidosis, 47
Ovarian carcinoma, metastasis to small
    bowel, 59, 62–64

P–Q

Palmaz stent, 380
Pancolitis, barium enema studies, 560
Pancreas
  mucin-hypersecreting tumors of the pancreatic duct, 353–59
  serous cystadenoma, 333–34, 340–48
  solid and papillary epithelial neoplasms,
      349–53
Pancreatic carcinoma. *See also* Neuroendocrine tumors of the pancreas
  metastasis to small bowel, 59, 62–64
  resectability rate, 43
Pancreatic inflammatory masses
  differential diagnosis
    duodenal hematomas, 29, 32–33
Pancreatic pseudocysts
  differential diagnosis
    pseudoaneurysms of the gastroduodenal artery, 301, 303
Pancreatitis
  abscess drainage, 271
  differential diagnosis
    duodenitis secondary to renal failure,
        109–10

Pancreatitis *(cont'd)*
  ischemic colitis and, 563
  mucin-hypersecreting tumors of the pancreatic duct and, 355
  pseudoaneurysms, 270, 310
Pancreatoblastoma
  differential diagnosis
    solid and papillary epithelial neoplasms, 352
Papillary cystic neoplasms. *See* Solid and
    papillary epithelial neoplasms
Papillary epithelial neoplasms. *See* Solid
    and papillary epithelial neoplasms
Parietal cells, removal after antrectomy, 537
Partial gastrectomy. *See also* Billroth procedures
  gastric and duodenal ulcer treatment,
      531–33
  gastric carcinoma and, 531–33
Pentamidine, aerosolized pentamidine prophylaxis, 286, 294
Peptic strictures. *See* Reflux-induced or peptic strictures
Percutaneous biliary drainage, 431
Percutaneous biopsies, and arteriovenous
    malformations, 301
Percutaneous drainage
  abscesses, **271–73**
    contraindications, **268–70**
    injection of contrast agent, 273–76
  ascitic fluid and, 268–69
  complications, 192
  follow-up CT or sonogram, 274–76
  pancreatic pseudocysts, 303
  periappendiceal inflammatory masses,
      190–93
  post-drainage imaging, 268
Percutaneous needle biopsy, serous cystadenomas, 348
Percutaneous transhepatic biliary drainage,
    246, **247–48**
Periappendiceal abscesses, **183**
  differential diagnosis
    mucocele of the appendix, 185–86
    phlegmon, 184–85
    ruptured cecal carcinoma, 183
    ruptured cecal diverticulum, 183
Periappendiceal inflammatory masses, **190–
    93**
Periportal adenopathy
  differential diagnosis
    cavernous transformation of the portal
        vein, 201
PET with F-18 fluorodeoxyglucose. *See*
    FDG-PET
Peutz-Jeghers syndrome, 38

Pharyngeal diverticula
  differential diagnosis
    new primary epidermoid carcinoma of the pharynx, 413
Pharyngeal necrosis, and laryngectomy, 322–23
Pharyngography
  new primary epidermoid carcinoma of the pharynx, 411
  recurrent or persistent carcinoma of the pharynx, 416–17
Pharynx after radiation therapy, **422–23**
Pharynx carcinoma. *See* New primary epidermoid carcinoma of the pharynx
Phlegmons
  definition, 191
  differential diagnosis
    mucocele of the appendix, 185–86
    periappendiceal abscesses, 184–85
  percutaneous drainage, 191–92
Pneumatosis cystoides intestinalis, 81
Pneumocystis carinii infection
  aerosolized pentamidine prophylaxis, 286, 294
  differential diagnosis
    AIDS-related lymphoma, 285–86
  lymphadenopathy in patients with HIV infection and, 288
  in patients with AIDS, **294–95**
Pneumoperitoneum, and jejunal perforation, 216
Polycythemia vera, and portal vein thrombosis, 461
Polyvinyl alcohol particles, gastrointestinal hemorrhage embolization, 527
Portal vein in liver transplant recipients, **432–33**
Portal vein occlusion, and benign perfusion defects, 491–92
Portal vein thrombosis, **206–10**, 448, 455, 461–64
  differential diagnosis
    cavernous transformation of the portal vein, 199, 201–2, 204
Post-transplantation lymphoproliferative disorder, **437–38**
Potassium chloride, esophagitis cause, 21
Preferential segmental arterial flow, 448, 457, 459
Prevalence
  Barrett's esophagus, 7
  cavernous hemangiomas, 89, 99
  diverticulosis, 57
  gastrointestinal angiodysplasias, 513
Primary or idiopathic achalasia
  differential diagnosis
    secondary achalasia, 479–82
Pseudoachalasia. *See* Secondary achalasia

Pseudoaneurysms of the gastroduodenal artery
  angiographic embolization treatment, 310
  differential diagnosis
    arteriovenous malformations, 299–301
    neuroendocrine tumors of the pancreas, 303–9
    pancreatic pseudocysts, 301, 303
    upper abdominal varices, 309–10
Pseudomembranous colitis
  barium enema studies, 552, 556, 567–68, 573–75
  CT evaluation, 575–76, 580
  differential diagnosis
    cytomegalovirus colitis, 171
  features, 556
  thumbprinting characteristic, 573
  ulcer characteristics, 567–68
Pseudomyxoma peritonei, 193–94
Psoriatic arthritis, and type AA amyloidosis, 47
PTBD. *See* Percutaneous transhepatic biliary drainage
PTLD. *See* Post-transplantation lymphoproliferative disorder
Pylephlebitis
  causes, 207
  differential diagnosis
    cavernous transformation of the portal vein, 200–201
  liver abscesses and, 266
Pyoderma gangrenosum, and ulcerative colitis, 556
Pyogenic granuloma, and bacillary angiomatosis, 290
Pyogenic liver abscesses
  amebic abscesses comparison, 282
  appearance, 282–83
  differential diagnosis
    greater peritoneal sac abscesses, 256
  human immunodeficiency virus and, 281
  risks of percutaneous therapy, 268

Quinidine, esophagitis cause, 21

R

Radiation colitis
  barium enema studies, 551, 552–55, 567
  CT evaluation, 578
  radiation dosage and, 552–53
  ulcer characteristics, 567
Radiation enteritis, bowel wall thickening, 81

Radiation esophagitis
  differential diagnosis
    esophageal intramural pseudodivertic-
      ulosis, 3–4
  ulceration cause, 161
Radiation-induced ulceration
  differential diagnosis
    new primary epidermoid carcinoma of
      the pharynx, 411, 412–13
Radiation therapy
  Candida esophagitis and, 157
  epidermoid carcinoma, 413–20
  pharynx following, 422–23
Radiocolloid hepatic scintigraphy, focal nodular hyperplasia, 94
Radiography
  Brunner's gland hyperplasia, 118–19
  duodenal hematoma, 29
Rashes, HIV esophagitis symptom, 162
Recurrent or persistent carcinoma of the
  pharynx
  differential diagnosis
    new primary epidermoid carcinoma of
      the pharynx, 411–12
  ulceration as sign of, 414
Reducible hernias, 67
Reflux esophagitis
  Barrett's esophagus and, 10
  distal esophageal ulcer cause, 22
  following Billroth procedures, 538, 540
  ulcer appearance, 22–23
  ulceration cause, 19, 161
  ulcer location, 23–24
Reflux-induced or peptic strictures
  differential diagnosis
    secondary achalasia, 482
Regenerative nodules, **131**
Renal failure, duodenitis secondary to, 109
Rendu-Osler-Weber syndrome, 513–14
Retained antrum syndrome, 546–47
Rheumatoid arthritis, and type AA amyloi-
  dosis, 47
Richter hernias, 67
Rochalimaea henselae, 290
Rose thorn ulcers, 570
Rotavirus, and gastrointestinal infections in
  Australian AIDS patients, 173
Roux-en-Y choledochojejunostomy, 427, 429,
  543
Ruptured cecal carcinoma
  differential diagnosis
    periappendiceal abscesses, 183
Ruptured cecal diverticulum
  differential diagnosis
    periappendiceal abscesses, 183

S

Sacroiliitis, and ulcerative colitis, 556
Salmonella infection, and colitis, 569
Sciatic hernias, 72
Scintigraphy. *See also specific types of scintigraphy by name*
  cavernous hemangiomas of the liver, 98,
    101
  focal nodular hyperplasia, 94
  islet cell tumors, 308–9
Scleroderma
  Barrett's esophagus and, 8
  differential diagnosis
    secondary achalasia, 483–84
Sclerosing cholangitis, 430–31
  cholangiocarcinoma and, 242
  ulcerative colitis and, 556
Secondary achalasia
  differential diagnosis
    esophageal carcinoma, 482–83
    primary or idiopathic achalasia, 479–
      82
    reflux-induced or peptic strictures, 482
    scleroderma, 483–84
Serous cystadenomas, **340–48**
  differential diagnosis
    adenocarcinomas, 338, 347
    islet cell carcinomas, 347
    mucin-hypersecreting tumors of the
      pancreatic duct, 339
    mucinous cystic neoplasms, 334–38,
      346–47
    solid and papillary epithelial neo-
      plasms, 339
Shigella flexneri infection
  differential diagnosis
    CMV colitis, 170
  drug resistance, 175
Shigella infection, and colitis, 569
Sinus tract formation after laryngectomy,
  321
Small bowel hematomas, 214–15, 217
Small bowel infections
  AIDS and, 174–75
  "toothpaste" appearance of mucosal
    sloughing, 174
Small bowel ischemia. *See also* Ischemic
  colitis
  differential diagnosis
    duodenitis secondary to renal failure,
      110
Small bowel obstruction. *See also* Diverticula of the small bowel; Jejunal perforation
  bezoars and, 535
  closed-loop obstruction, **78–83**
  diagnosis, 75–78

Small bowel obstruction *(cont'd)*
  differential diagnosis
    jejunal perforation, 214
  diverticulitis, 57
  hernias, 68, 71
  malignant peritoneal implants and, 194
  metastases to the small bowel, 59, 62–64
Solid and cystic acinar-cell tumors. *See* Solid
    and papillary epithelial neoplasms
Solid and cystic tumors. *See* Solid and papil-
    lary epithelial neoplasms
Solid and papillary epithelial neoplasms,
    349–53
  differential diagnosis
    duct cell adenocarcinoma, 352
    islet cell carcinoma, 352
    mucinous cystic neoplasms, 352
    pancreatoblastoma, 352
    serous cystadenomas, 339
  low-grade malignancy classification, 350
Somatostatin-receptor scintigraphy with In-
    111 octreotide, carcinoid tumors, 511
Sonography. *See also* Color Doppler sonogra-
    phy; Doppler sonography; Gray-scale
    sonography
  abscesses following laparoscopic cholecys-
    tectomy, 396
  adenomatous hyperplasia, 128
  AIDS-related lymphoma, 281
  appendicitis, 186–88
  biliary obstruction, 246
  candidal abscess patterns, 266–67
  cavernous hemangiomas of the liver, 96
  focal nodular hyperplasia, 92
  hepatic lymphoma, 291
  hepatocellular adenoma, 103
  hepatocellular carcinoma, 138
  intraperitoneal hematomas, 394
  mucin-hypersecreting tumors of the pan-
    creatic duct, 356
  mucoceles, 186, 193
  pancreatic pseudocysts, 301, 303
  Pneumocystis carinii infection, 294
  porta hepatis, 427
  pseudoaneurysms, 299
  pyogenic liver abscesses, 282–83
  serous cystadenomas, 343, 345–46
  small bowel obstruction, 76–77
  solid and papillary epithelial neoplasms,
    351
  upper abdominal varices, 309–10
SPECT, cavernous hemangiomas of the liv-
    er, 98, 101
Spigelian hernias, 69–70
Squamous cell metastases, **372**
  differential diagnosis
    carcinoma of the cardia, 369

Staphylococcus aureus, and pyogenic liver
    abscesses, 256
Steroids
  Candida esophagitis and, 157
  hepatocellular adenoma and, 103
  HIV esophagitis treatment, 162
Stomach cancer. *See* Gastric carcinoma
Stool cultures, gastrointestinal infections in
    AIDS patients, 173–74
Strangulated hernias, **55, 57**
  differential diagnosis
    adhesions, 64
    Crohn's disease, 65
    diverticulitis, 57, 59
    metastatic tumor, 59, 62–64
Strangulation. *See* Closed-loop small bowel
    obstruction; Small bowel obstruc-
    tion; Strangulated hernias
Streptococcus, and pyogenic liver abscesses,
    256
Stromal cell sarcomas. *See* Duodenal lei-
    omyomas; Duodenal leiomyosarco-
    mas
Stromal cell tumors. *See* Duodenal leiomyo-
    mas; Duodenal leiomyosarcomas
Superficial spreading carcinoma
  esophageal tumor appearance, 24
  ulcer appearance, 19–20
  ulcer location, 22
Superior vena cava obstruction, 448, 455,
    457, 459–60
Survival rates. *See also* Mortality rates
  duodenal tumors, 38, 43
  endoscopic catheterization drainage of
    biliary obstruction, 248
  epidermoid carcinoma of the head and
    neck, 413
  fibrolamellar hepatocellular carcinoma,
    138
  laryngopharyngeal carcinomas, 319
  mucin-hypersecreting tumors of the pan-
    creatic duct, 355
  pancreatic cancer, 43
  percutaneous transhepatic biliary drain-
    age of obstruction, 248
  surgical resection of metastases to the liv-
    er from a primary colorectal car-
    cinoma, 497
  transjugular intrahepatic portosystemic
    shunt, 382
  type AL amyloidosis, 46
Systemic lupus erythematosus, and duode-
    nal hematomas, 35
Systolic acceleration time, and hepatic ar-
    tery stenosis, 435

T

Tc-99m erythrocyte scintigraphy
gastrointestinal bleeding with no etiology found by endoscopy or conventional barium studies, 517
hematochezia, 521
Tc-99m pertechnetate scintigraphy
Meckel's diverticulum, 510
retained antrum syndrome, 546–47
Telangiectasias, 513–14
Tetracycline, esophagitis cause, 20, 161
THAD. *See* Transient hepatic attenuation difference
TIPS. *See* Transjugular intrahepatic portosystemic shunt
Tobacco use
epidermoid carcinoma of the pharynx and, 411
laryngopharyngeal carcinoma and, 319, 327
Toxic megacolon, 560, 562, 573
Transient hepatic attenuation difference, 449–50, 453
Transjugular intrahepatic portosystemic shunt
Child's-Pugh classification of severity of liver disease, 381
development of, 378, 380
frequency of shunt stenosis, 382
indications for use, 380–81
placement of, 381–82, 387
pseudointimal hyperplasia, 377, 382
recurrent variceal bleeding, 377–78
reversal of portal venous flow and, 377
success rate, 382
typical candidate, 381
Trauma
abdominal trauma evaluation, 215–17
arteriovenous malformations and, 301
colonic hematomas, 214–15
duodenal hematomas and, 35–37
greater peritoneal sac abscesses and, 255
hernias and, 67
jejunal perforation, 213
pancreatitis and, 35–37
pyogenic liver abscesses and, 266
small bowel hematomas, 214–15
superior vena cava obstruction and, 459
Tuberculosis, and amyloidosis, 47
Type AA amyloidosis, 47–48, 49–50
Type AF amyloidosis, 48
Type AH amyloidosis, 48
Type AL amyloidosis, 46–47, 49–50
Tyrosinemia, and hepatocellular adenoma, 103

U

Ulcerative colitis
barium enema studies, 551, 555, 556–62, 567, 572–73
cholangiocarcinoma and, 235
CT evaluation, 578, 580
mosaic tile appearance, 555
pattern of spread, 573
ulcer characteristics, 567
Ulcers. *See specific types by name*
Upper abdominal varices
differential diagnosis
pseudoaneurysms of the gastroduodenal artery, 309–10

V

Vagotomy
combined with antrectomy, 537–38, 540
incomplete vagotomy as surgical inadequacy, 543, 546
postoperative complications, 540–48
Varices. *See* Upper abdominal varices
Vascular ectasias. *See* Gastrointestinal angiodysplasias
Vasopressin
complications, 526–27
gastrointestinal hemorrhage treatment, 522, 524, 526–27
Venography, islet cell tumors, 308
Veno-occlusive disease, and duodenal hematomas, 35, 37
Vinyl chloride exposure, and hepatocellular carcinoma, 132
von Hippel-Lindau disease, and
serous cystadenomas, 342
solid and papillary epithelial neoplasms, 349
von Recklinghausen's disease. *See* Neurofibromatosis type 1

W–Z

Whipple's disease, 174–75

Yersinia infection, and colitis, 569

ZE. *See* Zollinger-Ellison syndrome
Zollinger-Ellison syndrome, 40, 41
erosive gastritis cause, 146–48
retained antrum syndrome and, 546